Judith Gerdin,
BSN, MS
Phoenix, Arizona

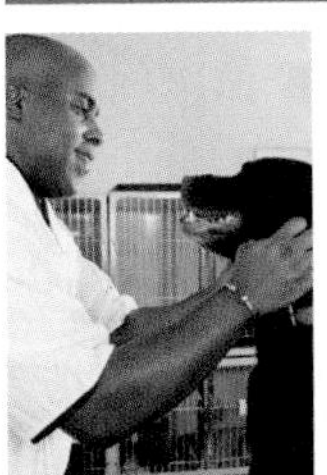
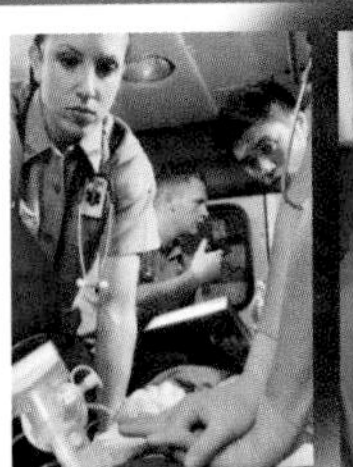
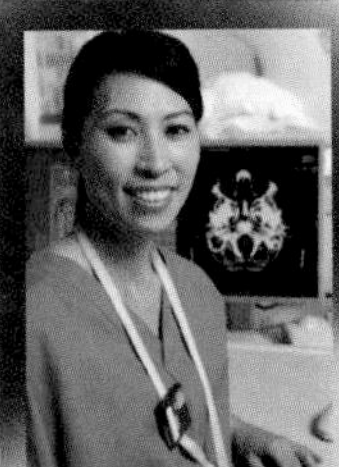

Fifth Edition

Health Careers Today

ELSEVIER
MOSBY

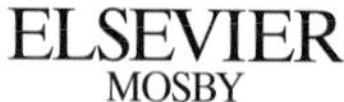

ELSEVIER
MOSBY

3251 Riverport Lane
St. Louis, Missouri 63043

HEALTH CAREERS TODAY, FIFTH EDITION ISBN: 978-0-323-07504-6

Library of Congress Cataloging-in-Publication Data or Control Number (in STL)
Gerdin, Judith A.
Health careers today / Judith Gerdin.—5th ed.
p. ; cm.
Includes index.
ISBN 978-0-323-07504-6 (hardcover : alk. paper)
1. Medicine—Vocational guidance. 2. Allied health personnel—Vocational guidance. I. Title.
[DNLM: 1. Health Occupations. 2. Allied Health Personnel. 3. Vocational Guidance. W 21]
R690.G47 2012
610.69—dc22

2011002153

Publishing Director: Andrew Allen
Managing Editor: Ellen Wurm-Cutter
Developmental Editor: Kristen Mandava
Publishing Services Manager: Julie Eddy
Project Manager: Jan Waters
Designer: Amy Buxton

Printed in the United States of America

Last digit is the print number: 9 8 7 6 5 4 3 2 1

Dedication

To my family and friends,
Always and forever.

Reviewers

Deborah A. Guyer, RN
Health Occupations and Nurse Aide Instructor
Cumberland High School
Cumberland, Virginia

Lisa J. Johnson, RD/LD, MBA, MEd
Advanced Health Occupations Specialist
Twin Falls High School
Twin Falls, Idaho

Michelle Merolla, RN
Page Unified School District
Page, Arizona

Preface

Health care is changing more quickly than I could ever imagine or document in this book. Researchers are finding new information that may be the cure or successful treatment for many of our health concerns and new concerns are emerging. New technological innovations can be seen on the news every day. It is clear that health care workers of the future will need to be able to find, evaluate, and learn to use new information and techniques.

Who Will Benefit From This Book?

Health Careers Today provides an overview to the basics of the health care environment and a specific overview of more than 45 of the most popular health careers. This is valuable information for students as they make choices based on their informed interest level and on their commitment to the educational and professional responsibilities that each health career requires. This preview into various health careers allows students to make more informed choices for their education and profession.

Organization

Health Careers Today is divided into three units: "Core Knowledge," "Anatomy and Physiology," and "Career Clusters." The "Core Knowledge" chapters provide the foundation from which all health care workers must operate. The "Anatomy and Physiology" chapters provide background information in health as they relate to the human body. The "Career Clusters" chapters provide a sampling of information about the jobs, knowledge, and skills in each cluster area. With this book, we hope that an educated decision may be made about a career path in the health care field.

Distinctive Features of this Book

Anatomy and Physiology

A separate unit covers all of the body systems. This text is one of only a few that covers anatomy and physiology. Application of anatomy and physiology to practice allows students to see the science in action within various career settings. Each anatomy and physiology chapter begins with a system terminology box and an abbreviation box. This gives the student a quick reference point for terms that involve each individual system.

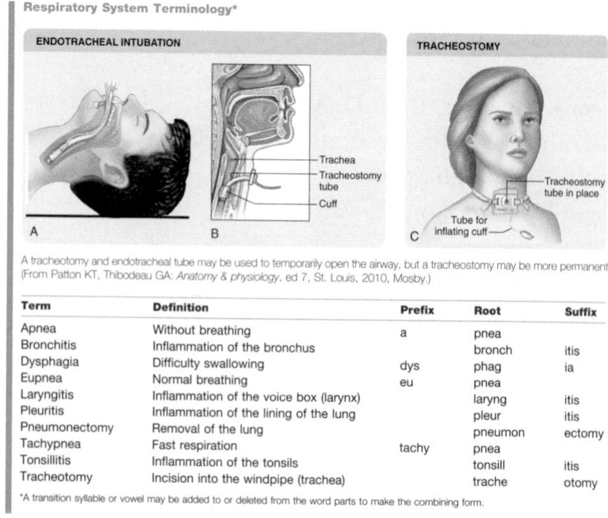
Respiratory System Terminology*

A tracheotomy and endotracheal tube may be used to temporarily open the airway, but a tracheostomy may be more permanent. (From Patton KT, Thibodeau GA: *Anatomy & physiology*, ed 7, St. Louis, 2010, Mosby.)

Term	Definition	Prefix	Root	Suffix
Apnea	Without breathing	a	pnea	
Bronchitis	Inflammation of the bronchus		bronch	itis
Dysphagia	Difficulty swallowing	dys	phag	ia
Eupnea	Normal breathing	eu	pnea	
Laryngitis	Inflammation of the voice box (larynx)		laryng	itis
Pleuritis	Inflammation of the lining of the lung		pleur	itis
Pneumonectomy	Removal of the lung		pneumon	ectomy
Tachypnea	Fast respiration	tachy	pnea	
Tonsillitis	Inflammation of the tonsils		tonsill	itis
Tracheotomy	Incision into the windpipe (trachea)		trache	otomy

*A transition syllable or vowel may be added to or deleted from the word parts to make the combining form.

Abbreviations of the Respiratory System

Abbreviation	Meaning
ABG	Arterial blood gases
BS	Breath sounds
CF	Cystic fibrosis
CO_2	Carbon dioxide
COPD	Chronic obstructive pulmonary disease
ENT	Ears, nose, and throat
TB	Tuberculosis
TCDB	Turn, cough, deep breath
Trach	Tracheotomy
URI	Upper respiratory infection

Skill Activities

Skill activities are integrated with the content of the chapters. Each skill provides detailed instructions on how to perform crucial tasks such as transferring a patient from a bed to a chair, performing CPR, moving a patient in bed, aseptic technique, assisting a patient with hygiene, and many others. These activities provide students the opportunity to obtain hands-on experience. A complete list of skill activities can be found on pp. ix–x.

SKILL LIST **2-1**
Assertive Behavior

1. Take a few long, deep breaths. Allow time to gain composure so that the message can be delivered in matter-of-fact, unemotional tones.
2. Describe the behavior you would like the other person to change. Be specific about one incident or action.
3. State the effect or how you feel when the behavior occurs.
4. State the positive behavior you would like to see rather than the one you do not like.
5. State the consequences that will occur if the behavior is not changed. These consequences must be timely, reasonable, enforceable, and clearly understood by the other person.
6. Follow through with the consequences if the behavior does not change.
7. Evaluate the success of the confrontation with the other person. Demonstrate appreciation for the change in the behavior.

Numerous Content Boxes throughout Each Chapter

More than 70 content boxes appear throughout the text, providing students with additional information to help reinforce key chapter concepts.

New to this Edition

Health Careers in Practice

Career chapters feature interviews of working health professionals in a specific health career. These short bios allow students to relate to a real world example and provide valuable information regarding the education, employment opportunities, and pros and cons of specific careers.

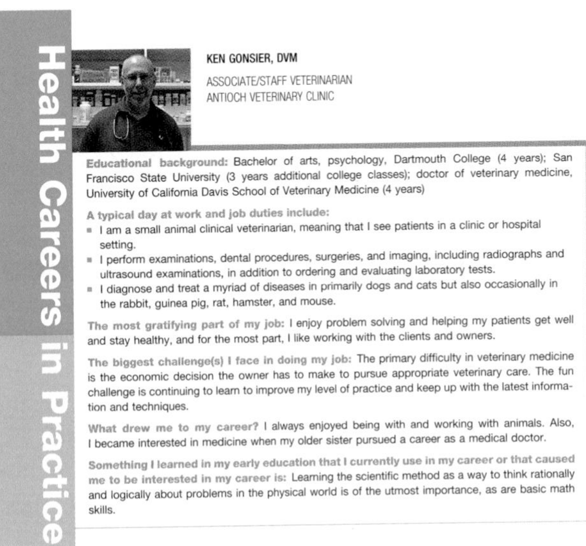

Health Careers in Practice

KEN GONSIER, DVM
ASSOCIATE/STAFF VETERINARIAN
ANTIOCH VETERINARY CLINIC

Educational background: Bachelor of arts, psychology, Dartmouth College (4 years); San Francisco State University (3 years additional college classes); doctor of veterinary medicine, University of California Davis School of Veterinary Medicine (4 years)

A typical day at work and job duties include:
- I am a small animal clinical veterinarian, meaning that I see patients in a clinic or hospital setting.
- I perform examinations, dental procedures, surgeries, and imaging, including radiographs and ultrasound examinations, in addition to ordering and evaluating laboratory tests.
- I diagnose and treat a myriad of diseases in primarily dogs and cats but also occasionally in the rabbit, guinea pig, rat, hamster, and mouse.

The most gratifying part of my job: I enjoy problem solving and helping my patients get well and stay healthy, and for the most part, I like working with the clients and owners.

The biggest challenge(s) I face in doing my job: The primary difficulty in veterinary medicine is the economic decision the owner has to make to pursue appropriate veterinary care. The fun challenge is continuing to learn to improve my level of practice and keep up with the latest information and techniques.

What drew me to my career? I always enjoyed being with and working with animals. Also, I became interested in medicine when my older sister pursued a career as a medical doctor.

Something I learned in my early education that I currently use in my career or that caused me to be interested in my career is: Learning the scientific method as a way to think rationally and logically about problems in the physical world is of the utmost importance, as are basic math skills.

Case Studies

Case studies have been added to all chapters, providing students the opportunity for critical thinking as they learn to solve questions and problems that occur in the various health professions. Answers to the case studies are provided on the Evolve website.

Brain Bytes

Facts and points of interest relating to chapter subject matter have been added to all chapters of the text.

Explore the Web

Internet sites have been added to each chapter to give students practice with online resources and research.

Explore the Web

Career Information

Bureau of Labor Statistics
http://www.bls.gov/

Salary.com
http://salary.com

Professional Associations

American Veterinary Medical Association
http://www.avma.org/

National Association of Veterinary Technicians in America (NAVTA)
http://www.navta.net/

Standards and Accountabilities

This section has been updated at the end of appropriate chapters. It provides the specific number and name of each national standard covered in that chapter, along with the page number on which that content can be found. This feature will provide both the instructor and the student quick access to National Health Care Skills Standards coverage.

Overall Content Update

The entire text has been updated so that all National Health Care Skills Standards are adequately covered.

Ancillaries

For the Instructor

Evolve Resources

The Evolve website for *Health Careers Today* features many helpful assets that instructors can use in planning and preparation. The Instructor's Resource Manual features Lesson Plans for each chapter in *Health Careers Today*, along with PowerPoint presentations specifically written for the content. In addition, the Evolve website includes all text and workbook answers, competency sheets, an image collection that includes all figures from the text (approximately 300), and nearly 800 test bank questions that include rationales, Bloom's taxonomy levels, and page references for the correct answers. The test bank is programmed in ExamView, a simple-to-use test generator program that helps formulate tests and quizzes quickly and easily. It is also easy to add additional questions.

For the Student

Evolve Resources

The Evolve website, *http://evolve.elsevier.com/Gerdin*, free to students who purchase a new text, reinforces information provided in the text and helps the student get a better grasp of the content. This website includes chapter-specific, self-grading, fill-in-the-blank and drag-and-drop quizzes, chapter-specific key term flashcards, anatomy and physiology animations, 20 skill videos, an audio glossary (more than 300 terms), answers to the text case studies, and chapter specific WebLinks.

Study Aids

Workbook

The Workbook to accompany *Health Careers Today* provides students with vocabulary practice exercises, key term puzzles, medical abbreviation practice exercises, concept application exercises, laboratory exercises, critical thinking exercises, and Internet exploration exercises, all organized by chapter. These exercises reinforce cognitive content and develop critical thinking skills.

Table of Contents

Unit I

Core Knowledge 1

Unit II

Anatomy and Physiology 155

Unit III

Career Clusters 345

Appendixes 574

Glossary 595

Skills

UNIT ONE

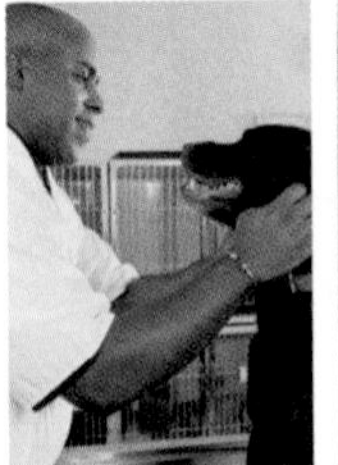
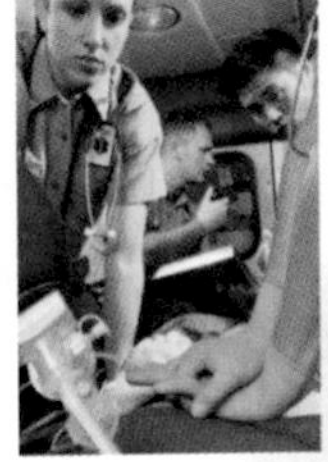
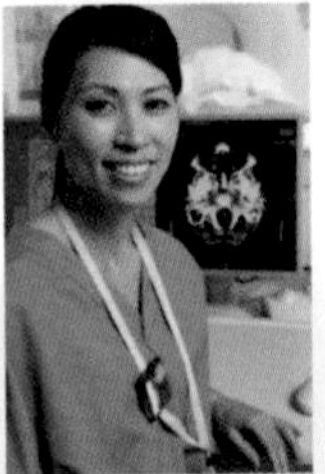

Core Knowledge

CHAPTER 1

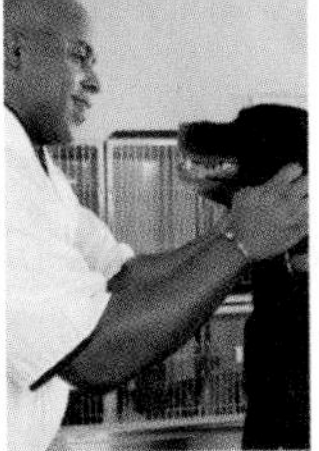
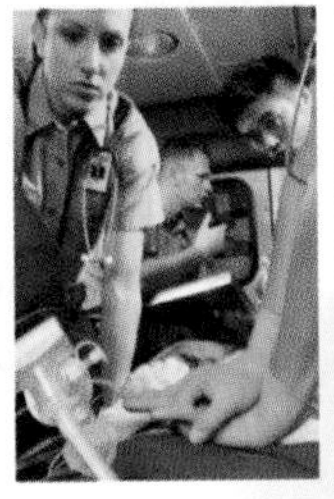
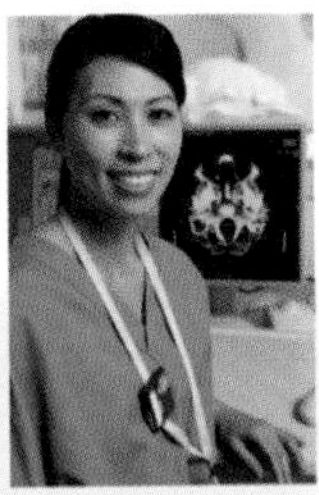

Health Care of the Past, Present, and Future

LEARNING OBJECTIVES

- Define at least 10 words relating to health care of the past, present, and future.
- Identify three socioeconomic factors that influence the health care industry.
- Describe at least three advantages to following a career in the health care field.
- Describe a career ladder for at least one health care occupation.
- List at least three factors to be considered when choosing an occupation.
- Identify at least five milestones in the advancement of health care.
- Describe at least two factors that have contributed to the rising cost of health care.
- Describe at least two methods being used to reduce health care costs.
- Describe at least three types of health care services.

KEY TERMS

Accreditation *(uh-kred-uh-TAY-shun)* Official authorization or approval

Career *(kuh-REER)* Occupation or profession

Certification *(sert-uh-fuh-KAY-shen)* Documentation of having met certain standards

Diagnosis-related grouping *(die-ug-NO-sis ree-lay-ted GROOP-ing)* Predetermined payment structure for health care services established by the federal government

Health *(helth)* State of optimal well-being, achieved through prevention of illness and injury

Insurance *(in-SHER-ens)* Payment for health care expenses, which may or may not occur, in return for a specified payment in advance

Licensure *(LISE-en-sher)* Legal authority to perform an activity

Litigation *(lit-uh-GAY-shen)* Legal dispute; lawsuit

Occupation *(ahk-yoo-PAY-shen)* Vocation, activity in which one participates

KEY TERMS cont'd

Pandemic *(pan-DEM-ik)* Epidemic that spreads over a wide geographical area, affecting a large part of the population

Paraprofessional *(par-uh-pruh-FESH-uh-nel)* Worker who assists a professional in the performance of duties

Profession *(pruh-FESH-un)* Occupation that requires specialized knowledge and, often, long and intensive academic training

Quackery *(KWAK-uh-ree)* Treatment that pretends to cure disease

Registration *(rej-is-TRAY-shun)* Official record of individuals qualified to perform certain services

Health Care of the Past

In the earliest civilizations health needs were met by a specific person or group. Ancient treatments were harmful in some cases and helpful in others. Some of the most helpful were the use of herbs and plants for medication. The World Health Organization (WHO) estimates that 80% of the world's population use plants or herbal treatments as part of their primary care. According to the American Association for the Advancement of Science (AAAS), about 118 of the 150 prescription drugs sold in the United States originate from plants, fungus, bacteria, and extractions from animals. Some of these remedies, such as quinine for malaria and digitalis for heart conditions, are still in use today (Box 1-1; also see Medical Milestones on pp. 21-22).

Hippocrates (460-377 B.C.) is considered the father of modern medicine. He initiated the oath of practice that, in adapted form, most physicians still adopt (Box 1-2).

In early times plagues or epidemics caused millions of deaths. Many of these diseases are now preventable through vaccination and improved methods of cleanliness and sanitation (Fig. 1-1). Although communicable diseases still cause many deaths in less-developed countries, new technological advances are being used to provide better health care throughout the world.

In the past, the "patient" of the health care industry was a passive recipient of the treatment recommended by the health care professional. The relationship was a dependent one, with the health care provider as the guiding force. The patient often accepted without question the treatment suggested by health care providers.

BOX 1-1

Remedies of the Past and Present

Past	Present
Bark of willow tree	Aspirin used to reduce inflammation
Citronella and garlic	Repel bugs; garlic to promote immune response
Eucalyptus	Clears airways in respiratory disorders
Foxglove	Digitalis, used to treat heart disease
Green tea	Antioxidant, used to lower enzyme levels and prevent cancer
Lavender oil	Treatment of cuts and bruises; promotes sleep and relaxation
Lemon oil	Purifies water; with honey to reduce cough
Pacific yew tree	Taxol used to treat cancer
Quinine	Treatment of malaria
Tea tree oil	Antiseptic

Society has traditionally accorded respect to health care providers. The ancient Egyptians, Greeks, and Chinese who **practiced** the art of surgery or were witch doctors or neighborly herbalists all enjoyed stature in their communities. The arts of the past have become the **professions** of today (Box 1-3). These health care professions have many educational and training requirements.

BOX 1-2

Hippocratic Oath

I swear by Apollo Physician, by Aesculapius, by Health, by Heal All, and by all the gods and goddesses, that, according to my ability and judgment, I will keep this oath and stipulation; to reckon him who taught me this art equally dear to me as my parents, and share my substance with him and relieve his necessities if required. To regard his offspring as on the same footing with my own brothers and to teach them this art if they should wish to learn it, without fee or stipulation; and that by precept, lecture, and every other mode of instruction I will impart a knowledge of my art to my own sons and to those of my teachers and to disciples bound by a stipulation and oath according to the law of medicine, but to none others.

I will follow that method of treatment which, according to my ability and judgment, I consider for the benefit of my patients, and abstain from whatever is deleterious and mischievous. I will give no deadly medicine to anyone if asked, nor suggest any counsel. Furthermore, I will not give to a woman an instrument to produce an abortion.

With Purity and with Holiness, I will pass my life and practice my art. I will not cut a person who is suffering with a stone, but will leave this to the practitioners of this work. Into whatever houses I enter I will go into them for the benefit of the sick and will abstain from every voluntary act of mischief and corruption; and further from the seduction of females or males, bond or free.

Whatever, in connection with my professional practice, or not in connection with it, I may see or hear in the lives of men which ought not to be spoken abroad, I will not divulge, as reckoning that all such should be kept secret.

While I continue to keep this oath inviolated, may it be granted to me to enjoy life and practice the art, respected by all men, at all times, but should I trespass and violate this oath, may the reverse be my lot.

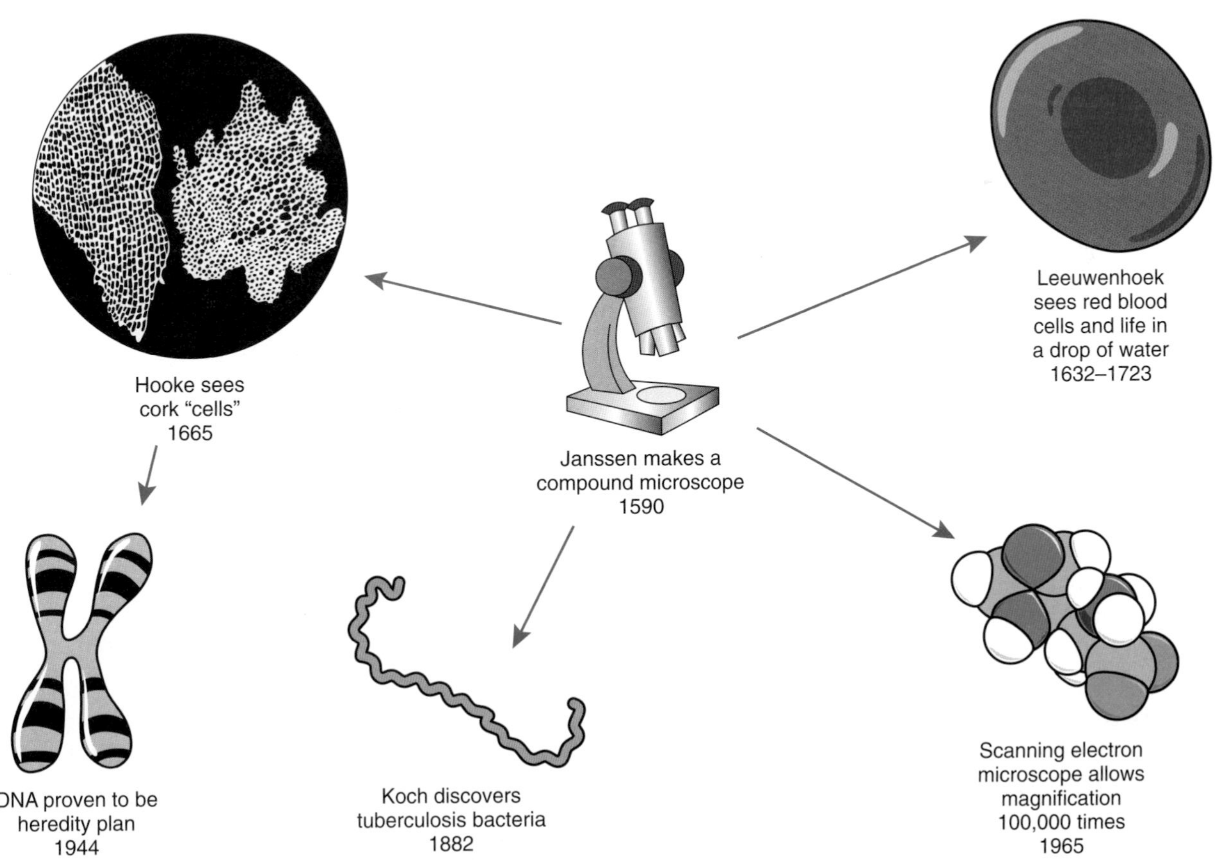
Hooke sees cork "cells" 1665
Janssen makes a compound microscope 1590
Leeuwenhoek sees red blood cells and life in a drop of water 1632–1723
DNA proven to be heredity plan 1944
Koch discovers tuberculosis bacteria 1882
Scanning electron microscope allows magnification 100,000 times 1965

FIGURE 1-1 Many health care innovations are possible because of prior discoveries.

BOX 1-3

Evolution of a Profession

Florence Nightingale is credited with raising nursing to the level of a profession. Nurses were trained before her time, but not with the strong educational background that increased the respect for nurses.

When Nightingale asked to attend nursing training, her parents refused to allow it. She continued to learn on her own by visiting hospitals and finally obtained 3 months of training. She became superintendent of a small hospital and was quickly offered a position in a larger institution because of her strong views on social welfare.

In 1854 Florence Nightingale led a group of 38 nurses to Turkey to care for soldiers injured in the war in which England was involved. Although doctors did not welcome the nurses because they were women, they improved the terrible conditions and organized and restructured the care greatly.

In 1860 the Nightingale School of Nurses opened with funding that was provided by the English government in appreciation for the service of these nurses. Nightingale believed that nursing was an art that must be founded on organized, practical, and scientific training. She taught that the person, not the disease, should be treated. Although in poor health, Nightingale lived to be 90 years of age.

Health Care of the Present

In the United States the focus of health care has shifted from the prevention of contagious diseases to those such as cancer, drug abuse, and heart disease, that are the result of lifestyles. Additionally, concerns relating to emergency response and preparedness services have become of primary concern to the health care industry (Table 1-1). Some communicable diseases are still a focus, including acquired immunodeficiency syndrome (AIDS), tuberculosis (TB), and flu. The WHO reported 33 million people living with AIDS worldwide in 2007. At the end of 2006, the Centers for Disease Control and Prevention (CDC) estimated that 1.1 million people were living with human

TABLE 1-1
CDC Categories of Emergency Preparedness and Response

Emergency	Example
Bioterrorism agents	Anthrax
	Botulism
	Plague
	Smallpox
	Tularemia
	Viral hemorrhagic fevers
Chemical emergencies	Biotoxins
	Blister agents, vesicants
	Blood agents
	Caustics (acids)
	Choking, lung, pulmonary agents
	Long-acting anticoagulants
	Metals
	Nerve agents
	Organic solvents
	Riot-control agents, tear gas
	Toxic alcohols
	Vomiting agents
Radiation emergencies	Dirty bombs
	Nuclear blasts
Mass casualties	Explosions and blasts
	Brain injuries
	Burns
	Injuries
	Emergency wound care
Natural disasters and severe weather	Earthquakes
	Extreme heat
	Flood
	Hurricane
	Landslide, mudslide
	Tornado
	Tsunami
	Volcano
	Wildfire
	Winter weather
Recent outbreaks and incidents (2009)	Multistate *Escherichia coli* outbreak
	Santa Barbara wildfire
	H1N1 flu outbreak
	Oklahoma-Texas wildfire
	Italian earthquake
	North Dakota floods
	Mount Redoubt volcano eruption
	Salmonella outbreak

From Centers for Disease Control and Prevention (CDC), retrieved September 2009, from http://www.bt.cdc.gov, Centers for Disease Control.

immunodeficiency virus (HIV) or AIDS in the United States. It also reported a total of 12,898 cases of TB in 2008, which shows a decline of 2.9% from 2007 and 54% from 1980. According to WHO, nine Asian countries reported outbreaks of the H5N1 avian flu in birds by February 2006, six of which reported cases affecting humans. More than half of the confirmed cases were fatal. An outbreak of H1N1 swine flu was detected in April 2009. By July 2009 the CDC reported 43,771 cases; 302 of these patients died. The government has allocated money and the CDC has established preparation guidelines for a possible flu pandemic. Table 1-2 provides an overview of the pandemics and pandemic scares.

TABLE 1-2
Pandemics and Pandemic Scares

Year	Name	Description
1918	Spanish flu	20%-40% of world population became ill; more than 20 million people died worldwide
1957	Asian flu	Appeared in two waves; 69,800 died in the United States
1968	Hong Kong flu	33,800 died in the United States
1976	Swine flu scare	Identified and stayed in Fort Dix, NJ, region; mass vaccination program enacted
1977	Russian flu scare	Appeared primarily in children
1997	Avian flu scare	Moved quickly from chicken to people; 18 died of the few hundred affected

Institutional health care is provided by general hospitals, convalescent care centers, health maintenance organizations, home health agencies, and public health agencies (Table 1-3). Voluntary organizations provide education and support to individuals with specific concerns. The organizational structure of the facility defines the role of the health care worker (Fig. 1-2).

The federal agency that oversees the nation's health care is the Public Health Services, which is

TABLE 1-3
Agency Health Care Providers

Agency	Service
General hospital	Provides short-term care, acute care, and diagnostic and rehabilitation services; may be for profit or nonprofit, teaching or nonteaching
Specialty hospital	Provides treatment for a specific condition such as tuberculosis, mental health disorders, or rehabilitation services
Practitioner office	Provides diagnosis, simple testing, treatments, and counseling services; may be independent or group practice
Long-term care center	Provides personal care for elderly and extended convalescent care
Outpatient care facility	Provides surgical, diagnostic, and ambulatory care
Clinic	Provides combination of practices, which may or may not be supported by public health care funding
Health maintenance	Provides health services at group rates
Home health care	Provides care in the home of the patient; may be publicly or privately owned
Hospice care	Provides medical and psychological care for the terminally ill, either in the home or at a hospice facility; may be private or part of another facility
Assisted living facility	Provides residents a way to live alone or with someone in an apartment; provides services as needed, including meals and health care
Day care	Provides care for the elderly or children and may include care for illness
Public health care	Provides care through federal, state, and local agencies for those who cannot afford to pay for health care and provides preventive services for the entire population
Voluntary organization	Provides research, education, and support for specific concerns; funded by donations and grants

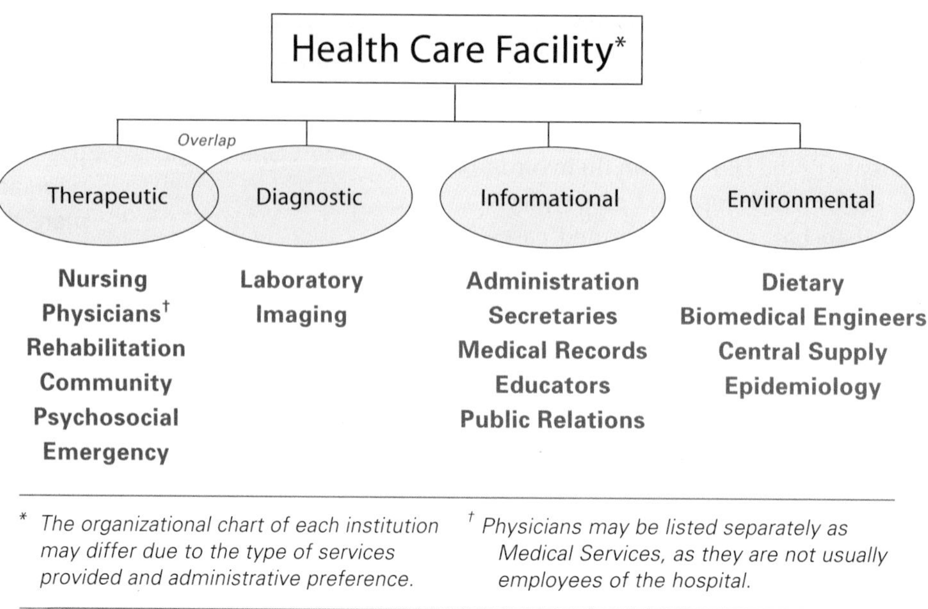

FIGURE 1-2 The organizational structure of a health care facility.

part of the Department of Health and Human Services. It was established in 1798 to provide care for the American merchant seamen but has expanded to cover many other facets of health care (Box 1-4). The Department of Labor also regulates some health concerns through the Occupational Safety and Health Administration.

Health care is one of the largest industries in the United States. Currently the supply of workers is less than the demand, creating opportunities and job security in many areas of health care. The cost of health care in the United States continues to increase much faster than do other factors in the cost of living. The Kaiser Family Foundation reported the expansion of health care to 16.2% of the gross domestic product (GDP) in 2007. Some of the reasons for rising health care costs are the advanced technological developments, malpractice litigation, increase in longevity, and disaster relief expenses.

In 2007 the Commonwealth Fund's annual survey found that the U.S. health care system to be the most costly and consistently underperforming, compared to the seven countries considered. According to the U.S. Treasury Department, a 2008 census report indicated that 15.4%, or 46.3 million of Americans, did not have health insurance.

In March 2010 the U.S. government passed the Affordable Care Act. Some provisions in the legislation took effect in 2010, with others becoming effective in 2014. For example, children with preexisting conditions will not be denied insurance on that basis beginning in 2010. Small business owners will receive a tax credit of up to 35% of their premiums to insure employees. The constitutionality of some provisions of the bill, such as the mandatory requirement for individuals to have health insurance, is being challenged.

Medicare is the federal health program for individuals 65 or older, certain younger people with disabilities, and people with end-stage renal disease. Since 1984 Medicare has reimbursed for services on the basis of the diagnosis instead of the actual cost. Diagnosis-related groupings (DRGs) have greatly affected the health care industry by shortening the time allowed for treatment. In 2005 Medicare began offering a prescription drug plan for applicants. Medicaid is a joint program between the federal and state governments. It helps provide health care coverage for individuals with low income and limited resources. Programs for Medicaid vary from state to state. The Social Security Act established both Medicare and Medicaid in 1965.

Insurance companies have established options designed to lower or tailor the cost of coverage to the individual need. These include managed care models,

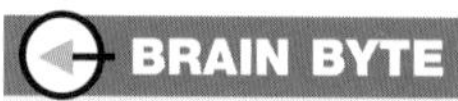

The Centers for Medicare & Medicaid Services (CMS) estimate that the United States will spend $3.1 trillion on health care in 2012.

BOX 1-4

Department of Health and Human Services Divisions and Functions

Administration for Children and Families (ACF): Responsible for programs that assist needy children and families, including administration of the state and federal welfare programs, such as Head Start

Administration on Aging (AOA): Provides services for elderly, including Meals on Wheels

Agency for Healthcare Research and Quality (AHRQ): Provides information through research to help people make better decisions about health care in the areas of safety, medical error, and effective service

Agency for Toxic Substances and Disease Registry (ATSDR): Conducts health studies, assessments, and education training to prevent exposure to hazardous substances in waste sites

Centers for Disease Control and Prevention (CDC): Monitors and prevents outbreaks of disease, including maintaining statistics and providing immunizations

Centers for Medicare and Medicaid Services (CMS): Provides Medicare and Medicaid services for aged and indigent populations, which include about one in every four Americans

Food and Drug Administration (FDA): Regulates safety of food, cosmetics, pharmaceutical, biological products, and medical devices

Health Resources and Services Administration (HRSA): Provides services for underserved populations, such as migrant workers, the homeless, and public housing residents. This division is also responsible for the organ transplantation system, infant mortality, and services to people with AIDS

Indian Health Service (IHS): Supports the hospitals and health centers that provide care to 557 federally recognized tribes of American Indians and Alaska Natives

National Institutes of Health (NIH): Supports more than 35,000 research projects in diseases such as cancer, diabetes, and AIDS

Program Support Center (PSC): Provides service-for-fee support services such as training and grant administration throughout the federal government

Substance Abuse and Mental Health Services Administration (SAMHSA): Works to improve substance abuse and mental health prevention and services

increased deductibles, coinsurance, copayments, and preventive care. Managed care insurance plans include health maintenance organizations (HMOs), preferred provider organizations (PPOs), and point-of-service (POS). In one type of HMO described as the staff model, the health care providers are employed by the organization and work in a designated facility. The independent-practice association model contracts physicians and other health care providers to provide care to the HMO members. POS plans generally allow members to select treatment either "in network" or, for a greater cost, "out-of-network."

The traditional model of insurance (fee-for-service) may also include cost-containment measures similar to those of managed care. The insured person may choose a plan that provides a percentage of the cost or a specified amount (Table 1-4).

Health care cost-containment measures have included the promotion of wellness and early detection by screening. In 2005 the National Committee for

TABLE 1-4
Sample Insurance Cost Comparison

Indemnity (Fee-for-Service)	Managed Health Care (HMO, PPO, POS)
Payment of a monthly fee	Payment of a monthly premium
Yearly deductible for individual and family	Co-payment for office visit
80%-20% split of care after deductible is met	Coinsurance (70%/30% or 80%/20%)
	Generally includes preventive care
	Yearly deductible for individual and family

Health Insurance

Indemnity

Reimbursement for care regardless of who provides the service; amount may be limited.

Reimbursement: Actual Cost	Reimbursement: Percentage of Actual Cost	Indemnity
Insurer reimburses actual cost of services.	Insurer reimburses a percentage of actual cost, often 80%.	Insurer pays specified amount per day for a specified amount of days.

Managed Care

A specified network of providers is selected for services.

Health Maintenance Organization (HMO)	Preferred Provider Organization (PPO)	Point of Service (POS)
Members pay a fixed monthly fee; care is usually given in network facilities by network providers.	Members pay for services as they are given. The sponsor (employer) reimburses the member for costs less the co-payment. Care is given by network providers, with increased fees for use of out-of-network providers.	Members pay minimal co-payment for services within the network. A primary physician in the network must make all referrals to specialists, with an increase in cost for services provided out of the network.

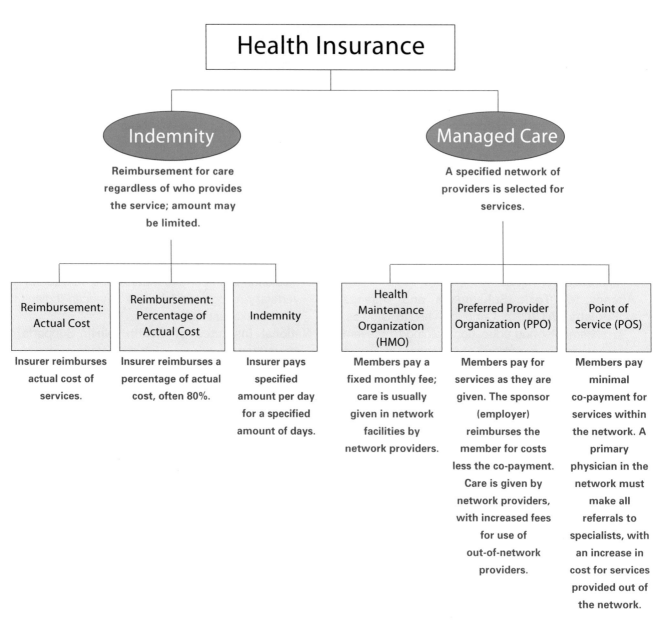

FIGURE 1-3 Health care insurance model.

Qualifying Assurance (the accrediting agency for managed care plans) and the *U.S. News & World Report* magazine ranked plans across the United States. One characteristic of the plans was the management of chronic health conditions. For example, a health professional focuses on a patient's overall health by monitoring a patient with a chronic condition such as diabetes or hypertension.

Employers have reduced benefits and shifted the cost of health care to the employee. According to the Kaiser Family Foundation's Employee Benefits Survey, premiums for health insurance rose 5% in 2007. Some insurance companies offer a "cafeteria-style" selection from which employees may choose various types of coverage up to a specified cost limit (Fig. 1-3).

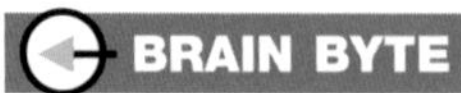

In 2008 the CDC estimated that 6.5% of the U.S. population did not get needed health care because of cost.

Other plans relating to health care include disability income insurance, long-term care insurance, medical savings accounts, and workers' compensation. Disability income insurance provides an income if a person becomes too sick, injured, or unable to work. When a chronic illness or disability prevents a person from working for an extended period, long-term care insurance offsets the expense of care. In a medical savings account, contributions are made to the account from one's salary before being taxed and then can be used to cover qualifying medical expenses. The fund withdrawals for medical coverage made from this account are not taxed. The first workers' compensation law in the United States was passed in 1908, but it covered only federal employees; now there are 55 such programs in the United States. Workers' compensation was designed to prevent litigation or lawsuits after the injury of an employee. Most programs pay medical expenses, lost earnings, and retraining costs when needed.

The Health Insurance Portability and Accountability Act (HIPAA) of 1996 allows employed individuals to maintain insurance coverage if they lose or change jobs. The act specifically limits exclusion of coverage caused by preexisting conditions, prohibits denial of coverage because of prior illness, and guarantees the insured individual's right to purchase insurance if unemployed. It also mandates the formats for electronic data interchange of information, such as patient and care identifiers. Chapters 2 and 4 provide more information about the HIPAA guidelines.

Hospitals are meeting the challenge of increased cost by becoming large corporate facilities and by forming partnerships with physicians for services such as extended care. Many smaller hospitals have been forced to close or sell to larger corporations, which because of their size have better buying power. Some hospitals have refused care for patients who have conditions or diagnoses for which treatment is not financially profitable.

The rise in professional malpractice insurance has contributed greatly to the increase in health care costs. To prevent the risk of liability, some physicians practice defensive medicine, such as ordering many tests and avoiding care for high-risk patients. In the field of obstetrics, the cost has led some physicians to stop delivering infants. In many states the obstetrician has been held financially responsible for children up to 18 or 21 years of age for damage that may have occurred at birth. Studies indicate that in most of the cases which have been taken to court, the abnormalities initiating the suit were not related to medical care.

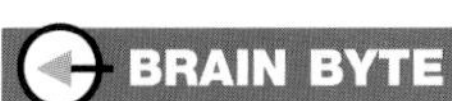

Several states, such as California, have passed laws that limit noneconomic damages from malpractice to $250,000.

Pharmaceutical companies are also using defensive economic strategies by reducing the manufacture of drugs that have a high risk of adverse affects. Concern about the liability of vaccine manufacture was addressed in the Homeland Security Act to encourage vaccine development. The Food and Drug Administration (FDA) requires extensive testing of drugs before allowing their use. The Orphan Drug Act allows the FDA to release some drugs early to meet needs of the ill when other medications have not been developed for the disease.

The state of the economy, the values of society, the law of supply and demand, and technological developments all influence health care in the United States. The industry, patients, and workers are currently adapting to the new technologies and challenges of an advanced society. Health is no longer considered to be just the absence of illness or injury. **Health** is a state of optimal well-being, achieved through prevention of illness and injury. The health care workers of today are concerned with the physical, emotional, and social needs of their patients.

Those who choose a career in the health field seek more than economic security. Other factors to consider include the nature of the duties, the working conditions, and the opportunities for advancement in health care **occupations**. Knowing the number and location of jobs, methods and qualifications for employment, and the psychosocial factors involved in the work is also important. Health care provides an opportunity to work with people, data, or things to complement the interests and abilities of the worker (Fig. 1-4).

Most health care **careers** provide workers with an opportunity to meet new challenges, enjoy a stable salary and employment, and move to new locations. The Bureau of Labor Statistics projects the health services as one of the top 10 growing industries to 2012. Jobs in health care offer a good working environment, and others respect these workers. Many people have reached top-level positions in health care through a series of occupations or a career ladder, both of which provide experience and support during the process. For example, an entry-level assistant or phlebotomist in the laboratory may become a medical technician, technologist, and pathologist with additional education. Career change might also occur on a horizontal level rather than a vertical one. For example, a medical radiology technician prepared in computed tomography (CT) might complete additional training to qualify to take magnetic resonance images (MRIs). Advancement is

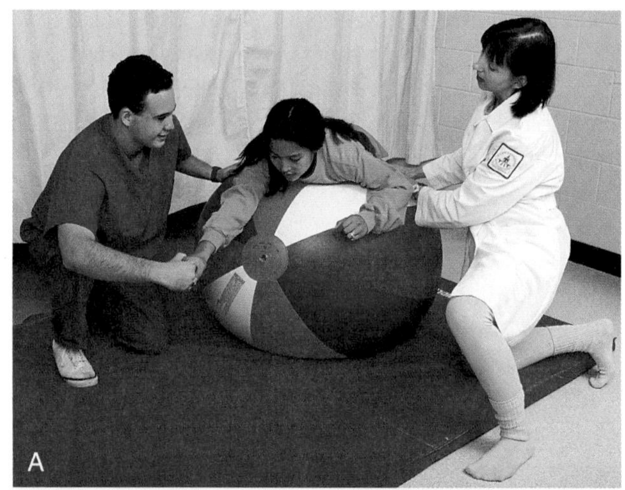

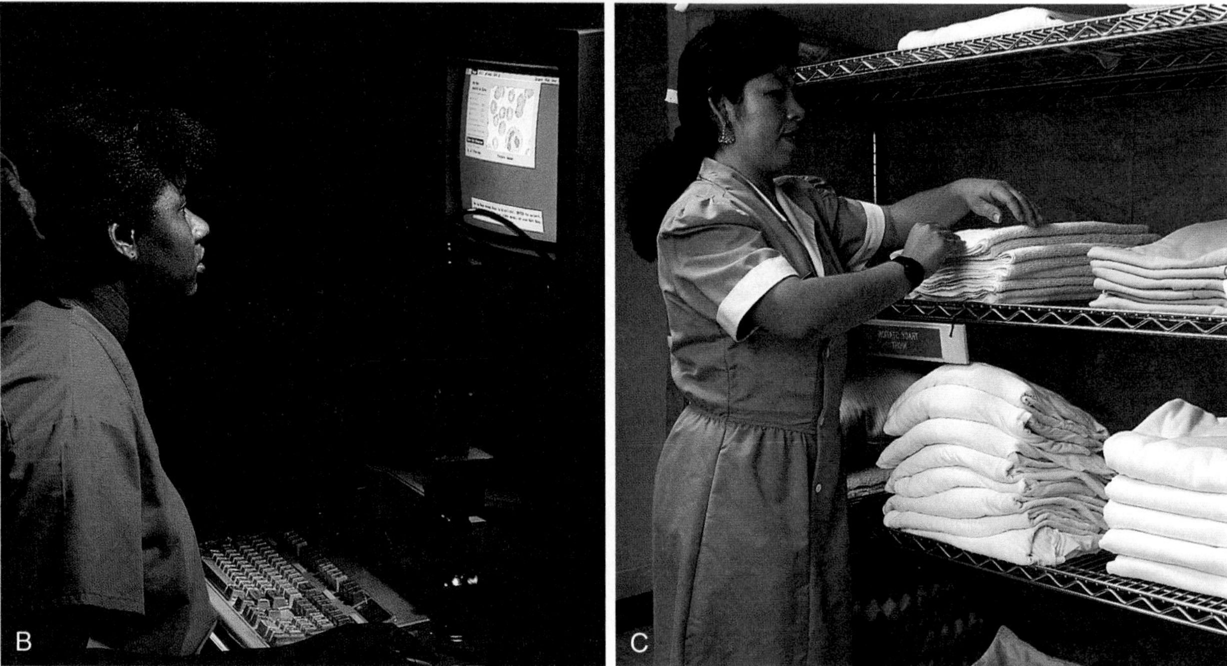

FIGURE 1-4 Health care today provides a variety of working conditions for employees who want to work with people **(A)**, data **(B)**, or things **(C)**.

TABLE 1-5
Career Ladder in Health Care

Title	Educational Requirement	Example
Aide	On-the-job training	Laboratory aide
Assistant	Up to 1 year of classroom and clinical preparation	Laboratory assistant
Technician	A 2-year community college or vocational training program	Laboratory technician
Technologist	A 3- to 4-year college program	Laboratory technologist
Professional	A 4-year degree, advanced degree, and clinical training	Pathologist (medical doctor)

usually based on additional experience, education, and training (Table 1-5).

With the advances in technology, the need for a strong academic background and continuing education is even more critical for the health care worker. Those in paraprofessional careers—for example, the physician assistant, nurse practitioner, and midwife—help provide more care than in the past to more people, especially in rural areas. Prehospital emergency care has become a new area of practice. The

BOX 1-5

Patient Rights

Key Areas of the Patient Bill of Rights

- Access to emergency services
- Choice of providers and plans
- Complaints and appeals
- Confidentiality (privacy) of health information
- Consumer responsibilities
- Information for patients
- Respect and nondiscrimination
- Taking part in treatment decisions

The Patient Care Partnership*

What to Expect during Your Hospital Stay:

- High-quality hospital care
- A clean and safe environment
- Involvement in your care
- Protection of your privacy
- Help when leaving the hospital
- Help with your billing claims

*The American Hospital Association (AHA) replaced the Patient Bill of Rights with a brochure that informs patients about their expectations, rights, and responsibilities. (http://www.aha.org/aha/issues/Communicating-With-Patients/pt-care-partnership.html)

BOX 1-6

The Resident's Bill of Rights

The Nursing Home Reform Act of 1987 requires nursing homes to provide an environment that promotes enhancement of the quality of life of each resident. Some specific rights of the Act include the following:

The resident has the right to freedom from abuse, mistreatment, and neglect.

The resident has the right to freedom from physical restraint.

The resident has the right to privacy and confidentiality.

The resident has the right to be fully informed in advance of health care and facility changes.

The resident has the right to communicate freely.

The resident has the right to voice grievances without discrimination or reprisal.

The resident has the right to visits with physicians, residents, and family groups.

The resident has the right to medical, physical, psychological, and social accommodations if necessary.

The resident has the right to be treated with dignity, respect, and freedom.

The resident has the right to exercise self-determination or autonomy and make independent choices regarding care.

knowledge and technology that make it possible to save many trauma victims have created many new career opportunities.

The patient of today has become a "client," or "consumer" of health care services. A shift in responsibilities has resulted in the client taking more responsibility for his or her own care. Today clients of health care are consumers with a greater awareness of the effect of their lifestyle on related health conditions. To avoid confusion, the term *patient* will be used throughout this text. Obtaining second opinions, shopping for the lowest health care costs, and seeking alternative and complementary providers have become common practice.

In 1972 the American Hospital Association (AHA) adopted the Patient's Bill of Rights, which describes the rights of the patient to participate in the system of care. This has now been replaced with a pamphlet to improve consumer understanding (Box 1-5). Congress enacted the Nursing Home Reform Act in 1987, which provides similar requirements to protect nursing home residents and places a strong emphasis on individual dignity and self-determination (Box 1-6).

As those seeking care have more critical needs, advanced skills are required of workers. Professional associations and government agencies set standards to ensure the quality of education and training. Agencies of **accreditation** have been established to determine whether a training program meets acceptable standards. The professional associations of the health care occupation provide most agencies of accreditation.

Many occupational areas are regulated by law to ensure that the quality of care is acceptable. Health care workers may need licensure, certification, or registration to practice. **Licensure** is controlled by the state and is usually based on successful completion of an examination. **Certification**, which may be given by an agency or a training program, indicates successful completion of a particular course. Individuals who have met a criterion of excellence or legal responsibility may be registered in some fields. **Registration** may be earned through the state or through an agency. Recently the federal government has required specific training for nursing assistants working in extended care facilities. Practicing without holding the proper credentials in the professions that are regulated is illegal.

Health Care of the Future

All people in the United States use the health care system during their lifetime. Health care of the future will continue to emphasize wellness and prevention instead of cure. Wellness services will include nutritional advice, stress-reduction counseling, habit-cessation management, and exercise instruction (Box 1-7). Concern for childhood obesity and related illnesses will also play a more central role. (In 2006, 17.6% of children ages 12 to 19 were reported to be overweight.) Technology will continue to drive the type and pace of changes in the industry.

One main area of service in the future will be care of the elderly. The population of the United States continues to age and live longer. With fewer children being born each year, the average age of an American has risen to 36.8 and will continue to increase. In 2008 it was reported that 38.9% of the U.S. population was 65 years or older, and it is projected that this number will rise to 12%; 5.7% of this group were 85 or older. Older people require three times the amount of health care as those in younger groups. Many older people experience at least one chronic disease, and about half have some type of limited movement. Health care of the future will provide rehabilitative services for the elderly population.

BOX 1-7

The Leading Health Indicators*

- Physical activity
- Overweight and obesity
- Tobacco use
- Substance abuse
- Responsible sexual behavior
- Mental health
- Injury and violence
- Environmental quality
- Immunization
- Access to health care

*The leading health indicators were selected to reflect the major health concerns in the United States at the beginning of the twenty-first century by the Healthy People 2010 project.

BRAIN BYTE

People under 20 make up 27.6% of the U.S. population, whereas 12.6% are over 65.

CASE STUDY 1-1 You are caring for a patient in a long-term care facility. The patient does not seem to be able to stay upright in a chair. You would like to tie some support around the patient. What should you do?

Answers to Case Studies are available on the Evolve website: ***http://evolve.elsevier.com/Gerdin***

More small hospitals will close their doors, and the number of large urban institutions and state-of-the-art intensive care units will increase. Hospitals will continue to provide care for only the severely ill and injured and will reduce the number of beds for other patients, who will be treated in other settings, especially home care.

Alternative providers and treatments will continue to develop. One alternative that has increased in popularity and acceptance is holistic health. In this type of care, patients are seen as unique individuals who are responsible for their own care. Holistic health care uses many methods of diagnosis and treatment, of which traditional medical practice is just one. The National Institutes of Health (NIH) is currently providing research money for unconventional therapies through the Office of Alternative Medicine. These therapies include the use of bee pollen to control asthma, acupuncture for depression, hypnosis to speed bone healing, yoga to control addiction, and shark cartilage to reduce tumors. However, development of alternative provisions may lead to an increase in the incidence of quackery as patients look for alternative treatments (Box 1-8).

In 2001 Congress considered a Patient Bill of Rights that would allow the consumer to hold HMOs legally responsible for treatment choices and practices. Other provisions of the law would have allowed health care patients to seek care at the nearest emergency department, obtain perinatal care without a referral, and use a pediatrician as the primary physician for children. Although the bill passed in the Senate and a similar one passed in the House, a committee was not appointed to consider it, so it died.

BOX 1-8

Twenty-Five Ways to Spot Quacks and Vitamin Pushers

How can food quacks and other vitamin pushers be recognized? Here are 25 signs that should arouse suspicion:

1. When talking about nutrients, they tell only part of the story.
2. They claim that most Americans are poorly nourished.
3. They recommend "nutrition insurance" for everyone.
4. They say that most diseases are caused by faulty diet and can be treated with "nutritional" methods.
5. They allege that modern processing methods and storage remove all nutritive value from our food.
6. They claim that diet is a major factor in behavior.
7. They claim that fluoridation is dangerous.
8. They claim that soil depletion and the use of pesticides and "chemical" fertilizers result in food that is less safe and less nourishing.
9. They claim you are in danger of being "poisoned" by ordinary food additives and preservatives.
10. They charge that the recommended dietary allowances (RDAs) have been set too low.
11. They claim that under everyday stress and, in certain diseases, your need for nutrients is increased.
12. They recommend "supplements" and "health foods" for everyone.
13. They claim that "natural" vitamins are better than "synthetic" ones.
14. They suggest that a questionnaire can be used to indicate whether you need dietary supplements.
15. They say it is easy to lose weight.
16. They promise quick, dramatic, miraculous results.
17. They routinely sell vitamins and other "dietary supplements" as part of their practice.
18. They use disclaimers couched in pseudo-medical jargon.
19. They use anecdotes and testimonials to support their claims.
20. They claim that sugar is a deadly poison.
21. They display credentials not recognized by responsible scientists or educators.
22. They offer to determine your body's nutritional state with a laboratory test or a questionnaire.
23. They claim they are being persecuted by orthodox medicine and that their work is being suppressed because it is controversial.
24. They warn you not to trust your doctor.
25. They encourage patients to lend political support to their treatment methods.

Courtesy Stephen Barrett, MD, Allentown, Pa. Written by Stephen Barrett, MD, and Victor Herbert, MD, JD.

The impact of technology in the future can only be imagined. Some innovations that may become common include the inventions of nanotechnology and telemedicine. A physician can now view the intestines from the inside after the patient swallows a small camera. Some forms of blindness will be cured with a microchip within 10 years. Some patients are receiving daily monitoring of health care conditions through remote data collection and consultations using computers. Distance surgery has been performed using similar technology. Recombinant deoxyribonucleic acid (DNA) techniques will allow new types of gene therapy and fetal stem cell research. Technology will stimulate controversy, such as the use of cloning of humans and their organs.

CASE STUDY 1-2 You use a personal digital assistant (PDA) to record vital signs digitally. One of your co-workers asks you to let him use your password to record his data because he cannot remember his. What should you do?

Answers to Case Studies are available on the Evolve website: ***http://evolve.elsevier.com/Gerdin***

The Internet provides the patient with a wealth of information about a condition or disease; however, the information may or may not come from a reputable health care practitioner. The Internet gives the consumer access to clinical trials and research results. It also provides a way to buy pharmaceuticals, which may or may not be effective. With the increasing use of computers and technology in health care, the issue of privacy of information will become a central concern of the future.

The health care team will become more responsible for relieving some of the ills of society, such as the "border babies" and other abandoned children. Border babies are well infants who are left in hospitals because their mothers are unable to care for them due to drug addiction or poverty. Some states have passed laws that allow a mother to abandon an infant at a site designated a "safe haven" without fear of legal repercussions. In 48 states a baby may be left at a fire station or hospital with no questions asked.

The health care worker of the future must be trained for a broad range of skills and know about many areas of care. Fig. 1-5 demonstrates the relationship of the clusters defined by a project led by WestEd, from 1992 to 1996, and their related academic content. The project included health care workers, industry representatives, and education participants. Box 1-9 provides more specific descriptions and skill standards for each of the clusters that have been established. The placement of career opportunities in the clusters as described by the National Consortium on Health Science and Technology Education is shown in Fig. 1-6.

Additionally, the worker must be flexible, know how to solve problems as they arise, and use independent judgment. He or she must be willing to continue to learn and adapt to new technologies. The health care workers of the future will be highly regulated to ensure the quality of care that is provided. Technicians will continue to be trained to become multicompetent so that they can offer more than one kind of service. Expanded skills for health practitioners will be used in many facilities, especially in small hospitals, as fewer professional and more technical staff members are employed.

BOX 1-9

National Health Care Skill Standards Clusters

- The therapeutic cluster includes occupations that maintain or change the health of the client over time. Careers might include dental assisting, home health, medical assisting, pharmacy, nursing, and similar occupations.
- The diagnostic cluster occupations create a picture of the health of the client at one point in time. Careers might include cardiology, radiology, laboratory technology, and similar occupations.
- Information services careers document client care and include records management, risk management, unit coordination, and similar occupations.
- Support services workers provide a therapeutic environment for health care and include facility maintenance, supply personnel, housekeeping, and similar occupations.
- Biotechnology and research professionals use bioscience to find cures, create tools and treatments for disease, and improve health and the human condition. Careers include genetics, molecular biology, and clinical trial research.

CASE STUDY 1-3 During conversation one of your assigned patients shares with you that she does not have health insurance and will have to pay the bill herself. She asks you to cut corners for her care. What should you do?

Answers to Case Studies are available on the Evolve website: ***http://evolve.elsevier.com/Gerdin***

On September 11, 2001, the World Trade Center and Pentagon were attacked by terrorists, killing more than 3000 people. After that date, several cases of anthrax occurred in various parts of the country. During 2005 natural disasters such as Hurricanes Katrina and Rita added new challenges to the industry. The health care team will need to make adjustments with the rest of society to deal with this new phase of American history. Emergency care providers and procedures will grow in number and specialization to deal with the reality of emergency response and bioterrorism. Additionally, security measures for all public facilities, including research and health care facilities, will be a concern.

CASE STUDY 1-4 While giving daily care, a patient asks you whether the doctor who is handling his case is a good physician. What should you do?

Answers to Case Studies are available on the Evolve website: ***http://evolve.elsevier.com/Gerdin***

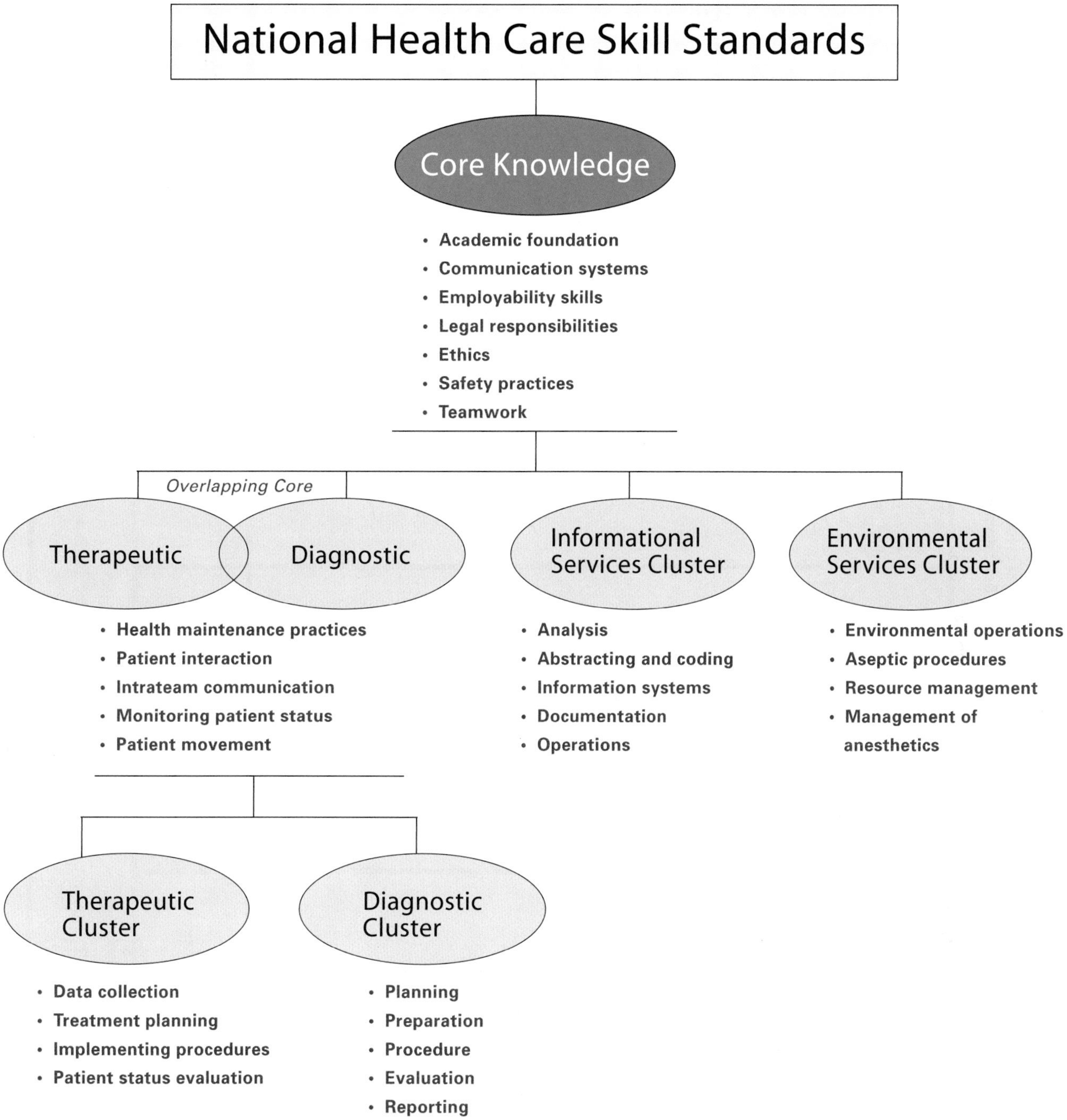

National Health Care Skill Standards

Core Knowledge

- Academic foundation
- Communication systems
- Employability skills
- Legal responsibilities
- Ethics
- Safety practices
- Teamwork

Overlapping Core

Therapeutic / **Diagnostic**

- Health maintenance practices
- Patient interaction
- Intrateam communication
- Monitoring patient status
- Patient movement

Therapeutic Cluster

- Data collection
- Treatment planning
- Implementing procedures
- Patient status evaluation

Diagnostic Cluster

- Planning
- Preparation
- Procedure
- Evaluation
- Reporting

Informational Services Cluster

- Analysis
- Abstracting and coding
- Information systems
- Documentation
- Operations

Environmental Services Cluster

- Environmental operations
- Aseptic procedures
- Resource management
- Management of anesthetics

FIGURE 1-5 National health care skill standard model. A biotechnology and research career pathway has been added to the model. (Courtesy WestEd, San Francisco, Calif.)

Summary

- The state of the economy, the values of society, the law of supply and demand, and technological developments influence the health care industry.
- Pursuing a health career offers several advantages, including economic security, an opportunity to meet new challenges, and mobility.
- An example of a career ladder in health care that may be followed with additional education and training is the transition of a nurse assistant to licensed practical nurse to registered nurse.
- Some of the factors that may be part of choosing an occupation include the working conditions, nature of the job, and opportunities for advancement.

Health Science Career Cluster

Planning, managing, and providing therapeutic services, diagnostic services, health informatics, support services, and biotechnology research and development.

Sample Career Specialties/Occupations	♦ Acupuncturist ♦ Anesthesiologist Assistant ♦ Art / Music / Dance Therapist(s) ♦ Athletic Trainer ♦ Audiologist ♦ Certified Nursing Assistant ♦ Chiropractor ♦ Dental Assistant / Hygienist ♦ Dental Lab Technician ♦ Dentist ♦ Dietitian ♦ Dosimetrist ♦ EMT ♦ Exercise Physiologist ♦ Home Health Aide ♦ Kinesiotherapist ♦ Licensed Practical Nurse ♦ Massage Therapist ♦ Medical Assistant ♦ Mortician ♦ Occupational Therapist / Asst ♦ Ophthalmic Medical Personnel ♦ Optometrist ♦ Orthotist/Prosthetist ♦ Paramedic ♦ Pharmacist/Pharmacy Tech ♦ Physical Therapist / Assistant ♦ Physician (MD/DO) ♦ Physician's Assistant ♦ Psychologist ♦ Recreation Therapist ♦ Registered Nurse ♦ Respiratory Therapist ♦ Social Worker ♦ Speech Language Pathologist ♦ Surgical Technician ♦ Veterinarian / Vet Tech	♦ Cardiovascular Technologist ♦ Clinical Lab Technician ♦ Computed Tomography (CT) Technologist ♦ Cytogenetic Technologist ♦ Cytotechnologists ♦ Diagnostic Medical Sonographers ♦ Electrocardiographic (ECG) Technician ♦ Electronic Diagnostic (EEG) Technologist ♦ Exercise Physiologist ♦ Geneticist ♦ Histotechnician ♦ Histotechnologist ♦ Magnetic Resonance (MR) Technologist ♦ Mammographer ♦ Medical Technologist / Clinical Laboratory Scientist ♦ Nuclear Medicine Technologist ♦ Nutritionist ♦ Pathologist ♦ Pathology Assistant ♦ Phlebotomist ♦ Positron Emission Tomography (PET) Technologist ♦ RadiologicTechnologist/Radiographer ♦ Radiologist	♦ Admitting Clerk ♦ Applied Researcher ♦ Community Services Specialists ♦ Data Analyst ♦ Epidemiologist ♦ Ethicist ♦ Health Educator ♦ Health Information Coder ♦ Health Information Services ♦ Healthcare Administrator ♦ Medical Assistant ♦ Medical Biller/Patient Financial Services ♦ Medical Information Technologist ♦ Medical Librarian/Cybrarian ♦ Patient Advocates ♦ Public Health Educator ♦ Reimbursement Specialist (HFMA) ♦ Risk Management ♦ Social Worker ♦ Transcriptionist ♦ Unit Coordinator ♦ Utilization Manager	♦ Biomedical / Clinical Engineer ♦ Biomedical / Clinical Technician ♦ Central Services ♦ Environmental Health and Safety ♦ Environmental Services ♦ Facilities Manager ♦ Food Service ♦ Hospital Maintenance Engineer ♦ Industrial Hygienist ♦ Materials Management ♦ Transport Technician	♦ Biochemist ♦ Bioinformatics Associate ♦ Bioinformatics Scientist ♦ Bioinformatics Specialist ♦ Biomedical Chemist ♦ Biostatistician ♦ Cell Biologist ♦ Clinical Trials Research Associate ♦ Clinical Trials Research Coordinator ♦ Geneticist ♦ Lab Assistant-Genetics ♦ Lab Technician ♦ Microbiologist ♦ Molecular Biologist ♦ Pharmaceutical Scientist ♦ Quality Assurance Technician ♦ Quality Control Technician ♦ Regulatory Affairs Specialist ♦ Research Assistant ♦ Research Associate ♦ Research Scientist ♦ Toxicologist
Pathways	**Therapeutic Services**	**Diagnostics Services**	**Health Informatics**	**Support Services**	**Biotechnology Research and Development**
Cluster K & S	**Cluster Knowledge and Skills** ♦ Academic Foundation ♦ Communications ♦ Systems ♦ Employability Skills ♦ Legal Responsibilities♦ Ethics ♦ Safety Practices ♦ Teamwork♦ Health Maintenance Practices ♦ Technical Skills♦ Information Technology Applications				

FIGURE 1-6 The National Consortium for Health Science Education lists a variety of career opportunities in health care. (From the Michigan Health Council: http://www.mhc.org.)

- A growing population of the elderly and the expense of technology are some of the factors influencing the cost of health care.
- Methods being used to reduce the cost include alternate forms of payment, including indemnity and managed care plans.
- Some places in which care services are provided include a hospital, clinic, or home. The types of services might be therapeutic, diagnostic, informational, or environmental.

Review Questions

1. Research does not support the claim that static magnets are effective in relieving pain. What term best describes the use and sale of such magnets?
2. Compare and contrast the meaning of the terms certification and licensure.
3. List three factors of society that influence the health care industry.
4. Describe five advantages to pursuing a career in the health field.
5. Describe the factors that should be considered in choosing an occupation.
6. The term that best describes the worker who assists the professional would be the ___________.
7. The term that describes an occupation that requires specialized education and training is ___________.
8. Draw a Venn diagram to compare and contrast indemnity and managed care insurance.
9. Describe the influence of advanced technology, malpractice coverage, and expanded roles of the health care industry on increased health care costs.
10. Compare the educational preparation and level of responsibility of the assistant, technician, technologist, and professional.
11. Identify at least three occupations in each area of the hospital organization.
12. Match each of the following milestones with the person credited with the event.

a. William Harvey	______	described poisoning of environment with pesticides
b. Jonas Salk	______	developed the laws of heredity
c. Rachel Carson	______	performed first successful heart transplant
d. Gregor Mendel	______	developed the smallpox vaccine
e. Christian Barnard	______	described the circulation of blood
f. Edwin Jenner	______	developed poliomyelitis vaccine

Critical Thinking

1. Defend or deny the idea that the microscope is the most important milestone in health care.
2. Investigate the cost of malpractice insurance for five health care professionals. Hypothesize reasons that the rates for some professions, such as neurosurgery and gynecology, are higher than others.
3. Use medical milestones (see Medical Milestones on pp. 21-22) to trace the development of a treatment modality in health care. For example, trace the development of transplantation of organs or gene therapy. Synthesize the information gained to predict the future of this type of health care treatment.
4. Investigate a person famous for a health care discovery. Using information gathered about the person's life, form a hypothesis as to the events that led the person to that discovery.
5. Investigate the use of advanced technologies such as cloning or stem cell research. Develop guidelines for the safe use of this technology.
6. Investigate a form of alternative or complementary treatment to determine its use and effectiveness. Design an experiment or research project that would prove or disprove the usefulness of the treatment.
7. Investigate the pandemics and pandemic scares of influenza in the United States. Create a Venn diagram that compares and contrasts the three major pandemics. Write a paragraph that describes the current state of avian influenza A (H5N1). Include your opinion as to whether it should be considered a real threat or a scare.
8. Investigate and write a paragraph that compares and contrasts health care insurance and automobile insurance. For example, how is the coverage determined, who provides coverage, and who gets coverage?
9. Investigate and write a paragraph that describes the outbreak of the H1N1 flu. Include statistics on the number of cases, methods of transmission, and means of prevention. Include a

personal opinion regarding the CDC decision in July 2009 to discontinue probable case counts for this flu.

10. Use the Internet to write a report or present an effective oral presentation that describes the health care reform bill provisions.

11. Use the Internet to research the impact of local, state, and national government on one aspect of the health care industry. Write an essay or present an effective oral presentation that compares the impact at each level of government.

Explore the Web

Health Care Reform Bill

HealthReform.gov
http://www.healthreform.gov/

Patient's Rights

National Association for Home Care & Hospice
http://www.nahc.org/home.html

Workers' Compensation

Wikipedia: Workers' Compensation
http://en.wikipedia.org/wiki/Workers_compensation

Insurance

HowStuffWorks: Health Insurance
http://health.howstuffworks.com/health-insurance.htm

HowStuffWorks: Car Insurance
http://auto.howstuffworks.com/car-insurance4.htm

Emergency Preparedness

CDC Emergency Preparedness
http://www.bt.cdc.gov/

Epidemics

Wikipedia: Epidemics
http://en.wikipedia.org/wiki/List_of_epidemics

Mayo Clinic: H1N1 Flu
http://www.mayoclinic.com/health/swine-flu/DS01144

WHO: Flu
http://www.who.int/topics/influenza/en/

CDC: H1N1 Flu
http://www.cdc.gov/H1n1flu/surveillanceqa.htm

STANDARDS AND ACCOUNTABILITY*

Foundation Standard 3: Systems

Healthcare professionals will understand how their role fits into their department, their organization and the overall healthcare environment. They will identify how key systems affect services they perform and quality of care.

Accountability Criteria

3.1 Healthcare Delivery Systems

3.11 Understand the healthcare delivery system (public, private, government, and non-profit).

3.12 Explain the factors influencing healthcare delivery systems.

3.13 Describe the responsibilities of consumers within the healthcare system.

3.14 Explain the impact of emerging issues such as technology, epidemiology, bioethics, and socioeconomics on healthcare delivery systems.

3.15 Discuss common methods of payment for healthcare.

*From the National Consortium for Health Science Education (2009). National Health Care Standards and Accountability Criteria. Available at http://www.healthscienceconsortium.org.

Medical Milestones

1518 College of Physicians is established in London.
1543 First anatomy textbook is published by Vesalius.
1590 Zacharis Janassen invents the compound microscope.
1628 William Harvey describes the circulation of blood.
1666 Anton van Leeuwenhoek uses the microscope to view microorganisms.
1670 Thomas Willis makes a connection between sugar in the urine and diabetes.
1796 Edwin Jenner develops the smallpox vaccine.
1816 Rene Laennec invents the stethoscope.
1818 James Blundel performs the first successful blood transfusion in humans.
1839 First dental school is founded in Baltimore.
1842 Crawford Long develops ether anesthesia.
1854 Florence Nightingale begins nursing soldiers and reforming the nursing profession.
1863 International Red Cross is established.
1865 Sir Joseph Lister uses asepsis in surgery.
1868 Thermometer is introduced to take body temperature.
1869 Gregor Mendel develops the laws of heredity.
1882 Robert Koch discovers that pathogens cause disease.
1887 Anne Sullivan helps Helen Keller communicate for the first time.
1893 Aspirin is developed.
1895 Wilhelm Roentgen discovers x-rays.
1898 Ronald Ross discovers that malaria is carried by mosquitoes.
1900 Blood groups are discovered.
1901 Jyokichi Takamine isolates the first hormone, adrenaline.
1910 Marie Curie isolates radium, later used to treat cancer.
1912 Sir F. Gowland Hopkins determines that some diseases are caused by lack of "accessory substances," later named vitamins.
1914 John B. Watson establishes the behaviorist theory of psychology.
1918 Francis Benedict develops a procedure to test basal metabolic rate.
1922 Frederick G. Banting treats diabetes with insulin.
1928 Sir Alexander Fleming discovers penicillin.
1937 First blood bank is established in Chicago.
1937 Alton Ochsner and Michael De Bakey link lung cancer to cigarette smoking.
1944 First kidney dialysis machine is developed.
1944 DNA is proved to be the hereditary plan.
1948 Philip Hench and Edward Kendall synthesize cortisone.
1952 Jonas Salk develops a vaccine to prevent poliomyelitis.
1953 First heart-lung machine is used for successful open-heart surgery.
1953 First successful kidney transplantation is performed.
1957 Alick Isaacs and Jean Lindermann discover interferon.
1961 First continuously operating laser is developed for surgical use.
1962 Rachel Carson, in *Silent Spring*, describes the poisoning of the environment by pesticides.
1963 Thomas Starzl performs the first human liver transplantation.
1964 James Hardy performs the first human lung transplantation.
1966 First hormone, insulin, is synthesized.
1967 Christian Barnard performs the first successful heart transplantation.
1967 First hospice is founded in England.
1967 First penicillin-resistant pneumococcal strain is reported.
1969 Denton Cooley implants the first temporary artificial heart.
1972 Computed tomography (CT scan) is introduced.
1975 Lyme disease is reported for the first time.
1976 Legionnaire disease outbreak occurs in Pennsylvania.
1977 Human growth hormone is produced by bacteria using recombinant DNA technology.
1978 The first "test tube" baby is born in England.

Continued

Medical Milestones—cont'd

1981 AIDS is identified as a disease.

1981 First successful surgery on a fetus is performed in California.

1984 First baby is conceived from a frozen embryo in Australia.

1984 Virus that causes AIDS is identified.

1990 Genetically engineered blood cells are used to treat immune disorders, first gene therapy.

1990 U.S. Congress passes Patient Self-Determination Act (PSDA), an amendment to the Omnibus Reconciliation Act.

1992 Method for detection of cystic fibrosis gene is developed in England.

1993 Embryos are screened for genetic abnormalities before implantation.

1993 Human embryo is cloned.

1993 Genes that cause glaucoma, amyotrophic lateral sclerosis, Mende syndrome, colorectal cancer, xeroderma pigmentosum, Hirschsprung disease, Canavan disease, and Wilms tumor are identified.

1994 Breast cancer gene (*BRCA2*) and 22 mutations are identified.

1994 Test is developed for detection of colon cancer caused by a mutant gene.

1994 Gene therapy is used to treat the inherited form of high cholesterol.

1994 Normal gene is transferred into the lungs of an individual with cystic fibrosis.

1994 Scientists in Boston devise an eye examination to detect Alzheimer disease.

1997 Dolly, a sheep, is introduced as the first mammal to be cloned from somatic cells.

1998 Stem cells are isolated from fetal tissues.

1999 Artificial bladder is grown from cells for implantation in humans.

2000 Human genome mapping project is completed.

2001 Human embryo is created through cloning.

2002 First robot-assisted coronary artery bypass surgery is performed.

2002 Josef Penninger and Peter Backx identify two genes, one that contributes to and one that protects against heart failure.

2003 First molecular diagnostic test for severe acute respiratory syndrome (SARS) is developed in Canada.

2003 Carlo Urbani of Doctors without Borders alerts WHO of threat from SARS, leading to effective response.

2004 First outbreak of polio in 26 years occurs in Minnesota.

2005 PillCam endoscopic camera pill receives the Technology Innovation Award.

2005 Jean-Michel Dubermard performs first partial face transplant.

2005 Marshall and Warren are awarded the Nobel Prize in Physiology and Medicine for the discovery of the bacterium *Helicobacter pylori* and its role in peptic ulcer disease.

2006 FDA approves over-the-counter sale of Plan B, a "morning after" emergency contraceptive, to women 18 and older.

2006 First human papilloma virus vaccine approved.

2007 Human skin cells used to create embryonic stem cells.

2008 Laurent Lantieri performs first full face transplant.

2009 U.S. President Obama signs Children's Health Insurance Reauthorization Act.

2009 WHO declares outbreak of H1N1 virus to be a global pandemic.

2010 U.S. Congress passes and President Obama signs Affordable Care Act.

KEY TERMS cont'd

Personality *(per-sun-AL-it-ee)* Set of traits, characteristics, and behaviors that make each person unique

Value *(VAL-yoo)* Rate of usefulness, importance, or general worth

Verbal *(VER-bul)* Relating to or consisting of words or sounds

Interpersonal Dynamics

To provide adequate care, the health care worker must be able to recognize and accept the values, attitudes, and beliefs unique to each person. The health care worker must consider the diverse cultural and religious background and special needs of individual patients. Some populations may need special care because of their **diversity** or differences. Examples of populations that need special care include pediatric, geriatric, obstetric, emergency, and disabled patients, and those with chronic or terminal illness. The health care worker also needs to be aware of the differences in culture and religion and how they affect the patient's view of health care.

Different beliefs about health care may result from **cultural** diversity. Factors that influence these beliefs include the age, gender, education, religion, ethnicity, and national origin. In Western culture, certain beliefs relate to health care. People generally believe health care can make an illness or injury better. They believe they can control nature and that it is better to do something as soon as possible rather than waiting. They also believe that something that is stronger or newer is better than something weaker or older. Most people of Western culture believe that authority figures are to be respected and trusted with health care decisions. People of other cultures of the world might not share these beliefs. The health care worker must be aware of and sensitive to differences in culture.

When working with a patient from a different culture, the health care worker should follow guidelines that are sensitive to diverse beliefs (Box 2-1). If n interpreter is necessary, the health care worker atches the patient, not the interpreter, when speakg. The health care worker should avoid the phrases ou must" or "you should" and offer reasonable options instead. Important information is repeated more than once.

The health care worker must be able to communicate effectively, provide leadership when necessary, and use technological equipment. The health care worker also must maintain the ethical code of the profession and be aware of the legal considerations of health care. More than any other single characteristic, the health care professional of the future must be flexible to adapt to the changing industry. The industry is changing daily because of new medical discoveries, technological advances, and evolving health concerns.

Interpersonal skills allow an individual to relate with friends, family, co-workers, and patients. Some

BRAIN BYTE

008 health care was the largest U.S. industry, employnore than 14.3 million workers.

BOX 2-1

Guidelines for Cultural Awareness

- Address patients by their formal names.
- Explain why personal information is necessary.
- Be aware that some cultures do not trust health care workers.
- Be aware that most, but not all, cultures prefer direct eye contact.
- Respect any cultural dietary preferences.
- Explain the need for tests and treatments.
- Respect the desire of the patient to include or exclude family members from treatment and health information.
- Respect the varied practices of religion by patients.

CASE STUDY 2-1 You are caring for a patient who often complains about pain. While you are giving daily care, the patient says you have hurt her arm by moving it. What should you do?

Answers to Case Studies are available on the Evolve website: ***http://evolve.elsevier.com/Gerdin***

CHAPTER 2

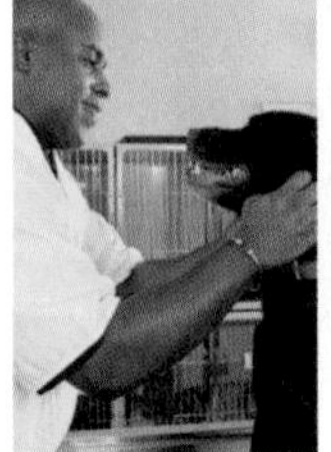

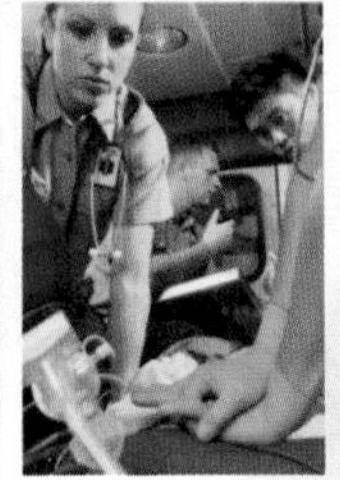

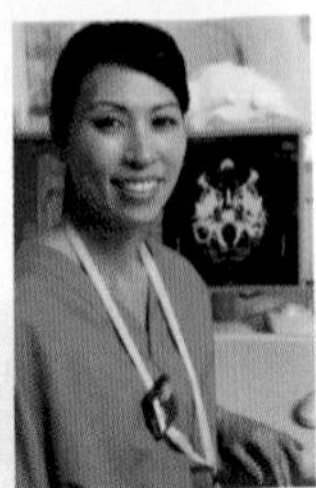

Interpersonal Dynamics and Communications

LEARNING OBJECTIVES

- Define at least 10 words relating to the health care worker's characteristics and abilities.
- Describe the relationship among values, attitudes, and behavior.
- Describe the hierarchy of needs established by Abraham Maslow.
- Identify at least five methods of maintaining good personal health and professional appearance.
- Use a problem-solving system to make a decision that involves identification of alternatives, risks, and evaluation of the outcome.
- Identify the elements of effective communication and at least three factors that might interfere with it.
- Describe at least one example of assertive communication that requests change in behavior.

KEY TERMS

Attitude *(AT-ih-tood)* Mental position or feeling with regard to a fact or situatic

Behavior *(be-HAY-vyer)* Manner of conducting oneself

Character *(KARE-ik-ter)* Distinctive qualities that make up an individual

Communication *(kuh-myoo-ni-KAY-shun)* Exchange of information

Culture *(KUL-cher)* Sum of the socially gained patterns that guide a per including values, beliefs, language, and thought

Diversity *(de-VUR-si-tee)* Quality of being different

Habit *(HA-bit)* Act performed voluntarily without conscious thought

Hierarchy *(HI-er-ark-ee)* Graded or ranked series

Nonverbal *(non-VER-bul)* Communicating without using languac

skills helpful in interpersonal relationships include the ability to communicate well, to act independently by making decisions, and to demonstrate sincere compassion for others.

Self-Awareness

Understanding and accepting the differences that exist among people of different backgrounds rely on an understanding of one's own values and motives. Understanding and accepting the self leads to development of high self-esteem. Psychologists believe that how a person thinks about an experience determines the feelings and behaviors that result from the event. Each mentally healthy person can choose the feelings that result from events that occur in life.

Personality is the sum of the traits, characteristics, and behaviors that make each individual unique. **Behavior** is the action of an individual that can be seen by others. Society prefers some behaviors to others. **Habits** are acts that are performed voluntarily but without conscious thought. Habits can be changed by repetitive behavior changes. Many behaviors result from habit and can be changed by the individual.

The behavior that an individual displays in a situation is seen as a reflection of an attitude. **Attitudes** are the mental views or feelings formed by an individual or group. With new information and experience, individuals can change their attitudes.

Attitudes are formed from personal values. **Values** make up the system each individual uses to measure or evaluate the worth of ideas, people, and things in the world. They are formed early in life as a result of the environment and experience. Values are difficult to change. An undesirable value such as prejudice might not even be recognized by the individual who holds it (Fig. 2-1). The sum of the behavior, attitudes, and values that a person exhibits to others is called **character**.

The patient and other caregivers expect certain characteristics, attitudes, and behaviors in the health care worker (Box 2-2). Undesirable behavior can be changed if it is recognized and the desired behavior is practiced.

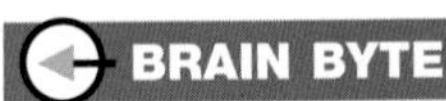

Most jobs in the health care industry require less than 4 years of college.

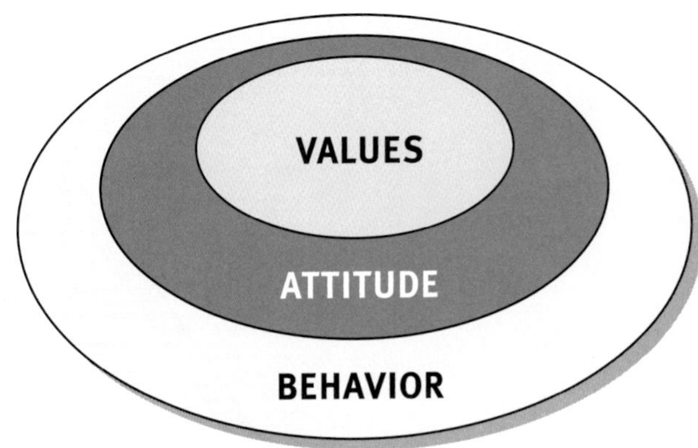

FIGURE 2-1 Values form the basis on which attitudes are formed. Attitudes are reflected by behavior. Behavior is made up of the actions seen by others.

BOX 2-2

Characteristics of the Health Care Worker

- Communicates concisely and accurately in a clear, well-modulated voice
- Dresses neatly and appropriately
- Maintains controlled and upright posture
- Promotes good health through lifestyle
- Shows patience and poise under pressure
- Remains tactful and courteous at all times
- Has sincere interest in and tries to understand others
- Takes responsibility for own actions
- Exhibits reliability, perseveres to accomplish tasks
- Is able and willing to follow directions
- Is flexible when changes in routine are necessary
- Displays humor but not at the expense of others
- Accepts criticism and makes an effort to improve
- Maintains ethical conduct including promptness, honesty, care of equipment, and respect for the organization's policies
- Shows initiative in tasks but knows the limits of practice and does not exceed them

Hierarchy of Needs

Psychologist Abraham Maslow created a **hierarchy** of human needs that is still widely used to understand behavior and motivation (Fig. 2-2). Maslow

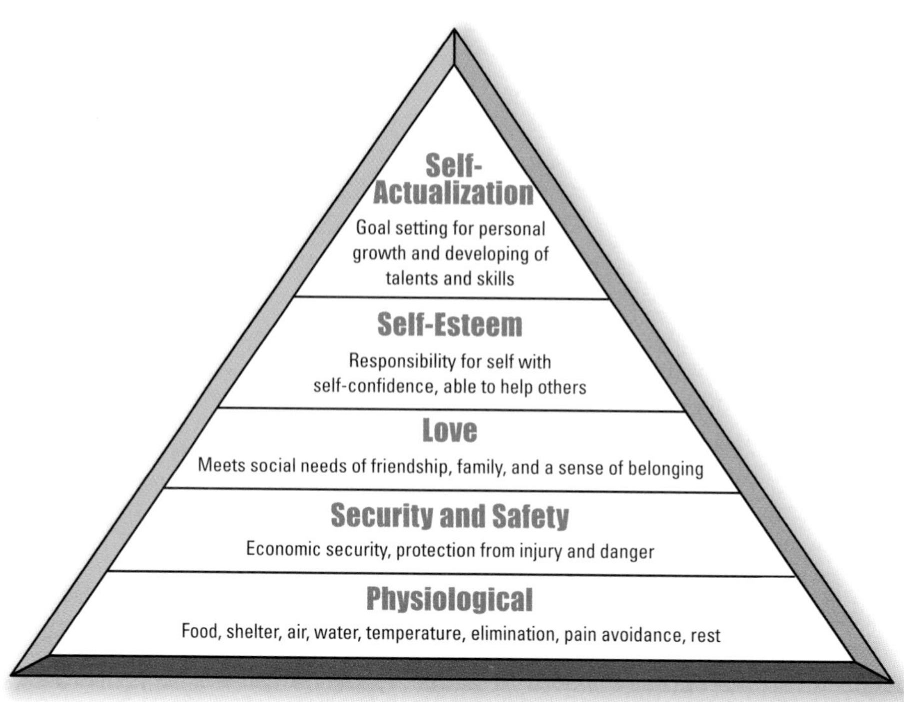

FIGURE 2-2 Maslow's hierarchy of needs.

stated that a person strives to meet the most basic needs first.

If the needs at the lower levels are not met, the higher needs cannot be reached. The first level describes the most basic needs, including phraseological concerns such as air, shelter, sleep, food, and water. The second level includes safety needs such as protection, order, security, and stability. Family, affection, relationships, and groups are included in the next level, described as "love or belongingness" needs. Esteem needs of the fourth level include achievement, status, responsibility, and reputation.

The fifth level of Maslow's hierarchy is called self-actualization and includes personal growth and fulfillment. Other people might describe a self-actualized person as self-motivated. Maslow later added three new levels. Between self-esteem and self-actualization, he added "understanding" and "aesthetic beauty." Understanding includes the need to know and learn. The need for aesthetic beauty describes the emotional need of the artist. Self-actualization was divided into two parts called "self-actualization" (self-potential) and "transcendence", or the ability to help other people reach their potential.

Task Achievement

Erik Erikson describes eight stages of psychosocial development with tasks that must be completed throughout life to develop an identity (Table 2-1). His theory of personality development states that achievement of a task, or crisis, may be complete, partial, or unsuccessful. The more the task is mastered or completed, the healthier the personality of the individual. A favorable resolution of the task is called a "virtue." Erikson states that the person must find a balance between the parts of a task. For example, a child who can get dressed independently demonstrates a balance between trust and guilt.

Personal Health

Good personal health is basic for an individual to establish high self-esteem. The World Health Organization defines health as a state of physical, mental, and social well-being. It is not just the absence of illness or injury. The foundation of good personal health, cleanliness, is maintained by a daily routine that includes bathing, using a deodorant, shampooing the hair, and cleaning the teeth (Table 2-2). Nutrition, exercise, sleep, posture, eye care, and good personal habits are also necessary to maintain good health. Some specific daily behaviors that indicate good personal grooming include the use of mouthwash, shaving, nail care, change of undergarments, and clean clothing that fits properly. Health care workers wear minimal jewelry to prevent both its loss and the spread of microorganisms.

TABLE 2-1
Erikson's Life-Stage Virtues

Psychosocial Stage	Virtue	Conflict
Infant	Hope	Trust vs. mistrust
Toddler	Will	Autonomy vs. shame and doubt
Kindergarten	Purpose	Initiative vs. guilt
Age 6 yr to puberty	Competence	Industry vs. inferiority
Teenager	Fidelity	Identity vs. role confusion
Young adult	Love	Intimacy vs. isolation
Midlife	Caring	Generativity vs. stagnation
Old age	Wisdom	Ego integrity vs. despair

TABLE 2-2
Good Grooming Habits for Health Care Workers

Habit	Action
Oral hygiene	Brush at least twice daily, and use mouthwash once daily
Hair care	Shampoo regularly, style hair away from the face and off the collar
Skin care	Cleanse regularly; treat rashes, blemishes
	Wear nylons or socks to prevent skin shedding (exfoliation)
	Use clear to no polish
	Use antiperspirant, no perfume
Nail care	Clean nails, trim close to fingertips
	Use clear or no polish
Clothing	Appropriate, modest
	Clean, pressed, well-fitting
	Mended, comfortable, allowing movement
	Undergarments changed daily, well-fitted, not visible through clothing
	Minimal or no jewelry
	Name pin and watch in place
Foot care	Socks or stockings clean daily
	Toenails trimmed regularly
	Shoes cleaned and polished
	Shoes sturdy, nonskid, low-heeled with closed toes

First impressions are often based on personal appearance. This impression is then modified by the behavior that is observed. Patients notice the personal appearance of the health care worker's face, hair, nails, dress, odor, skin, posture, and teeth. Appearance reflects self-esteem and how workers view themselves. The appearance of the health care worker is doubly important because it represents the employer and the worker.

Stress and Time Management

Health care is one of the most stressful occupations. The work affects the most fundamental part of the patient's and health care worker's lives. One of the first psychologists who studied stress-related disease was Claude Bernard. He proposed that the body has an "internal milieu," or need to maintain a consistent internal environment. Canon used the term *homeostasis* to describe the self-regulating processes of the body, including the "fight or flight" reaction to stress. Hans Seyle noted that many diseases share similar signs and symptoms, such as fatigue, weight loss, aches, and gastrointestinal problems. He stated that these result from a general stress reaction from increased adrenal gland secretions, shrinkage of lymphatic tissues, and increased secretion of hydrochloric acid in the stomach. Seyle proposed that illness results from too small or too large of a reaction by the body's stress adaptation mechanism (Table 2-3).

Some methods used to manage stress include proper nutrition, exercise, relaxation techniques, and personal behavior changes (Box 2-3). Stress is not the result of events that occur, but rather it is the result of attitudes that are formed about the events. Another stress management technique includes a method of time management.

Time management uses organization of a schedule to maximize effectiveness and productivity. The key to effective time management is planning. The basic tool for planning is a calendar. Learning and meeting

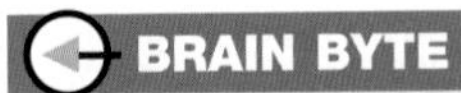

Analysts of the U.S. Department of Health & Human Services predict a shortage of 100,000 physicians, 1,000,000 nurses and 250,000 public health workers by 2020.

TABLE 2-3
Stress-Related Illness

Body Process	Effect of Stress
Cardiovascular system	Heart attack (myocardial infarction) High blood pressure (hypertension) Heart pain (angina) Migraine headache Stroke (cerebrovascular accident)
Digestive system	Ulcer Colitis Constipation, diarrhea
Skeletal system	Arthritis
Muscular system	Headache Backache
Respiratory system	Asthma
Endocrine system	Diabetes (Type II)
Nervous system	Accident proneness (decreased attention)
Immune process	Increased rate of infection Allergies Autoimmune disorders
Psychosocial process	Fighting and conflicts Alcoholism and drug abuse

BOX 2-3

Stress Management Techniques

- Plan and organize your workload. Use time management techniques.
- When possible, do things one at a time until they are completed.
- Occasionally plan to escape and have fun.
- Be positive about things, and avoid criticizing others.
- Avoid unnecessary competition. Learn to negotiate.
- Get regular exercise.
- Tolerate, forgive, and learn to accept others.
- Talk to someone about things that are troubling you.
- Use relaxation methods such as biofeedback or deep breathing.

the behavioral expectations of the setting help the worker concentrate on the task at hand.

Setting both short-term and long-term goals increases the probability of accomplishing them. Goals allow a person to establish step-by-step actions toward accomplishing something. Keeping focused on the goal helps one to complete the action steps necessary to reach it. Reaching a goal creates pride and self-confidence. Goals should be clearly defined, measurable, and tangible (Box 2-4).

Problem Solving

Problem solving is one method that can be used to make decisions (Box 2-5). It is based on evaluation of the factors involved in the decision, the risks, and possible solutions. The problem must first be well understood, clarified, and defined. Many people believe that a problem is the fault of someone else and that solving the problem requires a change in someone else's behavior. It may be necessary to identify the feelings that result from the problem and to stop laying blame for the situation before a solution is possible. These feelings might include fear, anger, or insecurity. The question, "How do I want this to turn out?" can be used to identify the real problem.

Once the problem is identified, brainstorming is one way to seek possible solutions. Brainstorming generates but does not evaluate the practicality of ideas. All possible ideas should be listed before any is chosen. The ideas can then be considered and possible solutions evaluated on the basis of the risks and consequences of each. Other methods of problem solving include making flowcharts or cause-effect diagrams. Resources such as co-workers may also be helpful, although gossip about problems is not. The problem may have more than one solution, and several possibilities may be chosen. When chosen, the solution can then be implemented. To implement a solution, specific steps or actions must be identified. The results of the plan can be evaluated for use in making future decisions. Most problems and decisions have more than one solution. If a problem is not resolved with the first action taken, an alternate step may be used. The merit or value of each decision can be evaluated only by its results.

Critical Thinking

Critical thinking has been identified as a necessary competency for workers in health care. Critical thinking is the ability to think independently and reflectively. It includes the ability to think creatively,

BOX 2-4

Setting Goals

Goal-Setting Guidelines

- State each goal as a positive statement, not as a negative criticism.
- Define a goal in a specific and precise manner, including dates and timelines.
- Set priorities for goals.
- Keep goals in written form.
- Make goals realistic.
- Revise goals as needed.

Goal-Setting Questions: Long-Term

- What is your goal for your career?
- What is your goal for your family relationships?
- What is your goal for your education?
- What is your financial goal?
- What is your health and physical goal?
- What is your goal for your spirit?

Goal Setting Questions: Short-Term

- What is your 10-year goal for each of your long-term goals?
- What is your 5-year goal for each of your long-term goals?
- What is your 1-year goal for each of your long-term goals?
- What is your monthly or weekly goal for each of your long-term goals?
- What is your daily "to do" list for each of your goals?

BOX 2-5

Model for Problem Solving and Decision Making

1. Recognize that a problem exists. Recognition may result from a feeling, observation, or conversation with others.
2. Describe the problem and clarify what the basic issue or question is and the factors that affect it. Identify who is involved, where the problem exists, and when and how it occurs.
3. Identify alternative methods of resolving the problem. Any alternative can be considered even if it is not immediately seen as practical.
4. Choose the best method for resolving the problem and implement it.
5. As the plan is being implemented, evaluate the results and adjust the method if necessary.

BOX 2-6

Elements of Critical Thinking

- Ask questions.
- Define a problem.
- Examine evidence.
- Avoid emotional reasoning.
- Analyze assumptions and bias.
- Avoid oversimplification.
- Consider other interpretations.
- Tolerate ambiguity.
- Think about one's own thinking.

make decisions, solve problems, visualize situational descriptions, learn new information, and reason (Box 2-6). Most formal definitions of critical thinking characterize it as the intentional application of rational, higher-order thinking skills. Critical thinking focuses on the application of logical concepts to everyday reasoning and problem solving. Critical thinking skills allow the health care worker to apply concrete information, such as facts of anatomy and physiology, and draw conclusions to determine the kind of care that would be best for a patient. Questioning techniques may be used to promote critical thought and clarify meaning (Box 2-7).

In 1990 the American Philosophical Association Delphi Report produced an international definition for *critical thinking*. They defined it as "purposeful, self-regulatory judgment that results in interpretation, analysis, evaluation, and inference, as well as explanation of the evidential, conceptual, methodological, criteriological, or contextual considerations upon which that judgment is based." They developed a list of critical thinking skills, including interpretation, analysis, evaluation, inference, explanation, and self-regulation.

BOX 2-7

Questions to Promote Critical Thought

- What do you mean by ...
- Could you say that another way?
- Can you give me an example?
- What is being assumed?
- Can this be tested?
- Is this always the case?
- Why do you feel this way?
- What is the effect of that?
- Is there another choice?
- Can someone else see this differently?

Leadership

In an organization, individuals join together to reach a goal through cooperation and division of tasks among themselves. Groups can accomplish goals faster and more easily than individuals can. An organizational chart shows the relationships among, and the roles of, the members.

Organizational frameworks may be planned by using management practices and theories. This is usually called organizational development. The goal of organizational development is to increase productivity, quality, and worker satisfaction. Models of organizational structures include hierarchical management or team-based approaches. The health care worker plays an important part in the health care organization by setting goals, meeting challenges, and implementing ideas.

The characteristics of the leader of a group should include honesty, the ability to communicate clearly, competence, and the ability to work well with others (Box 2-8). The leader of the group has responsibilities to the other members of the team as well as to management. These responsibilities include making decisions, giving direction, communicating change, and serving as a role model or representative of the institution. The leader should be available to allow workers to express their opinion, teach skills if necessary, and participate as a member of the team. The leader may also evaluate members of the team. Evaluation may be based on an objective set of performance indicators (Box 2-9).

BOX 2-8

Characteristics of the Effective Leader

- Both task- and people-oriented
- Confident
- Self-controlled
- Disciplined
- Intelligent
- Well-organized
- Detail-oriented
- Self-motivated
- Respectful
- Assertive
- Good communicator
- Good listener
- Responsible
- Maintains a vision and goals

BOX 2-9

Performance-Based Evaluation Indicators

- Knows and supports policies of the organization
- Performs skills in satisfactory manner
- Reports to work on time and follows procedures for notice in case of absence
- Communicates effectively with coworkers and patients
- Completes work as assigned in a timely manner
- Takes initiative to solve problems as needed
- Seeks assistance and direction as needed
- Recognizes and respects cultural and religious diversity

The Team

Health care workers participate as a team to provide care for the patient. Members of the team have different responsibilities. Some members provide direct care, working in contact with the patient, whereas others might not ever see the patient. Nevertheless, all members of the team are important in providing the best care possible.

BOX 2-10

Characteristics of the Good Team Member

- Works for consensus on decision
- Trusts co-workers
- Supports co-workers
- Displays genuine concern for others
- Takes responsibility for self and own actions
- Is a good listener
- Is a good role model
- Respects and speaks positively about others
- Is tolerant of differences
- Solves problems without blaming
- Understands and supports team objectives
- Encourages feedback on behavior and performance
- Does not participate in gossip
- Encourages other members

Some elements of effective teaming include a common purpose, specific goals, defined roles, and positive relationships. Leadership provides coordination and direction for the team. Team members are accountable for their individual roles. Teams may be influenced by the element of trust of each other. The value, competence, and contribution of each member should be recognized. Gossip, favoritism, and "backbiting" are examples of behaviors that result in an ineffective team (Box 2-10). The focus of the health care team is to provide good patient care.

CASE STUDY 2-2 You are listening to notes from the previous shift regarding patient care. After your assigned patients have been covered, a co-worker starts to talk with you. What should you do?

Answers to Case Studies are available on the Evolve website: ***http://evolve.elsevier.com/Gerdin***

The National Health Care Standards describe five pathway standards for careers in health occupations. The *diagnostic services* provide a picture of the patient's health status and include technicians in radiology, medical, dental laboratory, and cardiography. The *therapeutic services* provide treatment over time and include such providers as physicians, dentists, veterinarians, nurses, pharmacologists, and emergency personnel. *Health informatics* personnel process data and provide documents; these include administration, secretaries, and medical records personnel. *Support services* provide a supportive environment for the patient and include nutrition services, central supply, and facility management personnel. *Biotechnology research and development services* provide research in bioscience to develop new treatments, medications, and tests. These professionals include biochemists, bioinformatics scientists, cell biologists, and pharmaceutical scientists. Chapter 1 provides more information about the pathway standards.

Communication

Communication is the sharing of an idea or information that results in understanding. Reading, writing, hearing, touching, and seeing are various forms of communication. If it involves language, communication is said to be **verbal**, and if it does not, it is called **nonverbal**. Communication can take place on a one-to-one basis, in small groups, or with a large audience. Mass communication reaches large groups of people through television, radio, film, and newspapers.

In health care, communication between workers is completed in a professional and precise manner. The health care worker must determine to whom a message is being given before choosing the correct words to use. For example, the patient might not understand the medical term *hypertension*, but a colleague would immediately know that this word means *high blood pressure*. The goal of the health care worker's communication to other members of the team is to convey information concisely and accurately. The health care worker must be aware of the Health Insurance Portability and Accountability Act (HIPAA) and the laws regarding slander and libel when choosing when and how information is communicated. HIPAA guidelines require that protected health information or sensitive issues of health are kept confidential. Charts must be kept secure, the patient's modesty must be preserved, and information should be shared with other professionals only with the patient's consent. The organization may have a facility privacy officer who determines how information may be shared. Written notice of the privacy act is provided to patients each time they are admitted to the facility. Discussion of patient information in common areas such as elevators, restrooms, and eating areas or with an unauthorized person

BOX 2-11

Causes of Conflict

- Competition
- Cultural misunderstanding
- Lack of control of resources
- Miscommunication/misinformation
- Negative/destructive behavior
- Stereotyping
- Strong emotions
- Time constraint
- Unequal authority
- Value differences

constitutes a HIPAA violation. Telephone contact regarding the patient must be completed between authorized individuals. A patient may "opt out" of being included in a facility directory. In this case, the patient's name or treatment is not made available to others. More information about HIPAA is provided in Chapters 1 and 4.

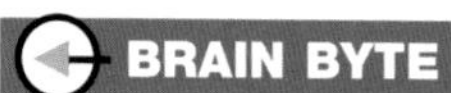

Jurors awarded a woman $3000 for invasion of privacy when the paramedic who treated her for an overdose told the woman's co-worker about it.

In the health care team, there is usually a "chain of command," or hierarchy of practitioners. The assistant, for example, may not report directly to the department head but through a team leader. This chain of command is structured to provide the department head with concise information and provide the assistant-level workers with immediate supervisory guidance as needed. Each organization has its own structure for communication and leadership that must be learned by each new health care employee.

Conflict

Conflict in teams is not necessarily a destructive force in the workplace. It can lead to new ideas and procedures. However, it can also cause a combative climate of distrust and reduced performance. Conflict results because of differences in individuals. Conflicts can occur in the health care work setting for numerous reasons (Box 2-11). Methods to manage team conflict vary with the issue in question and may be solved with changes in planning and communication (Box 2-12).

BOX 2-12

Methods to Resolve Conflict

- Bargaining/compromise/mediation
- Clarify responsibilities/allocation of resources
- Confront/acknowledge the issue
- Discuss/agree/commit to behavior change
- Enforcement of policy/rules
- Find area of agreement
- Listen for meaning/clarify perceptions
- Team meeting

CASE STUDY 2-3 One of your co-workers makes a complaint to you about the care being given to patients by a third co-worker. What should you do?

Answers to Case Studies are available on the Evolve website: *http://evolve.elsevier.com/Gerdin*

Verbal Communication

Effective communication may be defined as a shared understanding of a message. Effective communication consists of three parts: the sender, the message, and the receiver (Fig. 2-3). The English language is made up of about 100,000 words, of which most people use 30,000 to 60,000. Of these, 5000 have a double meaning. Estimates indicate that 7% of a message is conveyed by words, 38% by the tone of voice, and 55% by nonverbal behavior. The message also may be distorted because of interference from the sender, receiver, or environment. The quality of care given to a patient is often perceived on the basis of effective communication.

Feedback is a method to determine whether the message was received accurately. Feedback is a response by the receiver to indicate how the information was understood. One factor that may influence the communication process is the attitude of each person. Communication attitudes are based on previous knowledge, culture, and the communication skills of the sender and receiver. The complexity of the message is also a factor, as is interference, such as noise from the environment. Some attitudes may block effective communication (Box 2-13). Methods of communication that may lead to defensive responses from others include avoidance, unresolved anxiety, and poor self-esteem. Tone of voice, manner of speech, or the choice of words may be perceived as criticism or an attempt to control the other. Lack of interest or

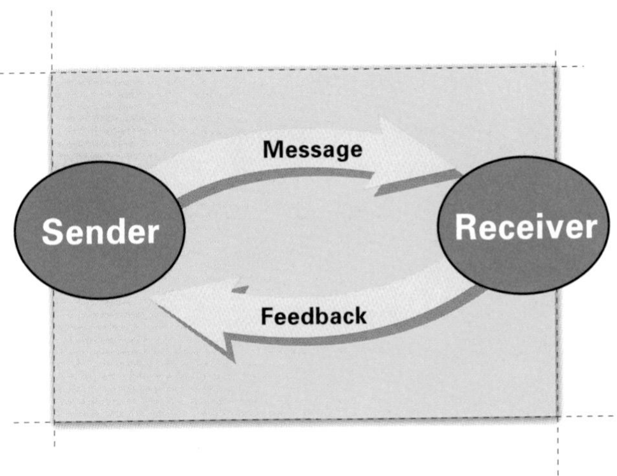

FIGURE 2-3 Feedback helps the receiver make certain the message was understood.

BOX 2-13

Attitudes and Behaviors That Act as Barriers to Effective Communication

- Advising
- Closed-mindedness
- Commanding
- Distracting
- Judging
- Lecturing
- Moralizing
- Name calling
- Offering solutions
- Off-on listening (tuning out)
- Ordering
- Preaching
- Prejudging
- Red-flag listening (reacting automatically to certain words)
- Speaker-centeredness instead of subject-centeredness
- Stereotyping
- Teaching
- Threatening
- Warning

dogmatism (certainty of rightness) also can result in a defensive response. Box 2-14 lists methods of communication to help avoid a defensive pattern of communication.

One technique that can improve communication is called assertiveness. Assertiveness is a learned skill that develops self-confidence and maintains individuality in stressful situations. The goal of assertiveness is to reduce the inner stress caused by inaccurate communication or lack of communication. The basis of assertiveness is that each person has a right to express feelings, opinions, and beliefs in a respectful and appropriate manner without feeling guilt. Aggressiveness results if the rights of others are violated during the communication. If either person's rights are overlooked, respect is lost and resentment results. (See Skill List 2-1, Assertive Behavior, p. 38).

BOX 2-14

Guidelines to Avoid Defensive Communication

- Be descriptive rather than critical of observed behaviors.
- Speak in terms of beliefs in viewpoints rather than certainties of rightness.
- Be spontaneous rather than manipulative. Do not have a preconceived outcome of the conversation.
- Communicate on an equal basis rather than as a superior.
- Approach the discussion with a goal of mutual problem solving rather than controlling the other person.
- Speak with empathy, showing concern for the other person.

Good listening skills can be learned (Box 2-15). Listening may be done on several levels. Social listening is for entertainment. It does not need to be completely attentive. Discriminating or critical listening helps analyze the information to form a judgment or to take notes. Faking attention to the message, having prejudice against the sender, and listening to only part of the information (selective listening) may distort the meaning. Other actions that may interfere with communication include showing boredom, criticizing, and distracting behavior.

Good listeners are usually people with good self-concepts. They are able to pay better attention to the speaker because they are not worried about what the speaker will think of them or what their response will be. Active listening is an important part of effective communication (Box 2-16). The receiver interacts with the sender and provides feedback to indicate understanding of the message. The health care worker must listen for feelings in addition to facts by observing nonverbal behavior (Fig. 2-4).

BOX 2-15

Good Listening Guidelines

- Allow the other person to talk more than half of the time.
- Listen thoughtfully. Try to see the other person's point of view.
- Speak your mind freely. Say what you mean. If you disagree, say so in a friendly manner.
- If you do not understand what is being discussed, ask for clarification. Use examples and paraphrasing as needed.
- Be prepared for the discussion. Bring notes if necessary to remember all points.
- Keep an open, friendly posture even when in disagreement.
- Do not argue if the dispute is over a fact or record. Have someone look it up.
- Evaluate the discussion for accomplishments and feelings.
- Be patient in allowing the other person time to form his or her thoughts.
- Do not display anger during communication.
- Find a quiet location to talk or remove distractions.
- Speak slowly, softly, and clearly.
- Look for the humor in negative situations if appropriate.

BOX 2-16

Active Listening Guidelines

1. Stop all other activities.
2. Look at the person speaking for nonverbal, as well as verbal, messages.
3. Focus attention on what is being said.
4. Confirm understanding with paraphrasing, clarifying, reflecting, validating, or encouraging.
5. Give own opinion only after listening.

CASE STUDY 2-4 You were asked to provide daily care for a patient who is in traction. You thought that you understood the directions about the special care needs, but when you enter the room, you do not know what you are expected to do. What should you do?

Answers to Case Studies are available on the Evolve website: *http://evolve.elsevier.com/Gerdin*

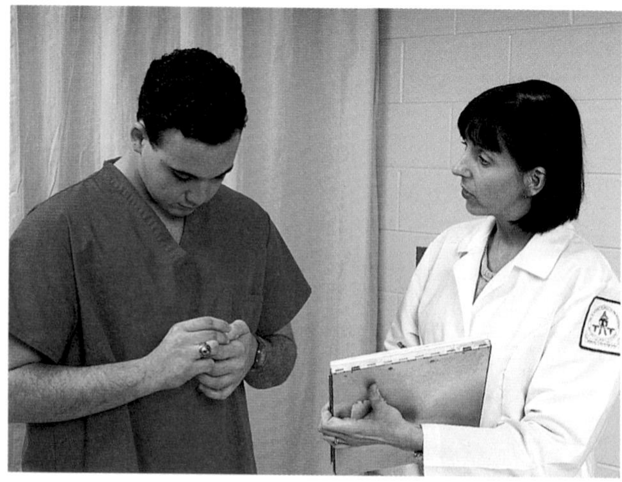

FIGURE 2-4 Body language may lead to varied interpretations of the message.

Videoconferencing over the Internet is used to allow the patient to communicate with a health care provider in a different location. Telemedicine or telehealth services may be used in rural and underserved areas. They are also used in home health, school settings, and nursing homes. They have also been used on cruise ships and on National Aeronautics and Space Administration space missions. Telehealth is the use of technology to provide health care over a distance. Telehealth is more than telemedicine because it provides nonclinical services such as education and research, as well as clinical care. Telemedicine can prevent delay in health care and reduce the expense of travel.

Nonverbal Communication

Messages are conveyed by appearance, facial expression, body motions (gestures), tone of voice, and the distance kept between the sender and receiver. These nonverbal methods of communication may be called body language and include eye and facial movement (oculesics), personal appearance, gestures (kinesics), spacing (proxemics), and time allowed for and pace of speech (chronemics). Use of touch (haptics), reaction to smells (olfactics), and pitch, inflection, tone, and volume of the voice also communicate a message. For effective communication, nonverbal and verbal messages to the patient should convey the same meaning (Fig. 2-5).

Reading and writing skills are used in the health care field to convey information such as the instructions for medication, treatment, and care. Records of health care (charting) must be precise, clear, and concise to record the activities of care (see Appendix II, Fig. II-1 *A* and *B*, pp. 582-583). Charts should include observations, nursing actions, safety precautions, responses to treatment, and unusual incidents. Communication or attempts to communicate with doctors are also part of the record. Each entry should be dated, timed, and in the order of occurrence. Each sheet of the chart includes the patient's name and identification number. Each entry is signed, and no blanks are left. Charting is not subjective. Instead, charting is objective and states the facts accurately using observations made using the senses. Charts are not altered, and errors are corrected with a single initialed line so that the original entry is not obliterated or blocked out. Only the health care worker giving the care may legally chart it (Fig. 2-6).

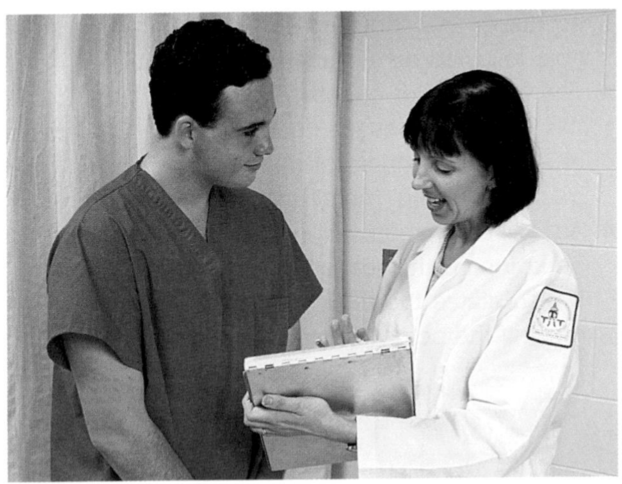

FIGURE 2-5 The nonverbal message should be the same as the verbal message.

Many records are now recorded and kept electronically by using computers or PDAs. Electronic data storage may be completed more quickly than handwritten notes. The information is immediately available to others using the system. However, the small screen on a PDA allows only a portion of the record to be seen at one time. The small screen and lack of a printed page might lead to an error that could be prevented by comparison of written records.

The security, privacy, and legal issues of the use of electronic medical records (EMRs) in health care are regulated by the HIPAA legislation, as well as by other laws. Records are protected by passwords to limit access to records and encryption of data. The Federal Electronic Signatures in Global and National Commerce Act allows signatures to be transmitted electronically. Rules for maintaining the integrity of the records, length of time, and method by which they are kept are established by the institution. The chart,

Date	Time	Nursing Margin / Other Depts Margin
7/18	1045	Requested assistance to lie down. States. "I don't feel well. I have a little upset stomach."
		Denies pain. VS taken. T-99(O). P-76 regular rate and rhythm. R-18 unlabored.
		BP 134/84 L arm lying down. Signal light within reach. Paula Jones, RN notified at 1040
		of resident's complaint and VS. Mary Jensen, CNA
	1100	Asleep in bed. Appears to be resting comfortably. Color good. No signs of
		discomfort or distress noted at this time. Paula Jones, RN
	1145	Refused to go to the dining room for lunch. Complains of nausea.
		Denies abdominal pain. Has not had an emesis. Abdomen soft to
		(Mistaken entry 4-10, PJ)
		palpation. Good bowel sounds. VS taken. T-~~98.2~~ 99.2. P-76 regular
		rate and rhythm. R-18 unlabored. BP-134/84. States she will try to
		eat something. Full liquid room tray ordered. Paula Jones, RN

FIGURE 2-6 Charts are the legal record of care given to the patient. (From Sorrentino SA: *Mosby's textbook for nursing assistants*, ed 7, St. Louis, 2008, Mosby.)

BOX 2-17

Guidelines for Charting Health Care Records

- Records are kept on all patients receiving care or treatment. The chart is considered the property of the facility.
- Written consent of the patient, or a legal representative, is necessary to release any information contained in the chart.
- The agency policy determines who can write in the chart or enter information in the computer.
- The professional status of the person charting (e.g., registered nurse) is clearly shown with all entries.
- All entries in the chart must be legible and written in ink (black ink is preferred) and in the order of occurrence.
- All entries must be dated, timed, and signed by the writer.
- No part of the record may be erased, altered, destroyed, or obliterated. Do not chart before an event occurs.
- Never leave a blank space in the chart and never chart for another person.
- Charting should be a concise, accurate report of the care given.
- Chart only the facts. This includes things that can be seen, felt, heard, or smelled.
- Use only appropriate symbols and abbreviations. The agency determines which symbols are approved.
- Remember that the chart is the legal record of the care given. If the care that is given is not charted, legally it may not have been provided.

whether handwritten or electronic, is the documentation that serves as the legal record of the care given to the patient (Box 2-17). When the information contained in the EMR is available to other facilities, physicians, and the consumer, it is called the electronic health record.

Summary

- Behaviors are the actions that reflect our attitudes or feelings that result from our basic values or worth that we place on something.
- Abraham Maslow designed a hierarchy of needs, which stated that more basic needs such as food and shelter must be met before higher-level ones such as self-esteem and the ability to help others can be met.
- Five methods of maintaining good personal health and professional appearance include maintaining good oral hygiene, hair care, skin care, nail care, and foot care.
- One problem-solving model involves recognizing and describing the problem, brainstorming for solutions, and choosing and implementing a solution, followed by evaluation of the results.
- The elements of effective communication include the sender, message, and receiver. Barriers to effective communication include advising, distracting, judging, moralizing, and threatening.
- Assertive communication describes the undesired behavior and the desired behavior without emotion. It also states the realistic consequences that will result if the behavior does not change.

Review Questions

1. Define and describe the interrelationship of values, attitudes, and behavior. Which is most easily changed? Which is the most difficult to change?
2. Describe the hierarchy of needs as described by Abraham Maslow.
3. Draw a figure that represents a well-groomed health care worker.
4. Describe an example of the decision-making process using a problem-solving method.
5. List the three elements necessary for effective communication.
6. Describe an example of assertive communication.
7. The type of communication that best describes the use of body language is ___________.
8. The sum of a person's values, attitudes, and behavior is called ___________.
9. Refer to Appendix II (Fig. II-2, *B*, p. 585) to list two types of intake.

Critical Thinking

1. Explain the statement made by psychologists that how a person thinks about an experience determines the feelings that result from it.
2. Describe some student behaviors that teachers prefer. Describe some that teachers find less

desirable. How would these behaviors relate to patients in the health care setting?

3. Choose one aspect of personal appearance on which to improve. Keep a daily log for 20 days, recording the activities used to improve appearance.
4. Develop a plan to change an undesirable habit. Keep a log for 20 days documenting the amount of repetition of the habit.
5. Refer to Appendix II (Fig. II-1, *A*, p. 582) to describe "charting by exception."
6. Compare and contrast the psychosocial models of Maslow and Erikson.
7. Investigate the critical thinking model designed by Linda Elder and Richard Paul. Describe the three parts of thinking and each of the eight elements of thought. Use the descriptions in the model to describe your own thinking.
8. Write a paragraph that describes an example of effective teaming and explain how the concept helps provide quality health care.
9. Write a paragraph that describes how effective communication techniques are used to integrate consensus-building.
10. Write a paragraph that evaluates the positive and negative effects of relationships with peers, family, and friends on physical and emotional health. How do positive relationships promote a healthy workplace and community?

Explore the Web

Critical Thinking

Critical Thinking Organization
http://www.criticalthinking.org/starting/Begin-CTModel.cfm

Insight Assessment—The Delphi Report
http://www.insightassessment.com/dex.html

Psychosocial Models of Behavior

Maslow
http://www.wisc-online.com/objects/index_tj.asp?objID=I2P401

Erikson
http://psychology.about.com/library/bl_psychosocial_summary.htm

STANDARDS AND ACCOUNTABILITY*

Foundation Standard 2: Communications

Healthcare professionals will know the various methods of giving and obtaining information. They will communicate effectively, both orally and in writing.

Accountability Criteria

2.1 Concepts of Effective Communication

2.11 Interpret verbal and nonverbal communication.
2.12 Recognize barriers to communication.
2.13 Report subjective and objective information.
2.14 Recognize the elements of communication using a sender-receiver model.
2.15 Apply speaking and active listening skills.

2.2 Medical Terminology

2.21 Use roots, prefixes, and suffixes to communicate information.
2.22 Use medical abbreviations to communicate information.

2.3 Written Communication Skills

2.31 Recognize elements of written and electronic communication (spelling, grammar, and formatting).

Foundation Standard 4: Employability Skills

Healthcare professionals will understand how employability skills enhance their employment opportunities and job satisfaction. They will demonstrate key employability skills and will maintain and upgrade skills as needed.

Accountability Criteria

4.1 Personal Traits of the Healthcare Professional

4.11 Classify the personal traits and attitudes desirable in a member of the healthcare team.
4.12 Summarize professional standards as they apply to hygiene, dress, language, confidentiality, and behavior.

4.2 Employability Skills

4.21 Apply employability skills in healthcare.

4.3 Career Decision-making

4.31 Discuss levels of education, credentialing requirements, and employment trends in healthcare.

Continued

STANDARDS AND ACCOUNTABILITY—cont'd

4.32 Compare careers within the health science career pathways (diagnostic services, therapeutic services, health informatics, support services, or biotechnology research and development).

4.4 Employability Preparation

4.41 Develop components of a personal portfolio.

4.42 Demonstrate the process for obtaining employment.

Foundation Standard 8: Teamwork

Healthcare professionals will understand the roles and responsibilities of individual members as part of the healthcare team, including their ability to promote the delivery of quality healthcare. They will interact effectively and sensitively with all members of the healthcare team.

Accountability Criteria

8.1 Healthcare Teams

8.11 Understand roles and responsibilities of team members.

8.12 Recognize characteristics of effective teams.

8.2 Team Member Participation

8.21 Recognize methods for building positive team relationships.

8.22 Analyze attributes and attitudes of an effective leader.

8.23 Apply effective techniques for managing team conflict.

*From the National Consortium for Health Science Education (2009). National Health Care Standards and Accountability Criteria. Available at http://www.healthscienceconsortium.org.

Note: See also Evolve Appendix: National Consortium for Health Science Education, National Health Science Career Cluster Models, Therapeutic Services Pathway Standards & Accountability Criteria; also available at http://www.healthscienceconsortium.org/healthcare_standards.php.

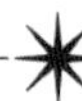

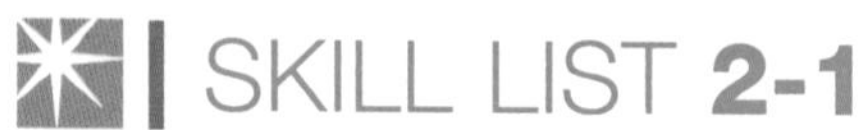

SKILL LIST 2-1
Assertive Behavior

1. Take a few long, deep breaths. Allow time to gain composure so that the message can be delivered in matter-of-fact, unemotional tones.
2. Describe the behavior you would like the other person to change. Be specific about one incident or action.
3. State the effect or how you feel when the behavior occurs.
4. State the positive behavior you would like to see rather than the one you do not like.
5. State the consequences that will occur if the behavior is not changed. These consequences must be timely, reasonable, enforceable, and clearly understood by the other person.
6. Follow through with the consequences if the behavior does not change.
7. Evaluate the success of the confrontation with the other person. Demonstrate appreciation for the change in the behavior.

CHAPTER 3

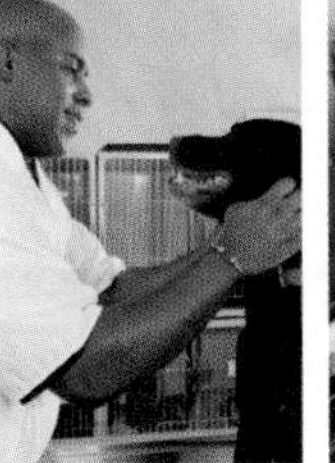
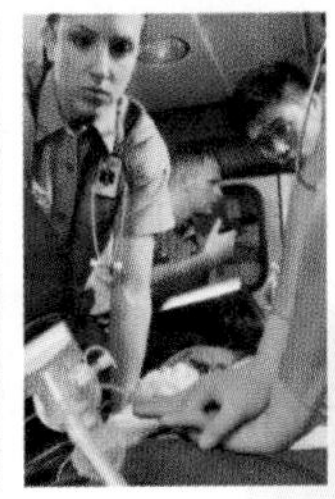
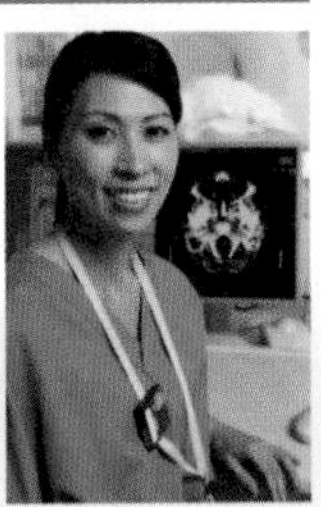

Safety Practices

LEARNING OBJECTIVES

- Define at least 10 terms relating to safety practices in health care.
- Describe the infectious process and methods to prevent infection.
- Describe the methods of Standard and Transmission-Based Isolation Precautions that prevent the spread of microorganisms.
- Describe three levels of medical asepsis.
- List at least three principles of surgical asepsis.
- Identify the functions of the Omnibus Budget Reconciliation Act (OBRA) and the Occupational Safety and Health Administration (OSHA).
- Describe the guidelines for using good body mechanics.
- Describe the signs and symptoms of general and localized infection.

KEY TERMS

Anthrax *(AN-thraks)* An infectious disease of warm-blooded animals (such as cattle and sheep) caused by a spore-forming bacterium (*Bacillus anthracis*) and characterized by external ulcerating nodules or lesions in the lungs

Antiseptic *(ant-uh-SEP-tik)* Substance that deters the growth of microorganisms

Asepsis *(a-SEP-sis)* Freedom from infection; the methods used to prevent the spread of microorganisms

Autoclave *(AW-toe-klaev)* Unit that uses steam under pressure to sterilize materials

Contaminated *(kon-TAM-in-ayt-ed)* Soiled, made unclean, or infected with pathogens

Disinfectant *(dis-in-FEK-tent)* Substance that kills microorganisms except viruses and spores

Ergonomics *(err-go-nom-iks)* Design of equipment for the workplace that maximizes productivity by reducing fatigue and discomfort

Local infection *(LOH-kuhl in-FEK-shun)* An infection limited to a small area of the body

OBRA *(OH-bra)* Law that requires training for nursing assistants including competency testing of skill performance

KEY TERMS cont'd

OSHA *(OH-shuh)* Federal agency that establishes and enforces standards of safety for the workplace

Pathogen *(PATH-uh-jen)* Disease-causing microorganism

Standard Precautions *(STAND-erd pre-CAW-shuns)* CDC guidelines for infection control that are applied to all body fluids of all patients all of the time

Sterile *(STARE-uhl)* Free from living microorganisms

Systemic infection *(si-STEM-ik in-FEK-shun)* An infection located throughout the body

Transmission-Based Precautions *(trans-MISH-un baest pre-CAW-shuns)* CDC guidelines for infection control applied to patients with known or suspected infections

Vector *(VEK-ter)* Organism that carries or transports a pathogen

Disease Transmission

The Infectious Process

The infectious process is the interaction of microorganisms that cause disease with the environment and the host. Infection requires several elements:

- A disease microbe (agent)
- A reservoir where the microorganism can live
- A way of exit or escape from the reservoir
- A way for transmission or transfer to the host
- A way of entry into the host
- A susceptible (vulnerable) host

The microbes or agents include anything that can cause communicable disease, such as bacteria, virus, fungi, protozoa (protists), or animals like worms. The source or reservoir for the microbe may be the patient, other people, or nonliving (inanimate) objects. Five main methods of transmission include contact, droplet, airborne, common vehicle, and vectors. Contact transmission may be direct or indirect (through an inanimate object). Common vehicle transmission includes items such as water, food, or contaminated equipment. **Vectors** or organisms that can spread the agent include mosquitoes, flies, rats, and other such vermin (pests). The host that does not have enough resistance to (i.e., is susceptible to) the infecting agent will become sick. Resistance may be lowered by poor nutrition, open wounds, invasive therapies such as an intravenous line, or a suppressed immune system. For infection to occur, all six of the elements of the infectious process must be present in order. The chain of infection or transmission can be broken and the infection prevented at any of the links (Fig. 3-1).

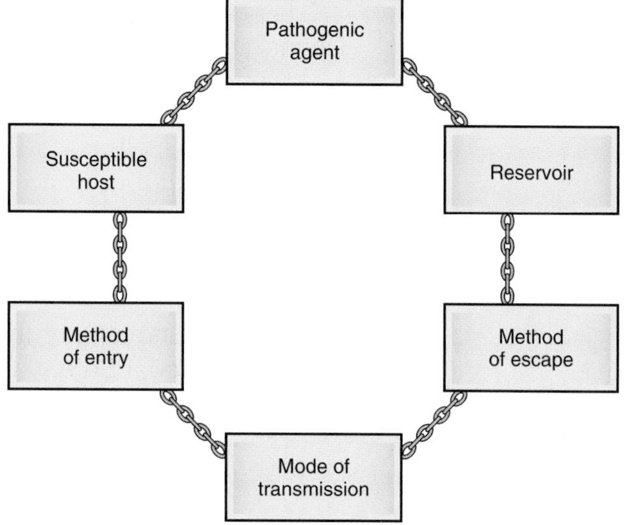

FIGURE 3-1 Infectious process.

Infection is a reaction caused by a microorganism. Infection may be symptomatic or asymptomatic (i.e., with or without expression of health). A **local infection** is an infection limited to a small area of the body. A **systemic infection** is an infection located throughout the body. Infection may occur in a general or local manner. Signs and symptoms of a general infection include a fever, chills, pain, an ache or tenderness, a general feeling of tiredness, and night sweats. A local infection in a wound or incision may be characterized by redness, heat, swelling, pain, or fluid that is white, yellowish, or greenish.

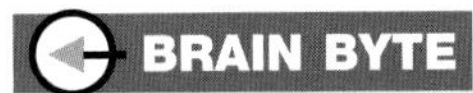

According to the Bureau of Labor Statistics, the rate of nursing home injuries and illness is 14.2%, compared with 10.8% for construction workers.

Infection Control

Isolation Precautions

In the past, isolation procedures and precautions were based on the patient's diagnosis (Box 3-1). Someone with an infection was separated from others to prevent the spread of the microorganisms. In 1996 the Healthcare Infection Control Practices Advisory Committee (HICPAC) of the CDC established a two-level set of guidelines for isolation precautions designed for acute care hospitals. The two levels are **Standard Precautions**, which are applied to all patients, and **Transmission-Based Precautions**, which are applied to patients with known or suspected infections. These guidelines also may be applied to other health care delivery systems (Table 3-1).

BRAIN BYTE

According to The Commonwealth Fund, one in five Americans report that they or a family member have experienced a medical error of some kind.

Standard Precautions combine features of the previously used Universal Precautions and Body Substance Isolation guidelines. They are applied at all times to all patients and all body fluids except perspiration. They are designed to prevent transmission of HIV, hepatitis B virus (HBV), and other bloodborne pathogens when providing first aid or

BOX 3-1

Evolution of Infection Control Procedures

1877	Hospital handbooks recommended patients with infectious conditions be placed in separate facilities.
1910	Cubicle system introduced in multiple bed wards, also known as barrier nursing, required washing of hands and disinfecting contaminating materials between patient contacts.
1950-1960	Infectious-disease hospitals, except those for tuberculosis, were closed.
1960-1970	Tuberculosis hospitals closed.
1970	Manual published by the CDC introducing a system of isolation procedures with seven categories: strict, respiratory, protective, enteric, wound and skin, discharge, and blood precautions.
1983	CDC manual for disease-specific isolation was revised to include strict contact, respiratory, tuberculosis, enteric drainage or secretions, and blood or body fluid precautions.
1985	Universal Precautions were instituted to combat the spread of HIV through needle sticks and skin contamination with patient blood. Emphasis was placed on applying infection precautions to each patient regardless of diagnosis. Hepatitis B vaccination of health care workers became a requirement.
1987	BSI was introduced to focus on all moist and potentially infectious body fluids regardless of diagnosis.
1989	OSHA published a ruling regarding bloodborne pathogens.
1990	CDC published Standard Precautions guidelines for all patients that combine Universal Precautions and BSI principles. It also combined the disease-specific categories into three sets of Transmission-Based Precautions.

BSI, Body substance isolation; *CDC,* Centers for Disease Control; *HIV,* human immunodeficiency virus; *OSHA,* Occupational Safety and Health Administration.

TABLE 3-1
Transmission-Based Precautions*

Type	Sample Infection	Precautions
Airborne	Measles, varicella, tuberculosis	Private room, respiratory protection (mask), special air handling and ventilation
Droplet	Diphtheria, pneumonia, pertussis, streptococcal pharyngitis, scarlet fever, adenovirus, influenza, mumps	Private room, mask, patients positioned at least 3 ft apart
Contact	Gastrointestinal, respiratory, skin or wound infections, diphtheria, herpes simplex virus, impetigo, pediculosis, viral or hemorrhagic conjunctivitis and infections (Ebola, Lassa, Marburg), methicillin-resistant *Staphylococcus aureus* (MRSA), vancomycin-resistant *Enterococcus* (VRE), vancomycin-resistant *S. aureus* (VRSA)	Private room, gloves, gowns, handwashing with antimicrobial soap after removal of gloves, cleaning and disinfecting equipment

*All Transmission-Based Precautions are used in addition to Standard Precautions.

BOX 3-2

Requirements of Standard Precautions

Handwashing
- Whenever visibly soiled
- Before and after patient contact
- After contact with body fluids or moist surfaces
- After removing gloves

Personal Protective Equipment and Attire
- Gloves
- Gowns
- Eye protection
- Head cover
- Footwear

Engineering and Work Practice Controls
- Leakproof sharps disposal
- No recapping of needles

Education
- Training records to be kept for 3 years

Housekeeping, Waste Disposal, and Laundry
- Surfaces cleaned and decontaminated
- Regulated or biowaste disposal
- Sharps disposal boxes
- Soiled laundry—minimum contact and agitation

Hepatitis B Vaccine
- Offered at no cost

Employee Exposure Protocol
- Injured employee seen and treated within 2 hours of incident
- Written exposure control plan

Records and Written Plans
- Employee medical records are kept confidential and maintained for 30 years

health care (Box 3-2). All body fluids of all patients are considered to be potentially infectious under the Standard Precautions guidelines. Body fluids that are included in the precautions include blood, semen, vaginal secretions, and tissues such as pleural, peritoneal, pericardial, cerebrospinal, amniotic fluids, and nonintact skin. Handling of feces, sweat, nasal secretions, urine, tears, and vomitus does not require Universal Precautions unless they contain visible blood. Contact with saliva only requires Standard Precautions when contaminated by blood and in the dental setting. Standard Precautions do not apply to breast milk except when contact is long such as in milk banking.

Protective barriers or personal protective equipment (PPE) used in the Standard Precautions include gloves, gowns aprons, masks, and protective eyewear. Gloves are worn when touching body fluids and when handling items or touching surfaces that are soiled with body fluids. They are changed after contact with each patient. The hands are washed immediately after removing gloves. PPE may also be worn when in contact with hazardous chemicals and some medicines. In some situations, protective hats and footwear may also be used. Disposable aprons, goggles, and masks are worn when there is the possibility of secretions splattering. The type of PPE used is determined by assessing the risk of transfer of microorganisms to and from the patient. Signs are placed outside the patient's room to indicate which type of PPE is needed.

Prevention of injury from needles, scalpels, and other sharp devices is also included in the Universal Precautions. Needles should not be recapped or removed from syringes by hand. Sharp instruments such as needles and scalpel blades should be disposed of in puncture-resistant containers.

CASE STUDY 3-1 While providing care for a patient, you find that someone has left an uncapped needle on the bedside tray. What should you do?

Answers to Case Studies are available on the Evolve website: ***http://evolve.elsevier.com/Gerdin***

Transmission-Based Precautions are used for patients with known or suspected infections. They are used in addition to Standard Precautions. The three categories of Transmission-Based Precautions guidelines are airborne, droplet, and contact precautions. Airborne precautions are used for infections spread through the air, such as chickenpox. Droplet precautions are used for infections spread in large droplets by coughing, sneezing, or talking, such as the flu. Contact precautions are used when an infection, such as the herpes simplex virus, can be spread via skin to skin contact or by contact with surfaces. The precautions are combined when the infection can be transmitted by more than one method.

CASE STUDY 3-2 You are using Transmission-Based Precautions to care for a patient. When care is completed, you notice that one of your gloves ripped sometime during the care. What should you do?

Answers to Case Studies are available on the Evolve website: ***http://evolve.elsevier.com/Gerdin***

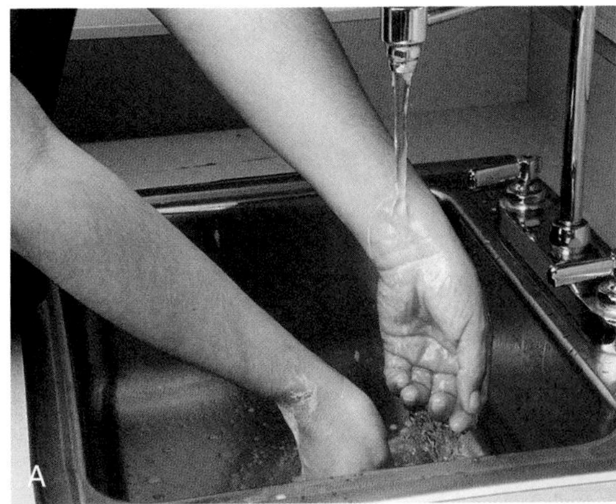

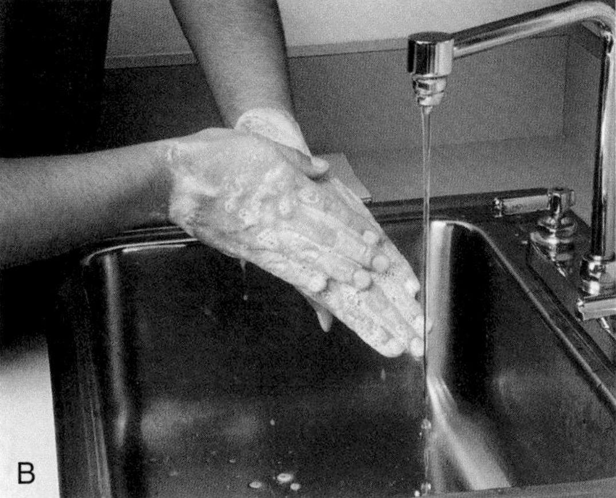

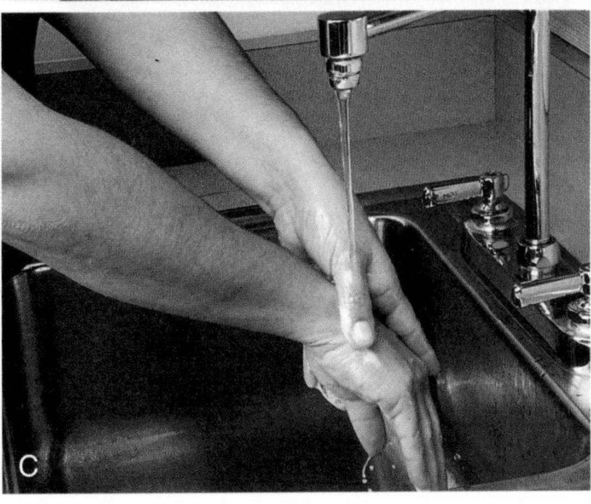

FIGURE 3-2 Handwashing technique. **A,** Keep the hands lower than the arms during the procedure. **B,** In addition to soap and water, friction or rubbing also cleans the skin. **C,** Rinsing hands thoroughly prevents skin irritation from soap. (From Kinn MF, Woods M: *The medical assistant,* ed 8, Philadelphia, 1999, Saunders.)

The primary method of protection from infection is good handwashing technique (Fig. 3-2). The hands are washed thoroughly at the beginning of the work period, between each patient contact, before and after eating, before and after using the restroom, and before

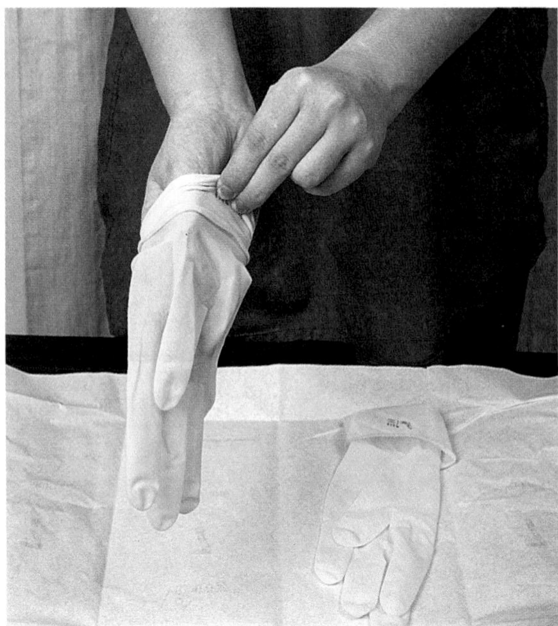

FIGURE 3-3 When applying sterile gloves, it is important not to allow the unsterile hand to cross over the sterile part of either glove.

leaving the work environment. Although state standards vary, the hands should be washed for a minimum of 20 seconds. Sterile gloves may be required to protect the patient during care or procedures (Fig. 3-3). Nonsterile gloves are worn when contact is made with body fluids, mucous membranes, or wet secretions. When removed, nonsterile gloves are placed directly in the designated receptacle to prevent contamination of any environmental surface. The hands are washed thoroughly immediately after removal of the sterile or nonsterile gloves. (See Skill List 3-1, Handwashing, and Skill List 3-2, Sterile Gloving, p. 56).

Infections acquired by the patient as a result of the care or as a result of pathogens in the facility are called nosocomial. In the United States, about two million people acquire a nosocomial infection while in the hospital each year. Epidemiology is a science devoted to studying health-related events in the human population. Principles of epidemiology are used to trace the source and minimize the risk of nosocomial and other infections. Of the infections acquired in the hospital, the CDC reports that 70% are resistant to at least one of the drugs commonly used to treat them. The most relevant nosocomial pathogen in the United States is *methicillin-resistant Staphylococcus aureus* (MRSA). The main mode of transmission of MRSA to patients is by the hands, usually of the health care worker. Box 3-3 provides more information about MRSA.

BOX 3-3

MRSA

According to the CDC, more than 90,000 Americans become infected with MRSA each year. In 2005 it was responsible for more deaths than HIV and AIDS. Bacteria are carried on the skin and spread with skin-to-skin contact. Although more than half of the cases are related to health care settings, more than one otherwise healthy high school student died of MRSA in 2007.

In the community, MRSA infections appear as pustules or boils. They may be red, swollen, painful, and with or without drainage-like pus. They usually occur in areas with skin trauma but may also be in areas covered with hair like the armpit.

Cleanliness is the best way to prevent MRSA. Some suggestions for students to avoid contact with it include the following:

- Frequent handwashing or using alcohol-based sanitizer
- Showering immediately after exercise
- Covering any skin abrasions or cuts with a clean dry bandage
- Avoiding sharing personal items that contact the skin, like razors or towels
- Avoiding sharing unclean equipment such as weight-training benches
- Maintaining a clean environment, including surfaces that directly touch the skin

When antibiotics are used to treat infection, there is a chance that microorganisms will develop resistance to them. Antibiotic-resistant microorganisms are created when some but not all of those being treated are killed. The few pathogens that survive an antibiotic treatment may develop resistance to it. That resistance is passed on to the generations of the pathogen that follow. Two factors associated with development of antibiotic resistance are overuse of antibiotic treatment and incomplete cycles of prescribed antibiotics. In 2005 the CDC listed eight diseases that have been connected to antibiotic resistance (Box 3-4). Special Transmission-Based Precautions or isolation may be used for antibiotic-resistant microorganisms

BOX 3-4

Diseases Connected to Antibiotic Resistance

- Gonorrhea
- Head lice
- Malaria
- MRSA
- Streptococcus pneumoniae
- Tuberculosis
- Typhoid fever
- Vancomycin/glycopeptide-intermediate *S. aureus*
- VRE

From the National Center for Preparedness, Detection, and Control of Infectious Diseases/Division of Healthcare Quality Promotion, http://www.cdc.gov/drugresistance/diseases.htm, Diseases, December 11, 2009.

BOX 3-5

Bioterrorism Agents*

Bacterial
- Anthrax
- Brucellosis
- Cholera
- Glanders (rare)
- Bubonic plague
- Pneumonic plague
- Tularemia
- Q Fever

Viral
- Smallpox
- Venezuelan equine encephalitis
- Viral encephalitis
- Viral hemorrhagic fever

Toxins
- Botulism
- Ricin
- T-2 Mycotoxins
- *Staphylococcus*, Enterotoxin B

*Plans for containment of bioterrorism agents include strategies for isolation, placement, transport of patients, cleaning and disinfection of equipment, discharge management, and post-mortem care.

(superbugs) and patients with immunosuppressed conditions. Isolation guidelines may also be used in the event of the use of bioterrorism agents such as anthrax (Box 3-5).

The most common method of transfer of pathogenic organisms that cause serious illness in the health care worker is contact with a contaminated needle or sharp instrument. To prevent contamination, needles should not be recapped but should be disposed of in a container specifically designed for that purpose. Other environmental risk factors are minimized with the use of hepatitis B vaccination and devices for cardiopulmonary resuscitation that eliminate mouth-to-mouth contact with mucous membranes during the procedure. Methods that are not considered effective include disposable eating utensils, "protective" isolation, disinfectant fogging, and double bagging for the removal of waste and linens. Waste and linen should all be disposed of according to individual agency specifications designed to prevent contact with secretions. More information regarding the infection process and disease transmission is found in Chapter 22.

Principles of Asepsis

Asepsis is the absence of disease-causing microorganisms (pathogens). Asepsis also includes the methods used to prevent the spread of microorganisms. Medical asepsis is a state of cleanliness or the use of clean technique. Some indications for the use of aseptic technique include the following:

- Open wounds
- Urinary catheters
- Insertion or dressing of intravenous lines
- Any procedure requiring the skin to be broken (invasive)

An area or object that becomes unclean is considered contaminated. Medical asepsis can be evaluated on three levels:

1. Antiseptic: Antiseptics inhibit the growth of bacteria. They can be used on the skin.
2. Disinfectant: Disinfectants are agents that destroy most bacteria and viruses. They can be caustic or harmful to the skin. Disinfection can be accomplished by boiling, as well as by using chemical agents.
3. Sterile: Surgical asepsis is a state of sterility or the use of sterile technique. Sterilization is the removal of all microorganisms including viruses and endospores. Sterilization can be accomplished by

using an **autoclave**. One type of autoclave is a pressure cooker that uses steam and pressure to destroy microorganisms. Other autoclaves use dry heat or chemical vapor to kill all microorganisms. Sterile technique also includes special methods of handling sterile equipment, maintaining sterile fields, changing dressings, and disposing of contaminated materials.

Clean technique does not require a sterile environment and equipment. It is also called nonsterile technique. Barriers are used to provide a "no-touch" or clean field by preventing contact with an infected area. Gloves and other protective equipment may be used to prevent the spread of microorganisms. Disinfectants are used to clean the environment and equipment. Clean technique is used in home care more often than in hospital care. Some indications for the use of clean technique in the health care setting include the following:

- Removing sutures
- Removing drains
- Dressing secondary wounds (wounds that will be left open, like stomas)
- Endotracheal suctioning

OBRA and OSHA Regulations

OBRA

In 1987 Congress passed a law that requires training for nursing assistants, including competency testing of skill performance. In addition to completing a written examination, the nurse assistant must demonstrate the ability to perform skills correctly. **OBRA** applies to all states and facilities in which nursing assistants are employed. Other requirements of OBRA include continuing education, periodic evaluation of performance, and retraining if the nursing assistant does not work in the field for 2 years or more at one time. In addition to training for nursing assistants, the act also requires long-term care and home health facilities to provide specific care for the residents. For example, it requires the provision of a doctor for each resident and limits the use of restraints.

OSHA

OSHA was established in 1970 as one of the agencies of the Department of Labor. OSHA's two functions are to establish standards of safety for the workplace and to enforce those standards. In 1971 the NIH established the branch called the National Institute of Occupational Safety and Health (NIOSH) to research and provide documentation to OSHA regarding the safe level of exposure to hazards in the workplace. OSHA must prove to the Office of Management and Budget that the health standards set are economically feasible for the industries to which they apply.

In 1985 regulations established by the federal government began requiring employers to tell employees of potential hazards in the workplace. This "right-to-know" information includes details of any health and safety hazards related to working with hazardous or toxic materials. The information is often described in the Material Safety Data Sheet (MSDS; Box 3-6). To reduce the incidence of needle sticks, OSHA defined "sharps" and reporting requirements in a broader manner in 2001.

There is always a risk of injury or loss due to hazards in the workplace (Box 3-7). Risk management works to identify the risks and develop methods to avoid or reduce them. Some risks cannot be removed and are accepted as part of the management plan. For example, nursing staff must use sharp needles to give medications. There is always a risk of puncture. Providing training and protective equipment reduces the risk of that injury.

Safe Movement

Body Mechanics and Ergonomics

Body mechanics is the way the body is moved to prevent injury to oneself and to others. It is accomplished by using knowledge of proper body alignment, balance, and movement. **Ergonomics** refers to the design of equipment for the workplace that minimizes fatigue and discomfort and maximizes productivity. Posture is the position of body parts in relation to each other. Balance is the ability to maintain a steady position that does not tip. Six principles of movement can be used to maintain good body mechanics (Fig. 3-4). Chapter 24 provides more information regarding positioning the patient. (See Skill List 3-3, Good Body Mechanics, p. 57).

In addition to the use of correct body mechanics, assistive devices can also be used to allow mobility while preventing injury. The gait belt is a safety device

BOX 3-6

Material Safety Data Sheet (MSDS)

Section I: Product Identification

Product Name	Windex Multi-surface Cleaner with Vinegar

Section II: Hazardous Ingredients

Ethylene glycol n-hexyl ether
Isopropanol
Water

Section III: Physical Data

Color	Clear
State	Liquid
Odor	Fragrant
pH 9.5-10.5	

Section IV: Fire and Explosion Hazard

Flash Point	129° F (does not sustain combustion)
Extinguishing Media	Foam, CO_2, dry chemical, Water fog

Section V: Health Hazards

LD50 (Acute oral toxicity)	Estimated to be greater than 5000 mg/kg (rats)

Section VI: Reactivity

Stable

Section VII: Spill and Disposal

No special requirements

Section VIII: Protective Measures

No special requirements under normal use conditions

Section IX: Special Precautions

None

MSDSs are often prepared by the product's manufacturer and provide only basic information.

BOX 3-7

Common Workplace Hazards

Mechanical Hazard

- Impact (collision, fall, hit, slip, trip)
- Confined space
- Puncture by sharp object
- Equipment (electrical, cutting)

Physical Hazard

- Noise
- Lighting
- Pressure
- Radiation
- Electrical
- Asphyxiation
- Temperature (cold, hot, dehydration)
- Fire
- Explosion
- Ergonomic (carpel tunnel)

Biological Hazard

- Bacteria
- Virus
- Fungi (mold)
- Bloodborne pathogen
- Airborne (tuberculosis)

Chemical Hazard

- Acid/base
- Heavy metal (mercury, lead)
- Particulates (asbestos, silica)
- Noxious fumes

Psychosocial Hazard

- Stress
- Violence
- Bullying
- Burnout

BRAIN BYTE

In 1998 the Bureau of Labor Statistics reported 90,000 days of work missed in health care as a result of musculoskeletal injury.

that may be worn by the patient when being transferred or ambulating. The gait belt is a strong cloth belt that provides a firm grasping area for the health care worker and protects the patient from trauma to the skin (Fig. 3-5). The health care worker may also use the gait belt to lower the patient gradually to the floor if necessary (Fig. 3-6). The health care worker may also wear this type of belt to prevent back injury.

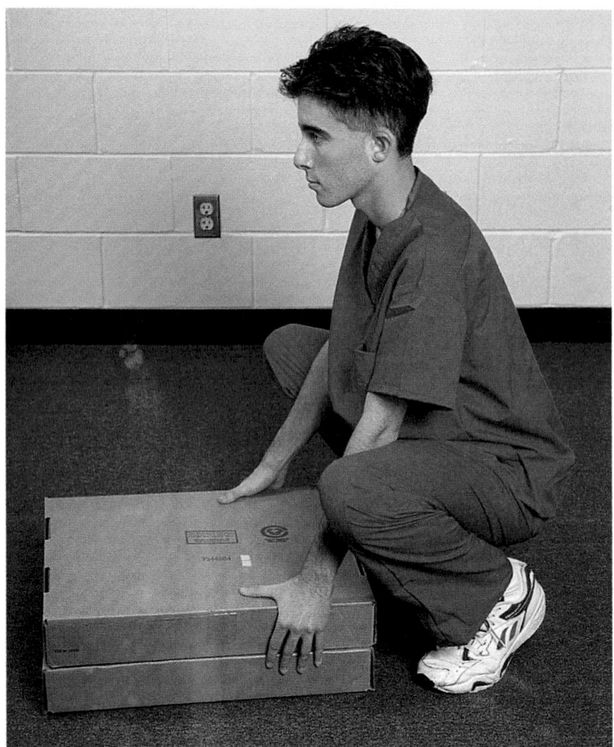

FIGURE 3-4 Principles of good body mechanics include keeping the back straight.

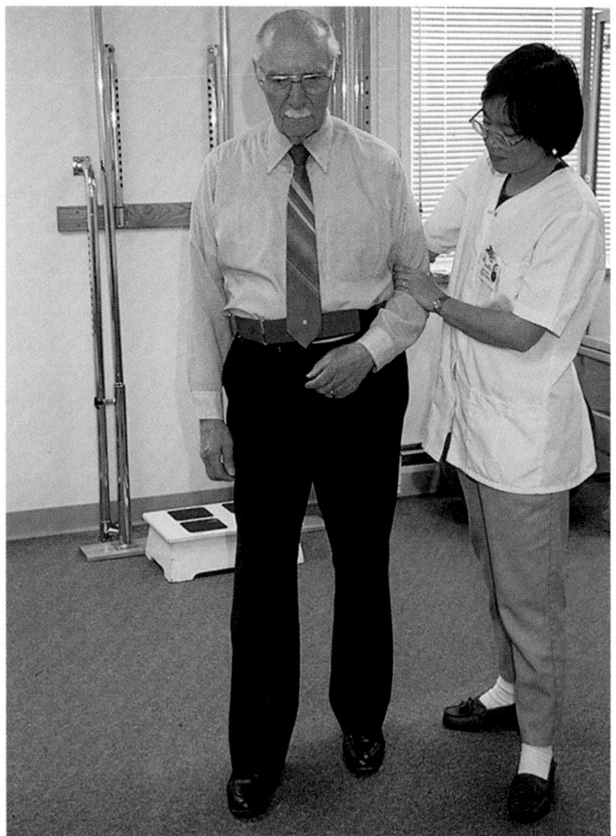

FIGURE 3-5 Injury to the patient and health care worker may be prevented by use of a gait or safety belt.

NIOSH reports that female nursing assistants and licensed practical nurses are more than twice as likely to suffer a back injury as other female workers. Other assistive devices include postural supports such as the pelvic holder, torso support, and elevated arm rests (Fig. 3-7). For moving patients, mechanical lifts, sliding sheets, and boards may be used (Fig. 3-8). It is the health care worker's responsibility to obtain and use assistive devices to prevent injury to the patient or worker. Chapter 24 provides more information regarding procedures for moving patients. (See Skill List 3-4, Ambulation with a Gait Belt; Skill List 3-5, Moving the Patient up in Bed; Skill List 3-6, Turning the Patient to the Side; and Skill List 3-7, Transferring the Patient from the Bed to a Chair, pp. 57-59).

BRAIN BYTE

Health care workers represent six of the top 10 occupations at risk for back injuries; nursing assistants are at the top.

CASE STUDY 3-3 As part of his daily care, you need to help an obese patient move from the bed to a chair. You ask one of your coworkers to help you. She responds that she moves that man by herself every day. What should you do?

Answers to Case Studies are available on the Evolve website: ***http://evolve.elsevier.com/Gerdin***

The international symbol of access in more than 60 countries indicates that a person with a disability can enter and use a building without being blocked by architectural design (Fig. 3-9). The symbol indicates, for example, that wheelchair ramps are available, doors are wide enough to accommodate a wheelchair, the elevators have Braille indicators, and telephones and drinking fountains are placed at a lower height. Physical devices that are used to provide better access by disabled individuals include the walker, cane, wheelchair, and crutches. Hydraulic mechanical lifts may be used so that a small force can lift a heavy object or person. With environmental adjustments and devices, the disabled individual may be able to perform activities of daily living such as eating, bathing, dressing, and moving about independently.

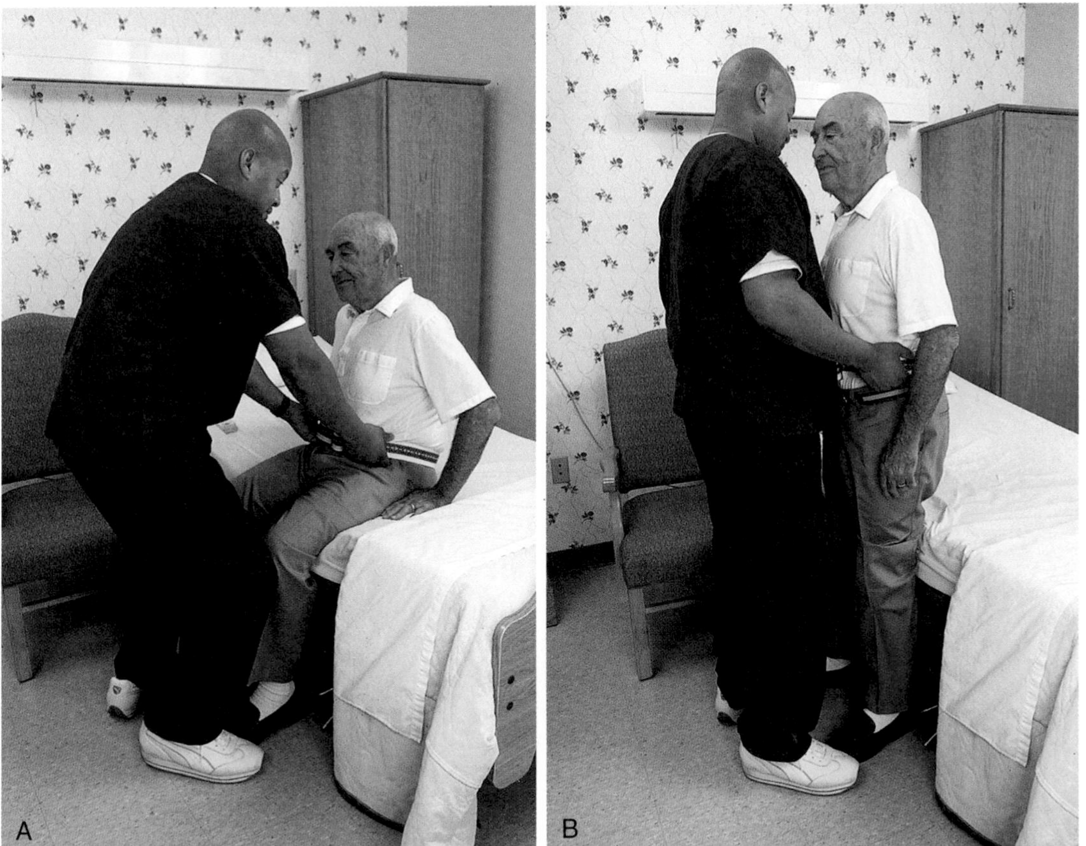

FIGURE 3-6 Transferring the patient to a chair by using a transfer belt. **A,** The patient's feet and knees are blocked by the assisting person's feet and knees. This prevents the patient from sliding or falling. **B,** The assisting person pulls the patient to a standing position and supports the patient by holding the transfer belt and blocking the patient's knees and feet.

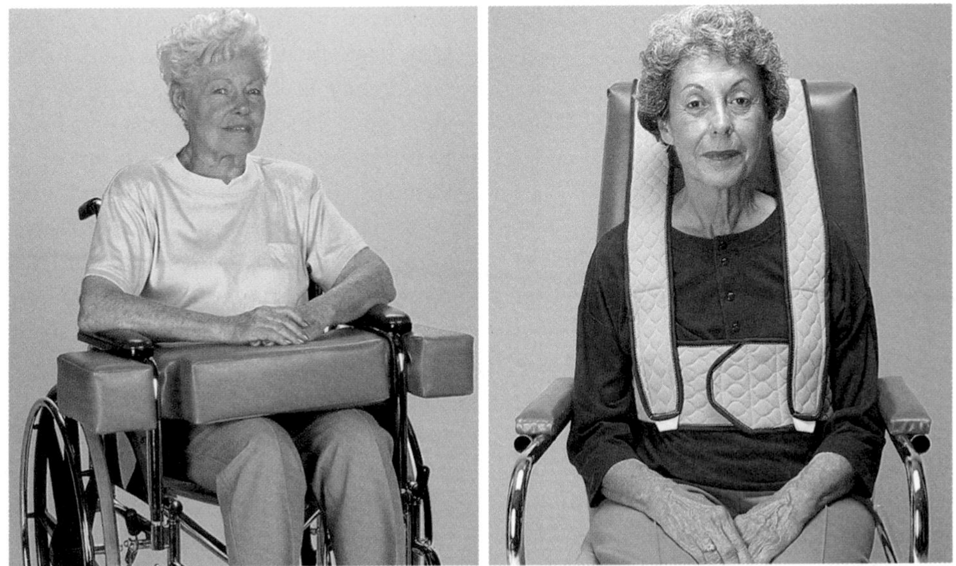

FIGURE 3-7 Postural supports help the patient maintain good alignment. (From Sorrentino SA: *Mosby's textbook for nursing assistants,* ed 7, St. Louis, 2008, Mosby. Images courtesy J.T. Posey Co., Arcadia, Calif.)

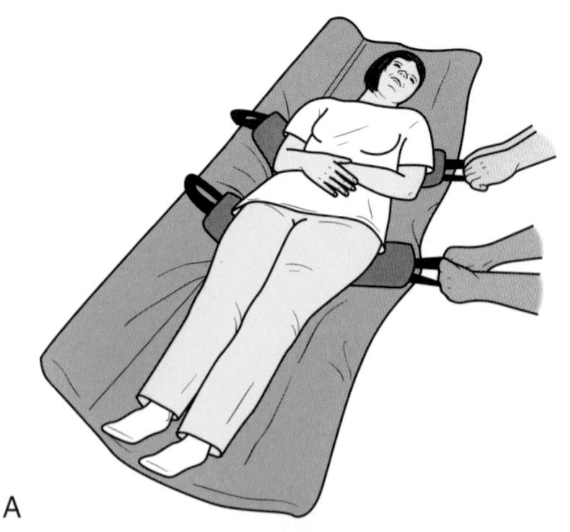

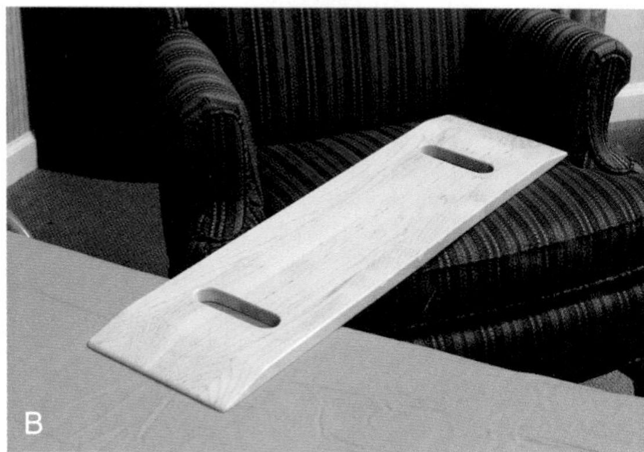

FIGURE 3-8 Assistive devices are used to move patients to prevent injury to the patient or worker. **A,** Slide sheet. **B,** Slide board for transferring to and from surfaces. (From Sorrentino SA: *Mosby's textbook for nursing assistants*, ed 7, St. Louis, 2008, Mosby.)

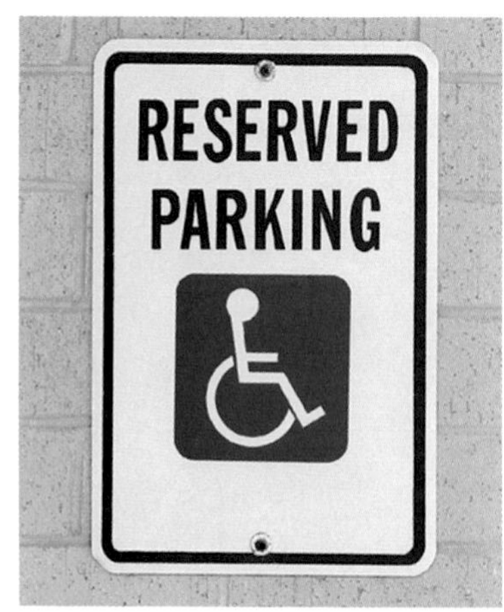

FIGURE 3-9 Parking sign designating parking space for persons with disabilities.

Identifying and Reporting Hazards

Fire and Electrical Hazards

Fire may occur in the home or health care facility as a result of equipment that is damaged or circuits that are overloaded. Smoking can also cause fires. For a fire to burn, it must have oxygen, fuel, and heat. A fire can be controlled or extinguished by removing any one of these elements. Health care workers are responsible for preventing and reacting to fires to protect their patients. Avoiding the accumulation of flammable materials and waste products may prevent hospital fires. Some facilities have fire sprinklers that activate when a fire occurs. Additionally, all employees should be familiar with the policy for fire response.

Although each facility has a procedure to follow in the case of fire, it is common practice to sound the alarm, notify the switchboard, and move any patient who is in danger first. If the fire is small, a fire extinguisher may then be used to extinguish it. To decrease the amount of air supply to the fire, all windows and doors should be closed and oxygen and electrical equipment turned off. Exits are kept clear at all times to allow patients and workers to leave if necessary. If smoke is present, the workers and patients should crawl or move close to the floor toward the exit because the smoke will rise. A damp towel or similar cloth can be used to cover the mouth and nose for breathing.

Each health care facility has a procedure for response to fire. The fire plan may vary and should be displayed in all departments and patient-care areas. One basic protocol that is used to respond to a fire emergency is known as RACE (Fig. 3-10). The "R" stands for "rescue." The first concern in case of fire is to move everyone from the point of origin of the fire. Critically ill patients are removed while in their beds. Ambulatory patients may walk to safety with supervision. Ambulatory and semiambulatory patients are removed from the area of the fire before the nonambulatory patients. Patient charts are moved with the appropriate patient. Evacuation may be either horizontal or vertical. Horizontal evacuation (used first) consists of moving patients through at least one set of fire doors on the same floor. Vertical evacuation consists of moving patients down stairs to a lower level or out of the building. Rescue may be performed simultaneously with the "A" of RACE, "alarm."

The fire emergency call box or pull station may be used to sound the alarm. In some institutions there is an emergency phone number to dial. The extent, origin, and location of the fire or smoke are reported

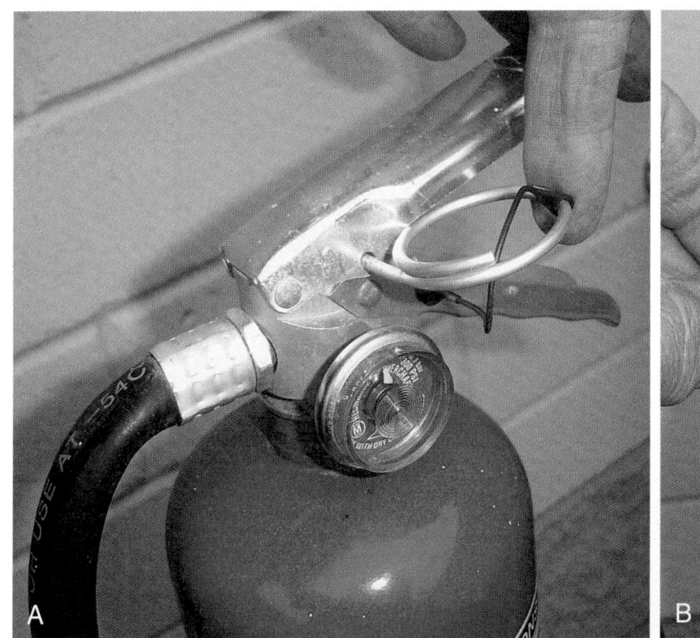

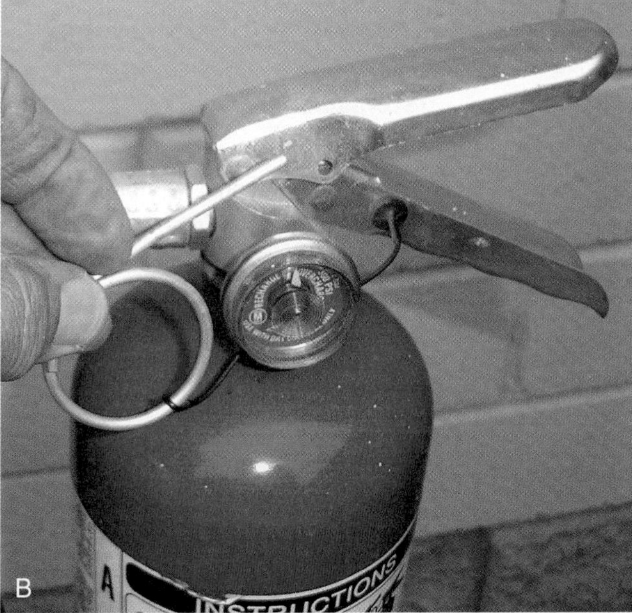

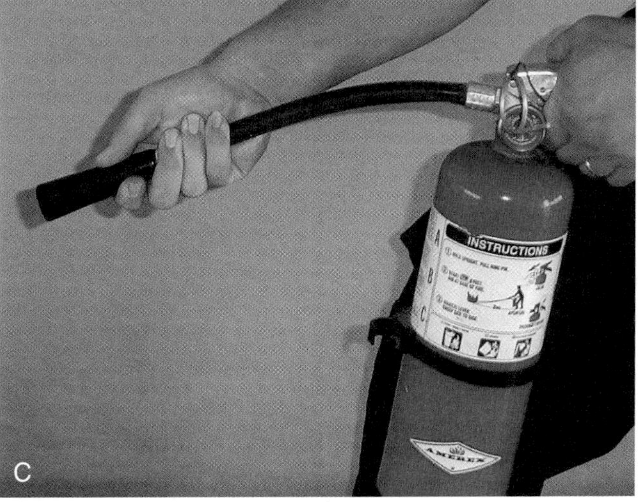

FIGURE 3-10 **A,** Hold the tank upright. **B,** Pull the pin. **C,** Aim at the base of the fire and spray side to side.

to an operator at this number. The sound of the fire alert allows health care workers in nearby areas to prepare for any action necessary in that area.

The "C" in RACE stands for "confine" or "contain." Burning and combustible materials should be contained or confined in one area if possible. By closing doors and windows, the smoke may be contained and the oxygen supply cut off from the fire.

The "E" in RACE stands for "extinguish." Handheld fire extinguishers may be used in case of a small, contained fire such as a wastebasket. This is attempted only after patients are removed from the area and the person using the extinguisher has a clear route of escape. Even if the fire is safely extinguished, the incident is reported to the emergency number.

Portable chemical fire extinguishers are useful in extinguishing small fires. Four classes of chemical fire extinguishers include the following:

- Class A: For use on paper, wood, trash, cloth, upholstery, rubber, and similar materials
- Class B: For use on fuel oil, gas, paint, solvents, and other flammable liquids
- Class C: For use on electrical equipment, fuse boxes, wiring, and appliances
- Class D: For use on metals

Some extinguishers are designed for multiple purposes. For example, an ABC extinguisher may be used for the home. Fire extinguishers are also rated by the size of fire that can be extinguished. All fire extinguishers operate the same way. When extinguishing

TABLE 3-2
PASS Guidelines for Fire Extinguisher Use

Action	Description
P = Pull	Pull the pin on the handle of the top fire extinguisher without squeezing the handle.
A = Aim	Take three steps back from the fire (8 to 10 ft from the fire). Aim the hose or nozzle at the base of the fire. Do not aim at the smoke or flames.
S = Squeeze	Squeeze the top handle toward the bottom handle to discharge the extinguisher contents.
S = Sweep	Sweep the nozzle from side to side across the base of the fire.

a fire, a person should aim the stream from the extinguisher at the base of the fire, not at the smoke or flames (Table 3-2).

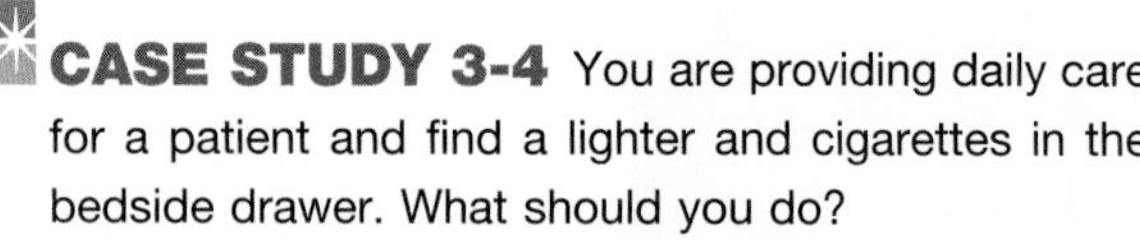

CASE STUDY 3-4 You are providing daily care for a patient and find a lighter and cigarettes in the bedside drawer. What should you do?

Answers to Case Studies are available on the Evolve website: ***http://evolve.elsevier.com/Gerdin***

Hazardous Waste

In health care, waste is divided into two categories: biomedical and general. Infectious and hazardous waste produced in health care facilities may sometimes be poured into the sewage system or disposed of by incineration. One concern that has been raised because of local incineration of wastes is the production of toxic gases containing dioxin, acid gases, and heavy metals. According to the federal Office of Technology Assessment, hospitals release 10 to 100 times more of these elements into the air than other incinerators found in a city.

In health care facilities, hazardous and infectious waste is usually placed in sealed bags before removing it from the area of use. The bag is labeled and sealed to indicate the kind of waste hazard that may exist and to alert other workers in the facility (Fig. 3-11). Some general guidelines for bagging waste for disposal include separating items into categories such as linens, plastics, glass, and wet or dry. If the bag is contaminated during loading, it may be double bagged.

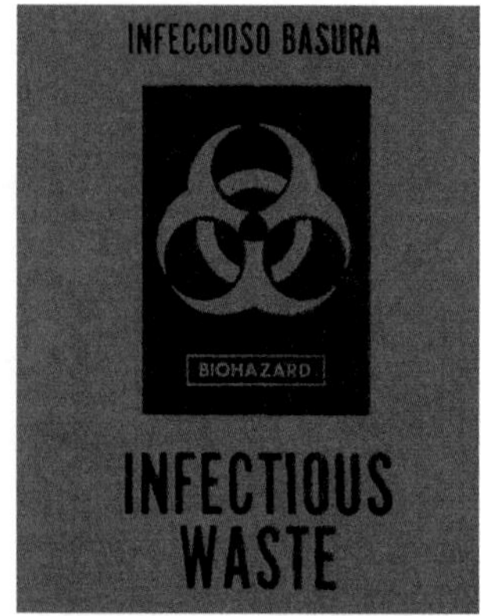

FIGURE 3-11 A biohazard symbol.

Chemical Safety

Chemicals in the health care workplace should be stored in a way that prevents exposure, property damage, and liability by the facility. Chemicals should be purchased and stored in amounts that will be used in a reasonable time. Some chemicals may change over time. The amount stored should also meet fire code limits. Containers used to store chemicals should be made of the correct material and clearly labeled with the contents. Workers using chemicals must be aware of the correct use, proper disposal, and risk associated with them. Additionally, emergency treatment and procedures should be known for improper exposure.

Equipment Maintenance

Equipment is routinely cleaned and maintained in the health care facility. Any equipment that is not working properly (malfunctions) or is defective in any way is reported to the supervisor. Some examples that should be reported include frayed or bent wires. If the defect is hazardous, the equipment is not used for patient care until it is replaced or repaired. The health care work area and equipment are kept clean to prevent the spread of infection. Equipment is returned to a designated storage area after use so that it can be located quickly. Emergency equipment is restocked immediately after use and checked routinely to ensure that all contents are ready for use when necessary. All personnel should be trained on the proper use of equipment that is unfamiliar to the worker.

Emergency Disaster Procedures

A disaster may be caused by nature or by humans and is considered to be any catastrophic event that injures or kills many people at one time. Some examples include tornadoes, explosions, plane crashes, and earthquakes. Policies and procedures for actions to be followed in a health care facility during a disaster depend on the type of facility. Some personnel may be asked to work in another area, such as the emergency department or at an unscheduled time. In hospitals some patients may be asked to go home or move to another facility.

Personnel from all areas of health care are asked to assist the community during a natural disaster or severe weather (Box 3-8). Additionally, incidents involving bioterrorism or outbreaks of contagious illness may activate emergency plans that include many health care workers. The Department of Homeland Security has established the National Response Plan to be implemented in the event of a domestic incident such as a bioterrorist attack. It provides a management structure that integrates the emergency responders, medical sector, law enforcement, private sector, and other agencies to help in a large-scale disaster. To provide medication to the public on a large scale, the plan includes points of distribution or designated places and personnel trained for that purpose. Individual preparedness for emergencies is also a focus of the plan. Items that an individual or family might need to survive in an emergency can be stored in a cool, dark place or central location for easy access (Box 3-9).

BOX 3-8

Types of Natural Disasters and Weather Events

- Earthquakes
- Extreme cold
- Extreme heat
- Floods
- Hurricanes
- Landslides and mudslides
- Power outages
- Tornadoes
- Tsunamis
- Volcanoes
- Wildfires

Summary

- Standard Precautions includes the procedures used to prevent the spread of microorganisms. The primary method used is good handwashing technique.
- Transmission-Based Precautions used in addition to Standard Precautions are determined by the type of infection present.
- Three levels of asepsis include antiseptic, disinfectant, and sterile.
- OBRA is the federal agency that regulates training of nursing assistants. OSHA establishes and enforces standards of safety for the workplace.
- Guidelines for maintaining good body mechanics include using bent knees, keeping a broad base, and keeping the back straight.
- A local infection is limited to a small area of the body and may cause redness or warmth at the site. A systemic infection may cause fever, chills, or a feeling of tiredness.

Review Questions

1. Describe the six elements of the infectious process.
2. Compare the signs and symptoms of localized and general infections.
3. Compare standard and transmission-based precautions.
4. List and describe three levels of asepsis.
5. Use the following terms in one or more sentences that correctly relate their meaning: asepsis, sterile, disinfect, contaminate, and antiseptic.
6. Describe the functions of OBRA and OSHA.
7. List the six guidelines for maintaining good body mechanics.
8. Describe the meanings of RACE and PASS in relation to fire emergencies.

Critical Thinking

1. Describe the type of precautions that might be used for a person with an infection of a surgical wound. Identify which of the elements of the infectious process is being broken.

BOX 3-9

Emergency Preparedness: Survival for 3 Days*

Medical
- Medication supply for 1 week to 1 month
- Medical records such as vaccinations and copies of prescriptions
- Medical contact such as doctor's names and numbers

Food
- Nonperishable canned and dry food supplies, including dry milk or juice
- Water for 3 days (1 gallon/person)
- Utensils including a can opener

Documents in Waterproof Bag
- Cash (including coins) and credit cards
- Birth certificates
- Credit card, insurance, and bank account numbers
- Memorabilia (e.g., photos, jewelry)
- Contact phone numbers
- Paper, pencils, or pens
- Map of area

Clothing
- Change of clothing
- Sturdy, closed-toe shoes and socks
- Blankets
- Rain gear
- Jacket or coat
- Heavy gloves
- Hat and sunglasses

Pets
- Records
- Food (2-week supply canned or dry)
- Litter box supplies
- Leash, collar, and travel cage

Tools
- Pliers, hammer, broom, and wrench
- Utility knife
- Plastic sheeting
- Duct tape
- Shovel
- Garbage bag with ties
- Dust mask

Other
- First aid kit including nonsteroidal antiinflammatory drugs, antibiotic cream, and antacid
- First-aid manual
- Whistle
- Clock or watch with extra batteries
- Signal flare
- Moist towelettes
- Disposable camera
- Plastic bucket with lid
- National Oceanic Atmospheric Administration weather radio with extra batteries
- Candles
- Flashlight with extra batteries
- Scissors
- Bleach
- Hygiene products (sanitary napkins, soap, toothbrush, toothpaste)
- Nail clippers, nail file
- Spare glasses, contact solutions
- Matches

*A 3-day supply may be placed in waterproof plastic bags and stored in portable, closed containers.

2. Describe the precautions that might be used for a person with an infectious cough. Identify which of the elements of the infectious process is being broken.
3. Describe the precautions that might be used for a patient with leukemia. Identify which of the elements of the infectious process is being broken.
4. Investigate the five C's or conditions in which MRSA is more likely to occur. Investigate the incidence of MRSA in infants and small children.
5. Investigate the local emergency disaster procedures including the closest point of distribution for medication in your community and local school district.
6. Use Box 3-9 to prepare a list of the items that would be necessary to take in case of an emergency that requires immediate evacuation.
7. Prepare a list of the MSDS requirements for a common household item.
8. Investigate and describe how forces including torque, tension, and elasticity influence movement and body mechanics.

Explore the Web

MSDS

http://www.fsafood.com/msds/MSDS_Products.asp?letter=W

MRSA

CDC

http://www.cdc.gov/mrsa/prevent/schools.html

Body Mechanics

You Tube

Search terms: body mechanics, caregivers, patient

http://youtube.com

Universal Precautions

You Tube

Search terms: universal precautions, health care

http://youtube.com

STANDARDS AND ACCOUNTABILITY*

Foundation Standard 7: Safety Practices

Healthcare professionals will understand the existing and potential hazards to clients, co-workers, and themselves. They will prevent injury or illness through safe work practices and follow health and safety policies and procedures.

Accountability Criteria

7.1 Infection Control

7.11 Explain principles of infection control.

7.12 Describe methods of controlling the spread and growth of microorganisms.

7.2 Personal Safety

7.21 Apply personal safety procedures based on OSHA and CDC regulations.

7.22 Apply principles of body mechanics.

7.3 Environmental Safety

7.31 Apply safety techniques in the work environment.

7.4 Common Safety Hazards

7.41 Comply with safety signs, symbols, and labels.

7.42 Understand implications of hazardous materials.

7.5 Emergency Procedures and Protocols

7.51 Practice fire safety in a health care setting.

7.52 Apply principles of basic emergency response in natural disasters and other emergencies.

Foundation Standard 10: Technical Skills†

Healthcare professionals will apply technical skills required for all career specialties. They will demonstrate skills and knowledge as appropriate.

Accountability Criteria

10.1 Technical Skills

10.11 Apply procedures for measuring and recording vital signs, including the normal ranges.

10.12 Apply skills to obtain training or certification in cardiopulmonary resuscitation, automated external defibrillator, foreign body airway obstruction, and first aid.

*From the National Consortium for Health Science Education (2009). National Health Care Standards and Accountability Criteria. Available at http://www.healthscienceconsortium.org.

†Additional technical skills may be included in a program of study based on career specialties.

Note: See also Evolve Appendix: National Consortium for Health Science and Technology Education, National Health Science Career Cluster Models, Diagnostic Services Pathway Standards & Accountability Criteria; also available at: http://www.healthscienceconsortium.org/healthcare_standards.php.

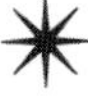

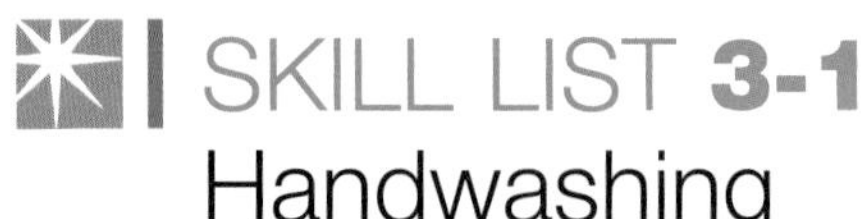

SKILL LIST 3-1 Handwashing

1. Maintain medical asepsis by using good handwashing technique and wearing gloves according to Standard and Transmission-Based Precautions.
2. Hands should be washed at the beginning of the workday, between each contact with a patient, and at the end of the day. They should also be washed before and after eating and using the restroom.
3. Wet the hands completely with water before applying the soap. Keep the hands lower than the arms during the procedure. The hands are washed and rinsed from the least contaminated area to the most (clean to dirty).
4. Rinse the soap bar before using it and replacing it in the dish. Soap can carry microorganisms to another person. In addition to the soap and water, friction or rubbing actually cleans the skin.
5. Using a circular motion, rub the surface of each wrist at least 2 inches above the hand. Friction helps to remove the dirt from the skin surface.
6. Wash the palms and back of the hands after both wrists are cleaned. After they are cleaned, the wrists are not retouched to prevent contamination by microorganisms from the less clean areas of the hands.
7. Clean each finger and thumb of each hand. Do not retouch the less clean areas (backs of the palms). The fingers are considered to have four sides. Special attention should be given to the area underneath the nails and between the fingers. The hands should be washed for at least 20 seconds.
8. Rinse each hand from the wrist to the fingers, keeping the hands below the level of the arms.
9. Using a circular motion, dry each hand thoroughly from the wrist to the fingertips. Use a separate towel or dry portion of the towel for each hand. Most skin irritations result from soap or moisture that remains on the skin after washing.
10. Use a dry towel to turn off the faucet handle and clean the sink area. Faucets and other metal fixtures (fomites) can also transmit microorganisms.

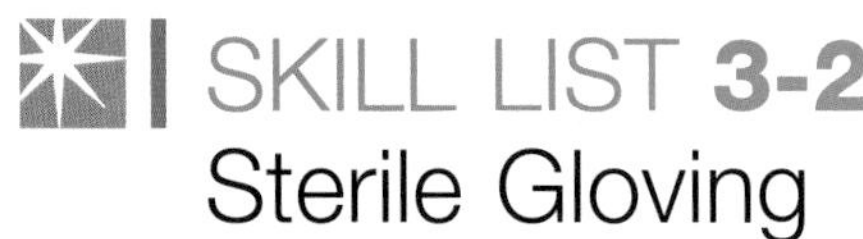

SKILL LIST 3-2 Sterile Gloving

1. Maintain medical asepsis by using good handwashing technique and wearing gloves according to Standard and Transmission-Based Precautions.
2. The hands can never be sterile. If any part of the hand touches the sterile outside of the gloves, the gloves are contaminated.
3. Touching only the outside and edges of the wrapper, open the sterile glove wrapper on a clean, dry surface. The inside of the wrapper creates a sterile field.
4. Remove one glove from the wrapper by grasping only the inside surface of the glove. Avoid touching the glove on the edges of the sterile field. Edges are considered contaminated. If the bare skin passes over the sterile part of the gloves, the gloves are contaminated.
5. With a smooth, upward motion, pull on the glove.
6. Using the gloved (sterile) hand, remove the remaining glove from the package, touching only the outside (sterile) surface.
7. Pull the remaining glove onto the ungloved hand in an upward motion without touching the outside (sterile) surface of either glove to the skin. Keep the hands above the level of the waist. Items below the waist and behind the back are considered contaminated.

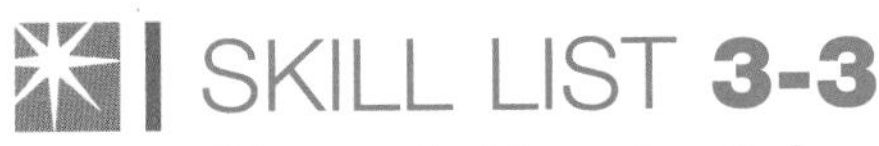

SKILL LIST **3-3**
Good Body Mechanics

1. Maintain medical asepsis by using good handwashing technique and wearing gloves according to Standard and Transmission-Based Precautions.
2. Identify the patient and explain the procedure.
3. Size up the load to be moved. Get help if necessary.
4. Keep a broad base of stance, with feet 12 to 18 inches apart.
5. Bring the object or patient close before attempting the move.
6. Squat by bending at the knees, and keep the back straight.
7. Do not lift anything that can be pushed or pulled.
8. Turn the body as a unit by pivoting the feet, not turning at the waist.

SKILL LIST **3-4**
Ambulation with a Gait Belt

1. Maintain medical asepsis by using good handwashing technique and wearing gloves according to Standard and Transmission-Based Precautions.
2. Select the correct gait belt for the patient. Gait belts may range from $\frac{1}{2}$ to 4 inches in diameter and 54 to 60 inches long.
3. Inspect the gait belt to ensure that it is clean and intact.
4. Place the gait belt around the patient's waist (over clothing) so that it fits snugly but allows room for your fingers under it.
5. Secure it in place by threading the belt through the teeth of the buckle. Thread the belt through openings to lock it in place.
6. If possible, instruct the patient to push with the arms while rising to a standing position.
7. Bend at the knees to use leg muscles, and keep the back straight while assisting the patient to stand.
8. Place one hand at the patient's back to grasp the gait belt and stabilize the patient.
9. Place the other hand under the patient's forearm to guide and provide support.
10. If necessary, draw the patient close with bent knees to lower the patient to the floor.
11. Assist the patient to the designated location.
12. Use correct body mechanics to lower the patient to a sitting or lying position.
13. Remove the gait belt and return it to the proper location for storage.

SKILL LIST **3-5**
Moving the Patient up in Bed

1. Maintain medical asepsis by using good handwashing technique and wearing gloves according to Standard and Transmission-Based Precautions.
2. Identify the patient and explain the procedure.
3. Remove the pillow and extra linens that might prevent easy movement.
4. Lower the head of the bed to a flat position.

Continued

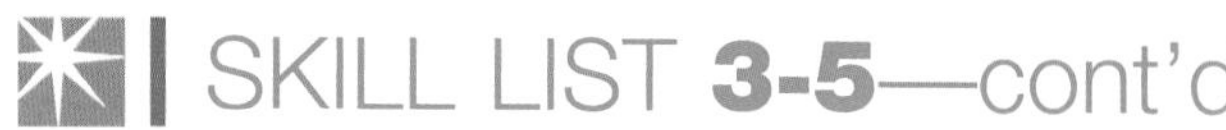

SKILL LIST 3-5—cont'd
Moving the Patient up in Bed

5. Lower the side rail on the near side.
6. Lower or raise the bed to a comfortable working height so that the back may be kept straight.
7. Place one arm under the patient's axilla and the other arm across the patient's back to guide the patient toward the top of the bed.
8. Allow the patient to assist, if possible, by bending the knees and pushing into the bed to lift the weight of the buttocks.
9. Glide the patient toward the top of the bed. Repeat if necessary.
10. Reposition the patient for comfort and safety. Raise the side rails.
11. Replace the pillow and call bell.
12. Practice good medical asepsis by washing the hands before leaving the area.

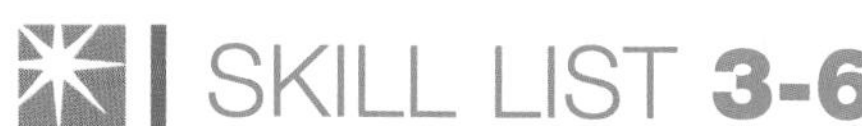

SKILL LIST 3-6
Turning the Patient to the Side

1. Maintain medical asepsis by using good hand-washing technique and wearing gloves according to Standard and Transmission-Based Precautions.
2. Identify the patient and explain the procedure.
3. Remove the pillow and extra linens that might prevent easy movement.
4. Lower the head of the bed to a flat position.
5. Lower the side rail on the near side.
6. Lower or raise the bed to a comfortable working height so that the back can be kept straight.
7. Place two arms under the patient's neck and back, and slide the upper torso toward the near edge of the bed.
8. Place two arms under the patient's back and upper legs, and slide the hips toward the near edge of the bed.
9. Place two arms under the patient's legs, and slide them into alignment with the head and hips.
10. Position the far arm above the patient's head.
11. Cross the patient's ankles.
12. Roll the patient onto one side toward the far edge of the bed.
13. Support the patient's back and cushion areas of pressure with pillows or linens.
14. Raise the side rail.
15. Replace the pillow and call bell.
16. Practice good medical asepsis by washing the hands before leaving the area.

SKILL LIST 3-7
Transferring the Patient from the Bed to a Chair

1. Maintain medical asepsis by using good hand-washing technique and wearing gloves according to Standard and Transmission-Based Precautions.
2. Identify the patient and explain the procedure.
3. Place the chair or wheelchair next to the head of the bed with brakes on.
4. Remove the pillow and extra linens that might prevent easy movement.
5. Lower the head of the bed to a flat position.

Continued

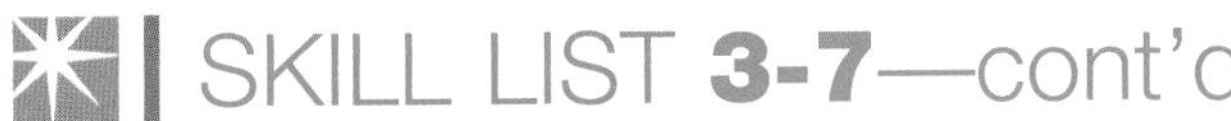

SKILL LIST 3-7—cont'd
Transferring the Patient from the Bed to a Chair

6. Lower the side rail on the near side.
7. Lower or raise the bed to a comfortable working height so that the back can be kept straight.
8. Place two arms under the patient's neck and back, and slide the upper torso toward the near edge of the bed.
9. Place two arms under the patient's back and upper legs, and slide the hips toward the near edge of the bed.
10. Place two arms under the patient's legs, and slide them into alignment with the head and hips.
11. Raise the head of the bed to a 45-degree angle.
12. Place one arm on the patient's back and one under the patient's knees.
13. Pivot the patient to a sitting position.
14. Face the patient while assisting him or her to stand.
15. When the patient feels steady, pivot him or her to the wheelchair.
16. If necessary, move the patient back in the wheelchair by placing an arm under each of the patient's axillae from the back of the chair and lifting him or her up and back.
17. Adjust the footrests and place the safety belt on the patient.
18. Practice good medical asepsis by washing the hands before leaving the area.

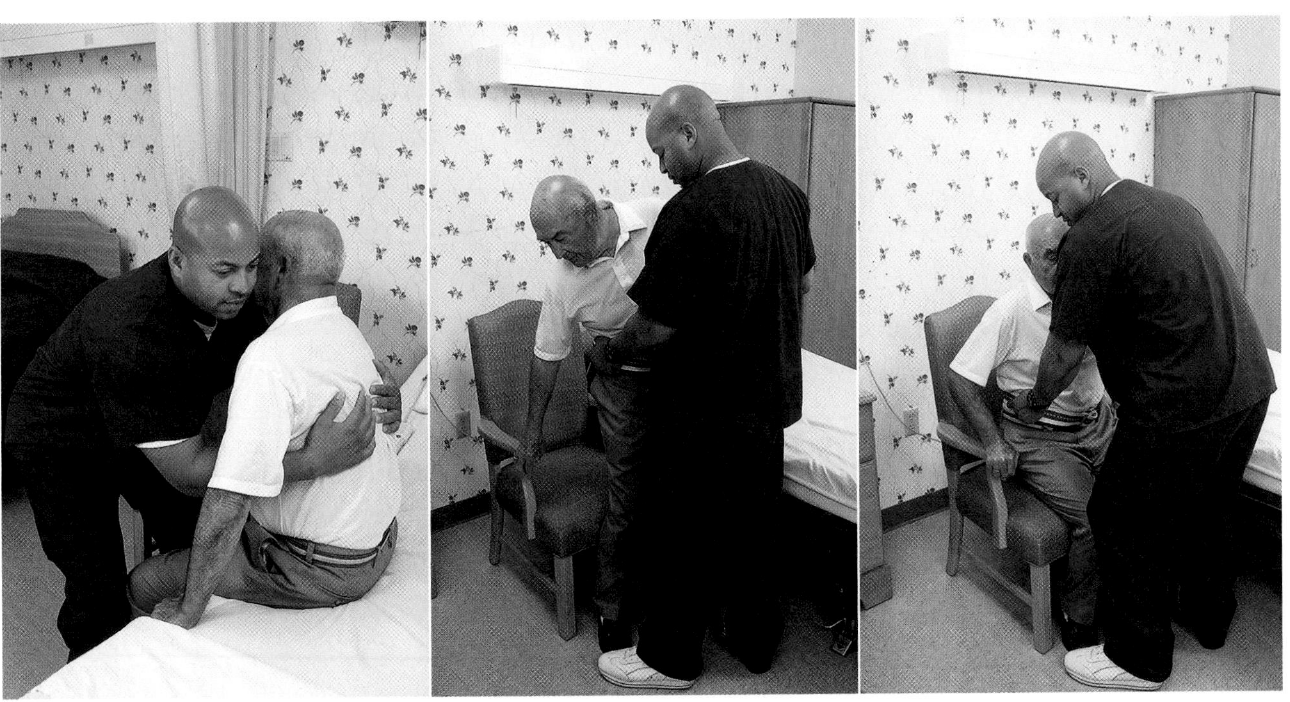

CHAPTER 4

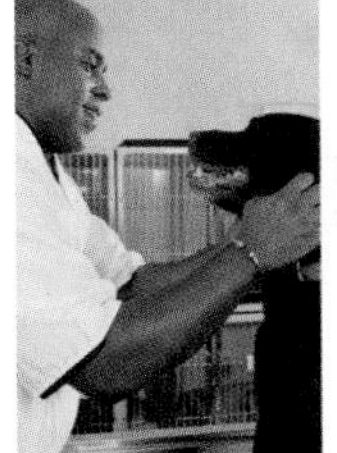
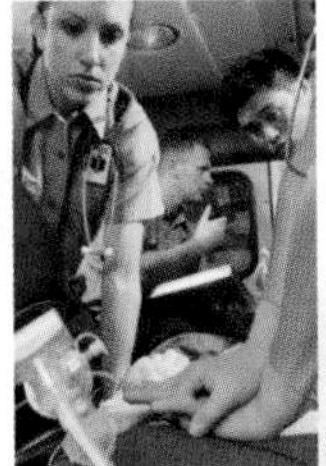
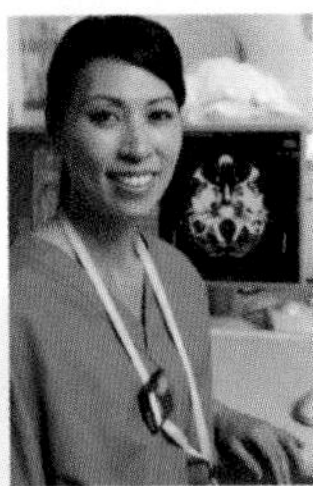

Legal and Ethical Principles

LEARNING OBJECTIVES

- Define at least 10 terms relating to legal and ethical principles.
- Describe at least five examples of ethical behavior for the health care worker.
- Identify at least five situations that show improper ethical or legal behavior.
- Explain the importance of confidentiality in health care, including privacy issues resulting from advanced technology.
- Describe at least two examples of rights of the health care patient.
- Describe the role of the health care worker regarding current legal issues, including advanced directives and telemedicine.

KEY TERMS

Confidential *(kahn-fuh-DEN-chel)* Private or secret

Ethics *(ETH-iks)* Dealing with what is good or bad, determining moral duty and obligation

Informatics *(in-fer-MAT-iks)* Study of information processing, computer science

Informed consent *(in-FORMD kuhn-SENT)* Agreement to surgical or medical treatment with knowledge of the facts and risks involved

Jurisprudent *(jur-is-PROOD-ent)* Understanding the science or philosophy of law

Legal *(LEE-gul)* Deriving authority from or founded on law

Liable *(LIE-uh-bul)* Legally responsible

Libel *(LIE-bul)* Communicating something untruthful and harmful about another person in writing

Malpractice *(mal-PRAK-tiss)* Failure of professional skill or learning that results in injury, loss, or damage

Moral *(MORE-ul)* Relating to principles of right and wrong

Negligence *(NEG-li-jens)* Failure to execute the care that a reasonable (prudent) person exercises

KEY TERMS cont'd

Slander *(SLAN-der)* Verbally communicating something untruthful and harmful about another person

Telehealth *(TEL-uh-helth)* Use of technology to deliver health-related services and information, including telemedicine

Telemedicine *(TEL-uh-med-uh-sin)* Use of telecommunications technology to provide, improve, or make health care services faster

Legal and Ethical Terminology

Which Term Best Fits with this Example?
Wanda Roberts was run over by a truck in 1992. After 6 weeks of treatment at a hospital, she was transferred to another facility. In *Roberts v. Galen* (1999), the U.S. Supreme Court considered her claim of "patient dumping." This practice was described as moving a patient without insurance to a publicly funded facility for care regardless of condition.

Term	Definition
Abandonment	Neglecting a patient or client under and in need of immediate professional care, without making reasonable arrangements for the continuation of such care
Assault	A threat or an attempt to injure another person in an illegal manner
Battery	Unlawful touching of another person without consent, with or without injury
Breach	Breaking the law, an obligation, or the terms of a contract
Civil law	Defines the legal relationships between individuals
Common law	Unwritten law; customs that may have authority or have been established by prior court decisions

Professional Codes of Conduct

Ethical and legal responsibilities are a central part of all health care occupations. The worker must understand and follow ethical practices, including respect for cultural, social, and ethnic differences of the patients and other workers. Legal responsibilities include practicing within the guidelines of laws, policies, and regulations established for each type of employment (Box 4-1).

BOX 4-1

Legal Issues in Health Care

- Abuse
- Fraud
- Insurance/managed care
- Medical records privacy
- Medicare/Medicaid
- Patient care bioethics

Health care workers must stay within a "scope of practice" or use the methods and procedures in which they are trained (Table 4-1). The Nurse Practice Acts (NPAs) are state laws that determine which tasks nurses may legally perform. Some common laws or traditional practices also influence nursing practice. Performing skills or tasks that are outside the health care worker's scope of practice is illegal as well as unethical. The health care worker who is supervising others may delegate some tasks. For example, the registered nurse or licensed physician may ask a licensed practical nurse to assess the patient's health by collecting, reporting, and charting data. The licensed practical nurse does not work independently. The nurse assistant works under the supervision of the registered nurse or licensed practical nurse (Fig. 4-1). The medical assistant works under the supervision of a licensed physician. The dental assistant works under the supervision of a licensed dentist. Dental hygienists may practice without the supervision of a dentist in some states.

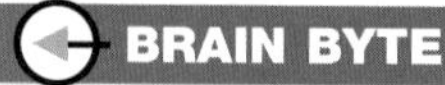

In some cases nurse assistants may assist a patient with medication in a home setting, but not in a hospital.

TABLE 4-1
Sample Scope of Practice

	Registered Nurse	Licensed Practical Nurse	Nursing Assistant
Assessment	Functions on own to: Assess and evaluate patients Collect objective and subjective data Analyze, report, and record data Update data	When directed by the registered nurse or physician, functions to: Contribute to assessment of patient Collect, report, and record data Observe condition of patient Recognize signs and symptoms that are not normal	When directed by the registered nurse or licensed practical nurse, functions to: Collect, report, and record basic data Recognize signs and symptoms that are not normal

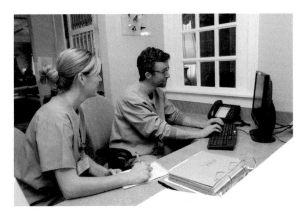

FIGURE 4-1 The nursing assistant may use handwritten notes to report to the supervising nurse to be charted electronically. (From Sorrentino SA: *Mosby's textbook for nursing assistants,* ed 7, St. Louis, 2008, Mosby.)

Health care has become an industry that involves many complex professions and technologies. The health care worker must make legal and ethical decisions daily. **Ethics** are the principles and values that determine appropriate behavior. An individual, community, or society adopts moral standards that distinguish right from wrong. **Morals** are based on the experience, religion, and philosophy of the individual and the society. The basis of ethical behavior in the health care field is the respect for the needs and rights of others.

CASE STUDY 4-1 You enter a room and find the patient is gone. You look all over the floor and then alert the rest of the staff of the absence. As you are contacting security, the patient reappears and states she had gone to the chapel. What should you do?

Answers to Case Studies are available on the Evolve website: ***http://evolve.elsevier.com/Gerdin***

Ethical codes are guidelines for the actions of people in a profession. They are established by the professionals to whom they apply, and they may not be legally binding. What is ethical in one society or profession might not apply to another and may change over time. In most health care professions, the rules of ethics are preserved in an oath or code of standards. Physicians established the first code of ethics for a profession. Lawyers followed them. The third and fourth professions to establish codes were pharmacists and veterinarians.

Ethical standards apply to relationships with fellow workers, patients, and the community. These are based on individual morals and society's expectations. Some ethical standards are the same for all health occupations (Box 4-2). Each profession may have an oath or pledge that states the basic beliefs and goals of the group (Box 4-3).

The health care worker must be **jurisprudent**, or aware of the laws that influence the industry. Workers in all occupations are legally responsible (**liable**) for their behavior and the care given. The employer also may be liable for the actions of the worker that are not reasonably prudent (**negligent**) or that reflect bad practice (**malpractice**). **Slander** means to communicate verbally something that is untrue and harmful about another person, and **libel** means to put it in writing. Inadequate charting is the cause of many incidences of liability for the health care worker. Another common concern is the violation of a patient trust that could result in invasion of privacy or illegal restraint.

Hospitals and other health care facilities may have an institutional or internal review board that meets to oversee the agency's guidelines for ethical conduct. The board also may decide issues relating to a worker's conduct, responsibility, and scope of practice when necessary. Many health care occupations

BOX 4-2

Code of Ethics

- The primary goals of the health care worker are to promote an optimal level of wellness, preserve life, and provide for a peaceful death when necessary.
- The health care worker respects the religious beliefs and cultural values of all patients.
- The health care worker provides adequate and continuous care for all patients regardless of age, gender, race, or nature of the illness or injury.
- The health care worker knows the limits of practice for which he or she is competent and stays within those limits.
- The health care worker maintains competence and current knowledge by pursuing continuing education.
- The health care worker practices jurisprudent behavior at all times by avoiding unethical or illegal practices.
- The health care worker respects the dignity and rights of each patient by maintaining confidentiality and a professional attitude regarding all information relating to the patient.
- The health care worker asks for clarification and assistance when unsure of any aspect of care.
- The health care worker participates in professional activities and organizations to provide better health care.
- The health care worker maintains a high standard of ethical and legal behavior in his or her private and professional life.

are regulated by state agencies. Some workers hold a license that determines which actions may be performed. Licensed professionals are legally responsible for their actions when performing as employees or in their own practice.

Malpractice and Liability

Health care workers are legally responsible or liable for the care that is given to their patients. There are several types of law that apply to health care. The health care worker is accountable for all of them (Table 4-2).

Legal and Ethical Terminology

Which Term Best Fits with this Example?

In *Hunter v. Mann* (1974), a doctor treated a man and a girl for injuries from a traffic accident. The doctor refused to disclose their identity to the police who were looking for a man and girl who had earlier run away from an accident.

Term	Definition
Conduct	Behavior or a person's actions
Consent	Permission granted by a person voluntarily and in sound mind; written consent is most easily proved
Crime	Performing an act that is forbidden or omitting a duty required by public law, making the offender liable for the action
Criminal law	Defines the legal obligation between an individual and the state or society
Custom	An accepted behavior or common practice
Duty of care	By law, health care workers must perform services in a manner that meets common standards of practice
Ethics	Standards of behavior and practice that are established by a professional organization for its members

The scope of duties that may be legally performed by a health care worker depends on the level of training and education of the worker. Some functions, such as giving medications, are regulated by laws and require a license. The health care worker must understand the limits or scope of his or her practice. A written job description helps define the scope of practice for a job.

CASE STUDY 4-2 You are working on a floor that is very busy. A nurse asks you to change an intravenous (IV) bag for a patient because she has to give medications in another room. You have never changed an IV bag, although you have seen it done many times. What should you do?

Answers to Case Studies are available on the Evolve website: ***http://evolve.elsevier.com/Gerdin***

TABLE 4-2
Types of Law Affecting Health Care

Type of Law	Description	Examples
Administrative	Enforce statutory law, code-regulating bureaucracies	OSHA, NPA
Civil	Dispute between individuals	Assault, false imprisonment (restraint)
Common	Decisions made by judges, based on earlier court decisions	Protect disoriented patient, exemptions from immunizations
Constitutional	Supreme law of the land	Freedom of speech
Criminal (penal)	Legal punishment for public concerns (Common or statutory) (Local, state, or federal) (Felony or misdemeanor)	Falsification of patient records, fraud, theft
Statutory	Rules passed by government (local, state, or federal)	DRG law, NPA

DRG, diagnosis-related grouping; OSHA, Occupational Safety and Health Administration. NPA, Nurse Practice Act.

BOX 4-3

Nightingale Pledge

I solemnly pledge myself before God, and in the presence of this assembly, to pass my life in purity and to practice my profession faithfully.

I will abstain from whatever is deleterious and mischievous and will not take or knowingly administer any harmful drug.

I will do all in my power to maintain and elevate the standard of my profession, and will hold in confidence all personal matters committed to my keeping and all family affairs coming to my knowledge in the practice of my profession.

With loyalty I will endeavor to aid the physician in his work and devote myself to the welfare of those committed to my care.

Performing skills that are beyond the level of health care worker's education and training is considered malpractice. Neglecting to do something that is considered common practice, such as leaving the patient in an unsafe situation, is also malpractice. Malpractice or liability insurance may be purchased by the health care worker for financial protection in the event that a patient questions the quality or scope of care. The cost of the insurance varies with the level of responsibility of the position and may be included as part of the worker's compensation or benefit package.

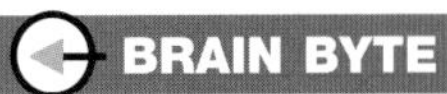

In some specialties, such as obstetrics, up to 50% of the cost of medical services goes to pay the physician's malpractice insurance cost.

Confidentiality

Information regarding the patient in health care is considered **confidential**, or private. The health care worker is ethically and legally responsible for maintaining the patient's privacy. The health care worker must share information regarding the patient with only the appropriate personnel involved in the care. Confidentiality is important so that the patient may tell the health care worker personal information related to health without fear of it being shared with someone who is not involved in the patient's health care.

CASE STUDY 4-3 You are eating lunch in the cafeteria and a co-worker joins you. The co-worker begins talking about one of the patients for whom you both provide care. What should you do?

Answers to Case Studies are available on the Evolve website: *http://evolve.elsevier.com/Gerdin*

Legal and Ethical Terminology

Which Term Best Fits with this Example?
In 1998 the Washington King County Medical Examiner's Office donated parts of Bradley Gierlich's brain to a research institute investigating bipolar and schizophrenic disorders. Although he did not leave a will, the sister of Mr. Gierlich stated that he did not want his body parts donated.

Term	Definition
Felony	A serious crime for which the penalty is imprisonment for more than 1 year
Ideal	Standard of perfection or excellence
Illegal restraint	Holding or detaining a person against his or her will
Invasion of privacy	Unlawfully making known to the public any private or personal information without the consent of the wronged person
Liable	Legally responsible for own actions
Libel	Communicating something untruthful and harmful about another person in writing

BOX 4-4

HIPAA Patient Protections

- Access to medical records includes the ability to see and obtain copies.
- Notice of privacy practices must be provided to patients by the provider.
- Limits on use of personal medical information allow only for information to be shared with others for treatment purposes.
- Prohibition on marketing requires specific authorization by the patient for release of information for marketing purposes.
- Stronger state laws are not affected.
- Confidential information directed to a specific phone or person.
- Complaints may be filed with the provider and the Office for Civil Rights.

In 1996 Congress passed the Health Insurance Portability and Accountability Act (HIPAA) to try to reduce the administrative cost of health care and ensure the ability of the patient to change insurance plans, even with preexisting conditions. HIPAA Privacy Rules were issued in 2000. They standardize and protect individually identifiable health information that might be accessible through use of electronic technology. HIPAA requires that only authorized workers may see health care information. For example, a direct health care provider may be allowed to see health information but not billing information. In April 2003 standards for the "Privacy of Individually Identifiable Health Information" went into effect (Box 4-4).

Protected health information (PHI) includes any individually identifiable health information that is transmitted or maintained in any way. This includes electronic, written, and verbal communication (Fig. 4-2). The rule applies to all agencies sharing or transmitting personal health information, whether it is paper, oral, or electronic. It covers people who are insured privately or those covered by public programs or who are uninsured. The standards protect medical records and personal health information. Life insurance and workers' compensation programs are not covered by the regulations. These providers are allowed to use and reuse patient information without prior consent. An exception to the patient's right to privacy is when there is imminent danger to another

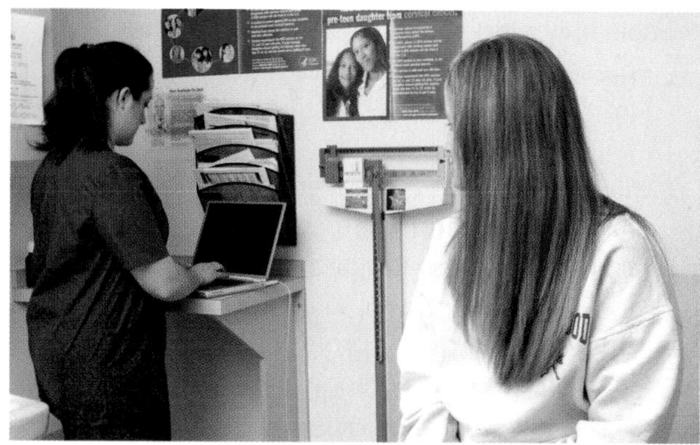

FIGURE 4-2 Electronic documentation is rapidly becoming available for use by all health care workers. This medical assistant is entering a patient's symptoms into an electronic medical record program using a computer. (From Bonewit-West K, Hunt S, Applegate E: *Today's medical assistant: clinical and administrative procedures*, St. Louis, 2009, Saunders.)

BOX 4-5

Examples of HIPAA Complaints*

- Covered entity refused to note a patient's request to correct the patient's medical record or did not provide complete access to a patient's medical records to that patient.
- Covered entity used health information for marketing purposes without first obtaining the individual's permission.
- Medical workers accessed hospital records of a famous person or public figure.
- Patient information was visible to anyone on provider's appointment-scheduling website.
- Patient's laboratory test results were faxed to the newspaper instead of to the hospital.
- Pharmacy allowed workers with different roles to use the same login ID and password.

*A "covered entity" is a health care provider, clearinghouse (such as a billing service), or health plan.

individual that can be foreseen by the practitioner. This "duty to warn" requires the health care practitioner to disclose the patient's relevant personal health information when such a threat exists.

The U.S. Department of Health and Human Services (HHS) Office for Civil Rights (OCR) is responsible for oversight and enforcement of HIPAA privacy regulations. The OCR may impose penalties on health care entities (workers or organizations) up to $100 per violation or $25,000 per year. Criminal penalties can be up to $250,000 and 10 years in prison if the PHI is sold, transferred, or used commercially, for personal gain, or for malicious harm. Box 4-5 lists some examples of violations of HIPAA. More information regarding HIPAA may be found in Chapters 1 and 2.

Legal and Ethical Terminology

Which Term Best Fits with this Example?
Cynthia Collins made several visits to the Cook County Hospital and clinic between 1986 and 1987. At that time, a nurse felt a lump on Ms. Collins's breast. After further evaluation, Ms. Collins was instructed to return in 3 months, which she did not do. Later in 1987, Ms. Collins was treated for abdominal cramps, vaginal discharge, and pain. In 1988 Ms. Collins was diagnosed with breast cancer that had spread to her neck and arm. She died of breast cancer in 1989. Ms. Collins's estate sued Cook County hospital (and the health care personnel).

Term	Definition
Licensure	Authorization by the state to perform the functions of an occupation for which educational and examination standards are specified
Litigation	A lawsuit or legal action
Malpractice	Bad or harmful practice that injures another person
Misdemeanors	Crimes that are less serious than felonies and result in imprisonment for less than 1 year
Negligence	Failure to perform duties in a reasonable and customary way
Privileged communication	Personal or private information relating to the care given by health care personnel
Reasonable care	Services given in a manner appropriate to the level of education and experience of the health care worker

Patient Rights

In 1998 the Advisory Commission on Consumer Protection and Quality in the Health Care Industry issued a report designed to protect consumers. The report had three goals and listed specific rights and responsibilities for the patient (Box 4-6). The report stated that consumers of health care have the right and responsibility to participate or have a representative in making treatment decisions. The patient is responsible for maintaining healthy habits and working with health care providers in treatment plans. The patient is also responsible for communicating honestly and showing respect for health care providers. The health care consumer is also responsible for making a "good-faith" effort to pay for care and follow the procedures of the health care plan.

BOX 4-6

Consumer's Bill of Rights and Responsibilities

Objectives

- Provide the consumer of health care with ways to address concerns and participate in their health, leading to greater confidence in the health care system
- Support a strong relationship between health care professionals and patients
- Establish rights and responsibilities for all participants in heath care

Patient's Bill of Rights

- Information disclosure
- Choice of providers and plans
- Access to emergency services
- Participation in treatment decisions
- Respect and nondiscrimination
- Confidentiality of health information
- Complaints and appeals

Modified from Consumer Protection and Quality in the Health Care Industry, Appendix A, http://www.hcqualitycommission.gov/final/append_a.html, July 1998.

The American Hospital Association (AHA) adopted a Patient's Bill of Rights in 1973 and revised it in 1992. In addition to the rights described by the Advisory Commission Report and the AHA, the patient also has the rights of any citizen of the United States and the state. Some of these rights include confidentiality and personal privacy. All patients must be given quality care without mistreatment, neglect, or abuse. The patient also has the right to voice grievances without fear of retaliation. The patient's personal possessions must be cared for and secured while care is being given. Chapter 1 provides more information regarding the rights of patients and extended-care facility residents.

CASE STUDY 4-4 You change a patient's bed, remove the sheets, and give personal care. When finished you cannot find the patient's dentures. The patient informs you they were on the bed. What should you do?

Answers to Case Studies are available on the Evolve website: ***http://evolve.elsevier.com/Gerdin***

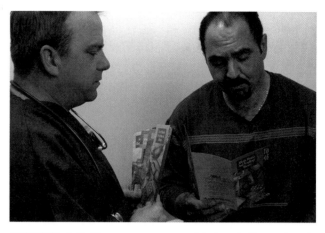

FIGURE 4-3 The nurse may need to teach the patient in order to obtain an informed consent. (From Hunt SA: *Saunders fundamentals of medical assisting,* St. Louis, 2007, Saunders.)

Informed Consent

Informed consent to a medical or surgical procedure means that the risks and medical information involved have been fully explained to the patient (Fig. 4-3). The patient has both the legal and ethical right to make decisions about what is done to his or her body. The health care facility determines which procedures and treatments require written consent, but the health care worker should ask permission (consent) before completing even simple tasks such as assessment of vital signs. Exceptions to informed consent laws may be made in emergencies, when the patient is not mentally competent, and for minors (decisions may be made by family or a medical representative). For example, a qualified health care provider does not need informed consent to provide first aid or perform cardiopulmonary resuscitation (CPR) on an unresponsive patient.

Informed consent includes the following elements:

- Description of the treatment or procedure (purpose and nature)
- Description of alternatives that are available (regardless of cost or insurance coverage)
- Risks, benefits, and unknown factors of each alternative
- Risks, benefits, and unknown factors of not receiving treatment
- Patient questions
- Assessment of the patient understanding
- Agreement by the patient for the treatment or procedure

Legal and Ethical Terminology

Which Term Best Fits with this Example?
In 1982 Caroline Eli worked at the Griggs County Hospital and Nursing Home as a nurse's aide. During her afternoon break in the dining room, she made offensive and derogatory remarks about her supervisor and Griggs. The residents and visitors were offended by her remarks. Ms. Eli's employment was terminated. She sued for reinstatement, back pay, and damages.

Term	Definition
Slander	Verbally communicating something untruthful and harmful about another person
Statutory law	Law established by the legislative branch of government that determines what is legal
Tort	Civil wrong
Unethical	Action that does not represent ideal behavior but might not be illegal
Value system	Ideals and thoughts that determine what is considered worthwhile or meaningful, right or wrong
Will	Written document that allows a person to distribute property after death

BOX 4-7

Elements of the Advanced Directive

I. Health Care Agent
This section designates a person to make medical decisions if the patient is unable to do so independently. This person is given a durable power of attorney for the health care of the patient. It may also include a second person in case the first is unavailable.

II. Treatment Preferences: Living Will
This section indicates what type of care is important to the patient in a life-threatening condition. For example, the patient may prefer to be pain free or to be able to recognize relatives.

If the condition is terminal, the patient may want artificial nutrition and hydration or not. The person may want life-sustaining measures such as CPR started or stopped in certain circumstances.

In the case of a persistent vegetative state or end-stage conditions such as Alzheimer disease, the patient may make the decision for CPR, nutrition, and hydration in another manner. The patient may designate someone to be a guardian if necessary.

III. Organ Donation
The patient may wish to donate part, all, or no tissues or organs.

IV. Autopsy
The patient may refuse or allow an autopsy.

V. Signatures
The signatures include the patient and witnesses who are not relatives, health care workers, or named in the will.

Legal Directives

Advanced directives and living wills are legal documents that allow patients to express their wishes about their health care and treatment. Parts of advanced directives include the living will, power of attorney (health care proxy), the do-not-resuscitate (DNR) order, and organ donor cards. Advanced directives vary from state to state but have similar components (Box 4-7). An advanced directive takes effect only when a patient loses the ability to make his or her own decisions.

A living will allows a person to state in advance which life-support procedures to use if the person is terminally ill or permanently unconscious. A durable power of attorney for health care allows another person or agent to make medical decisions if the patient is unable. The person does not need to be terminally ill or permanently unconscious for the durable power of attorney to take effect. Advanced directives do not necessarily mean "that a patient is not to be resuscitated." DNR orders are written by doctors to indicate that the patient is not to be resuscitated or revived after a cardiac arrest. The health care worker is responsible for knowing about and respecting the patient's legal directives.

Allowing organ donation may be part of the advanced directive. Regulation of organ donation is controlled by each state within the limits of the 1968 National Organ Transplant Act. In the United States, donation of organs requires an affirmative or positive statement. Although this "affirmative statement" may be included on the driver's license or in a living will, relatives can still prevent organ donation.

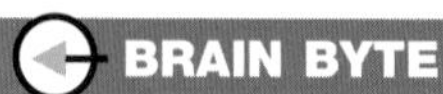

BRAIN BYTE

In most states, the Good Samaritan Act protects you from liability for emergency care within the limits of first aid.

Health Care and the Internet

Use of the Internet to access health care information and products has introduced a new set of issues and concerns. Patients can find information, join chat groups, purchase drugs and other medical items, and consult a health care practitioner online. **Informatics** is the term used to describe the development and use of information technology. Clear legal jurisdiction for health care that is provided over the Internet does not exist because it may cross state or even country boundaries. In the fall of 2000, the Joint Commission on Accreditation of Healthcare Organizations (now referred to as The Joint Commission) adopted new credentialing standards for hospitals that are using telemedicine.

Telehealth, which includes **telemedicine**, began in the 1960s when physicians provided health care treatment by phone to patients living in remote locations. Telehealth is a broader term than telemedicine and includes prevention, promotion and cure. Examples of current uses of telehealth include remote patient monitoring (electrocardiography, lung capacity), patient consultation via videoconference, transmission of images for diagnosis, and robotic surgery (telesurgery).

Documentation

Records of health care (charting) must be precise, clear, and concise to record the activities of care. The chart is the main technique used for health care workers to communicate about the patient's care. The chart is the written documentation that serves as the legal record of the care given to the patient. It is divided into sections according to the service being provided for easy reference. Policies of the facility determine who records each type of treatment and the acceptable method for charting. Two general guidelines for good charting include charting only for oneself and not for another person and keeping any information contained in the chart confidential.

Reporting (telling) and recording (charting) observations and vital or life signs are the methods by which communication about the patient's status is made. Accurate and timely communication is necessary to ensure the best care possible. Abnormal vital signs should be reported immediately to the appropriate supervising personnel. Vital signs are recorded on graphic sheets and flow sheets (see Appendix II, Fig. II-2 *A-C*, pp. 584–586). The handwriting on graphic sheets must be easy to read, and the information must be accurate. Information should be written on paper soon after the assessment is made so that it is not forgotten. Documentation also may be entered directly into a computer, providing rapid information access. Patient information in a digital form is called the electronic health record (EHR) or electronic medical record (EMR). The use of electronic records may provide a more efficient system and prevent duplication of services.

BRAIN BYTE

For legal purposes, if care is not recorded, it has not been done. In charting by exception, only changes in a patient's condition or abnormal findings are recorded.

Summary

- Six examples of ethical behavior are to promote wellness, preserve life, provide adequate and continuous care for all patients, know and do not exceed the limits of practice, maintain competence by continuing education, and practice jurisprudence.
- Five situations that show improper ethical or legal behavior include disrespecting a patient's religion, assault, libel, slander, and malpractice.
- Confidentiality in health care is important to ensure that the patient will share personal information regarding health without fear of it being told to someone not involved in health care.
- Two examples of rights of the health care patient are the right to voice grievances and the right to security of personal possessions.

- The role of the health care worker regarding legal issues such as advanced directives is to be aware of and respect them.

Review Questions

1. List two examples of patient's rights based on all citizens' rights.
2. Describe three elements or parts of an advanced directive.
3. Describe the role of the health care worker with advanced directives.
4. Use the following terms in one or more sentences that demonstrate their relationship to each other: legal, malpractice, and negligent.
5. Use the following terms in one or more sentences that demonstrate their relationship to each other: ethics and moral.
6. Use the following terms in one or more sentences that demonstrate their relationship to each other: libel and slander.

Critical Thinking

1. Investigate the code of conduct or rules of ethics for a health care profession.
2. Explain why each of the following is a legal or ethical consideration of health care.
   a. The patient is restrained in a wheelchair without a physician's order.
   b. The patient requests to attend church services in the hospital chapel and is permitted to go.
   c. The health care worker charts that the patient is "an old battle-ax."
   d. The health care worker does not change the linen for two patients as assigned.
   e. The health care worker eats leftovers from a patient's dinner tray.
   f. The patient requests a room change to a non-smoking area.
3. Describe the importance of confidentiality in health care.
4. Investigate the extent of use of computers for documentation in a local health care facility.
5. Investigate one of the five court cases described in the Legal and Ethical Terminology boxes. Write a paragraph that completely describes the participants of the lawsuit, the charges of the plaintiff, and the outcome of the dispute.
6. Use the HHS website to find a local informatics project. Describe the project in a paragraph.
7. Use the Internet to prepare an effective oral presentation describing an example of breech of confidentiality and its consequences.
8. Use the Internet to compare the professional code of ethics and scope of practice of two health care occupations.

Explore the Web

Research/News

WebMD

http://webMD.com

Telemedicine

Search Terms: nurse abandonment patient

Informatics

HHS Projects – AHRQ-Funded Projects

http://healthit.ahrq.gov

Case Studies

Search Terms: malpractice case studies

STANDARDS AND ACCOUNTABILITY*

Foundation Standard 5: Legal Responsibilities

Healthcare professionals will understand the legal responsibilities, limitations, and implications of their actions within the health care delivery setting. They will perform their duties according to regulations, policies, laws, and legislated rights of clients.

Accountability Criteria

5.1 Legal Implications

5.11 Analyze legal responsibilities.

5.12 Apply procedures for accurate documentation and record keeping.

Continued

STANDARDS AND ACCOUNTABILITY—cont'd

5.2 Legal Practices

5.21 Apply standards for Health Insurance Portability and Accountability Act (HIPAA).

5.22 Describe advance directives.

5.23 Summarize the Patient's Bill of Rights.

5.24 Understand informed consent.

5.25 Explain laws governing harassment, labor, and scope of practice.

Foundation Standard 6: Ethics

Healthcare professionals will understand accepted ethical practices with respect to cultural, social, and ethnic differences within the healthcare environment. They will perform quality healthcare delivery.

Accountability Criteria

6.1 Ethical Boundaries

6.11 Differentiate between ethical and legal issues impacting healthcare.

6.12 Recognize ethical issues and their implications related to healthcare.

6.2 Ethical Practice

6.21 Apply procedures for reporting activities and behaviors that affect the health, safety, and welfare of others.

6.3 Cultural, Social, and Ethnic Diversity

6.31 Understand religious and cultural values as they impact healthcare.

6.32 Demonstrate respectful and empathetic treatment of all patients/clients (customer service).

*From the National Consortium for Health Science Education (2009). National Health Care Standards and Accountability Criteria. Available at http://www.healthscienceconsortium.org.

CHAPTER 5

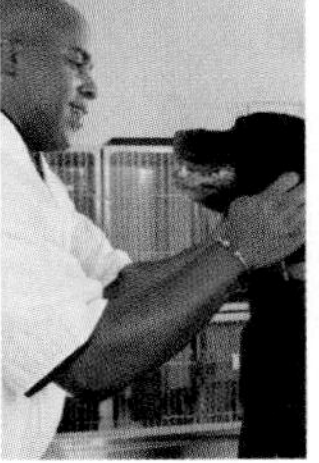

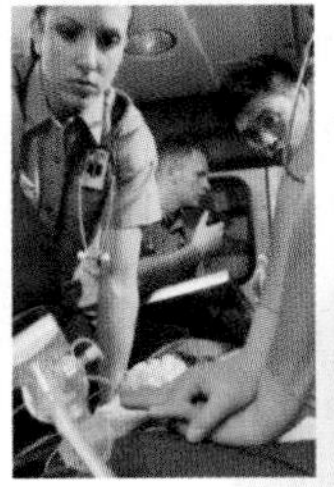

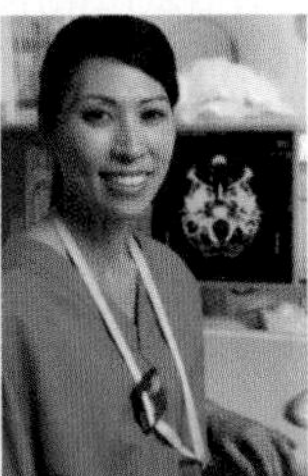

Culture and Health Care*

LEARNING OBJECTIVES

- Spell and define the key terms.
- Discuss eight specific examples of how cultural differences affect patient care.
- Describe five signs that may indicate a potential cultural barrier exists.
- List seven actions that can overcome cultural obstacles.
- List at least three culturally sensitive questions for patient care. Explain why each might be sensitive to a patient's culture.
- Describe at least five guidelines to follow when using an interpreter.

KEY TERMS

Acculturation *(uh-KUL-chir-AY-shun)* The process of learning cultural behaviors from one group or person

Assimilation *(uh-sim-uh-LEY-shun)* The merging of cultural traits from different cultural groups

Culture *(KUL-chir)* The act of belonging to a designated group

Cultural competence *(KUL-chir-uhl COM-puh-tense)* The ability to meet the health care needs of patients while meeting and adhering to their cultural values, beliefs, and practices

Emotive *(i-MOH-tiv)* Expressing or exciting emotion

Ethnocentrism *(eth-no-SEN-triz-uhm)* The belief that one's own culture is superior to another

Ethnography *(eth-NAH-gruh-fhee)* A branch of anthropology that studies and records various human culture

Matriarchal *(MEY-tree-ahrk-el)* Society or group with a female as head of the family or tribal line

Stereotype *(STER-ee-uh-tahyp)* Simplified image used to characterize or describe a group

Stoic *(STOH-ik)* Free from passion, without complaint

---

*We would like to acknowledge Elizabeth Molle, RN, MS, Nurse Educator, Middletown, Conn., who initially wrote this chapter in the fourth edition.

Cultural Overview

The United States is rich with cultures, ethnic customs, and traditions. The patient's culture plays a large role in his or her health. The health care worker's own cultural background will also affect health care career choices. The importance of cultural values and connections cannot be underestimated.

Culture is the act of belonging to a designated group. It comes from the Latin word *colo*, which means "to cultivate." Culture refers to the norms and practices of a particular group that are learned, shared, and transcended through generations. They guide our thinking, decision making, and actions. Although culture fills a large part of our lives, its effect is unconscious. The actions are usually subtle, and thus most people are unaware of them. Culture provides security and reassurance. All humans have a great need to feel connected and bonded with other people. When bonds are weak and we do not feel connected or safe, it affects our health and wellness.

Culture is not biologically inherited. It is learned behaviors transmitted from generation to generation by family members and close friends (Fig. 5-1). These behaviors can be reinforced through social, religious, and school activities. The process of learning the behaviors occurs by osmosis. In other words, the behaviors become absorbed through repetition and positive reinforcement. Parents offer praise to their child when they demonstrate appropriate behavior.

Culture is reflected in many aspects of our lives. No aspect of our lives is free from cultural input. Our culture is expressed daily in the following:

- Eating habits
- Language
- Dress
- Hobbies
- Living patterns
- Occupation choices
- Education
- Religious affiliations
- Political points

It also affects our interpersonal relationships, including marriages, communication patterns, and sexual habits.

Acculturation

When people with different cultural backgrounds meet, learning and growth occur. **Acculturation** is the process of learning cultural behaviors from one group or person. It is an unconscious fusion of attitudes and beliefs. This does not occur quickly; rather, it occurs over years. Because the United States is a melting pot of many different cultures, acculturation is always occurring. Each cultural group contains many subcultures, which can be as broad and varied as the whole group. The U.S. Census Bureau collects data every 10 years about the population in the United States. Besides population statistics, the bureau also collects

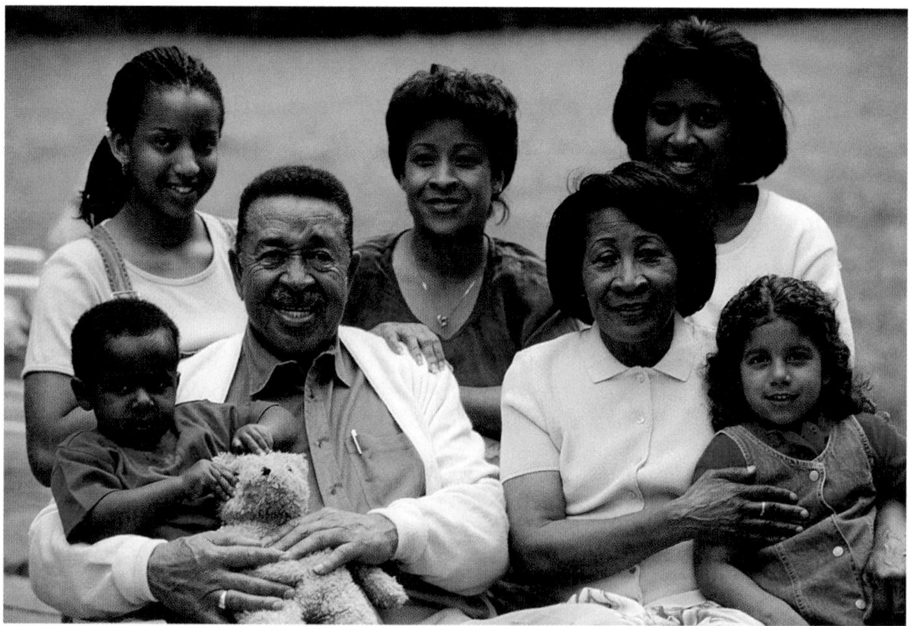

FIGURE 5-1 Culture comprises learned behaviors passed from generation to generation.

TABLE 5-1
Ethnic Groups in the United States

Ethnic Group	Description	% of U.S. Population*
White or Anglo-American	Refers to Western European countries such as England, France, Ireland, and Germany.	75.0
Hispanic or Latino (of any race)	Refers to Puerto Rico, Cuba, Mexico, and South and Central America. The term *Chicano* generally refers to Mexican descent, and the term *Hispanic* refers to other Spanish-speaking ancestry.	15.4
Black or African American	Refers to ancestry from any of the countries within the African subcontinent.	12.4
Asian American	Among the 17 Asian subcategories are Bangladeshi, Chinese, Filipino, Hmong, Indonesian, Japanese, Korean, Laotian, Malaysian, Sri Lankan, Taiwanese, Thai, and Vietnamese.	4.4
American Indian (Native American)	The 2000 census data identified 36 tribes in this category, including Apache, Cherokee, Cheyenne, Houma, Navajo, Ottawa, Pueblo, Seminole, and Sioux.	0.8 (Includes Alaskan Native)
Arab American	Includes Egyptian, Iraqi, Jordanian, Lebanese, Moroccan, Palestinian, and Syrian.	*Classified as white American by ACS† 0.3
Native Hawaiian (Pacific Islander)	Refers to Hawaii, Samoa, Guam, and other Pacific Islands.	9.1
Alaskan Native	Includes four main subgroups: Alaskan Athabaskan, Aleut, Eskimo, and Tlingit-Haida.	Included with Native American by ACS
Two or more races		2.3

*U.S. Census Bureau, 2005-2007 American Community Survey (ACS).
†U.S. Census, 2000

data about various races, religions, and ethnic groups in the United States (Table 5-1).

Defining each culture's characteristics in a simple box is impossible because of acculturation. Patients cannot be put into culturally specific boxes or given labels on the basis of race, religion, or ethnic background. Health care workers should not assume that one criteria or belief of a certain cultural group is true for every patient in that bracket. However, some consistent beliefs and attitudes exist. Being aware of those beliefs and attitudes and being willing to accept the patient's beliefs to care for him or her are important. Health care providers may not always agree with a patient's beliefs, but it is important to understand that various beliefs exist and to find ways to work within those belief systems.

Ethnography

Ethnography is a branch of anthropology that studies and records various human cultures. Health care educators look at the research information from ethnographic studies and teach providers to become culturally competent. **Cultural competence** is the ability to meet the health care needs of patients while meeting and adhering to their cultural values, beliefs, and practices. It requires sensitivity to the patient's needs and wants and a deep understanding of their views and values.

Cultural Impact on Health Care

Each interaction with a patient will have cultural implications. Below are some examples of conflicts that can occur. Health care workers should keep in mind that these are examples from decades of ethnographic studies and that each patient must be viewed independently (Box 5-1).

BOX 5-1

Culturally Sensitive Questions

- How does your sickness work?
- What do you think caused your sickness?
- Why do you think your sickness started when it did?
- How long do you think you will have the sickness?
- What do you call your sickness?
- What about your sickness makes you afraid?
- What about the treatment makes you afraid?
- What are the biggest problems your sickness is causing?
- Whom do you know with the same problem?
- What have you done to treat your sickness, and how has it worked?
- Who else should be asked about or involved with your care?

BOX 5-2

Western Health Care Culture

- Activism (do something)
- Healing (make it better)
- Aggressiveness (stronger is better)
- Orientation (newer and sooner is better)
- Consistent (treat everyone the same)
- Individualism and autonomy (nature can be controlled)

Wellness and Health Prevention

Americans are focused on healthy living and disease prevention (Box 5-2). The general view is that it is important to eat right, get enough sleep, exercise, and have preventive medical visits (e.g., annual Pap tests, mammograms, immunizations). An illness is seen as interference with one's schedule, and thus it must be overcome quickly. Other cultures disagree with these beliefs. For example, some American Indian tribes view weight gain as a normal occurrence in adulthood; jogging and aerobic activities are seen as senseless.

Many cultures view thinness as a sign of wasting away and sickness. What may be considered overweight to one group is healthy and normal for another.

Various national organizations have studied ethnic groups and cultures to see the differences in their approach to preventive medicine. Breast cancer mammography screening is known to be effective against early detection, but Chinese Americans are reluctant to make visits for such preventive care. Studies suggest that cultural beliefs warn against "looking for trouble" and see it as senseless medical care.

Some cultures do not value immunizations, and other cultures perceive immunizations as injecting poison or harm into the body. According to the CDC, 60.6% of whites receive the pneumococcal vaccination, but only 23.8% of Hispanics and Latinos have that immunization. Most Americans view immunizations as basic preventive health care.

BRAIN BYTE

Telling a story is a therapeutic method of teaching and healing in some cultures.

Touch and Physical Space

In some cultures, close touching and human contact is a sign of respect and friendship. A simple handshake with a smile and "Hi, I am going to be your nurse today," shows warmth and caring. Yet in other cultures direct hand contact is not welcomed and is seen as an invasion of privacy. For example, Muslim women cannot be touched by men who are not immediate family members. Always ask permission first before touching any patient, regardless of cultural differences.

Most Americans prefer to keep a physical distance of 3 feet between peers and acquaintances. Yet other cultures see that distance as lack of personal caring and closeness. They may view distance as "cold." Be alert to positive or negative signs that tell whether the patient is comfortable with the amount of physical space allowed.

Communication

Communication is vital to our survival. Obviously language barriers affect our ability to communicate. According to the U.S. Census Bureau, 82% of households speak only English, but 10% of Spanish households do not speak English at all, and 18% speak English in only small amounts. Language is a form of cultural connection. It ties a group of people together.

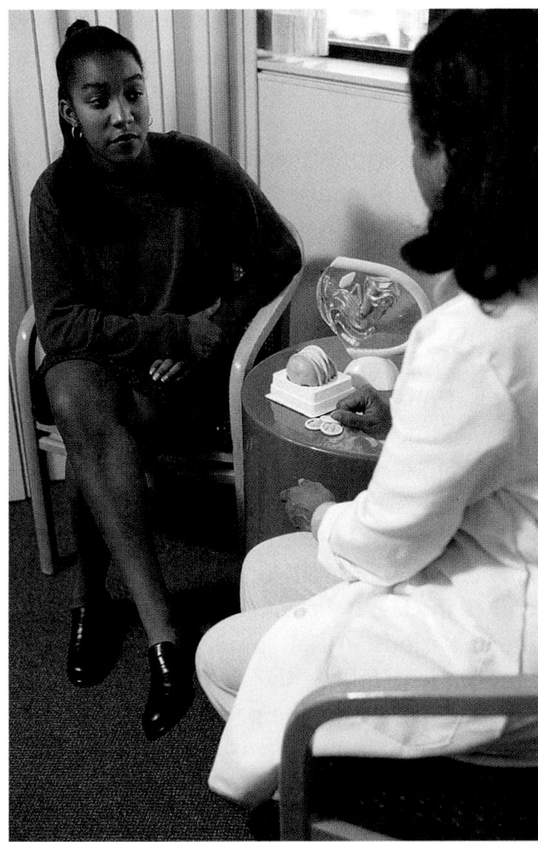

FIGURE 5-2 Discussions about sexual activity may be considered taboo and insulting to certain cultural groups, whereas other cultures may discuss these ideas freely.

Volunteer interpreters may help translate, but they also can help with cultural assimilation. **Assimilation** is the process of accepting and exchanging cultural information.

The ability to communicate has far more importance than language alone. For example, discussions about sexual activity may be considered taboo and insulting to certain cultural groups (Fig. 5-2). Yet other cultural groups, like Americans, are willing to discuss sexual habits and activities more freely. Asking a patient, "When did you have your last bowel movement?" may be appropriate in the United States, but to some cultures discussing elimination patterns is inappropriate.

Asking young women about menstruation may be viewed as intruding and inappropriate in some cultures. Yet in other cultures women willingly and openly discuss it and even joke about it.

In **matriarchal** societies and cultures, the oldest woman in the home makes all the decisions, including health care choices, but in patriarchal societies, the oldest male makes the decisions. Most Americans have a strong cultural belief in their independence and make solo decisions. It may seem peculiar or even upsetting to see a woman look to her husband for permission to speak or act. Respecting such beliefs and traditions, and not interfering with them, is important.

CASE STUDY 5-1 You enter a patient's room to ask how she feels. Her husband repeatedly interrupts you and answers for the patient. What should you do?

Answers to Case Studies are available on the Evolve website: ***http://evolve.elsevier.com/Gerdin***

General Procedures

Inpatients and outpatients are often asked to remove their clothing and wear a hospital gown for examinations. Patients do not like this procedure, but most will accept it as routine. However, it is important to be sensitive to patients who are not comfortable with this. For example, women who follow the hijab (traditional Muslim dress) cannot be seen unveiled. They will don a gown but will place a veil back on. Mexican Americans are uncomfortable changing in front of members of the opposite sex.

Before entering any patient room, all health care team members should announce their arrival and wait a few moments before entering. This allows patients to apply veils or blankets to prepare to be seen.

Some cultures fear invasive procedures. For example, many Hmong people may resist blood draws and lumbar punctures because removing these fluids will upset the body's harmony. In addition, Hmong people may fear operations because of the potential for impaired spiritual health. They fear that surgical incision may frighten the soul and cause it to leave the body.

CASE STUDY 5-2 You are caring for a patient who always wears a traditional amulet or talisman around his neck. You are asked to take him to radiology for a radiograph. What should you do?

Answers to Case Studies are available on the Evolve website: ***http://evolve.elsevier.com/Gerdin***

Dietary Needs

Food is a universal item that plays a huge role in people's lives. Food is a social tool as well as a biological need. Food has many ethnic and religious implications. All attempts should be made to meet a hospitalized patient's nutritional needs in conjunction with his or her requests. For example, Americans view meat and milk products as staples, but in India these foods may be considered taboo. In Islam, only specially prepared (halal) meats are permitted; alcohol and pork are forbidden. American Indians prefer to eat foods that are indigenous. Asians prefer to follow traditional oriental cooking patterns over fast food cooking patterns (Box 5-3).

In working with a patient who has high cholesterol, before explaining what foods should be avoided, the health care worker should take time to listen to the patient's dietary preferences and history of eating patterns. If the patient was never taught to eat fruits as a child, the health care worker should slowly introduce them into the diet. Dietary changes take a long time to implement.

If socializing within the culture depends on large family meals with many heavy dishes, cutting down on fats and calories may be an insult to the family structure and traditions.

Some medications, such as insulin (which treats diabetes) and heparin (an anticoagulant), have pork ingredients. Alcohol is often found in cough syrups. Pork and alcohol are considered taboo in some cultures. Instead of using a pork-based insulin, a different type could be selected that is made through chemical processing. An alcohol-free cough syrup should be selected.

Many cultures and religions require fasting rituals. Sometimes the fasting lasts one day, or it may extend for longer periods. All attempts should be made to help the patient follow the fasting regimen. If the health care team thinks the patient is at risk for malnutrition or dehydration, consultations with a dietician may offer some options. An example of an option would be to start an intravenous line (IV) and give the patient fluids. Some cultures aim to maintain a hot-cold balance in their bodies. Thus they will not drink cold beverages.

BOX 5-3

Yin and Yang Foods

For more than 3000 years, traditional Chinese beliefs have followed in the philosophy of Tao. Tao is the balance of yin and yang elements to maintain harmony and balance in the body. It believes that when food is digested, it turns into air that is either yin or yang. Although many people refer to yin as cold and yang as hot, this is incorrect terminology. The balance of yin and yang foods is essential for good health. Excess of either side will cause harm and illness. Here is a list of common yin and yang foods:

Yin	Yang
Bean sprouts	Beef
Bland foods	Catfish
Broccoli	Chicken
Cabbage	Eggplant
Carrots	Eggs
Celery	Fatty foods
Cucumber	Fried foods
Fish (some types)	Garlic
Melon	Leeks
Milk	Mushrooms
Pork	Peanuts
Potatoes	Red foods
Spinach	Shellfish
Water	Tomatoes

Spirituality

For many ethnicities, the spiritual component is essential for recovery and strength. Regardless of the health care provider's belief in God, prayer, or a higher being, the patient's belief should be accepted and assistance offered when requested. Patients often ask and want visits from their spiritual leaders while hospitalized. The health care worker should always use the correct terminology when referring to a clergyman. Using incorrect terminology is a sign of great disrespect and is insulting.

For example, Catholics use terms like *father* or *priest*, Muslims use the term *imam*, and Jews refer to leaders as *rabbis*. It could be insulting to say to a Catholic patient, "May I call your rabbi?" or to a Muslim patient, "May I call a priest?" If it is not obvious which term to use, one can use generic terms such as spiritual leader or clergyman.

Western medicine providers have mixed feelings about the effects of prayer on health recovery. Recent large studies have shown that prayer is powerful and may provide balance and harmony to the patient. Some religions require daily prayers at certain hours with specific rituals (kneeling, bending, interlocking of fingers, facing Mecca, or looking into the sky). Patients may prefer to pray quietly and alone. All attempts should be made to give patients privacy during these times.

Death

Views on death and dying vary greatly. Some cultures welcome death and see it as "advancing to the next stage." Other cultures see death as finality, and thus life should be extended for as long as possible even if artificial life-sustaining equipment is required. The rituals surrounding death vary. For example, Muslim patients should have their heads slightly elevated after death and turned to face Mecca if possible. Mexican Americans prefer to be in the room with the patient, whereas Japanese Americans prefer not to be in the room. Asian immigrants may offer to wash the body and prepare it for cremation or burial.

Deaths from suicide have many cultural implications. Some cultures believe that suicide brings shame to the entire family, and in other cultures it is strictly forbidden. Family members who have these beliefs will react differently in hospital emergency departments when they are called with such news. They may refuse to listen to any information, whereas other family members from other cultures will ask numerous questions and request to see the body.

Medications

The actions and side effects of some medications vary on the basis of patient ethnicity (Fig. 5-3). The FDA and the Institute for Safe Medication Practices have conducted and released many studies showing drug differences on the basis of ethnicity.

For example, some antilipemic drugs (used to lower cholesterol) have an increased potential to cause rhabdomyolysis (a serious muscle condition) when given to patients with Japanese or Chinese ethnicity.

In 2006 the FDA approved a combination of isosorbide and hydralazine drugs specifically to treat congestive heart failure in black patients. The drug combination is marketed under the trade name of BiDil. It is the first drug specifically targeted to one ethnic group.

In other cases, sometimes the dosages of the medications will be lowered for a particular ethnic group. Here are six other specific examples:

1. Women from Islamic and African cultures with vaginal yeast infections often prefer oral drugs to vaginally inserted medications. Inserting such drugs into the vaginal cavity is not culturally correct.
2. Latin Americans prefer injections to oral medications. They perceive oral medications as less effective.
3. Some cultures practice religious fasting, which can affect medication schedules or interfere with drug absorption.
4. Mexican and Puerto Rican patients' concern about potential addictive effects of medications can lead to reluctance to take long-term medications.
5. Vietnamese patients may take only half of their prescribed medication, believing that too much is wrong.
6. Hmong patients often have concerns about the effects of long-term medications, especially when medications are prescribed for a condition that does not cause the patient to feel ill (e.g., hypertension, diabetes).

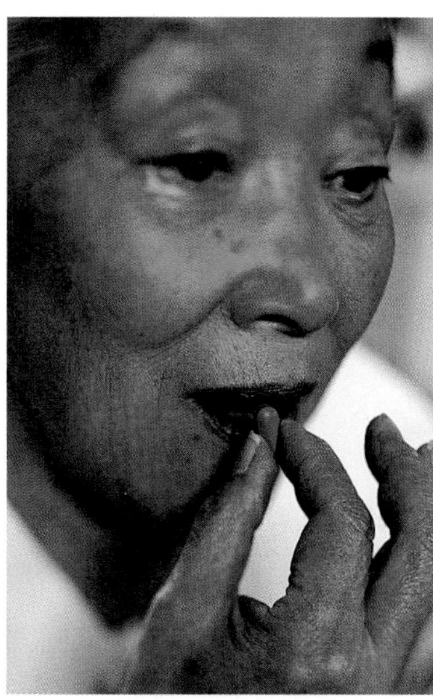

FIGURE 5-3 Some cultures believe that pills for conditions such as high blood pressure are harmful and not needed because there is no illness.

Pregnancy

Many beliefs about pregnancy and childbearing exist (Fig. 5-4). Some beliefs have lessened through acculturation and technological advances in Western medicine. Male partners in North America may be involved in prenatal care visits, whereas other cultures do not encourage such involvement. Box 5-4 lists some restrictive and taboo beliefs.

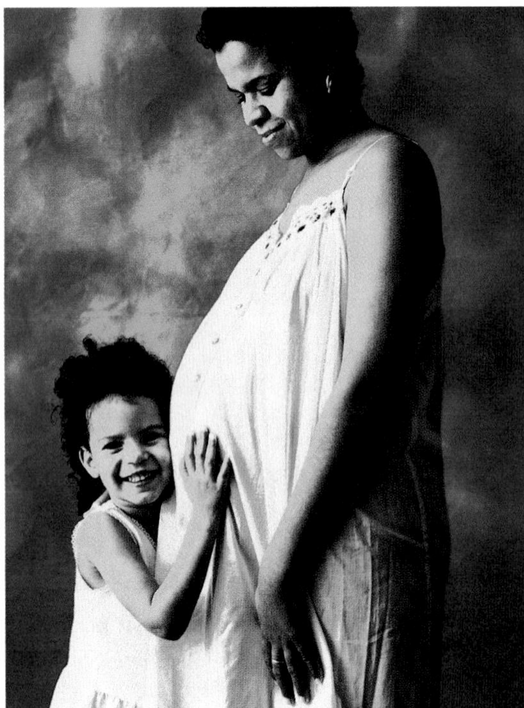

FIGURE 5-4 Beliefs about pregnancy and childbirth vary greatly.

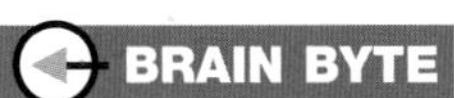

Some cultures practice "pica," which is eating nonnutritive substances during pregnancy.

BOX 5-4

Pregnancy Beliefs

Restrictive beliefs and taboos about pregnancy exist, but not everyone in a particular group will believe all of these, and it is important to realize that acculturation also exists.

Examples of restrictive beliefs:

- Avoid cold air during pregnancy. (Mexican, Haitian, Asian)
- Do not reach over your head: It will cause the umbilical cord to wrap around the baby's head. (Hispanic, Asian)
- Avoid funerals and weddings: It will bring bad luck to the baby. (Vietnamese)
- Do not tie knots or allow the father to do so: It will cause difficult labor. (Navajo Indians)

Examples of taboos:

- Avoid lunar eclipses and direct moonlight: It will cause deformities. (Mexican)
- Do not join in dances such as the Squaw: It will cause harm to the baby. (Navajo Indian)
- Do not engage in talk with people who cast spells: It will cause the baby to be eaten in the womb. (Haitian)
- Do not say the patient's name before the naming ceremony: Harm may come to the baby. (Orthodox Jewish)

In some cultures, specific postplacenta delivery rituals are followed. Some families will hold ceremonies with the placenta after birth. It must be buried in the ground to celebrate the new life. Placing the placenta in the earth honors the child's birth. Often a year later a tree or flower is planted in the same spot to allow the placenta to nourish its growth. In Chinese medicine, the placenta is known as a great life force and is highly respected in terms of its medicinal value.

Some cultures participate in placentophagia, which is eating of the placenta. Americans often allow health care providers to dispose of the placenta and do not even want to look at it or touch it.

Pain Management

Pain is subjective, and cultural beliefs about pain vary. Research has shown that unrelieved pain may slow recovery. The response to pain may be stoic or emotive. A **stoic** patient does not express pain or may deny that pain is present. Asian, Native American, Pacific Islander, and East Indian cultures may be stoic. Asian patients may not accept pain medication until asked twice in order to be polite. **Emotive** patients express their pain and want assistance with their suffering from others. Hispanic, Arabic, and Mediterranean patients may be emotive. Anglo-Americans might not express pain openly but accept pain medication.

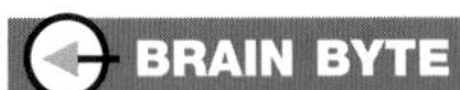

In some cultures, the patient and family might express themselves loudly and dramatically, whereas others may be stoic about pain.

Some cultures believe pain is caused by demons and is a sign from above that the spirits are upset. Thus the patient may refuse to admit to pain and see it as "something that I deserve and will go away on its own." Other cultures see pain as a symptom of an illness that should be treated and totally eliminated.

The health care worker should use listening and assessment skills to look for nonverbal cues of pain. Asking a patient to describe the pain on a scale of 1 to 10 may give the health care provider an idea of how intensely the pain is felt. Pain may also be identified by a facial expression (grimace or eye squeeze), perspiration, or "guarding" the affected area. Regardless of the pain assessment, the health care worker must honor the patient's beliefs and values about pain management.

Other

Cultural differences affect patient care in many other ways, including the following:

- Refusal to give blood or to get blood transfusions
- Refusal to donate or receive organ transplants
- Refusal to place aging parents into nursing homes despite the inability to care for them at home
- Fertility control
- Mental illnesses

When health care workers ignore cultural differences, patient care suffers, resulting in the loss of trust and respect. Patients and family members who lack a sense of trust or respect with their health care professionals will not follow treatment regimens.

Interpreters and Translation

Federal and state laws protect people with limited-English proficiency from discrimination. The provisions for health care workers are based on Title VI of the 1964 Civil Rights Act.

Many health care facilities provide interpreters to translate instructions when there is a language barrier or hearing impairment. The translation might be completed using a telephone translation service. If the interpreter is not an employee of the health care facility, the patient must give permission for the interpreter to participate. In some cases, a family member or member of the community may act as interpreter. In some cultures, such as the Arabic community, a member of the same sex might be preferred for translation. In all cases, the interpreter should be aware of confidentiality of patient information.

A professional interpreter or another health care worker may be more objective than a family member or friend of the patient. If the interpreter is not a health care worker, he or she might not understand the vocabulary used. The health care worker should provide clear instructions and speak in simple language to make sure that the patient understands (Box 5-5).

BOX 5-5

Guidelines for Using an Interpreter

- Speak slowly and clearly.
- Use short sentences.
- Use simple terms without jargon or slang.
- Use visual aids when appropriate.
- Repeat important information more than one time.
- Use language that identifies the interpreter as a messenger or go-between, not the authority (i.e., the doctor says or has ordered...).
- Talk to the patient, not to the interpreter, when speaking.
- Make eye contact with the patient as appropriate.
- Watch body language for understanding or confusion.
- Pause for the interpreter to translate.
- Before beginning, identify factors that might influence the translator's interpretation; ask the interpreter to report anything that is difficult to translate.
- Explain to the interpreter to repeat everything that the client and health care worker say without paraphrasing, judging, or omitting anything.
- Ask the interpreter to share personal cultural insights as his or her own opinion.
- Interrupt and ask the interpreter to explain what is being said if the translation seems long or off topic.
- Make sure the patient is aware of everything that is being discussed, even if it does not directly involve him or her.
- Provide key points in writing, such as appointment times, directions, and medication names.
- Ask the patient to repeat key points in his or her own words.

Signs of Cultural Barriers

Identifying a patient's cultural beliefs or attitudes by simply looking at the patient is impossible. Listening to the patient closely and looking for nonverbal cues that something is wrong are important. The following are a few signs that may indicate a cultural barrier:

- Resistant to change
- Uncooperative

- Argumentative
- Overly agreeable and flaccid
- Noncompliant after multiple teaching attempts

For example, a patient refuses to drink a cold glass of water with medications. He or she may say, "I'll take the pills later." A patient who is seen in a physician's office for uncontrolled high blood pressure may say, on questioning, "I stopped taking those pills. I feel fine." Misinterpreting such action as uncooperative is easy. The action may appear to be noncompliance, but it may be due to cultural beliefs that pills are harmful and not necessary unless one is really sick.

A patient who is informed that she needs a mammogram may smile and shake her head in agreement. She may appear agreeable and pleasant, yet when pushed to schedule the appointment, various reasons arise for the inability to schedule it. Some cultures view health care professionals as superiors and thus may avoid any form of disagreement or discussion. When patients are pushed to do something that they are against, they may opt to discharge themselves without explanation.

Obstacles to Cultural Competence

Ethnocentrism is the belief that one's own culture is superior to another. The belief is often unconscious but may be seen in daily activities. Ethnocentric approaches are ineffective in a health care setting. Although cultural heritage and beliefs are always present, the health care provider cannot allow them to interfere with providing care.

CASE STUDY 5-3 While you are providing daily care for a young woman, she mentions that she does not date because her parents have arranged her marriage. What should you do?

Answers to Case Studies are available on the Evolve website: ***http://evolve.elsevier.com/Gerdin***

Stereotyping

Stereotyping refers to seeing or viewing patients in one ethnic group all "molded together" as one. It assumes conformity. For example, it would be a stereotype to say that all Americans love hot dogs and baseball. Hasty generalizations cause alienation and lack of trust and respect. An example of a health care stereotype may be, "Herbal medicines are a form of quackery." Many cultures have strong beliefs in herbal and folk medicine. To ignore or dismiss their beliefs can cause problems.

For instance, Mr. Xyia uses garlic to remedy an illness. He knows that his doctor does not believe or trust in herbal medicines, so he decides not to talk about it. However, Mr. Xyia is taking a medication that interacts with garlic. Because he did not feel safe in his doctor's perception and stereotyping of such practices, he becomes sicker. Patients need to feel trusted and safe.

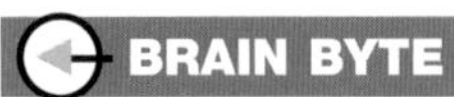

The Pacific-Islander culture views illness as an imbalance of self, ancestors, and the environment.

Prejudice and Discrimination

Stereotyping can lead to prejudice, which leads to discrimination. For example, a health care provider may have decided that a particular ethnic group of patients does not care about patient education and learning. Because of this stereotype, the health care provider might decide not to give this ethnic group any materials. This action is a form of discrimination. All health care providers must agree to care for patients regardless of race, age, color, sex, or ethnic origin. Some providers will actually be required to take this oath at graduation events.

Overcoming Obstacles

Among the many methods to overcome cultural obstacles are the following:

- Explore personal ideas and perceptions about different cultures. Understanding personal heritage and beliefs is vital to understanding and accepting others.
- Learn as much as possible about the cultures represented locally. Research and ask questions about their beliefs and practices. For example, how does this culture respond to pain? Does this culture have dietary habits or restrictions?
- Always use the patient's family name unless given permission to use first names only. Some cultures view not calling people by their full names as rudeness and a sign of great disrespect.
- Direct eye contact is viewed as important in American culture. Lack of eye contact indicates betrayal

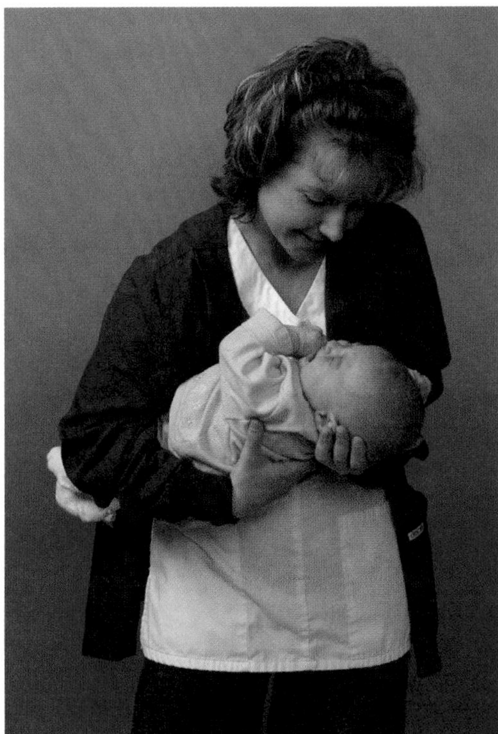

FIGURE 5-5 Some cultures believe that an infant should be touched when complimented to prevent an "evil eye." (From Sorrentino SA: *Mosby's textbook for nursing assistants,* ed 7, St. Louis, 2008, Mosby.)

and secretiveness. Many Asian populations, Native Americans, Arabs, and certain Hispanic groups consider it rude and disrespectful to make eye contact. For instance, Latino women are taught that downcast eyes are a proper response to authority. Latinos, as well as people of other cultures, believe that admiring a baby without touching it shows envy and brings bad luck by casting an "evil eye" (Fig. 5-5).

- Encourage patients to talk about their illnesses and look for areas of misunderstanding between cultural beliefs and the current diagnosis.
- Look for confusion and fear; watch for cues and respond with compassion. Do not belittle or dismiss culture-based anxiety.
- Treat all patients with respect, concern, and compassion.
- Recognize that other cultures are not as time sensitive as Americans. A patient may arrive for an 11:00 AM appointment at 11:45 AM and consider it normal. Not all cultures are time dependent.
- Many cultures are intensely involved with the supernatural and may believe that spirits or hexes cause illness. In these cultures, the supernatural being must be appeased, or soothed, before healing can begin. In extreme cases they perform rituals in the hospital setting to rid the body of the demon.

CASE STUDY 5-4 You enter a patient room and find the patient huddling on the floor and mumbling incoherently. What should you do?

Answers to Case Studies are available on the Evolve website: ***http://evolve.elsevier.com/Gerdin***

Summary

- Cultural differences can have an effect on health care. Examples of these differences include differences in beliefs regarding preventive measures, preferences in close touching and physical space, communication, beliefs regarding general procedures (e.g., blood draws, undressing), dietary practices, spiritual beliefs, views on death, beliefs about medications, beliefs about pregnancy and childbearing, and beliefs about pain.
- Cultural barriers may exist if the patient is resistant to change or appears uncooperative or argumentative, overly agreeable, or noncompliant after multiple teaching attempts.
- Although cultural heritage and beliefs are always present, the health care provider cannot allow stereotyping, prejudice, or discrimination to interfere with providing care. Many methods are available to help the provider to overcome cultural obstacles.
- An example of a culturally sensitive question would be to ask the patient if there is someone else who should help. The patient may want a priest, rabbi, shaman, family member, or some other person to participate in their care. Another is to ask the patient if someone else has the same problem to allow the patient to "tell as story" if preferred. Another culturally sensitive question is to ask the patient what treatment causes fear to allow the patient to describe concerns about care.

Review Questions

1. Describe how a patient's cultural background affects his or her health care.
2. List at least seven ways that a person's culture is expressed on a daily basis.

3. How does a patient's culture or ethnic background affect the taking of medications?
4. How does a patient's culture affect dietary beliefs?
5. Name five potential signs that may indicate the existence of a cultural obstacle. Give an example showing how these signs may be misinterpreted.
6. Discuss at least five steps that you can take to overcome or prevent a patient's culture from interfering with his or her health care needs.
7. List five culturally sensitive questions.
8. List five guidelines for using an interpreter.
9. Which cultures would be less likely to participate in immunization for the seasonal and H1N1 influenza?

Critical Thinking

1. Describe your cultural background. How has your background evolved or changed from that of your parents and grandparents? How much acculturation has occurred in your family's culture?
2. Describe a cultural barrier that you have experienced between yourself and a friend, peer, physician, or teacher. How did you feel about the encounter?
3. Use the Internet to investigate the Tuskegee syphilis experiment. Write a paragraph that describes the event and how it might affect how an African American patient views health care.
4. Use the Internet to describe the measures taken to inform people of various cultures about the H1N1 vaccination.
5. Use the Internet to describe a case study or story about the affect of culture on health care.
6. Use the Internet to investigate the Indian Health Care System. Describe how the system came into place and to whom the services are available.

Explore the Web

H1N1

Flu.gov
http://www.pandemicflu.gov/

CDC Facebook
http://www.facebook.com/CDC?ref=search&sid=1056483420.4133318816..1

HHS Office of Minority Health
http://www.omhrc.gov/templates/browse.aspx?lvl=2&lvlid=192

Tuskegee Syphilis

CDC
http://www.cdc.gov/tuskegee/timeline.htm

Indian Health Services

HHS
http://info.ihs.gov/Profile09.asp

Case Studies

Transcultural Nursing
http://www.culturediversity.org/cases.htm

CLAS Standards

HHS
http://thinkculturalhealth.org
https://www.thinkculturalhealth.org/Documents/CLAS_Standards.pdf

STANDARDS AND ACCOUNTABILITY*

Foundation Standard 6: Ethics

Healthcare professionals will understand accepted ethical practices with respect to cultural, social, and ethnic differences within the healthcare environment. They will perform quality healthcare delivery.

Accountability Criteria

6.1 Ethical Boundaries

6.11 Differentiate between ethical and legal issues impacting healthcare.

6.12 Recognize ethical issues and their implications related to healthcare.

6.2 Ethical Practice

6.21 Apply procedures for reporting activities and behaviors that affect the health, safety, and welfare of others.

6.3 Cultural, Social, and Ethnic Diversity

6.31 Understand religious and cultural values as they impact healthcare.

6.32 Demonstrate respectful and empathetic treatment of all patients or clients (customer service).

*From the National Consortium for Health Science Education (2009). National Health Care Standards and Accountability Criteria. Available at: http://www.healthscienceconsortium.org.

CHAPTER 6

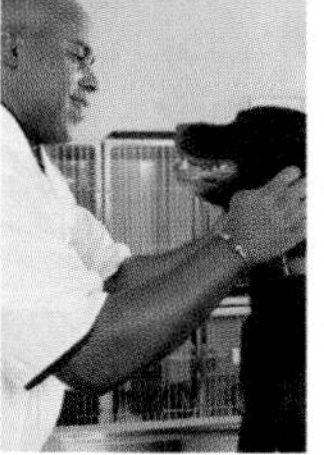
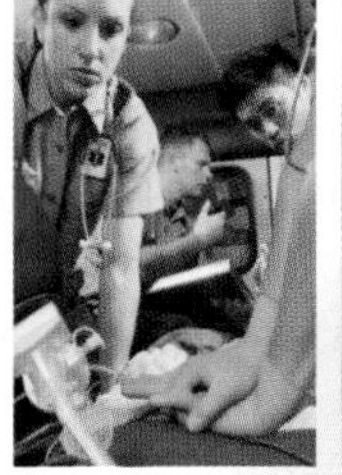
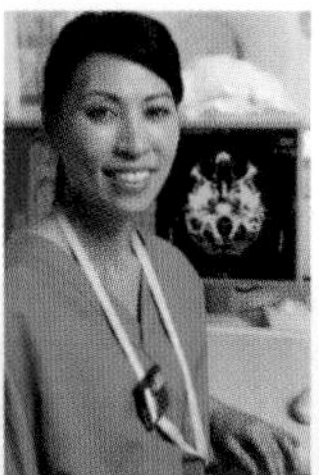

Employability Skills

LEARNING OBJECTIVES

- Define at least 10 terms relating to seeking a career in health care.
- Describe the purpose of a professional organization.
- List three benefits of membership in a student organization.
- List at least three reasons to use parliamentary procedure during an organization meeting.
- Identify the use of three motions of parliamentary procedure.
- Describe the purposes of the job application, resumé, portfolio, interview, and resignation letter.
- List at least five rules for completing a job application form.
- Provide a positive response for at least five questions that might be asked in a job interview.
- Complete a job application.
- Prepare a resumé or personal data sheet.
- Identify the components of a personal budget.

KEY TERMS

Adjourn *(uh-JERN)* To suspend a session to another time or permanently

Agenda *(uh-JEN-duh)* List of things to be done or considered, program of work

Budget *(BUD-jit)* Summary of projected income and expenses

Debate *(di-BAYT)* Discuss a question

Harassment *(huh-RAS-ment)* To disturb persistently, torment, bother, or persecute

Initiative *(in-ISH-uh-tiv)* Energy or aptitude for action, enterprise

Motion *(MO-shen)* Proposal for action

Organization *(or'guh-ni-ZAY-shun)* A structure through which individuals cooperate systematically to conduct business

Resumé *(REZ-oo-may)* Brief summary of professional and work experience

Tax *(taks)* Contribution to the support of government, fee, or dues of an organization to pay its expenses

Professional Organizations

In an organization, a group of individuals unites to achieve a goal by cooperation and division of tasks among themselves. Groups can accomplish goals faster and more easily than individuals. An organizational chart shows the relationships among and the roles of the members (Fig. 6-1).

Management practices and theories may be used to plan the framework of organizations. This is usually called organizational development. The goal of organizational development is to increase worker satisfaction and lead to increased productivity and quality. The health care worker plays an important part in the health care organization by setting goals, meeting challenges, and implementing ideas.

Work is a means of self-fulfillment and a method to earn a salary and establish economic security. Careful examination of the type of occupation may determine whether it will be satisfying and meet the needs and goals of the prospective health care worker. The choice of a career should be based on an individual's interests, abilities, and character.

Student Organizations

Student organizations provide a means to learn the behavior and skills necessary to succeed in school, on the job, and as citizens. Each student member is responsible for the effectiveness and success of the student organization. Two national organizations that may be part of a health careers program include the Health Occupations Students of America (HOSA) and SkillsUSA (Fig. 6-2). SkillsUSA is open to students in

STUDENT ORGANIZATION FRAMEWORK*

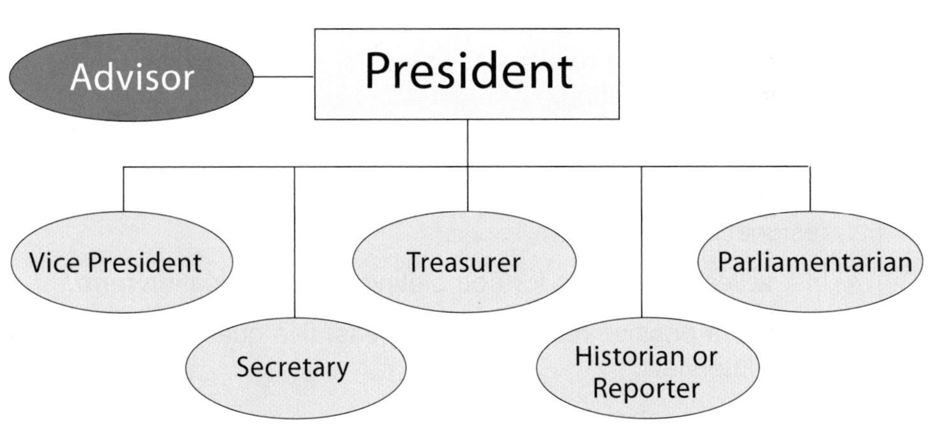

*The leadership of student organizations may vary.

Officer Responsibilities

President: Chairs the meetings. Prepares the agenda with the assistance of the secretary.

Vice President: Chairs the meeting in the absence of the President. Co-chairs all committees.

Secretary: Takes the minutes of the meetings. Prepares the agenda with the assistance of the President.

Treasurer: Maintains the financial books for the organization.

Historian/Reporter: Provides historical records and publicity for the organization using print and photographic media.

Parliamentarian: Ensures that parliamentary procedure is used during meetings. Answers procedural questions.

Advisor: Provides assistance as needed for organizational activities. Not a voting member.

FIGURE 6-1 As with health care facilities, student organizations maintain levels of organization to protect each member's rights and expedite business.

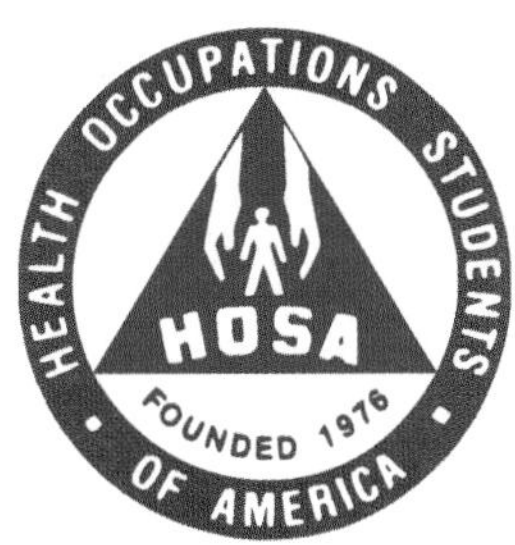

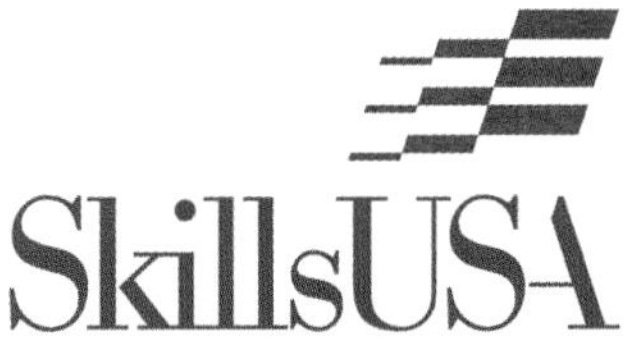

FIGURE 6-2 The HOSA motto: "The hands of HOSA mold the health of tomorrow." The SkillsUSA motto: "Preparing for leadership in the world of work." (HOSA motto and emblem used courtesy of HOSA, Flower Mound, Tex.; SkillsUSA motto and logo used courtesy of SkillsUSA, Leesburg, Va.)

BOX 6-1

SkillsUSA

SkillsUSA prepares America's high-performance workers. It provides quality education experiences for students in leadership, teamwork, citizenship, and character development. It builds and reinforces self-confidence, work attitudes, and communications skills. It emphasizes total quality at work, high ethical standards, superior work skills, lifelong education, and pride in the dignity of work. SkillsUSA also promotes understanding of the free enterprise system and involvement in community service activities.

SkillsUSA is a partnership of students, teachers, and industry representatives working together to ensure America has a skilled workforce. It helps each student to excel.

From http://www.skillsusa.org.

all trade and industrial programs. SkillsUSA has chapters in all 50 states, four territories, and the District of Columbia (Box 6-1). HOSA is open only to students in health science (occupations) programs.

Benefits of membership in a student organization include the exchange of information with others who have similar interests, an opportunity to sharpen skills through competition, and a way to develop leadership ability. Health care workers need leadership skills to provide better care. Many styles of leadership may be effective in different situations and may be practiced in student organization meetings (Table 6-1). Through organization membership, students develop programs and activities that build character, good citizenship, and a respect for ethical practices (Fig. 6-3). Confidence gained by assuming responsibility may lead to self-actualization. Student organizations promote and recognize individual and group achievements.

TABLE 6-1
Leadership Style

Style	Description
Autocratic	Leader makes all the decisions, discourages creativity, and allows quick decision making and decisive action.
By example	Leader is a role model for participants.
Coaching	Leader explains decisions, asks for suggestions, and supervises projects.
Delegating	Responsibility for decisions is given to others.
Democratic	Participation is encouraged, decisions are made jointly, and everyone is considered equal; this may result in "tyranny of the majority" in which the minority never gets its way.
Directing	Leader provides instruction and supervision.
Laissez-faire	Nobody is in charge. Decision making is scattered. Creativity is encouraged. This style may lead to lack of action.
Situational	Leader adapts and changes styles depending on the matter at hand.
Supporting	Leader assists and shares decision making.

One of the elements of an effective group is a clear understanding of its purposes and goals. The group must be flexible in the methods used to meet the goals. The members need to practice good communication skills and be able to initiate and carry out effective problem solving. An effective group shares the

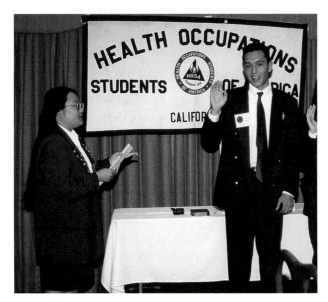

FIGURE 6-3 Officers of student organizations swear an oath of office as a sign that they understand the responsibilities and importance of their positions.

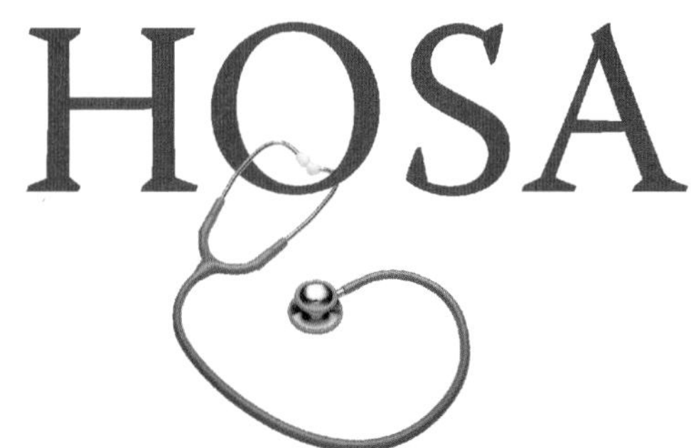

FIGURE 6-4 HOSA is 100% health care. (Courtesy of HOSA, Flower Mound, Tex.)

leadership responsibilities among its members and uses the abilities of all members.

In meetings members make decisions and develop a sense of belonging to the organization. A good meeting develops a sense of pride and enthusiasm for activities. Good meetings are possible when all members feel a sense of ownership of the decisions. Leadership ensures that the meeting is planned, organized, and conducted to cover all ideas in a fair manner. Following through with plans after the meeting is also important to reach goals and develop a sense of community within the group.

BOX 6-2

HOSA

- The professional association led by students
- The mission is to promote career opportunities in the health care industry and enhance the quality of health care to all people
- Open to secondary, postsecondary adult, and collegiate students enrolled in health science and technology programs (HSTE)
- Leadership development programs as well as competition
- Competition is held in five categories, including health occupations skills, health occupations-related skills, individual leadership skills, team leadership skills, and recognition

From http://www.hosa.org.

HOSA

Founded in 1976, HOSA is a student-led organization in 47 states and Puerto Rico with more than 110,000 members (Fig. 6-4). HOSA is open to all students at the secondary and postsecondary or collegiate levels who are interested in a career in the health professions. HOSA is an integral part of many health science programs, providing students with an opportunity for leadership development and service learning (Box 6-2). HOSA allows students to connect with the health care community while preparing them for entry-level certification and further education. HOSA is only open to health occupations students.

The HOSA National Competitive Events program provides a means of recognizing student knowledge and skills learned through health science education. Students compete in regional, state, and national competition in 57 areas (Box 6-3). Awards for competitors include scholarships for further education. Additionally, HOSA hosts leadership academies, including a Washington Leadership Academy to train state officers in leadership and advocacy.

SkillsUSA

SkillsUSA is a national organization of students, teachers, and representatives of industry. It helps students in high school, vocational centers, and 2-year colleges prepare for careers in trade, technical,

BOX 6-3

Health Occupations Students of America (HOSA) Competitive Event Categories*

Health Science Events

- Dental Spelling
- Dental Terminology
- Medical Spelling
- Medical Terminology
- Medical Math
- Knowledge Tests
  - Human Growth and Development
  - Pathophysiology
  - Concepts of Health Care
  - Pharmacology
  - Nutrition

Health Professions Events

- Biotechnology
- Clinical Nursing
- Clinical Specialty
- Dental Assisting
- Home Health Aide
- Medical Assisting
  - HOSA Medical Office
  - Centers for Medicare & Medicaid Services (CMS) 1500
- Medical Laboratory Assisting
- Nursing Assisting
- Personal Care
- Physical Therapy
- Sports Medicine
- Veterinary Assisting

Emergency Preparedness Events

- CPR/First Aid
- Emergency Medical Technician
- First Aid/Rescue Breathing
- Community Emergency Response Team (CERT) Skills
- Public Health Emergency Preparedness
- Epidemiology
- Medical Reserve Corps (MRC) Partnership

Leadership Events

- Extemporaneous Health Poster
- Extemporaneous Speaking
- Extemporaneous Writing
- Medical Photography
- Job-Seeking Skills
- Prepared Speaking
- Researched Persuasive Speaking
- Interviewing Skills
- Speaking Skills

Teamwork Events

- Community Awareness
- Creative Problem Solving
- Forensic Medicine
- HOSA Bowl
- Parliamentary Procedure
- Career Health Display
- Biomedical Debate
- Medical Reading
- Health Education
- Public Service Announcement

Recognition

- Outstanding HOSA Chapter
- National Recognition Program
- Kaiser Permanente Health Care Issues Exam
- National Service Project
  - School Publication: HOSA
- Barbara James Service Award
- Outstanding Alumni Member
- Outstanding State Leader
- Chapter Newsletter
- HOSA Week
  - HOSA Week Proclamation

*Event information may be updated on the HOSA website, http://www.hosa.org.

and skilled service occupations, including health occupations. It was formerly known as Vocational Industrial Clubs of America. The organization places an emphasis on total quality at work, including leadership, teamwork, citizenship, and character development. It has been cited by the U.S. Department of Labor as a "successful model of an employer-driven youth development training program." SkillsUSA holds yearly skills and leadership competitions on local, state, and national levels.

Parliamentary Procedure

Parliamentary procedure is a set of rules for conducting a meeting in an organized and efficient manner. Robert's Rules of Order is the basis for these rules and serves as the guide or authority for business procedures in many groups and organizations. Parliamentary procedure maintains a sense of order during meetings and ensures that all members have a chance to participate equally. The procedure is designed to simplify matters by allowing only one person to speak at a time and by discussing only one idea at a time. Decisions are reached through a process of motions, **debate**, and voting that ensures all members can be heard (Table 6-2). The vote of the majority determines the course of action, but the minority also has the right to be heard.

The **agenda** lists activities for the meeting (Box 6-4). The agenda for the first meeting should include establishing a yearlong calendar of activities on the basis of goals set by the group. **Motions** are made to propose action for the group. Types of motions used in parliamentary procedure include main, subsidiary, privileged, and incidental ones. The type of motion determines when a person may speak. When the meeting is finished, a motion to **adjourn** ends it. Election of officers is determined by the constitution and bylaws of the organization. Parliamentary procedure can be learned by practice.

BOX 6-4

Agenda

I. Call to order
II. Invocation
III. Pledge of allegiance
IV. Roll call and establish quorum
V. Minutes of previous meeting
VI. Treasurer's report
VII. Officers' reports
VIII. Committee reports
  A. Standing
  B. Special
IX. Unfinished business
X. New business
XI. Program
XII. Announcements
XIII. Adjournment

TABLE 6-2
Parliamentary Procedure: Motions Used to Conduct Meetings

Motion	Can Interrupt Speaker?	Second Required?	Debatable?	Amendable?	Type of Vote Required	Purpose
Main	No	Yes	Yes	Yes	Majority	To introduce business
Refer to committee	No	Yes	Yes	Yes	Majority	To refer the matter to a committee
Approve minutes	No	Yes	Yes	Yes	Majority	To accept the minutes of a previous meeting
Amend a main motion	No	Yes	Yes	Yes	Majority	To change a motion
Table a motion	No	Yes	No	No	Majority	To wait to consider the matter
Adjourn	No	Yes	No	No	Majority	To end the meeting
Question of privilege	Yes	No	No	No	No vote	To give immediate attention to a problem
Division	No	Yes	No	Yes	No vote	To call for the vote to be verified
Point of order	Yes	No	No	No	No vote	To raise a parliamentary question

Career Planning

Each person seeks different things from a job (Fig. 6-5). Approximately one third of a person's life is spent working, so the job should meet as many of the person's needs as possible. After deciding on the type of job preferred, the applicant must apply for available positions. Available jobs may be found through online services and searches, newspaper advertisements, employment agencies, and friends. Other resources for job opportunities may include teachers, counselors, professional journals, and job posting boards at the place of employment. Employers look for the best person to fill the vacancy. They use the application, resumé, and interview to determine the best applicant.

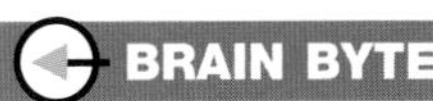

Allied health providers make up 60% of the health care workforce.

Application

Some positions may require a letter of application (Fig. 6-6). The letter of application requests a chance to apply for a position and should be brief. (See Skill List 6-1, Preparing a Letter of Application, p. 105).

Applications are often used to determine which candidates get an interview. The prospective employee should consider the application to be an example of the work the employer might expect (Fig. 6-7). It should be filled in neatly, leaving no blank spaces. The application must be honest but should present the applicant in the best light possible (Box 6-5). If possible, the applicant should obtain two blank application forms for the position. The first should be completed in pencil and then proofread and corrected. The final application can then be recopied in ink or typed, proofread, and returned to the employer. It may, however, be necessary to complete the application at the time it is obtained, so the applicant should have all necessary information at hand. (See Skill List 6-2, Completing a Job Application, pp. 105-106).

CASE STUDY 6-1 You go into a health care facility to pick up an application. The receptionist tells you that you cannot take it with you but must complete and turn it in onsite. What should you do?

Answers to Case Studies are available on the Evolve website: *http://evolve.elsevier.com/Gerdin*

BOX 6-5

Application Guidelines

- Print or type all items accurately and neatly. Read every line carefully. If possible, have someone review the application for errors.
- Do not leave any blank spaces or lines. The phrase "not applicable," "N/A," or a dash indicates that the question was read but does not apply.
- Account for any periods you were not working or termination of employment in a positive manner. For example, a termination might have been caused by a "reduction in force" or "seeking better employment opportunity."
- Answer the question of salary as "open" if an amount is not known.
- Use a phone number that will be answered promptly. That may be the number of a family member or a friend who would take a message.

Resumé

The personal data sheet, or **resumé**, provides additional information that is not found on the application (Fig. 6-8). The resumé includes educational and work experience, skills, achievements, and other activities presented in an easily read and neat format. As with the letter of application and application form, the resumé should be without error and concise and present the prospective employee in the best manner. The resumé should be typed on good-quality paper and limited to one page. The applicant should take at least three copies of the resumé to the job interview (Box 6-6). (See Skill List 6-3, Preparing a Resumé, p. 106).

Personal Portfolio

Personal and professional commitment may be demonstrated by providing an employer or scholarship committee with a portfolio (Box 6-7). A portfolio is a sample of a person's work, achievements, and experiences. The content of a portfolio includes the resumé, a writing sample, a description of work experience, and a list of skills. It may also include verification of participation in community or volunteer projects. Documentation of job shadowing or observation of a health care professional at work can be included to indicate a real knowledge of the occupation. Evidence of special skills, such as a computer-generated

Text continued on p. 97

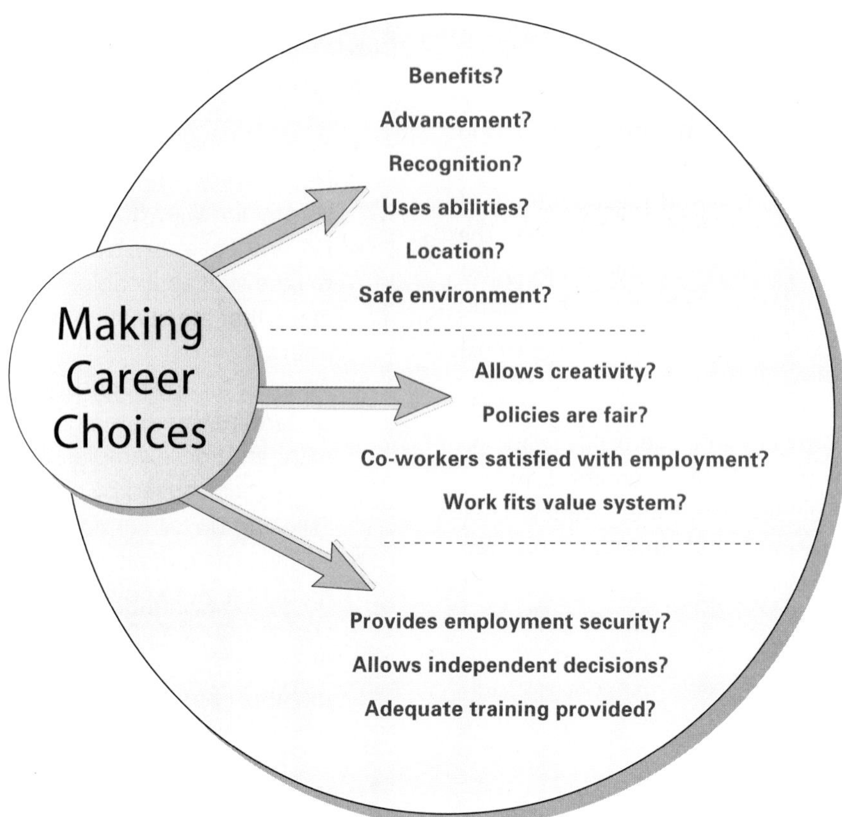

FIGURE 6-5 Career choice considerations.

BOX 6-6

Resumé Tips

- Include job objective.
- Change the resumé to fit the job description.
- Analyze the job description to find key words to describe experience.
- Avoid personal pronouns such as I, me, or my.
- Do not make any handwritten notes or marks.
- Limit to one side of one page.
- List most important information first.
- Redo the application instead of making corrections.
- Do not include photos or graphics.
- Use **bold** print or CAPITAL letters to draw attention to information.
- Use clear, conventional font such as 12-point Times New Roman.
- Use past tense to describe past events.
- Use plain white or off-white paper.

BOX 6-7

Health Occupation Students of American (HOSA) National Recognition Program Portfolio Criteria*

1. Letter of Introduction: Introduction of the participant including career goal
2. Resume: Professional resumé including education, work experience, activities, and awards
3. Project: Description and evidence of a classroom or community activity that required problem solving and hands-on application of health care knowledge and skills
4. Writing Sample: Example of ability to follow instructions effectively and answer questions in written form
5. Work-Based Learning: Detailed summary of work-based learning experience, such as job shadowing, internship, or volunteering experience

*Details and information about all HOSA Competitive Events may be found on the website, http://www.hosa.org.

Date

Ms./Mr.______________
Human Resources Manager
Agency Name
Address
City, State, Zip Code

Dear Ms./Mr. ______________

Mr./Ms.__________________ , my health occupations education teacher, suggested that I contact you about the position you currently have open in the area of__________________ . Please consider me an applicant for this position.

I will graduate from __________________ High School in June of this year. My courses have included training and work that support my desire to be employed in the health care field. I have reached competency levels in many of the basic health care skills, such as assessing vital signs and understanding medical terminology. I am enclosing a personal data sheet that lists these courses and competencies.

I plan to continue my education by taking classes during the hours I am not working. May I have an interview at your convenience? Please call the number noted below at any time, and a message will be taken for me. Thank you for your time and consideration of my application.

Sincerely,

Student Name
Address
City, State, Zip Code

Phone Number

enclosure

FIGURE 6-6 Letter of application.

Application for Employment

Date ______________________

Name ______________________ Social Security # ______________________

Address ______________________ Zip __________ Telephone Number ______________

If employed and you are under 18 can you furnish a work permit? ❑Yes ❑No

Are you legally eligible for employment in the U.S.A.? ❑Yes ❑No

Have you worked here before? ❑Yes ❑No If Yes, when?______________________

Are there any hours, shifts, or days you cannot or will not work?______________________

Are you willing to work overtime if required? ❑Yes ❑No

List friends or relatives working here.______________________

Have you ever been convicted of a crime? ❑Yes ❑No (A conviction record will not necessarily be a bar to employment)

EDUCATION

Circle Highest Grade Completed	Grade School 1 2 3 4 5 6 7 8	High School 9 10 11 12	College 1 2 3 4	Graduate 1 2 3 4	Degree Received	Course of Study
High School	*Name and Address*					
College(s)						
Graduate/Professional						
Specialized Training, Apprenticeship, Skills						
Honors and Awards and Accreditations						

MILITARY SERVICE RECORD Have you served in the U.S. Armed Forces? ________ Dates of duty ________

POSITION(S) APPLIED FOR: 1) ______________________ 2) ______________________

You must indicate a specific position. Applications stating "ANY POSITION" will not be considered.

Wage or salary requirements $ ______________ When can you start? ______________

Continued

FIGURE 6-7 Application for employment.

Application for Employment—continued

WORK HISTORY

If presently employed, may we contact your employer? ❑ Yes ❑ No

(1) Present or Most Recent Employer	Address	Phone
Date Started	Starting Salary	Starting Position
Date Left	Salary on Leaving	Position on Leaving
Name and Title of Supervisor		
Description of Duties		Reason for Leaving
(2) Previous Employer	Address	Phone
Date Started	Starting Salary	Starting Position
Date Left	Salary on Leaving	Position on Leaving
Name and Title of Supervisor		
Description of Duties		Reason for Leaving
(3) Previous Employer	Address	Phone
Date Started	Starting Salary	Starting Position
Date Left	Salary on Leaving	Position on Leaving
Name and Title of Supervisor		
Description of Duties		Reason for Leaving

Continued

FIGURE 6-7, cont'd

ADDITIONAL INFORMATION

OTHER QUALIFICATIONS

Summarize special job-related skills and qualifications acquired from employment or other experience.

____

____

____

SPECIALIZED SKILLS (CHECK SKILLS/EQUIPMENT OPERATED)

____ Keyboarding 45 wpm	____ Fax	Other (list):
____ PC	____ Microsoft Office, MedSoft, AltaPoint EMR	______________
____ Calculator	____ CPR Certification	______________
	____ Fluent in Spanish	______________

State any additional information you feel may be helpful to us in considering your application.

____

____

____

____

Note to Applicants: DO NOT ANSWER THIS QUESTION UNLESS YOU HAVE BEEN INFORMED ABOUT THE REQUIREMENTS OF THE JOB FOR WHICH YOU ARE APPLYING.

Are you capable of performing in a reasonable manner—with or without a reasonable accommodation—the activities involved in the job or occupation for which you have applied? A description of the activities involved in such a job or occupation is attached. ❑ Yes ❑ No

REFERENCES

1. ____
(Name) Phone #
____
(Address)

2. ____
(Name) Phone #
____
(Address)

3. ____
(Name) Phone #
____
(Address)

UNDER MARYLAND LAW, AN EMPLOYER MAY NOT REQUIRE OR DEMAND, AS A CONDITION OF EMPLOYMENT, PROSPECTIVE EMPLOYMENT, OR CONTINUED EMPLOYMENT, THAT AN INDIVIDUAL SUBMIT TO OR TAKE A LIE DETECTOR OR SIMILAR TEST. AN EMPLOYER WHO VIOLATES THIS LAW IS GUILTY OF A MISDEMEANOR AND SUBJECT TO A FINE NOT EXCEEDING $100.00.

By my signature below, I certify that I have read the above and understand it completely.

____
Signature Date

FIGURE 6-7, cont'd

Personal Data Sheet

Student Name
Address
City, State, Zip Code

Phone number

Personal data:

Date of birth	Weight
Marital Status	Height

Course work:

Typing	Health Occupations I
Computers	Health Occupations II

Activities:

President, Health Occupations Organization
Chairperson, March of Dimes Walk-a-Thon

Skills:

Have knowledge of medical terminology
Able to assess vital signs
Certified in cardiopulmonary resuscitation
Able to apply body mechanics safely

Work experience:

Volunteer at hospital weekly, 3 years
Student assistant in science, 1 year

References:

List three in alphabetical order. Include name, address, and telephone number. A reference should be asked prior to including the name.

FIGURE 6-8 Personal data sheet.

presentation, may be included. Certification such as first aid, special awards, and other forms of recognition is also part of a portfolio. Other items that might be included are a graduation certificate, transcripts, standardized test scores, and a self-reflection essay. The items chosen for the portfolio should emphasize the positive qualities of the person.

Interview

Many prospective employees do not recognize that the first interview occurs when the application is obtained from the receptionist. The appearance and behavior of the applicant during this part of the procedure may determine whether an interview is granted with the person who actually makes the hiring decision (Box 6-8).

The interview provides the employer a chance to evaluate the applicant. It also provides the applicant

BOX 6-8

Interview Questions

Interviewer

1. What are your future goals?
2. What can you tell me about yourself?
3. Why did you choose our company for possible employment?
4. For which type of position are you applying?
5. Have you ever been dismissed from a job?
6. Why did you leave your last place of employment?
7. Why do you feel qualified for this position?
8. What do you feel are your strong points?
9. What do you feel are your weak points?
10. Do you have any plans for further education?
11. How many days of school/work did you miss last year?
12. What skills do you have that would be useful in this position?
13. Who is your favorite teacher, and why?
14. How do you get along with your family?
15. What do you like to do in your free time?
16. Why do you think you are a better applicant than the others applying for this position?
17. What motivates you?
18. How well do you do in school?
19. How do you rate yourself as a leader?
20. What would you say are your most important accomplishments to date?

Interviewee

1. How is the department or company organized for supervision?
2. With whom would I be working?
3. Are there opportunities for advancement in this position?
4. What is the performance evaluation procedure?
5. Is additional on-the-job-training possible?
6. Does the supervisor encourage initiative and creativity?

with an opportunity to find out more about the job and employer. The applicant should prepare for an interview by anticipating questions and forming answers that are clear and concise (Box 6-9). (See Skill List 6-4, Interviewing, pp. 106-107).

Some employers use a behavioral-based interview technique. The prospective employee is asked to describe a specific situation from the past that demonstrates desirable traits such as leadership or teamwork (Box 6-10). The goal of the behavioral interview questions is to predict the future actions of the employee. Techniques that may be used to answer behavioral interview questions include the SHARE, STAR, and PAR models (Box 6-11).

BOX 6-9

Guidelines for the Interview

1. Know the name of the interviewer and his or her position within the organization.
2. Know about the organization and the position desired.
3. Bring all information regarding references, social security number, past employment, and education needed to complete the application form. If permitted to complete the application away from the site, take two to use one for practice.
4. Present yourself for the interview in a positive and confident manner.
5. Arrive 5 minutes early for the appointment, not earlier or later.
6. Do not chew gum, eat candy, or smoke before or during the interview.
7. Wear appropriate clothing for the position desired. Be neat and clean.
8. Shake hands firmly with the interviewer when introduced. If you must introduce yourself, call the interviewer by title and name.
9. Remain standing until the interviewer asks you to sit down.
10. Place any personal items such as a purse on the floor. Keep a pencil and some paper at hand.
11. Be enthusiastic but not overbearing. Answer all of the questions in a positive manner without criticizing yourself or others.
12. Think about each question before responding to it. Look at the interviewer when speaking.
13. After the interviewer has completed his or her questions, ask any questions that remain unanswered for you.
14. Thank the interviewer for his or her time. Ask when the decision regarding the position will be known.

BOX 6-10

Behavioral Interview Questions

- How do you describe your former co-workers, bosses, or teachers?
- Give an example of how you handled change.
- Give an example of how you have worked as a team member.
- Describe an idea or project that you initiated and implemented.
- Describe a situation when you went beyond the normal expectations to complete a job.
- Describe how you have met a past goal that you set for yourself.
- Give two or three examples of things that you have done that show you are willing to work hard.
- Give an example of how you used critical thinking and good judgment to solve a problem.
- What are the key ingredients to maintaining a good working relationship?
- Give an example of when you have demonstrated initiative.
- Describe a conflict that you were able to resolve.
- Give an example of when you have had to deny a request of a co-worker or friend.
- Describe an example of when you were able to communicate an idea effectively.
- How do you prepare written communications?
- Describe the most difficult person that you've worked with and how you handled the situation.
- Describe an example of when you were asked to keep information confidential.
- Give an example of when you have worked as the leader of a group.
- Give an example of when you did and when you did not listen well.
- Describe a situation when you were criticized about your work and how you handled it.
- Give an example of how you handle stress.
- Describe an example of how you have shown cultural sensitivity to someone.

BOX 6-11

Behavioral Job Interview Models

SHARE

S – Describe a situation.

H – Describe any obstacles (hindrances) to your actions.

A – Explain what you did (your actions).

R – Describe the results of your actions.

E – Summarize the outcome with a positive evaluation.

STAR

S – Describe the situation.

T – Describe the tasks you were asked (or asked) to do.

A – Describe your action that demonstrated leadership or teamwork.

R – Describe the positive result.

PAR

P – Describe the problem or task.

A – Describe the action you took to solve the problem.

R – Describe the results of your actions.

BRAIN BYTE

Past performance is the best predictor of future performance.

CASE STUDY 6-2 The interviewer asks you to tell him or her about an incident in your past that demonstrates your leadership ability. What should you do?

Answers to Case Studies are available on the Evolve website: ***http://evolve.elsevier.com/Gerdin***

Before the interview, the applicant should gather as much information as possible about the prospective employer. Minimally, the applicant should know the name and position of the interviewer, the basic job expectations, and a little about the employing agency. When the employer has finished questioning the applicant, it is appropriate to ask questions. These questions should reflect a real interest in knowing about the position.

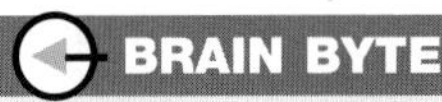

BRAIN BYTE

An interview is a two-way conversation.

Job Satisfaction

One criterion or need for job satisfaction is the ability to pay for the wants and needs of life. To determine whether an employment opportunity will provide for these needs, a personal **budget** may be used to determine whether these financial goals can be met (Fig. 6-9). The gross income is the money earned as a salary or wage. The net income is the amount that actually appears in the check after **taxes**, social security, and other deductions are made. A budget is a plan for the use of resources and expenditures. Once a budget is established, it can be adjusted as needed.

When income is received, a checking and savings account may be the best way to store and distribute money (Fig. 6-10). Banks and other financial institutions provide varied incentive programs for their accounts and may offer "free" services, interest, or checks for investing with their company (Table 6-3).

A personal financial statement is also a tool that can be used for planning a budget (Fig. 6-11).

Some taxes are taken directly from the check before it is received. This may include city, county, state, and federal taxes. Social security taxes, or Federal Insurance Contributions Act (FICA) wages, are taken out of the check as well. Social security is a retirement fund that was established to provide funds for the disabled, elderly, and unemployed. Other taxes, such as property tax, must be sent or paid annually to an agency such as the state. Indirect taxes are those paid every day, such as sales taxes and those on gasoline, cigarettes, and liquor. All citizens of the United States must prepare a federal income tax statement each year if the income reaches the specified amount.

Insurance costs may be deducted from the paycheck as well. Some types of insurance include health, life, unemployment, personal property, automobile, and worker's compensation. The employer may pay costs or share them with the employee.

Earning an income and becoming self-supporting increases an individual's understanding of money management and conservation of resources. Cost containment is also a growing concern for the health care industry. Each worker is responsible for limiting costs by using the resources of the workplace wisely and without unnecessary waste.

Health occupations job dissatisfaction results from the same factors that are attractions to it. The workload may be long and varied. The responsibilities can be unexpected, changing, and stressful. In large facilities, women fill most of the patient care jobs such as nursing. This can lead to verbal or physical abuse or

Cost-of-Living Budget

Regular or Fixed Monthly Payments*

Mortgage or rent	$
Automobile payment	$
Automobile insurance	$
Appliances	$
Loan	$
Health insurance	$
Personal property insurance	$
Telephone	$
Utilities (gas or electric)	$
Water	$
Other non-emergency expenses	$

Discretionary or Variable Payments

Clothing, laundry, cleaning	$
Medicine	$
Doctor and dentist	$
Education	$
Dues	$
Gifts and donations	$
Travel	$
Subscriptions	$
Automobile maintenance and gas	$
Spending money and entertainment	$

Food Expenses

Food—at home	$
Food—away from home	$

Taxes

Federal and state income tax	$
Property	$
Other taxes	$

Other

Other	$

Total Monthly Payments $

Sample Recommended Budget Expenditures

Shelter (Rent or mortgage)	20%
Food	25%
Clothing	12%
Transportation	12%
Medical and dental	6%
Dues and charities	9%
Education and entertainment	10%
Savings	6%*

* Financial advisors recommend that savings should cover expenses for at least 3 months.

FIGURE 6-9 A personal budget ensures that money earned will meet the needs of life.

CHECK NO.	DATE	CHECK ISSUED TO OR DEPOSIT RECEIVED FROM	AMOUNT OF CHECK	AMOUNT OF DEPOSIT	BALANCE
1	1/1	Apartments R Us	500.00		250.00

FIGURE 6-10 Accurate records for income and expenditures are made easier with written records.

TABLE 6-3
Types of Financial Institutions

Institution	Services	Regulation/Responsibility
Bank	Manage money (deposit/withdraw/save) Credit/check/loan money Mortgage property	For-profit FDIC insured (national banks)*
Credit union	Manage money (deposit/withdraw/save) Credit/check/loan money	Not-for-profit Owned by members FDIC insured*
Insurance companies/ pension funds	Insurance/securities/retirement funds Real estate/mortgage loans Credit/check/loans Tax-deferred savings	May be company created by employer, union, or state
Internet bank	Online banking services	May or may not have a building May or may not be FDIC*
Savings and loan	Real estate financing Save money	May have depositor membership

*The Federal Deposit Insurance Corporation (FDIC) is an independent agency created by Congress. It insures deposits, supervises financial institutions, and manages receiverships.

Personal Financial Statement

Assets

Cash	$
Securities (stocks, bonds, CDs)	$
Real Estate	$
Automobile	$
Furniture	$
Receivables (money owed to you)	$
Other	$

Value should be determined by the amount that could be obtained from a "quick" sale.

Total Owned $

Debts

Household bills unpaid	$
Installment payments:	
Automobile	$
Appliances	$
Loans	$
Real estate payments	$
Other	$
Insurance:	
Automobile	$
Personal property	$
Health	$
Other	$
Taxes	$
Other debts	$

Total Owed $

Total Owned Minus Total Owed = Total Worth $

FIGURE 6-11 A person's financial standing is determined by the difference between the amount owned (assets) and the amount owed (debts).

harassment from not only fellow workers but also from patients. Sexual harassment is action of a sexual nature that is not wanted or welcome by the recipient. This can be a verbal action such as sexual comments about appearance, innuendo, or ridicule. It may also be actions such as showing offensive visual materials or unwanted physical contact. The Civil Rights Act of 1964 legally protects both patients and health care workers from sexual harassment.

CASE STUDY 6-3 You are scheduled to work for an upcoming holiday. You have worked for all of the holidays for the last 6 months. You feel this is unfair and think you are being scheduled on holidays because you are not married. What should you do?

Answers to Case Studies are available on the Evolve website: ***http://evolve.elsevier.com/Gerdin***

CASE STUDY 6-4 You are caring for a patient who repeatedly makes remarks of a sexual or demeaning nature. You are embarrassed and angry over the remarks. What should you do?

Answers to Case Studies are available on the Evolve website: ***http://evolve.elsevier.com/Gerdin***

Resignation

Performing well and showing the favorable characteristics of a health care worker helps an employee keep the job. Some of these favorable characteristics include a positive attitude, enthusiasm, an open mind, and constant efforts to improve performance. Poor interpersonal relations, lack of technical knowledge, and lack of dedication to work ethics such as promptness, honesty, and good grooming are often reasons for job termination. Reporting on time (punctuality) and regular attendance are important aspects of keeping a job. Most people who lose a job after being hired do so because of attitude rather than the ability to do the job.

Job advancement is earned by doing the job better and more quickly than others and by showing the attributes of initiative, loyalty, and responsibility. Improvement in performance is expected over time from a new employee.

When a better opportunity or other personal considerations cause termination, there is a proper way to end the association. Ending employment is not advisable until another job has been secured. The time necessary to "give notice" of termination depends on the level of responsibility of the job. Two weeks is usually long enough for the employer to make arrangements to fill the vacancy. A letter of resignation is submitted to the employer before telling other employees or patients (Fig. 6-12). The letter should contain the date on which the employment will end and express appreciation for the opportunity of having worked with the establishment. Giving the reason for termination is not necessary if this information might leave bad feelings.

If dismissed, fired, or laid off from a job, the worker is at a disadvantage in finding new employment. Respectfully determining the reason for termination is important. In future interviews for employment, the applicant can use this information to demonstrate an effort to improve. Most employers will hire a person who has made a mistake but is willing to learn from it and improve.

BRAIN BYTE

According to the Bureau of Labor Statistics, jobs for Personal and Home Care Aides have a projected 51% increase by 2016.

Continuing Education

Continuing education refers to the training, courses, and study completed after the health care worker begins to practice. In many of the health care professions, continuing education is required for the health care worker to continue to practice or be relicensed.

Summary

- The purpose of a professional organization is to allow individuals to join together to reach a goal.
- Three benefits of membership in a student organization are exchange of information, opportunity to sharpen skills, and development of leadership ability.
- Three reasons to use parliamentary procedure during an organizational meeting are to maintain a sense of order, provide each member a chance to participate, and simplify matters.
- Motions used in parliamentary procedure include the main, amendment, and point of order.

Letter of Resignation

Date

Ms./Mr.________________
Supervisor
Agency Name
Address
City, State, Zip Code

Dear Ms./Mr.________________

It is now necessary for me to terminate my employment with the_________ __________________________________ agency. I have learned a great deal from my association with the organization and appreciate having had the opportunity to work with you and the other staff members.

To allow 2 weeks for hiring a replacement, I will be glad to work until_______ __________________________________. If there is any way I can help with the transition, please let me know.

Sincerely,

Employee Name
Address
City, State, Zip Code
Phone Number

FIGURE 6-12 Letter of resignation.

- The purpose of the job application, resumé, portfolio, interview, and resignation is to find and obtain a job that matches the needs of the employee and employer.
- Five rules for completing a job application are to use black ink, check spelling, do not leave blanks, use positive language, and provide a reliable contact number.
- The components of a personal budget are shelter, food, clothing, transportation, medical, dues, charities, education, entertainment, and savings.

Review Questions

1. Explain two purposes of a professional organization.
2. List three advantages of using parliamentary procedure during organizational meetings.
3. Use Table 6-2 to determine the correct way to interrupt a speaker during a meeting.
4. List at least five important items of information needed on a job application.
5. Compose at least five questions that might be asked during a job interview, and outline appropriate responses.
6. Answer at least three behavioral interview questions from Box 6-10 using the STAR, SHARE, or PAR model.
7. List two reasons why an employee might be offered advancement on a job.
8. List two reasons why an employee might be dismissed from a job.
9. Make a personal budget for both 1 month and 1 year.

Critical Thinking

1. Use the Internet to take a career inventory to choose an occupation.
2. Use the Internet to investigate and write a paragraph that describes your present choice in a career and its benefits.
3. Prepare a resumé.
4. Describe two ways that a person might think about being rejected for a job.
5. Write a paragraph that describes the benefits of one type of leadership style.
6. Attend a meeting of a professional organization or legislative body to view the procedures used and behavior of group members. Write a paragraph that describes whether the behavior was beneficial for conducting business.
7. Practice using parliamentary procedure by holding a meeting of the student organization.
8. Conduct a mock interview with a class member.
9. Use the Internet to research, compare, and contrast investment opportunities.
10. Describe how healthy relationships influence career goals.

Explore the Web

Student Organizations

HOSA
http://hosa.org

SkillUSA
http://www.skillsusa.org/

Resume Template

About.com
http://jobsearch.about.com/od/teenstudentgrad/a/studentresume.htm

Career Information

American Medical Association
http://www.ama-assn.org/ama/pub/education-careers/careers-health-care/directory.shtml

Career Inventory

Career Link
http://www.mpcfaculty.net/CL/cl.htm

STANDARDS AND ACCOUNTABILITY*

Foundation Standard 4: Employability Skills

Health care professionals will understand how employability skills enhance their employment opportunities and job satisfaction. They will demonstrate key employability skills and will maintain and upgrade skills, as needed.

Accountability Criteria

4.1 Personal Traits of the Health Care Professional

4.11 Classify the personal traits and attitudes desirable in a member of the health care team.

4.12 Summarize professional standards as they apply to hygiene, dress, language, confidentiality, and behavior.

4.2 Employability Skills

4.21 Apply employability skills in health care.

4.3 Career Decision-making

4.31 Discuss levels of education, credentialing requirements, and employment trends in health care.

4.32 Compare careers within the health science career pathways (diagnostic services, therapeutic services, health informatics, support services, or biotechnology research and development).

4.4 Employability Preparation

4.41 Develop components of a personal portfolio.

4.42 Demonstrate the process for obtaining employment.

*From the National Consortium for Health Science Education (2009). National Health Care Standards and Accountability Criteria. Available at: http://www.healthscienceconsortium.org.

SKILL LIST 6-1
Preparing a Letter of Application

1. Address the letter to the person who will conduct the interview or make the hiring decision.
2. Type the letter using a standard business correspondence format.
3. Proofread and correct any errors of spelling or grammar.
4. Include three paragraphs. Express interest in applying for the position, supply brief information regarding qualifications, and provide a method by which you may be reached to schedule an interview.
5. Include your name, mailing address, phone number, and e-mail address in the closing.
6. Include a personal data sheet or resumé with the letter.

SKILL LIST 6-2
Completing a Job Application

1. Obtain the application form from the employing agency. If applications do not need to be completed on-site, take two. The first may be completed as a draft and reviewed by another person before submitting a final version.
2. Print in black ink or type all items on the application accurately and neatly. Be consistent with the type of lettering used.
3. Do not leave any blanks or spaces to demonstrate thoroughness in the application completion. Draw

Continued

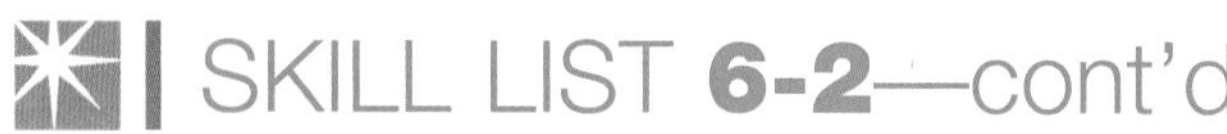

SKILL LIST **6-2**—cont'd
Completing a Job Application

a single line "em dash" or write "not applicable" or "N/A" if the item does not apply to you.

4. Use positive language to account for any periods of not working or attending school.
5. Account for any employment termination in a positive manner. For example, "reduction in force" or "better employment opportunity" would be more positive than "laid off" or "quit."
6. Answer questions on acceptable salary as "open" if the amount is negotiable or unknown.
7. Provide a phone number that will be answered by someone promptly. The employer will not make many attempts to contact a new applicant for an interview or to offer employment.
8. Submit the application before the deadline or closing of the position offering.

SKILL LIST **6-3**
Preparing a Resumé

1. Use only the information that presents you in the best light for the personal data sheet or resumé.
2. Head the resumé with your name, address, phone number, and e-mail address.
3. Divide the resumé into categories of information. For example, categories may include coursework, activities, skills, work experience, awards, and career goals. Use only one side of one sheet of paper.
4. List any chronological information, such as work dates, in order with the most recent listed first.
5. Type the resumé neatly without any errors. Center the information from the top to the bottom of the paper.
6. Include three references in alphabetical order by last name. Include name, address, telephone number, and e-mail address.
7. Make additional copies of your resumé to send with letters of application and to take to interviews.

SKILL LIST **6-4**
Interviewing

1. Dress appropriately for the interview. The type of dress will depend on the job being sought but should be neat, clean, and conservative. Come prepared with information such as social security number and employment history to complete the application form.
2. Arrive 5 minutes early to the interview. The interviewer may have other appointments scheduled. If the application must be completed at the time of the interview, allow additional time for that before the scheduled interview time.
3. Greet the receptionist politely. Many employers consider the receptionist's opinion of applicants in making a hiring decision.
4. Present yourself in a positive and confident manner. Always go alone to the interview.
5. Remain standing until asked to sit down. Shake hands firmly with the interviewer during

Continued

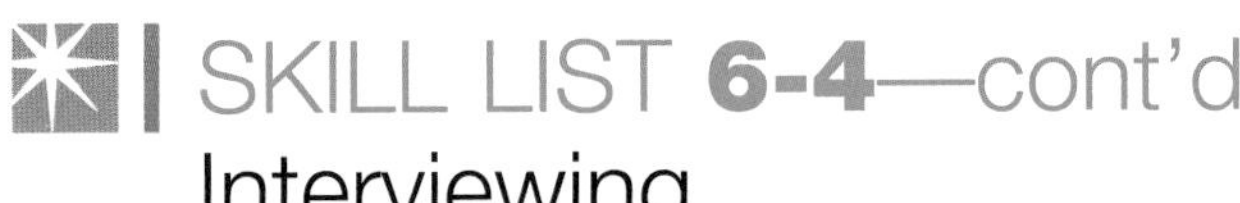

SKILL LIST 6-4—cont'd
Interviewing

introductions. Place any materials on the floor or on your lap, not on the interviewer's desk.

6. Sit comfortably but conservatively, with a straight back and feet on the floor or legs crossed at the ankles.
7. Answer questions completely, in a positive manner, using more than one-word responses. The interview allows the applicant to demonstrate the ability to communicate well.
8. Maintain eye contact when answering questions. Be enthusiastic but not overbearing.
9. Ask questions if some were unanswered during the interview. Questions show the interviewer that the applicant is interested and has been thinking during the interview. Before leaving, ask when the position will be determined and how you will be notified.
10. Thank the interviewer for his or her time, and shake hands on leaving.
11. When the interview is finished, leave the building. The interviewer may be expecting other applicants.

CHAPTER 7

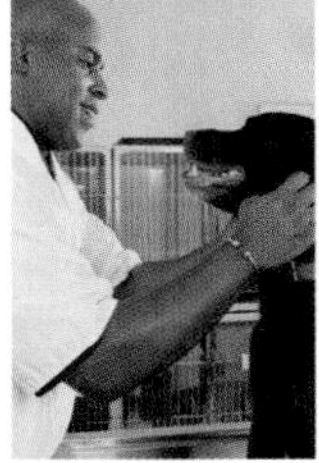

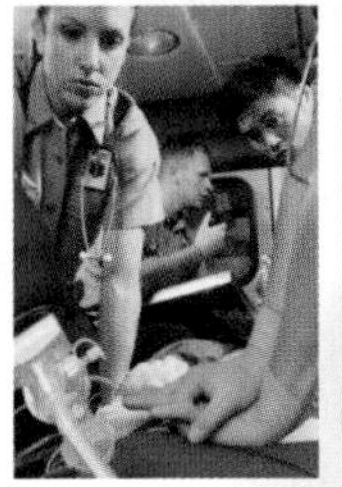

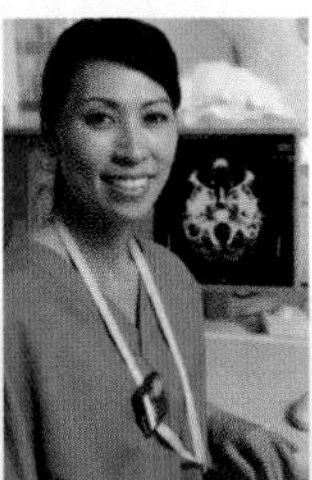

Foundation Skills

LEARNING OBJECTIVES

- Spell and define the key terms.
- Describe the elements of basic health assessment.
- Identify normal and abnormal vital sign values.
- Describe the importance of the values for normal vital signs.
- Perform basic mathematical skills related to health care.
- Use basic medical terminology and abbreviations.
- Identify risk factors for cardiac arrest.

KEY TERMS

Apical *(AYP-i-kul)* Pertaining to the apex or pointed end of the heart

Auscultation *(os-kuhl-TAY-shen)* Act of listening for sounds within the body

Blood pressure *(blud presh-er)* Pressure of circulating blood against the walls of the arteries

Cardiac arrest *(KAR-dee-ak uh-REST)* Sudden stopping of heart action

Diastolic *(die-uh-STAHL-ik)* Blood pressure during ventricular relaxation

Integer *(IN-te-jer)* Whole number, positive or negative, and zero

Palpation *(pal-PAY-shen)* Technique used to feel the texture, size, consistency, and location of parts of the body with the hands

Percussion *(per-KUSH-en)* Technique of tapping with the fingertips to evaluate size, borders, and consistency of internal structures of the body

Rational *(RASH-a-nal)* Number that can be shown as an integer or fraction

Systolic *(sis-TOL-ik)* Blood pressure during ventricular contraction

Vital *(VY-tul)* Necessary to life

Health Assessment

Patient Interview and Examination

The basic health assessment may include an interview and physical examination to determine functional, cultural, spiritual, and physical characteristics (Table 7-1). Basic health assessment may be the responsibility of many health care workers and is an ongoing process. The type and extent of assessment are determined by the role of the worker and the type of care being given. Some health care workers, such as the nurse assistant and licensed practical nurse, may collect data that will be analyzed and evaluated by another health care worker, such as the registered nurse.

TABLE 7-1
Physical Assessment

Assessment	Observations
Appearance	Physical, developmental, social development; general health; significant features; height, weight, posture; communication skills; grooming and hygiene
Hair	Color, texture, cleanliness, distribution
Nails	Color, texture, markings, shape, size
Skin	Color, temperature, turgor, lesions, mucous membranes, injury, edema
Neurological	Pupil reaction to light; motor and verbal responses; reflexes, gait, orientation
Musculoskeletal	Range of motion, gait, posture, injury
Cardiovascular	Heart rate and rhythm, peripheral pulses, temperature
Respiratory	Rate, rhythm, quality, breath sounds, sputum production or cough
Gastrointestinal	Abdominal contour, bowel sounds, nausea or vomiting, defecation frequency and consistency
Genitourinary	Urine color, amount, frequency, odor, clarity

The initial patient interview may include the health history, nature of the current complaint, and medication record. The medical or health history gathers subjective information about the patient's health. The physical assessment uses techniques of inspection, auscultation, palpation, percussion, and smell (Table 7-2). Visual observations are used for inspection. **Auscultation** means listening to sounds, often with a stethoscope (Fig. 7-1). **Palpation** is using the hands to observe structures by touch (Fig. 7-2). **Percussion** is striking the body to assess the sound made (Fig. 7-3). The patient is positioned according to physician orders and for comfort during assessment (Fig. 7-4). Information that is gathered during the initial or admission health assessment is used to develop a nursing care plan (see Fig. II-3 in Appendix II on pp. 587–588). (See Skill List 7-1, Admitting, Transferring, and Discharging the Patient; and Skill List 7-2, Recording Observations, pp. 125–126).

CASE STUDY 7-1 While giving daily care to a patient, you notice the odor of alcohol from the patient's mouth. What should you do?

Answers to Case Studies are available on the Evolve website: ***http://evolve.elsevier.com/Gerdin***

Vital Signs

Vital signs or life signs are values that can be used to measure changes in body function, general health,

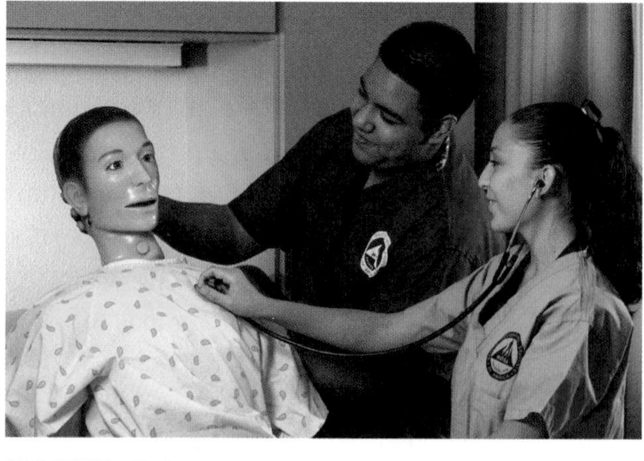

FIGURE 7-1 Students use manikins to demonstrate assessment skills during Health Occupations Students of America (HOSA) competition. (Photo courtesy National HOSA, Flower Mound, Tex.)

TABLE 7-2
Characteristic Odors*

Area	Smell	Possible Cause
Mouth	Alcohol	Drinking alcohol
	Bad breath (halitosis)	Poor dental hygiene, gum disease
	Fruity, sweet	Diabetes acidosis, medication
	Feces	Intestinal obstruction
	Acid breath	Peptic ulcer
	Rotten eggs, garlic	Cirrhosis, medication
	Ammonia	Kidney failure
Rectal area	Feces	Incontinence
Skin (under arms and breasts)	Foul, body odor	Poor hygiene, excessive sweating
	Stale urine	Uremic acidosis
Skin (under cast)	Musty	Infection
Tracheostomy	Sweet, fetid	Bacterial infection (*pseudomonas*)
Urine	Ammonia	Urinary tract infection
	Foul	Urinary tract infection
Vomit	Feces	Bowel obstruction
Wound site	Feces	Abscess
	Sweet, heavy	Bacterial infection (*pseudomonas*)

*Odor may also be due to food eaten, medication, and hygiene practices.

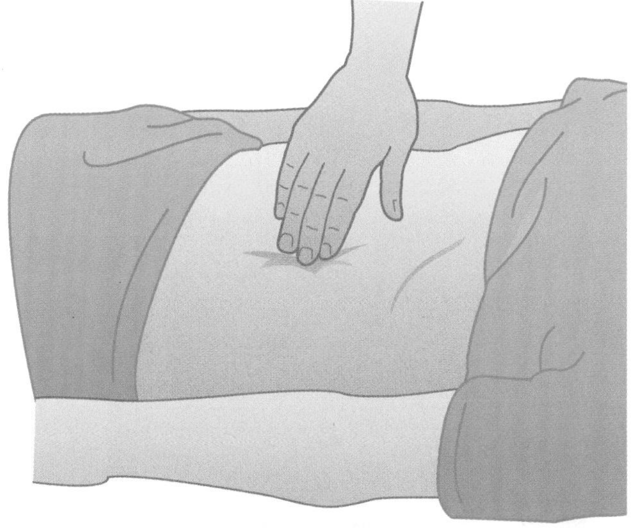

FIGURE 7-2 Touch or palpation is used during the health assessment. (From Bonewit-West K, Hunt S, Applegate E: *Today's medical assistant: clinical & administrative procedures,* St. Louis, 2009, Saunders.)

and the response to treatment. Vital signs include blood pressure (BP) and temperature, pulse, and respiration (TPR). The value of vital signs is affected by many factors, including age, activity, nutrition, emotion, fitness, medication, and illness. Height (ht), weight (wt), and fluid balance or intake and output (I&O) also may be used to assess the patient.

Vital signs are ordered with different frequency depending on the type of service being provided. Common orders for assessment include twice a day (bid), three times a day (tid), four times a day (qid), or routinely once a day (qd). Vitals may be ordered at regular intervals such as every 4 hours (q4h) or every 15 minutes (q15m).

CASE STUDY 7-2 You notice a patient is scratching her arm repeatedly while you complete daily care. What should you do?

Answers to Case Studies are available on the Evolve website: ***http://evolve.elsevier.com/Gerdin***

Blood Pressure

Blood pressure (BP) is a measurement of the force of the blood against the walls of the arteries as it circulates through the body. It reflects the effort the heart exerts to circulate the blood to the tissues. Two units or values for BP are measured: the maximum pressure at which the pulse can be heard (**systolic**) and the minimum pressure at which it is audible (**diastolic**). The systolic reading occurs while the ventricles of the heart are contracting. The diastolic reading occurs during relaxation of the ventricles. Instruments that

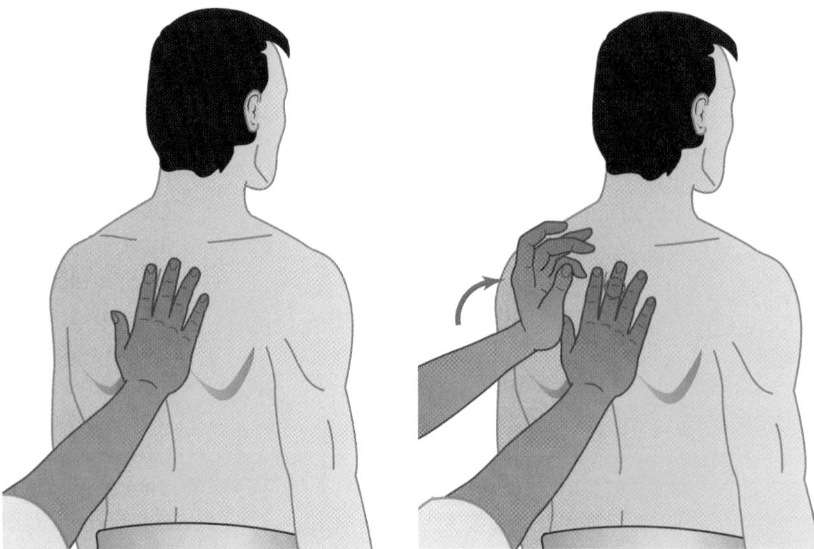

FIGURE 7-3 Assessment by percussion involves evaluating the sound produced by tapping the patient. (From Bonewit-West K, Hunt S, Applegate E: *Today's medical assistant: clinical & administrative procedures,* St. Louis, 2009, Saunders.)

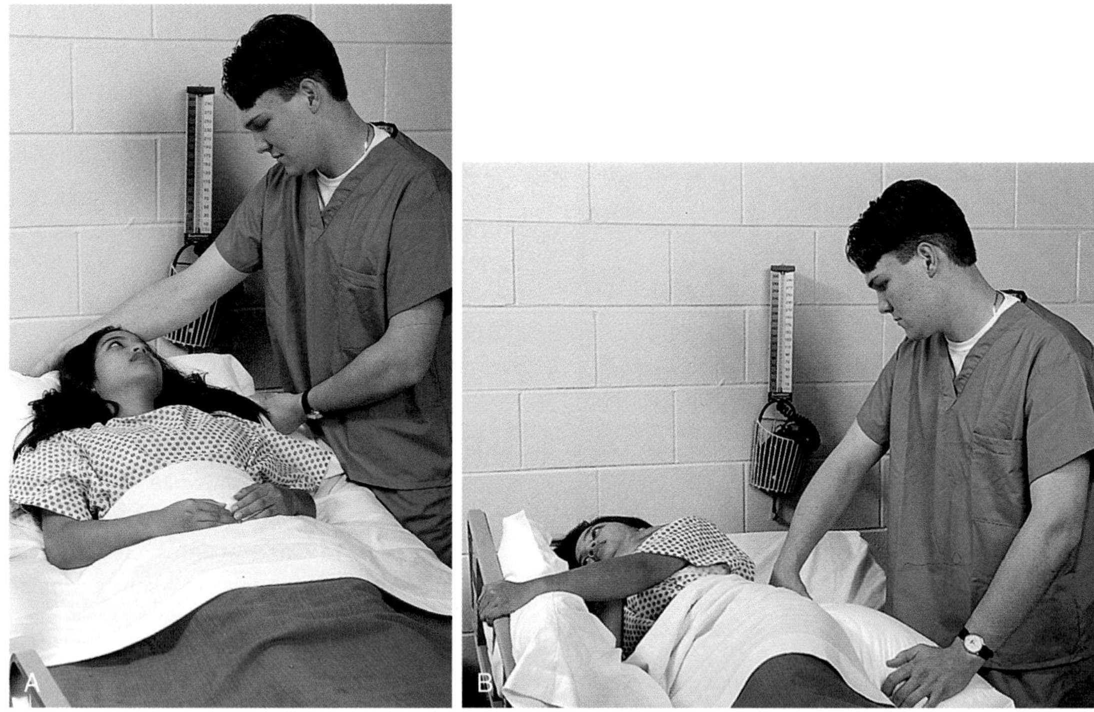

FIGURE 7-4 **A,** The procedure is explained to the patient before being performed. **B,** The bed is raised to a comfortable working height while assisting the patient to turn but returned to the lowest level when done.

are used to determine the blood pressure are the stethoscope and sphygmomanometer (Fig. 7-5). The stethoscope amplifies the sound. The sphygmomanometer is an inflatable cuff that uses air (aneroid) or a liquid to measure pressure. Automated cuffs may be used to measure BP using the radial artery of the wrist (Fig. 7-6). Mercury is no longer used in thermometers because of its environmental and safety risks, but sphygmomanometers containing mercury are still in use.

Blood pressure varies greatly among people. It is affected by the diameter and flexibility (elasticity) of the blood vessels, force of the heart contraction, and amount of blood in the vessels. Pressure on the area

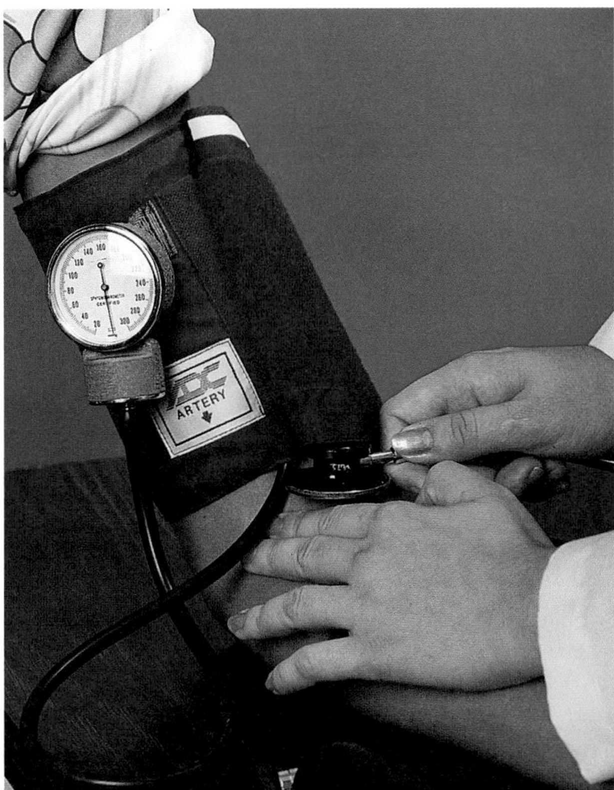

FIGURE 7-5 The brachial artery is found to determine the correct placement of the stethoscope.

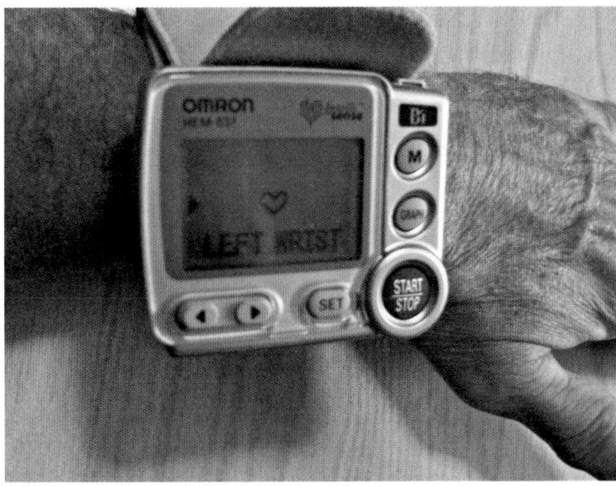

FIGURE 7-6 Blood pressure can be measured using several pulse points including the radial artery.

of the brain that controls BP can also change its value. Limits of the usual blood pressure for most individuals have been set. "Normal" blood pressure is commonly said to be 120/80 (systolic/diastolic) (Box 7-1). The range of BP is acceptable with a systolic pressure less than 119 and a diastolic pressure less than 80. (See Skill List 7-3, Taking a Blood Pressure, pp. 126–127).

BOX 7-1

Recommended Blood Pressure Levels

■ Normal value	119/79 or below
■ Prehypertension	120-139/80-89
■ High	140/90 or above

From the Joint National Committee (JNC7) on Prevention, Detection, Evaluation, and Treatment of High Blood Pressure, DHHS, 2003.

BRAIN BYTE

According to the CDC, about a fifth of the people with high blood pressure do not know it.

CASE STUDY 7-3 You are taking vital signs on patients during morning rounds. You assess a blood pressure of 184/144 for one patient. What should you do?

Answers to Case Studies are available on the Evolve website: ***http://evolve.elsevier.com/Gerdin***

Temperature

Temperature is the measurement of the balance between the heat produced and lost by the body. Several methods are used to measure temperature. They include the mouth (oral), armpit (axillary), rectum (rectal), ear (temporal), and by infrared radiation (Fig. 7-7). Temperature may be measured with the Fahrenheit or Celsius (Centigrade) scale. The normal reading for temperature depends on the location used to assess it (Table 7-3). An elevation of temperature (fever) may indicate infection or inflammation in the body.

Several types of thermometers are available for measuring temperature. The most common type is made of glass with an expandable liquid filling. Glass thermometers are designed differently for oral or rectal use. The bulb of the rectal thermometer is rounded to prevent injury to the tissues of the rectum. The tip of the stem of the rectal thermometer is red, and that of the oral thermometer is blue or silver for easy identification (Fig. 7-8). Rectal thermometers should never be used in the mouth. Mercury thermometers are not commonly used because of environmental and health hazards resulting from the possibility of spilling mercury. Electronic and disposable chemical thermometers are used. (See Skill List

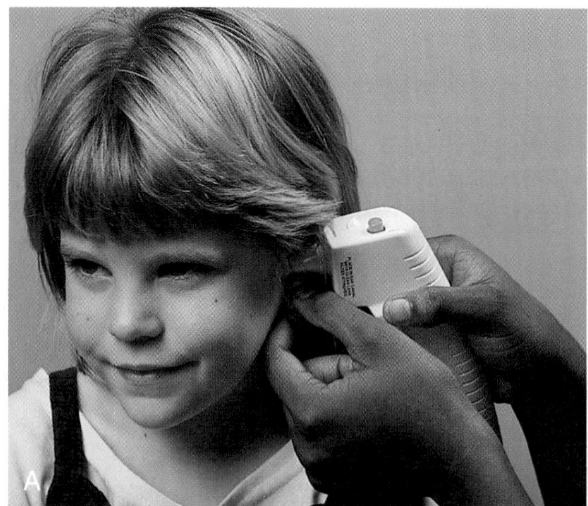

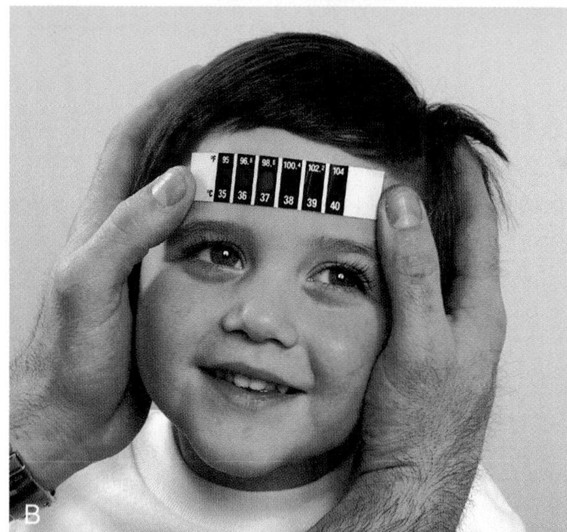

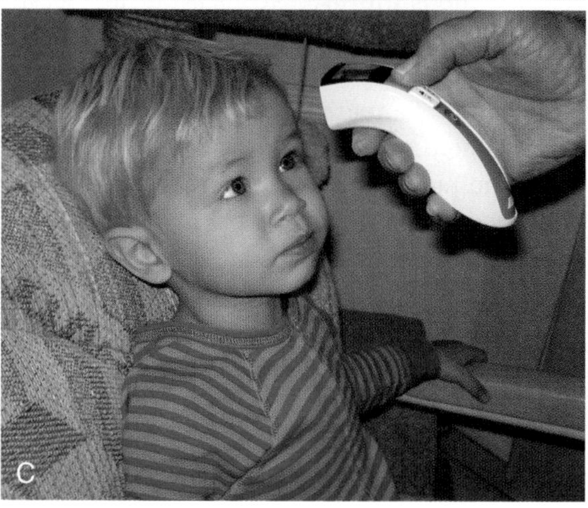

FIGURE 7-7 **A,** A tympanic thermometer may be used to assess temperature. **B,** Temperature strips may be used for young children. **C,** Infrared thermometers measure temperature without touching the patient.

TABLE 7-3
Temperature

Method	Time	Normal
Oral	3 min*	97.6°-99.0° F (98.6° F = 37.0° C)
Axillary	10 min*	96.6°-98.0° F (97.6° F = 36.4° C)
Rectal	3-5 min*	98.6°-100.0° F (99.6° F = 37.5° C)
Temporal	*	96.4°-100.4° F (98.4° F = 36.9° C)
Infrared	*	97.6°-99.0° F (98.6° F = 37.0° C)

*Time required to take temperatures may vary with the electrical instruments and is usually signaled by a sound from the device.

7-4, Taking an Oral Temperature; Skill List 7-5, Taking an Axillary Temperature; Skill List 7-6, Taking a Rectal Temperature; and Skill List 7-7, Taking an Infrared Temperature, pp. 127–130).

Pulse and Respiration

Pulse is the heartbeat that can be felt (palpated) on surface arteries as the artery walls expand. The pulse rate is usually counted using the radial artery near the wrist, but it may be found in other locations (Fig. 7-9).

The rate of the heartbeat must be adequate to supply blood and its nutrients to all parts of the body. The pulse of an infant is significantly faster than that of an adult (Table 7-4). The normal adult pulse rate can range between 60 and 100 beats per minute. In addition to the rate, it is important to assess the rhythm and character of the pulse. A regular rhythm is evenly paced. An irregular pulse may be fast or slow or may skip beats. Character, describing the force of the pulse, may be strong, weak, bounding, thready, feeble, or fleeting. (See Skill List 7-8, Taking a Radial Pulse and Measuring Respiration, p. 130).

The pulse can be counted by listening to the heart through a stethoscope placed on the chest. This pulse is called an **apical** pulse (Fig. 7-10). The apical pulse may differ from the radial pulse in some conditions that affect the peripheral blood flow. (See Skill List 7-8, Taking a Radial Pulse and Measuring Respiration, p. 130).

One respiration includes the inspiration and expiration of a breath. The normal rate for respiration is more rapid in infants than adults (Box 7-2). The rhythm and character of respiration are important

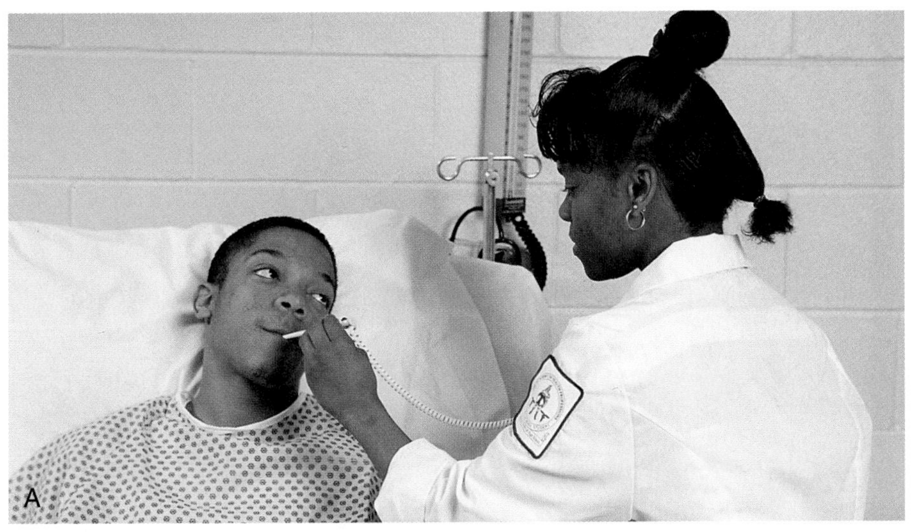

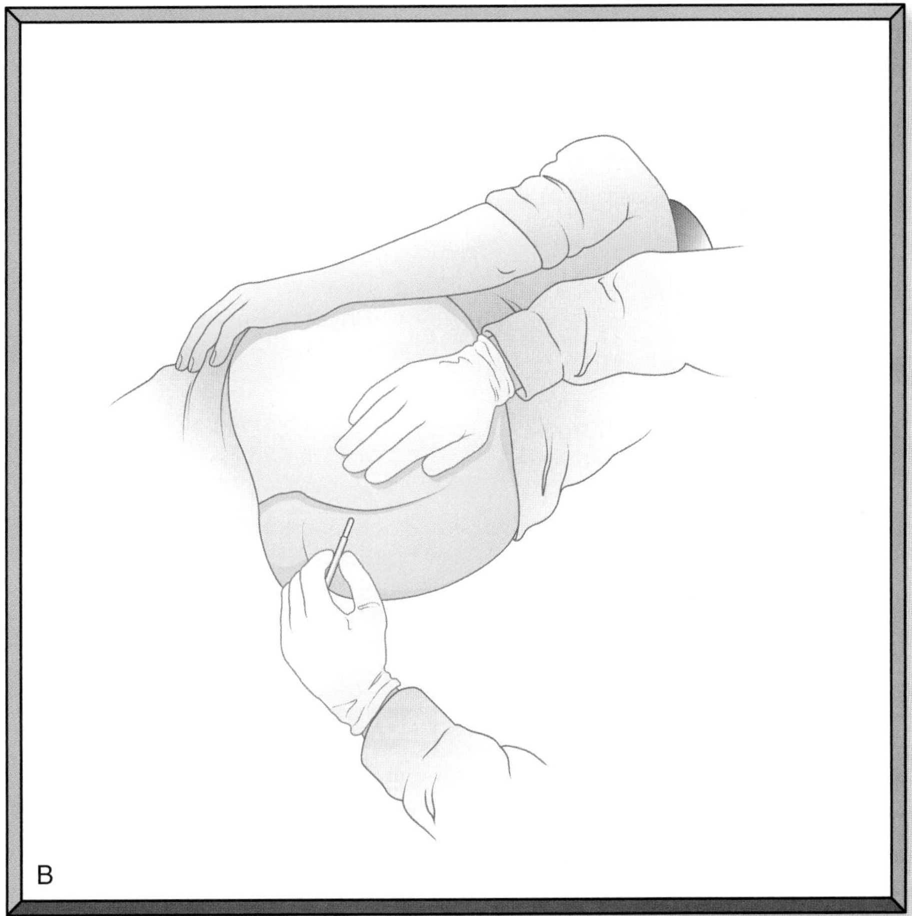

FIGURE 7-8 **A,** During the assessment of an oral temperature, the mouth should remain closed. **B,** Privacy is a primary consideration during assessment of the rectal temperature.

observations. The rhythm of respiration describes its regularity. Character describes the depth and quality of the sound. Respirations that are difficult to see may be assessed by feeling the rise (expansion) and fall (contraction) of the chest or by using the stethoscope to listen for the respiratory or breath sounds.

Height and Weight

Health professionals use charts that are developed by insurance companies to determine healthy weight (Fig. 7-11). The insurance companies determine at which weight for a specific height an individual is

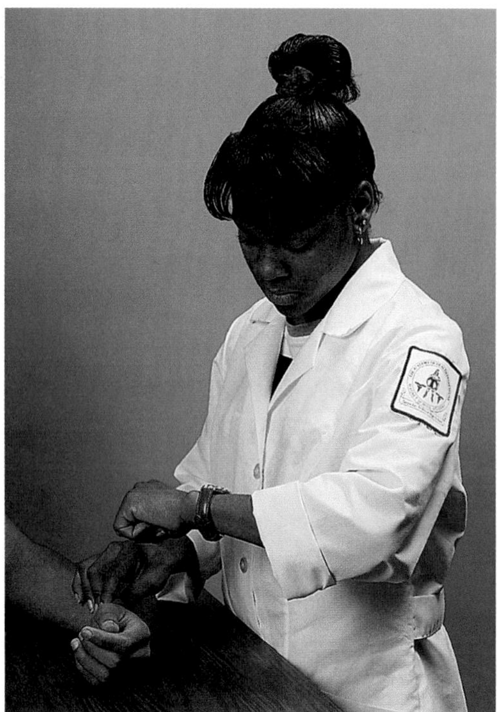

FIGURE 7-9 Pulse and respiration are assessed at the same time.

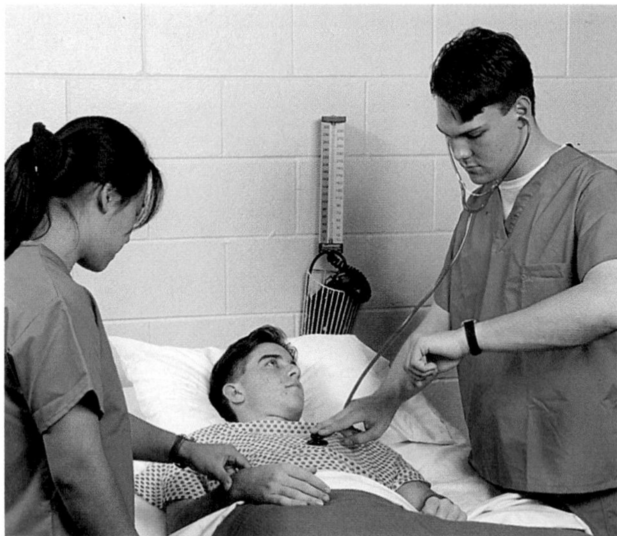

FIGURE 7-10 Taking of an apical and radial pulse at the same time may be necessary with some circulatory disorders.

TABLE 7-4
Pulse Ranges by Age Group

Age Group	Normal Pulse Rates (Beats/Min)	Abnormal Pulse Rates (Beats/Min)
Newborn	70-170	
Infant	80-130	
School age	70-110	
Adult	60-100	<60 (bradycardia) >100 (tachycardia)

BOX 7-2

Respiration in Adults

- Rate per minute: 14-20
- Rhythm: Regular
- Character: Effortless, deep, quiet
- Abnormal parameters
  - Tachypnea >24
  - Bradypnea <10
  - Shallow
  - Stertorous (snoring)
  - Apnea
  - Cheyne-Stokes

predicted to live the longest (Fig. 7-12). According to the National Heart, Lung, and Blood Institute, an ideal weight is having a body mass index between 18.7 and 24.9 (Box 7-3). More information about weight and nutrition may be found in Chapter 8.

BOX 7-3

Body Mass Index Formula

Weight (lb)/height (in)^2 × 703

CASE STUDY 7-4 You are asked to take a patient's vital signs. When you enter the room, the patient is eating breakfast. What should you do?

Answers to Case Studies are available on the Evolve website: ***http://evolve.elsevier.com/Gerdin***

Information Exchange

Basic Math

Many of the procedures performed by the health care worker include mathematics. For example, the conversion of medication dosages to calculate the correct dosage may be one of the responsibilities of the

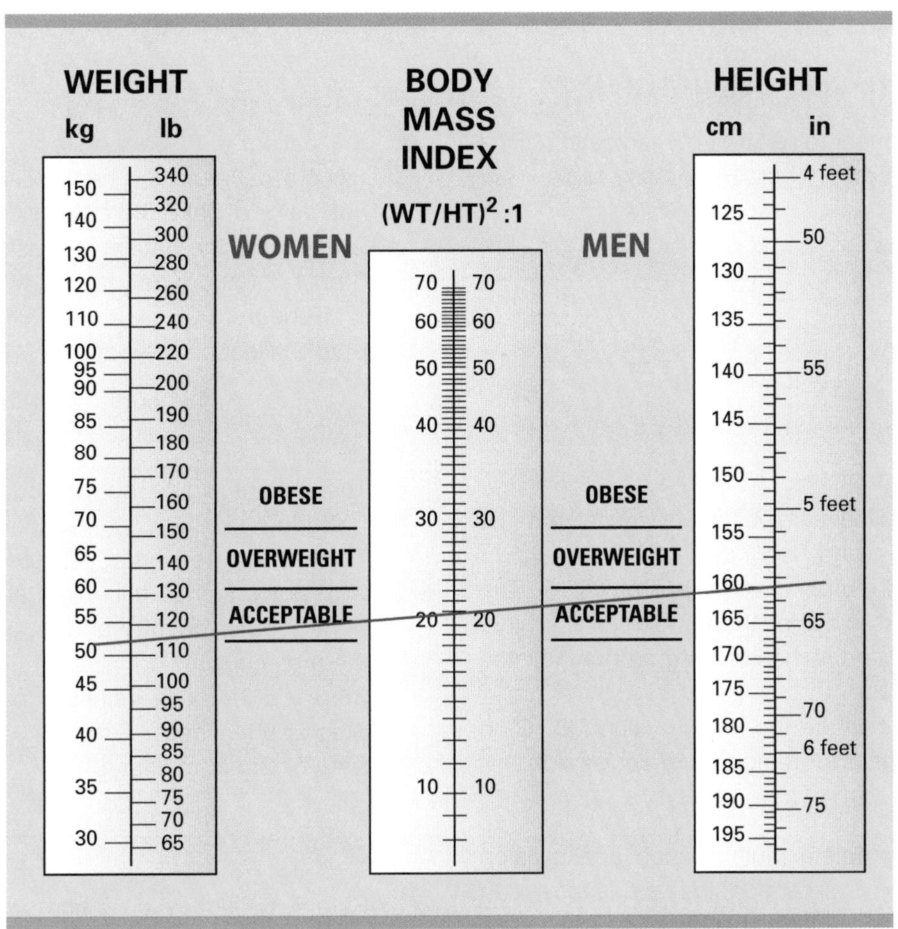

FIGURE 7-11 A height and weight chart including body mass index.

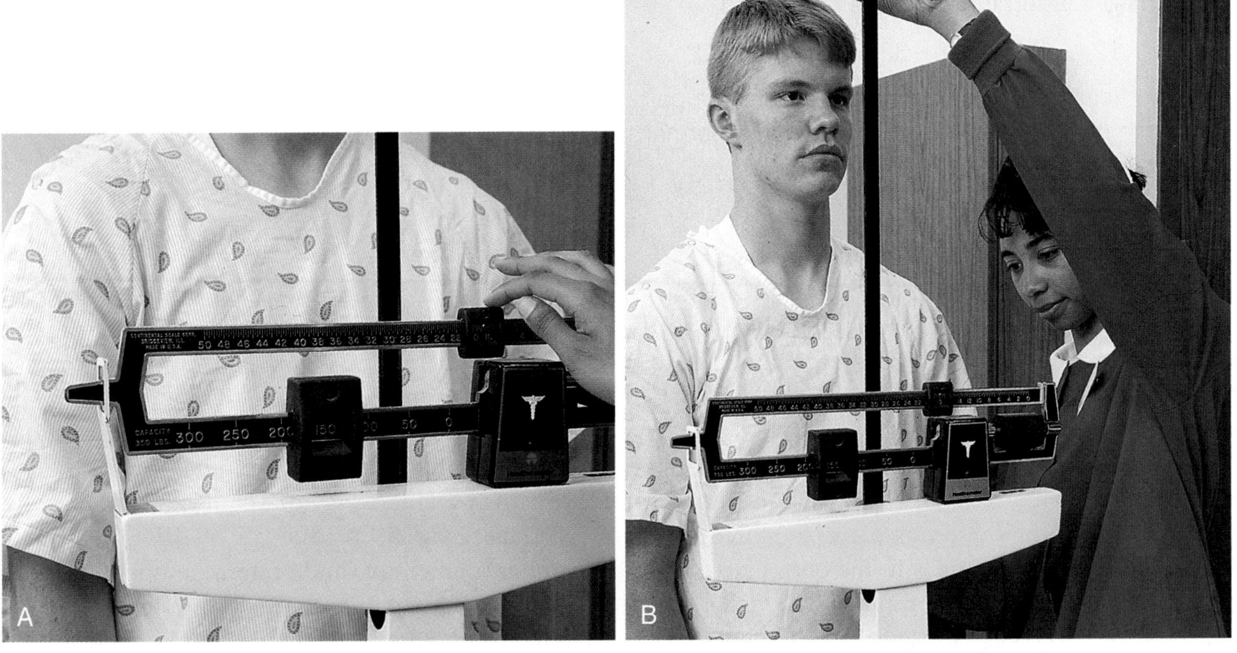

FIGURE 7-12 This patient is being measured for weight **(A)** and height **(B)**.

BOX 7-4

Metric Conversion Using Ratios

1. A tablet is marked as "5 gr of medication." The order is to give 15 gr. How many tablets are given?

   Step 1: $\frac{5\text{ gr}}{1\text{ tab}} = \frac{15\text{ gr}}{?\text{ tab}}$

   Step 2: Multiply each fraction by ? tab

   $$5\text{ gr} \times ? = 15\text{ gr}$$

   Step 3: Divide each fraction by 5 gr

   $$? = 3$$

   The dose would be 3 tablets. (Note that the units "gr" and "tab") cancel.
2. A patient's temperature is read as 36° C. The patient asks whether the temperature is high. What should the health care worker tell the patient?

   Step 1: Substitute the known value (36° C) in the formula for temperature conversion.

   $$F = 9/5\,(36) + 32$$

   Step 2: Complete multiplication and division functions before addition and subtraction unless the addition or subtraction is in parentheses.

   $$(9 \times 36)/5 = 64.8$$

   Step 3: Complete addition after multiplication and division functions are completed.

   $$F = 64.8 + 32 = 96.8$$

   The health care worker should assure the patient that the temperature is within normal limits.
3. If a patient is to be assisted to walk qid (four times a day) and the health care worker does not want to wake the patient during the night, when could the patient be assisted to walk?

   Step 1: 24 hours per day – 8 hours per night = 16 hours

   Step 2: Reduce the fraction.

   $$\frac{16\text{ hours}}{4\text{ walks}} = \frac{4\text{ hours}}{1\text{ walk}}$$

   The patient would be walked every 4 hours during the day.
4. The health care worker tells the patient that he is 5 feet 9 inches tall. The patient says he is from another country and would like to know the metric value.

   Step 1: 5 feet × 12 inches/1 foot = 60 inches

   Step 2: 60 inches + 9 inches = 69 inches

   Step 3: Cross-multiply

   $$\frac{69\text{ inches}}{?\text{ cm}} = \frac{1\text{ inch}}{2.54\text{ cm}}$$

   Step 4: 69 inches × 2.54 cm = 175.26 cm
5. The health care worker tells the patient that he weighs 160 lb. The patient says he is from another country and would like to know the metric value.

   Step 1: Cross-multiply

   $$\frac{160\text{ lbs}}{?\text{ kg}} = \frac{1\text{ lb}}{0.45\text{ kg}}$$

   Step 2: 160 × 0.45 = 72 kg

personnel administering them. The health care worker must be able to use the traditional, apothecary, and International System of Units (SI, metric) to measure time, temperature, distance, capacity (volume), and mass.

The place value or position of a digit or **integer** determines its value. For example, in the number 234, the two is in the hundreds place, the three is in the tens place, and the four is in the ones place. The number is the sum of two hundreds, three tens, and four ones, or 234. Numbers that can be shown as a whole number or a fraction are called **rational** numbers.

Addition and subtraction are methods for counting, resulting in a sum or difference between amounts. Multiplication and division perform addition and subtraction more quickly and result in a product or quotient. A fraction is a comparison of part of a whole to the entire unit. For example, ¼ indicates that the quantity being considered is 1 of 4 equal parts of the whole. Fractions may be "reduced" by dividing the top number (numerator) and bottom number (denominator) by the same number. For example, ²⁄₄ is equal to ½. In health care, fractions or ratios often are used to calculate medications, determine temperature, or determine a schedule for the patient's care (Box 7-4).

Three systems of measurement are used in health care. They are the apothecary, SI (metric), and household units. The health care worker should be familiar with all three systems to be able to convert from one to another when necessary (Table 7-5).

Military Time

Some countries, the military, and the health care industry use a 24-hour system to measure time. In this system the hours are numbered from 0 to 24, with noon being 12:00 (Fig. 7-13). Using the morning (AM) and evening (PM) designation is unnecessary because there are no times with the same number. For example, 15:00 is the same as 3:00 PM. The use of a 24-hour time system in health care eliminates many chances for error in treatment.

Graphing

Graphs may be used to interpret data visually. Four types of graphs are the bar graph, pie chart, pictograph, and line graph (Fig. 7-14). The line graph is commonly used to chart vital signs in health care. To read a graph, it must first be analyzed. The title tells what information is being depicted in the graph. The value or scale of each of the measurements is shown on the vertical and horizontal axes of the graph. (See Skill List 7-9, Constructing a Line Graph, pp. 130–131.)

Computer Literacy

Computers are electronic equipment that store, manipulate, and retrieve information according to a program (software). The software may allow the computer user to create a document of words, change images, play a game, and use many other applications. Some special applications are designed to input and retrieve information that is used in health care. The program is placed or loaded into the working space (memory) of the equipment. Computer hardware is the physical equipment including the keyboard, central processing unit, viewing screen (monitor), disk drive, and disks. Different operating systems in computers interpret and display the data. They are some variation of Microsoft's Windows, Apple's Mac, or Unix/Linux.

The computer may have two types of memory available to store information (data): read only memory (ROM) and random access memory (RAM). Magnetic recording devices include internal or external disks. Internal disks are called the hard drive. External devices can be used to store information outside of the computer and include USB (thumb drives), CDs, and other drives. When connected to a printer, computers can output paper files. The

TABLE 7-5
Liquid and Solid Systems of Measurement

Metric	Apothecary	Household
Liquid Measurement		
0.06 mL	1 minim (min)	1 drop (gtt)
5 mL	1 fluid dram	1 teaspoon (tsp)
15 mL	3 fluid dram	1 tablespoon (tbs)
30 mL	1 fluid ounce (fl oz)	2 tbs
240 mL	8 fl oz	1 glass or cup
473 mL	16 fl oz	1 pint (pt)
1 liter (L)	32 fl oz	1 quart (qt)
	15 grains (gr)	15.4 grains (gr)
Solid Measurement		
1 gram (g)		
28.35 g	480 gr	1 ounce (oz)
31 g	1 ounce (oz)	437.5 gr
373 g	1 pound (lb)	0.75 pounds (lb)
454 g (0.454 kg)	1.33 lbs	1 lb
1 kg	2.7 lbs	2.2 lbs
Distance Measurement		
1 meter (m)		39.37 inches (in)
2.54 centimeter (cm)		1 in
1 cm		0.394 in

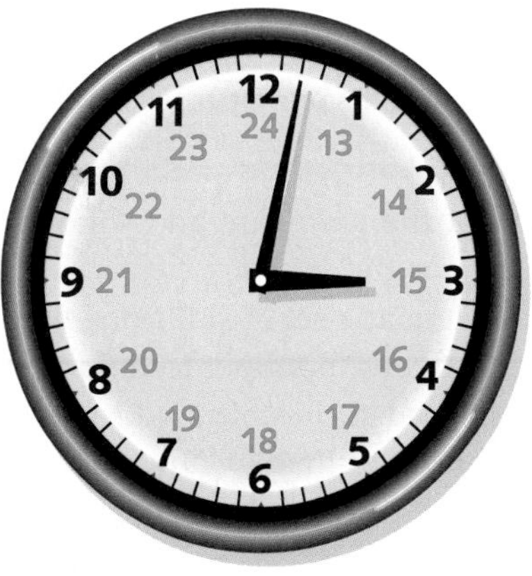

FIGURE 7-13 Using the 24-hour clock helps prevent confusion regarding the time when care is given.

AVERAGE GROWTH IN BOYS AND GIRLS

Growth in girls		Growth in boys	
Age	Growth in cm	Age	Growth in cm
2-3	8.6	2-3	8.3
3-4	7.6	3-4	7.4
4-5	6.8	4-5	6.8
5-6	6.4	5-6	6.4
6-7	6.1	6-7	6.0
7-8	5.9	7-8	5.8
8-9	5.7	8-9	5.4
9-10	5.8	9-10	5.2
10-11	6.7	10-11	5.1
11-12	8.3	11-12	5.3
12-13	5.9	12-13	6.8
13-14	3.0	13-14	9.5
14-15	0.9	14-15	6.5
15-16	0.1	15-16	3.3
16-17		16-17	1.5
17-18		17-18	0.5

A

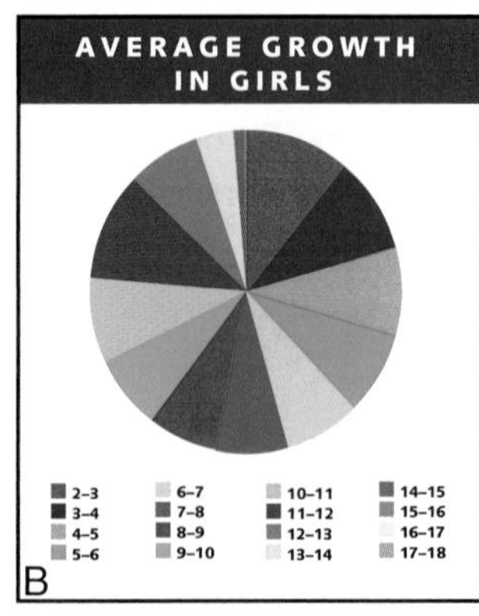

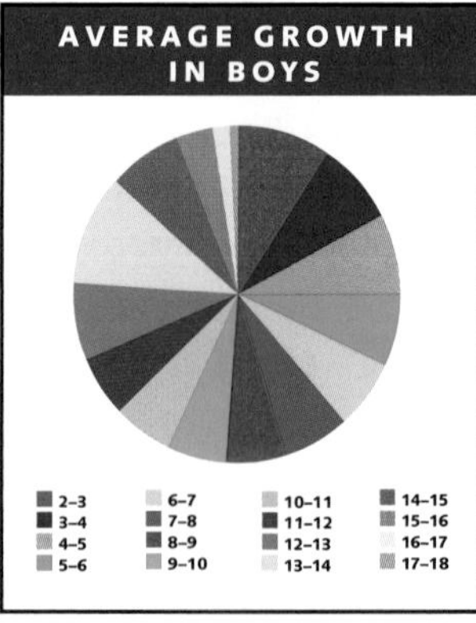

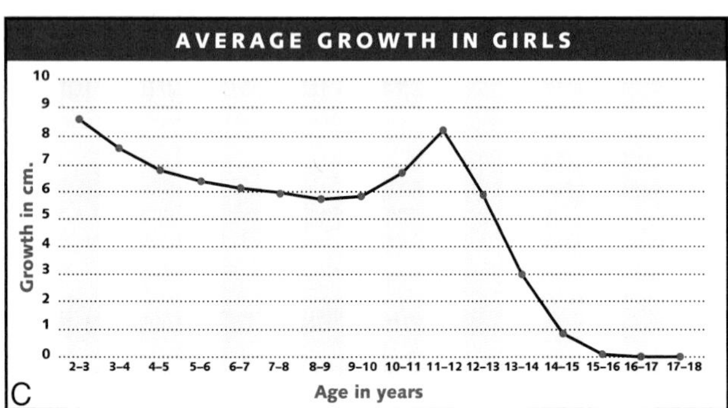

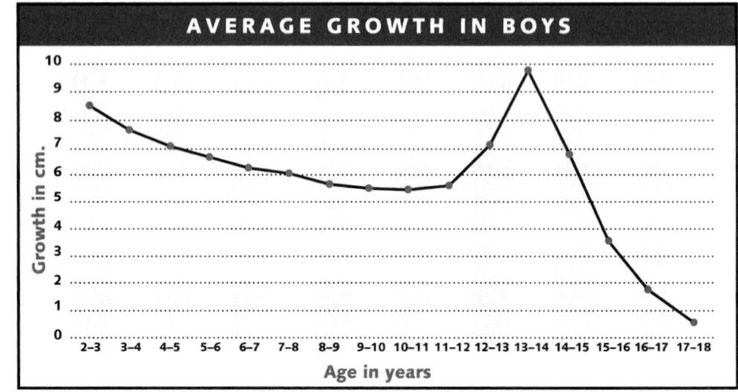

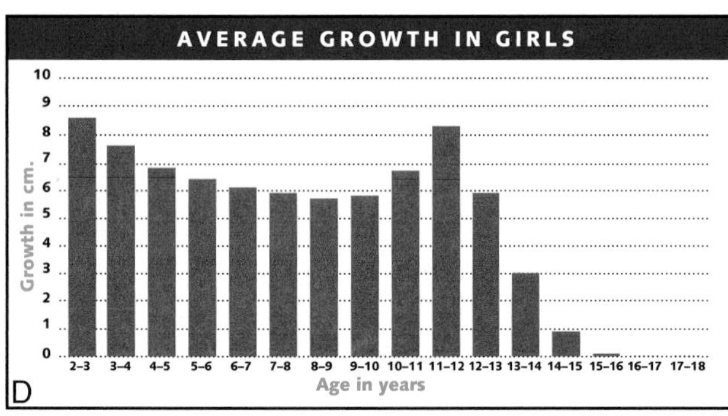

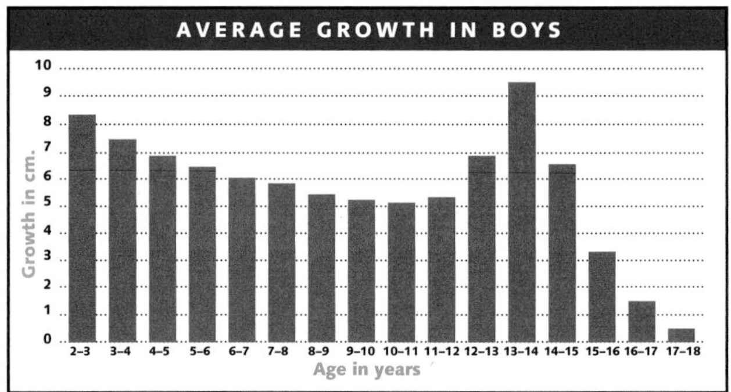

FIGURE 7-14 Graphs provide an easy way to show trends in data. **A,** Data chart. **B,** Pie chart. **C,** Line graph. **D,** Bar graph.

combination of the hardware and software is generally referred to as the *computer system.*

Keyboarding is the set of skills one needs to use a computer effectively. Improper technique in using the computer can lead to mistakes and repetitive strain injury (RSI) and eyestrain. Many different methods are available for learning keyboarding skills. Some keyboards are designed for teaching, such as those with color-coded keys. Free and commercial software is available to help learn the placement of the keys and improve typing speed and accuracy.

Computers are used in all aspects of health care. Laboratory tests and respiratory ventilators are run by computerized equipment. Magnetic resonance imaging (MRI) and heart monitoring equipment are computer driven. Information about patient services and charges for services are maintained on computer systems in most facilities. The health care worker must be able to enter and retrieve data from the computer to provide efficient care. Although each computer system has its own specifications for use, some basic rules apply to all units and programs (Box 7-5).

Personal digital assistants (PDAs) are handheld or mobile computers. They are increasingly being used in health care to record patient care and vital signs (Box 7-6). They can be used to research medical information or drug interactions. Benefits of PDA use include faster access to information and fewer billing errors. They also reduce the number of prescription errors caused by handwriting confusion. Often the information on a PDA is transmitted or "beamed" to another device, such a printer, wirelessly (Fig. 7-15). PDAs must meet HIPAA guidelines for privacy. They

BOX 7-5

Guidelines for Computer Users

- Computers use very little electricity. If the interval between periods of use is only 20 to 30 minutes, it is better to leave the hardware on than to turn it off.
- Computers and liquid do not mix. Beverages should be restricted from the computer area.
- Although computers may be shut down or turned off with the power switch, it is better to use the system program for shutdown.
- Compact disks must be handled with care. The information stored on the disk may be damaged by:
  - Excessive heat or cold
  - Fingerprints on the recording surface or imprints made by writing on the disk label
  - Bending
  - Magnets placed close to the surface
  - Dust, lint, and electrical static
  - Removing the disk from the drive when the light indicates that it is being read or written on

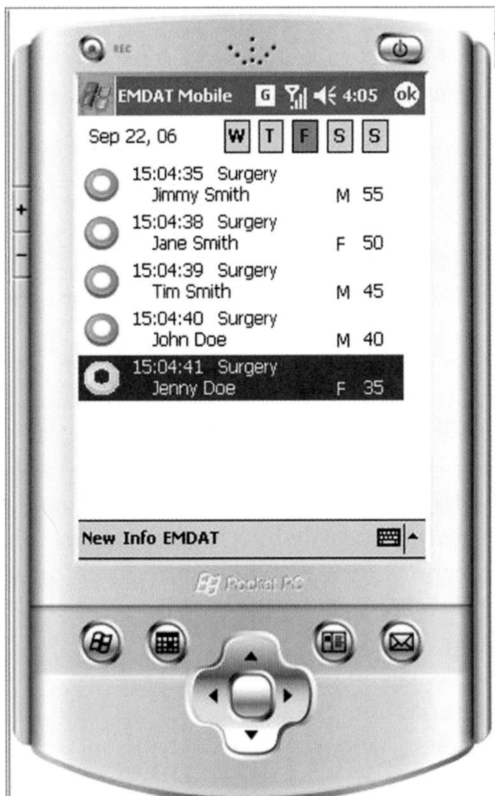

FIGURE 7-15 Collection of electronic data must comply with HIPAA privacy regulations. (Photo courtesy of Emdat, Inc.)

BOX 7-6

Use of Personal Digital Assistants in Health Care

- Patient tracking
  - Patient care notes
  - Medical records
  - Scheduling
  - Contact information
  - Billing record
- Laboratory test entry
- Checking laboratory results
- Accessing reference materials
- Mathematical calculations
- Prescription orders
- Billing

also must be guarded against unauthorized use (password protection). (See Skill List 7-10, Using the Computer, p. 131).

Medical Terminology

Medical terminology as it is used today dates to 300 B.C. in the writings of Hippocrates and Aristotle. The vocabulary is based on Latin and Greek roots for common words. Medical terminology allows health care workers to communicate in a precise and clear manner, so accurate pronunciation and correct spelling are important.

At first medical terminology appears difficult and confusing. However, each word can be divided into parts that are reused to form new terms. The parts are word roots and combining vowels, prefixes, and suffixes. The root is the central part and determines the main meaning. The root is usually modified by a prefix or suffix to make it more specific. The prefix is the first part, and the suffix is the last part. Not all medical terms have all three parts. Using a combining vowel between the parts of the term may be necessary for easier pronunciation. By memorizing the parts, many word combinations can be formed (Fig. 7-16). For example, the word root for "joint" is *arthro-*. Combined with the suffix that means "plastic reconstruction," it becomes *arthroplasty*. It could be combined with *-otomy* to make the term *arthrotomy*, which is an incision into the joint. The word root for "abdomen" is *laparo-*, so a laparotomy is an incision into the abdomen. A rhinoplasty is a plastic reconstruction of

NEPHR + ECTOMY

Prefix = Kidney | Suffix = Removal of

Nephrectomy = Removal of the kidney

FIGURE 7-16 Nephrectomy means removal of kidney.

the nose. Therefore, *rhino* must be the word root for "nose."

Abbreviations and symbols are used by health care workers to save time in conveying information. Some abbreviations are considered standard and are used in all areas of care. Others may be used in only one facility, and they may cause confusion. Abbreviations are learned most easily by use. They may be divided into categories for easier reference. Some categories of abbreviations that may be used include the following:

- Treatments and tests
- Conditions and diagnoses
- Titles (associations and personnel)

Common word roots, prefixes, suffixes, abbreviations, and symbols used in health care are found in Appendix I of the textbook.

Most of the communication among health care professionals involves the use of medical terminology. To provide safe and accurate care to the patient, all health care workers must have knowledge of the basic terms of anatomy and physiology and of tests and treatments.

Knowing the type of care or precautions that are necessary when a specific test or treatment is ordered by a physician may also be necessary. Some diagnostic tests require special diets or physical preparations before the test can be performed. For example, a barium enema (BE) allows the health care provider to view the large intestine, and the patient must have nothing to eat or drink (NPO) for several hours before the test.

Physician Orders

Most descriptions of the care that is to be given are written by the physician. These directions for care are called the physician orders and are written in the chart. Some examples of physician orders follow:

ac & cl ½ hr ac and hs

"Perform Acetest and Clinitest one-half hour before meals and at bedtime." The order probably would include directions for the administration of insulin if sugar or ketone is present in the urine test.

MOM 30 cc hs po PRN constipation

This order allows the patient to have 30 mL of milk of magnesia by mouth at bedtime, as needed, to relieve constipation. Although medications may be given (administered) only by licensed personnel, the health care assistant may be able to help by knowing what the order means.

Upper GI, GB series in am

The patient will have radiographs, or x-rays, of the gallbladder, stomach, and upper part of the intestine in the morning. The test may require some physical preparation such as dietary restrictions or special treatments to clear the intestines.

pt scheduled for TAH, BSO in am. NPO $\bar{p}$ MN

Surgery is scheduled for the patient in the morning. The patient is not to have anything to eat or drink after midnight. The procedure will be a total abdominal hysterectomy with a bilateral removal of the fallopian tubes and ovaries. It is much quicker to write "TAH, BSO" than the words that mean the same thing. The correct terminology for the procedure is "total abdominal hysterectomy, bilateral salpingo-oophorectomy."

Emergency First-Aid

First-aid is the immediate care given to the victim of injury or sudden illness. The purpose of first aid is to sustain life and prevent death. It includes the prevention of permanent disability and the reduction of time necessary for recovery. First-aid provides basic life support and maintenance of vital functions.

Certification in first aid is awarded by several accredited agencies including the American Red Cross (ARC) and the American Heart Association. The ARC course includes basic first aid for injuries, illness, and CPR procedures. In 2008 the American Heart Association, which teaches only CPR procedures, added "hands-only" (chest compressions only) guidelines for use by untrained bystanders for adults with sudden cardiac arrest. In 2010 it revised all of the guidelines (Box 7-7). Chapter 32 provides more information about first aid. (See Skill List 7-11, Performing

BOX 7-7

Major Changes in Guidelines for CPR*

- Airway-Breathing-Compressions (ABC) sequence changed to Compressions-Airway-Breathing (CAB)
- Emphasis is placed on effective chest compressions:
  - Hard, fast (at least 100/min)
  - At least 100/min
  - Minimum interruption
  - Full chest recoil
- For untrained lay rescuers continue compressions only
- For trained health professionals, begin mouth to mouth after 30 compressions and continue sets of 30:2 ratio
- Automated external defibrillators (AEDs) may be used with infants

*The 2010 American Heart Association guidelines for CPR and emergency cardiovascular care replace the previous guidelines.

Cardiopulmonary Rescue; Skill List 7-12, Performing Foreign-Body Airway Obstruction Rescue, and Skill List 7-13, Hands-Only CPR, pp. 131–133).

Cardiac Arrest

More than 15 million people worldwide have learned how to perform CPR. CPR is a combination of mouth-to-mouth breathing and chest compressions that supply oxygenated blood to the brain (Fig. 7-17). CPR may be necessary when cardiac arrest, drowning, respiratory failure, electrical shock, head injury, or drug overdose occur.

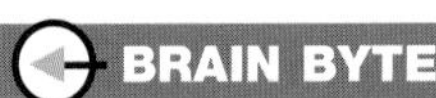

BRAIN BYTE

CPR doubles a person's chance of survival after a sudden cardiac arrest.

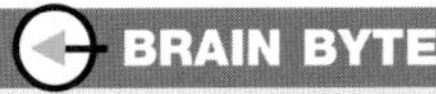

BRAIN BYTE

According to the CDC, in 2004, an average of nine people per day drowned in the United States.

Cardiac arrest also may result from blockage of an artery that supplies the heart or from insufficient supply of oxygen to the heart tissue. Signs and symptoms of a heart attack vary greatly. There may be more than one symptom present or none at all (Box 7-8). Risk factors for cardiac arrest have been identified (Box 7-9). The presence of more than one factor multiplies the risk greatly. Some risk factors can be changed through a prudent lifestyle, which includes regular exercise and a low-fat diet. Other risk factors such as heredity, gender, and age cannot be changed.

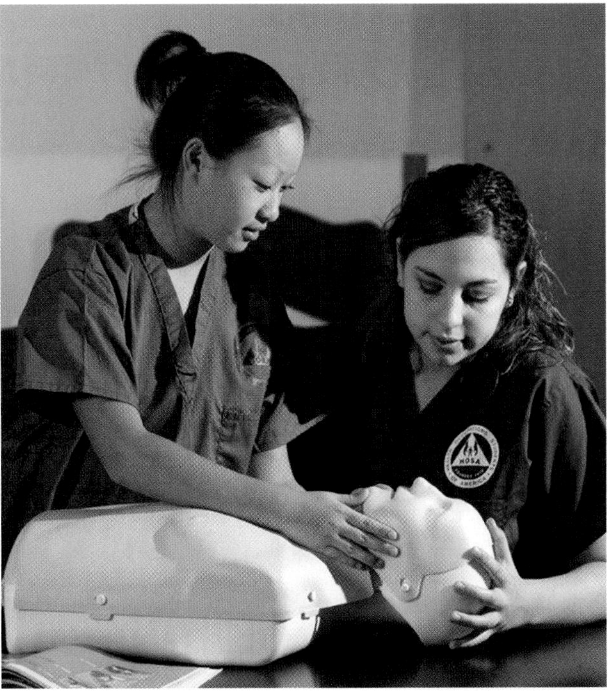

FIGURE 7-17 Students demonstrate the head-tilt, chin-lift movement used in CPR. (Photo courtesy of National Health Occupations Students of America, Flower Mound, Tex.)

BOX 7-8

Early Warning Signs of a Heart Attack

- Anxiety
- Chest pain
- Denial
- Dizziness
- Dyspnea (shortness of breath)
- Fatigue
- Indigestion
- Nausea
- Pale, clammy skin
- Perspiration
- Sensation of bowel movement

BOX 7-9

Risk Factors for Developing a Heart Attack

The most significant risk factors are smoking, high cholesterol levels, and high blood pressure. Each additional risk factor multiplies the risk of heart attack greatly.

- Age
- Diabetes
- Diet high in fat
- Family history of cardiovascular disease
- Gender
- High blood pressure
- High cholesterol level
- Lack of exercise
- Previous heart attack
- Race
- Smoking
- Stress

Additional information about emergency care can be found in Chapters 3 and 32. CPR information can also be found in Chapter 32.

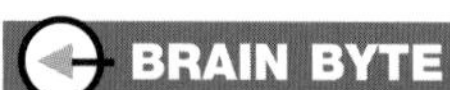

Sudden cardiac arrest is the leading cause of death in the United States.

Summary

- The elements of basic health assessment include an interview and physical assessment.
- Normal vital signs for an adult include a BP of 120/80, a pulse rate of 60 to 100, a respiration rate of 14 to 20, and a temperature of 98.6° F.
- The normal values of vital signs can be used to measure changes in body function, general health, and the response to treatment.
- Risk factors for cardiac arrest include diabetes, high-fat diet, high BP, and high cholesterol level.

Review Questions

1. Describe the elements of a health assessment.
2. Describe the normal parameters for vital signs, indicating what each measures.
3. Describe the risk factors for developing a heart attack that can be reduced by lifestyle change.
4. Explain the meaning of each of the numbers in 6543.
5. Use Appendix I to complete each of the following phrases of medical terminology:

Meaning	Root	Example	Meaning
Abdomen		Laparotomy	
Skull		Craniotomy	
Bladder		Cystoscopy	
	adeno		Tumor of the gland
Sun			Sun treatment
Vertebrae			Tumor of the vertebrae
	pnea	Tachypnea	
	pharyng	Pharyngitis	
		Tympanitis	
		Hydrophobia	

6. Use Fig. 7-14 to determine at what age girls and boys show the largest growth spurt.
7. Use Fig. 7-13 to determine at what time you wake up and go to bed using military time.
8. Use the following terms in one or more sentences that correctly relate their meaning: blood pressure, diastolic, and systolic.
9. Use the following terms in one or more sentences that correctly relate their meaning: auscultation, palpation, and percussion.

Critical Thinking

1. Describe a personal action or lifestyle change that might be taken to eliminate each of the risk factors for cardiac arrest.
2. Describe three activities that might change a person's vital signs.
3. Use the abbreviations in the appendix to write physician orders that would indicate that the patient was not supposed to eat after midnight because of surgery scheduled in the morning for a total abdominal hysterectomy.
4. Make a poster or brochure designed to teach the steps of CPR by the untrained bystander, layperson, or health professional.

5. Use the Internet to research and describe the difference between CPR rescue when it is done by one or by two health professionals.
6. Use the Internet to research and view videos of head-to-toe patient assessment techniques. Make a video or slide show that demonstrates a patient assessment.
7. Use the Internet to research and view videos of vital-sign assessment. Make a video or slide show that demonstrates vital-sign assessment.

Explore the Web

CPR/First Aid

AHA
http://americanheart.org

Red Cross
http://redcross.org

Assessment

Search Key Terms: head-to-toe assessment video
Search Key Terms: vital signs assessment video

STANDARDS AND ACCOUNTABILITY*

Foundation Standard 10: Technical Skills†

Health care professionals will apply technical skills required for all career specialties. They will demonstrate skills and knowledge as appropriate.

Accountability Criteria

10.1 Technical Skills

10.11 Apply procedures for measuring and recording vital signs including the normal ranges.

10.12 Apply skills to obtain training or certification in cardiopulmonary resuscitation (CPR), automated external defibrillator (AED), foreign body airway obstruction (FBAO), and first aid.

*From the National Consortium on Health Science Education (2009). National Health Care Standards and Accountability Criteria. Available at http://www.healthscienceconsortium.org

†Additional technical skills may be included in a program of study based on career specialties

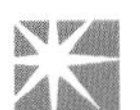

SKILL LIST 7-1 Admitting, Transferring, and Discharging the Patient

1. Maintain medical asepsis by using the guidelines provided in the Standard and Transmission-Based Precautions, including good handwashing technique and use of gloves as needed.
2. Gather the necessary equipment and supplies, including clean linens, an admission kit, an admission checklist, and a pen.
3. Prepare the room as needed with clean, appropriate equipment and supplies.
4. Greet the patient by name (Mr., Mrs., etc.), explain your role, and give your name. A nurse usually admits patients to the unit of the hospital, but other personnel may be assigned this duty if the patient does not need immediate care.
5. Assist the patient as needed to put on a gown or pajamas.
6. Complete the admission checklist.
7. Explain the facility's routine procedures and policies. The patient might not understand such regulations as the use of side rails for safety, removal of jewelry for safe storage, or use of a signal light to summon someone.
8. If transfer of the patient is necessary, explain the reason for the change. The patient may feel disoriented and insecure because of being moved to another location.
9. Transport the patient in a wheelchair, on a stretcher, or in a bed.

Continued

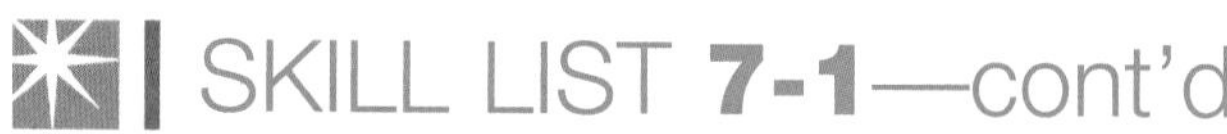

SKILL LIST 7-1—cont'd
Admitting, Transferring, and Discharging the Patient

10. When discharge from the facility is ordered, assist the patient to gather belongings in containers for transport.
11. Assist the patient to dress for discharge.
12. Accompany the patient to the car or other method of transport. The patient may need assistance to arrange adequate transportation to the home or another facility.

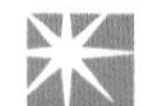

SKILL LIST 7-2
Recording Observations

1. Report any unusual findings to a supervisor before charting observations.
2. Use black ink and print information legibly.
3. Chart observations promptly after making them.
4. Follow all the rules for good charting.
5. Return the chart to the designated location when finished.

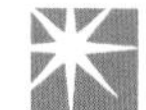

SKILL LIST 7-3
Taking a Blood Pressure

1. Maintain medical asepsis by using the guidelines provided in the Standard and Transmission-Based Precautions, including good handwashing technique and use of gloves as needed.
2. Gather all necessary equipment, including a stethoscope, sphygmomanometer, alcohol pledget, pen, and paper.
3. Identify the patient, and explain the procedure. Identification of the correct patient and explanation of the procedure prevents errors and misunderstanding.
4. Position the patient in either a sitting or lying position with the upper arm exposed and supported above the level of the heart. Clothing must allow exposure of the upper arm completely without binding. Privacy should be provided if necessary. Either arm may be used, but arms with injuries, IV lines, or other treatments should be avoided, because the procedure may cause injury or pain or the reading may be inaccurate.
5. Wrap the cuff of the sphygmomanometer around the arm 1 inch above the bend of the elbow (antecubital space). The cuff should be tight enough that two fingers may be placed under the edge comfortably. If the cuff is too tight or too loose, the reading will be inaccurate. The cuff is placed 1 inch above the level of the bend of the elbow to allow room for the flat placement of the stethoscope.
6. While palpating the radial artery, tighten the thumbscrew of the sphygmomanometer, and inflate until the pulse disappears. This reading is an approximate systolic pressure.
7. Deflate the cuff completely and allow the arm to rest for 30 seconds.
8. Clean the earplugs of the stethoscope with alcohol, and place them into the ears with the opening pointing toward the nose.
9. Locate the brachial pulse with the tips of two fingers and place the flat part (diaphragm) of the stethoscope on the location of the pulse.

Continued

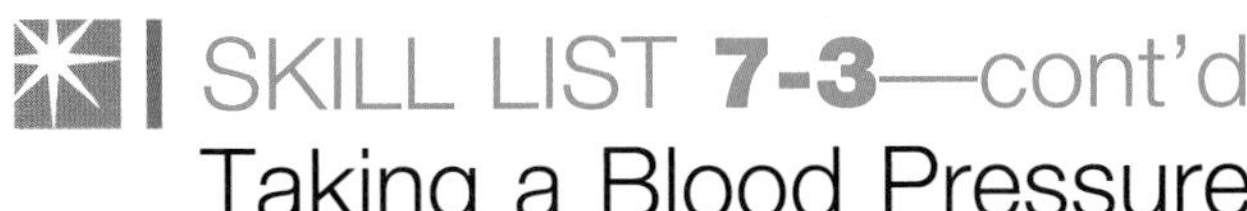

SKILL LIST 7-3—cont'd Taking a Blood Pressure

Placement over the brachial artery allows the pulse to be heard more easily (audible) when the cuff is inflated.

10. Tighten the thumbscrew valve by turning it clockwise, and inflate the cuff to 20 to 30 mm Hg above the approximate systolic value.
11. Deflate the cuff, slowly noting the location on the scale at which the first (systolic) and last (diastolic) pulse are heard. The last distinct beat is considered to be the diastolic pulse. Soft muffled or thumping sounds are not counted.
12. Deflate the cuff completely after the blood pressure is assessed, and remove the cuff from the arm. The blood pressure can be reassessed using the same arm a second time. If a third reading is necessary, the cuff should be removed briefly between readings or moved to the other arm because tightening the cuff repeatedly may change the pressure.
13. Record the results. Report any unusual findings to the supervisor immediately. An elevated or low blood pressure may signal an emergency situation.
14. Store equipment in the designated area and discard the alcohol pledget in an appropriate container.

SKILL LIST 7-4 Taking an Oral Temperature

1. Maintain medical asepsis by using the guidelines provided in the Standard and Transmission-Based Precautions, including good handwashing technique and use of gloves as needed.
2. Gather necessary supplies and equipment, including a thermometer, tissue, alcohol swab or pledget, pen, and paper.
3. Clean an oral thermometer with disinfectant solution before use. Wash it with cool, soapy water and rinse to remove the disinfectant. The disinfectant may irritate the tissues of the mouth.
4. Shake the liquid in the thermometer down with a sharp movement of the wrist until the reading is 96.0° F or lower. The shaking movement causes the liquid to fall to the bulb end of the thermometer. Activate the electronic thermometer if it is being used. Mercury is no longer used in thermometers because of its environmental and safety risks, but other nontoxic liquids may be used safely.
5. Cover the thermometer with a plastic sheath or wipe with alcohol from stem to bulb. The stem is considered cleaner than the bulb.
6. Identify the patient and explain the procedure. Determine that the patient has not consumed any hot or cold food or beverage or smoked for at least 5 minutes before taking the temperature. The temperature of the food or beverages and smoking will affect the reading.
7. Place the bulb end of the thermometer under the patient's tongue and instruct the patient to keep the lips closed for 3 minutes, taking care not to bite on the thermometer. If bitten, the thermometer could break and harm the patient. Electronic thermometers are held in place for 45 seconds. The mouth must be closed to obtain an accurate reading.
8. Remove the thermometer by holding it by the stem, and wipe it with alcohol from stem to bulb to prevent the spread of microorganisms. Discard alcohol pledget or swab in the proper container immediately. If a sheath or cover is used, remove it and discard it in the proper container immediately.
9. Read the thermometer by holding it at eye level and twisting the stem until the liquid can be seen. Record the result on paper. Readings that

Continued

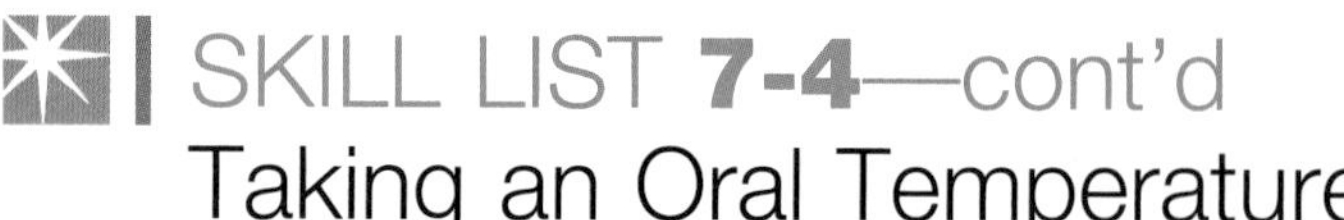

SKILL LIST 7-4—cont'd
Taking an Oral Temperature

are between two lines on the thermometer are considered to be the higher reading.

10. Report any unusual findings to the supervisor immediately.
11. Clean the thermometer with disinfectant and store it in the designated area. Deactivate an electronic thermometer and place it in the recharging element.
12. Maintain medical asepsis by washing your hands when the procedure is completed.

SKILL LIST 7-5
Taking an Axillary Temperature

1. Maintain medical asepsis by using the guidelines provided in the Standard and Transmission-Based Precautions, including good handwashing technique and use of gloves as needed.
2. Gather the necessary supplies, including an oral thermometer, tissue, dry wash cloth, alcohol pledget or swab, pen, and paper.
3. Clean an oral thermometer with disinfectant solution before use. Wash it with cool, soapy water and rinse to remove disinfectant. The disinfectant may irritate the skin.
4. Shake the liquid level of the thermometer down with a sharp movement of the wrist until the reading is 96.0° F or lower. Activate an electronic thermometer if it is to be used. Mercury is no longer used in thermometers because of its environmental and safety risks, but other nontoxic liquids may be used safely.
5. Cover the thermometer with a plastic sheath or wipe with alcohol from stem to bulb.
6. Identify the patient and explain the procedure. Provide for privacy.
7. Position the patient so that the area under the arm (axilla) is exposed. Pat the axilla dry with a clean cloth. Patting the area dry removes moisture and excess heat. Avoid rubbing and creating friction that may raise the temperature.
8. Place the thermometer with the end bulb in the middle of the axilla, and cross the patient's arm on the chest to keep the thermometer in place for 10 minutes.
9. Remove the thermometer and wipe it with alcohol from stem to bulb. Discard the alcohol swab and any sheath or covering in an appropriate container.
10. Read the thermometer by holding it at eye level and twisting the stem until the liquid can be seen. Record the result on paper. Readings that are between two lines on the thermometer are considered to be the higher reading. Report any unusual findings to the supervisor.
11. Reposition the patient for comfort and privacy.
12. Clean the thermometer with disinfectant solution and store it in the designated area. Deactivate an electronic thermometer and replace it in the recharging element.

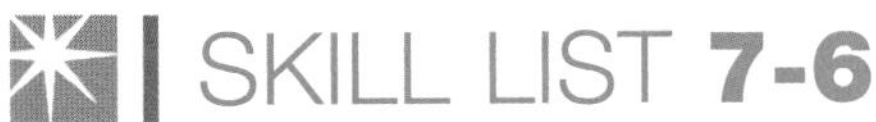

SKILL LIST 7-6
Taking a Rectal Temperature

1. Maintain medical asepsis by using the guidelines provided in the Standard and Transmission-Based Precautions, including good handwashing technique and use of gloves as needed.
2. Gather all necessary equipment and supplies, including a rectal thermometer, lubricating jelly, toilet tissue, disposable gloves, pen, and paper.
3. Clean a rectal thermometer with alcohol from stem to bulb, or cover with a protective sheath. Rectal thermometers may be tipped with red and have rounded bulbs. Confusing oral with rectal thermometers is not sanitary and may cause illness.
4. Shake the liquid level of the thermometer down with a sharp movement of the wrist until the reading is 96.0° F or lower. Activate an electronic thermometer if it is to be used. Mercury is no longer used in thermometers because of its environmental and safety risks, but other nontoxic liquids may be used safely.
5. Lubricate 2 inches of the bulb end of the thermometer with lubricating jelly.
6. Identify the patient and explain the procedure. Arrange the unit to provide privacy.
7. Wear disposable gloves to prevent the spread of microorganisms.
8. Position the patient on one side, and raise the patient's upper leg slightly toward the head.
9. Expose the anus by raising the upper buttocks. Gently insert the thermometer 1½ inches if the patient is an adult. The rectum of a child is shorter than that of an adult, and special care is necessary when taking a rectal temperature.
10. Remain with the patient while holding the thermometer in place for 3 to 5 minutes. Accidental injury may occur if the patient is left alone with a rectal thermometer in place.
11. Remove the thermometer and wipe with tissue from stem to bulb to remove any fecal material. Discard the tissue and any cover used on the thermometer in the appropriate container immediately.
12. Reposition the patient for comfort, privacy, and safety.
13. Read the thermometer by holding it at eye level and twisting the stem until the liquid can be seen. Record the result on paper. Readings that are between two lines on the thermometer are considered to be the higher reading. Report any unusual findings to the supervisor.
14. Clean the thermometer with disinfectant and store it in the designated area. Deactivate an electronic thermometer if in use and replace it in the recharging unit.
15. Discard gloves in an appropriate container.

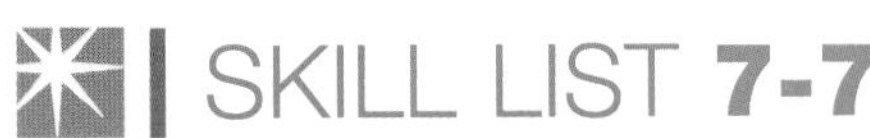

SKILL LIST 7-7
Taking an Infrared Temperature

1. Maintain medical asepsis by using the guidelines provided in the Standard and Transmission-Based Precautions, including good handwashing technique and use of gloves as needed.
2. Gather all necessary equipment and supplies, including a thermal thermometer, alcohol swab (pledget), pen, and paper.
3. Press the power button to activate the thermometer.
4. Check that the thermometer is set for the preferred mode (Fahrenheit or Celsius).
5. Press and hold "scan" until the image "00" appears on the screen.
6. Hold the thermometer about 2 to 3 inches away from and in the middle of the forehead.
7. While holding the "scan" button, move the thermometer toward and away from the forehead until it beeps continuously and the light flashes.

Continued

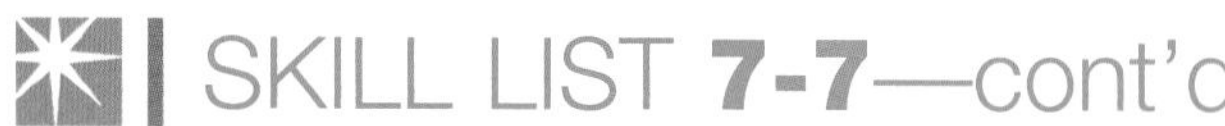

SKILL LIST 7-7—cont'd Taking an Infrared Temperature

8. When the beeping is continuous, release the "scan" button. The thermometer will beep once and show the temperature.
9. The thermometer will automatically shut off.
10. Use an alcohol swab to clean the thermometer lens. Store it in the designated area.
11. Discard the alcohol swab in an appropriate container. Maintain medical asepsis by washing your hands for a minimum of 20 seconds.

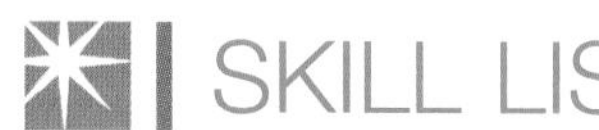

SKILL LIST 7-8 Taking a Radial Pulse and Measuring Respiration

1. Maintain medical asepsis by using the guidelines provided in the Standard and Transmission-Based Precautions, including good handwashing technique and use of gloves as needed.
2. Gather the necessary supplies and equipment, including a watch with a second hand, pen, and paper.
3. Identify the patient and explain the procedure.
4. Place the tips of your first two fingers over the radial artery. The thumb is not used because it has a pulse of its own, which may cause confusion.
5. Using a watch with a second hand, count the pulse beats for 1 minute. The pulse may instead be assessed for 30 seconds and doubled. An assessment less than 30 seconds can lead to error of four beats per minute or more. An irregular pulse must be counted for the complete 1 minute.
6. While still palpating the radial artery, count respirations for 1 minute. If the wrist is held, the patient will remain quiet so that respirations may be assessed. If coughing, talking, or other verbal reaction occurs during the counting of respirations, the count must be reassessed. The result may be affected if the patient is aware that the respirations are being counted.
7. Record the time, rate, and character of pulse and respirations.
8. Report any unusual findings to the supervisor immediately.

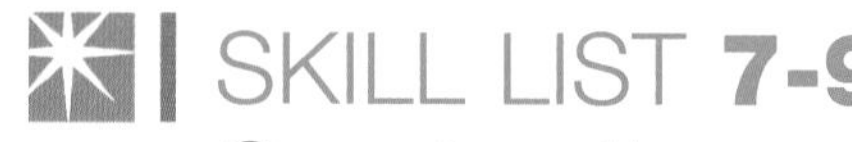

SKILL LIST 7-9 Constructing a Line Graph

1. Draw a vertical axis and a horizontal axis.
2. Determine which of the two types of data to be compared varies the least. Place this information on the horizontal axis.
3. Label the point of intersection of the two axes as zero for each.
4. Divide each axis of the graph into portions that will include all of the data.
5. Chart the first point where the value of the first data intersects on the graph.
6. Chart the second point where the next value intersects on the graph.

Continued

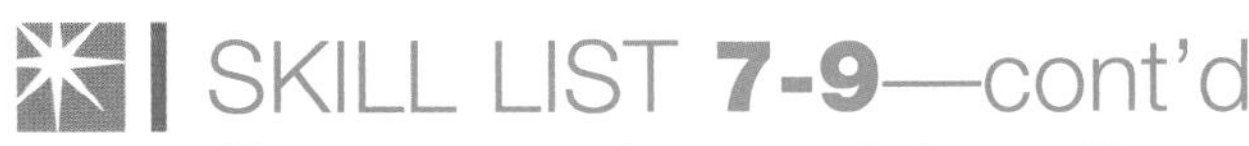

SKILL LIST 7-9—cont'd
Constructing a Line Graph

7. Draw a straight line to connect the two points.
8. Chart the third point where the third set of data intersects on the graph.
9. Join the second point to the third point with a straight line.
10. Continue charting and joining points on the graph until all data have been noted.
11. Label each axis with the units of measurement.
12. Label the graph.

SKILL LIST 7-10
Using the Computer

1. Identify the monitor, central processing unit, and disk drive for the computer. Information can be obtained in the central processing unit or on a CD.
2. Turn the computer on as indicated by the manufacturer's directions.
3. Initiate or "boot" a program according to the manufacturer's instructions.
4. Enter log-in and password information as needed according to the program instructions.
5. Enter information by patient.
6. Save information to the disk according to the program instructions.
7. Turn the computer off according to the manufacturer's instruction.

SKILL LIST 7-11
Performing Cardiopulmonary Resuscitation (HCP)*

1. Maintain medical asepsis by using the guidelines provided in the Standard and Transmission-Based Precautions including a CPR mask, eye protection, good handwashing technique and use of gloves as needed.
2. Check to see if the person is responsive by gently shaking him or her, rubbing the sternum with your knuckles and shouting.
3. If the victim does not respond or is gasping only, call 911 or have someone else do it.
4. Palpate for pulse for 10 seconds.
5. If pulse is absent, use an AED† if available.
6. If AED is not available, begin chest compressions. Place the heel of one hand in the middle of the victim's chest and the other hand on the top.
7. Compress the chest at least 2 inches (adults and children) and then allow it to reexpand or recoil completely. Compress about 1 ½ inches in infants.
8. Use the head-lift, chin-lift method to open the airway.

Continued

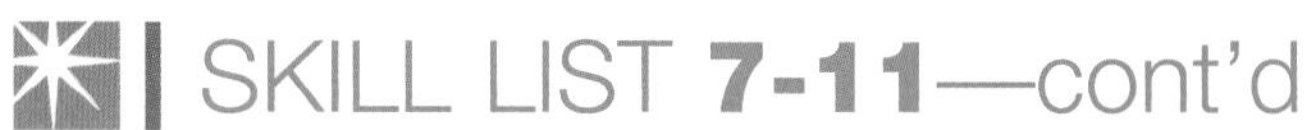

SKILL LIST 7-11—cont'd
Performing Cardiopulmonary Resuscitation (HCP)*

9. Pinch the nose closed and give two slow mouth-to-mouth breaths. Breaths should be about one second long or one breath every 6-8 seconds.
10. Perform compressions and breaths at a ratio of 30:2.
11. Rotate compressors every 2 minutes when two HCP are present.
12. If the victim recovers and there are no other signs of injury to the back or neck, turn the victim to his or her side.
13. Continue monitoring breathing until instructed to stop by advanced emergency personnel.

*These are general guidelines for trained health care professionals (HCP). Two-rescuer CPR may be performed using a modified ratio of 15:2 compressions to ventilations for children and infants.
†Automated External Defibrillators (AEDs) can be safely used by lay rescuers with a few hours of training. When the device is attached to the victim with two adhesive pads, it analyzes the heart activity and determines whether shock is necessary.

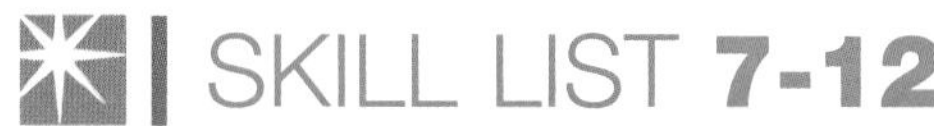

SKILL LIST 7-12
Performing Foreign-Body Airway Obstruction Rescue

1. Maintain medical asepsis by using the guidelines provided in the Standard and Transmission-Based Precautions, including good handwashing technique and use of gloves as needed.
2. Assess whether assistance is necessary. Ask the person if he or she is choking.
3. If the victim cannot speak or cough forcefully, perform abdominal thrusts until the object is dislodged.
4. Lower the victim to the ground if unresponsiveness occurs.
5. Call 911 or have someone else do it.
6. Attempt cardiopulmonary resuscitation.

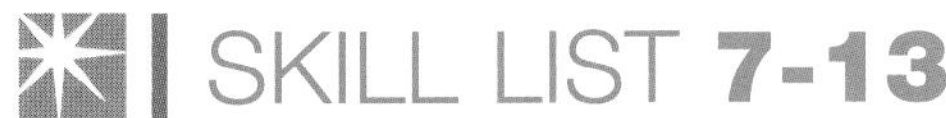

SKILL LIST 7-13 Hands-Only Cardiopulmonary Resuscitation (CPR)*

1. Maintain medical asepsis by using the guidelines provided in the Standard and Transmission-Based Precautions including a CPR mask, eye protection, good handwashing technique and use of gloves as needed.
2. Check to see if the person is responsive by gently shaking him or her, rubbing the sternum with your knuckles and shouting.
3. If the victim does not respond or is gasping only, call 911 or have someone else do it.
4. Use an AED† if available.
5. Begin chest compressions. Place the heel of one hand in the middle of the victim's chest and the other hand on the top of the first hand.
6. Compress the chest at least 2 inches (adults and children) and then allow it to reexpand or recoil completely. Compress about 1 ½ inches in infants.
7. Perform compressions at a rate of at least 100/minute.
8. If the victim recovers and there are no other signs of injury to the back or neck, turn the victim to his or her side.

*These are general guidelines for untrained rescuers. A course given by the AHA or ARC is available, as well as training materials for the layperson.

†Automated External Defibrillators (AEDs) can be safely used by lay rescuers with a few hours of training. When the device is attached to the victim with two adhesive pads, it analyzes the heart activity and determines whether shock is necessary.

CHAPTER 8

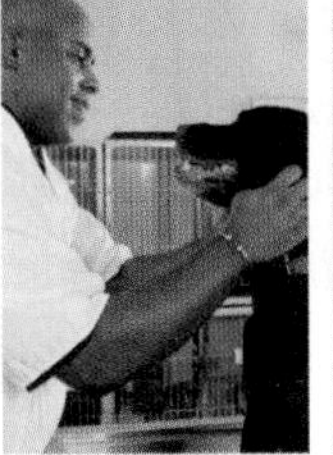
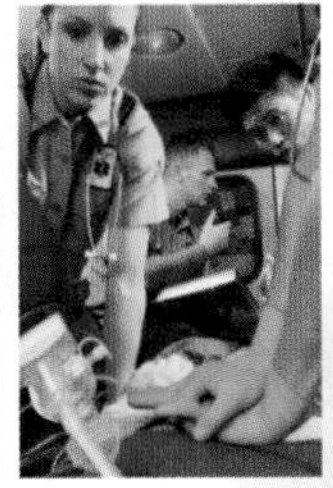
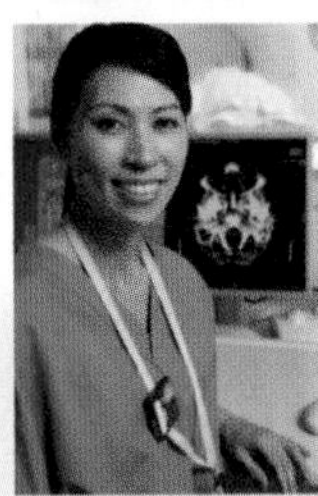

Wellness, Growth, and Development

LEARNING OBJECTIVES

- Define at least 10 terms relating to wellness, growth, and development.
- List at least three factors that may be used to determine a level of wellness.
- Describe three categories of disease prevention.
- List the function of each of the five nutrients.
- Construct a personalized U.S. Department of Agriculture (USDA) food pyramid and number of recommended daily servings for each category.
- Describe the relationship of calories to weight loss and gain.
- Describe at least five types of therapeutic diets used to meet individual nutritional needs.
- Identify at least five events that may lead to a reaction of stress.
- Describe at least five health conditions that may result from stress.
- Describe at least four methods that may be used to manage stress.
- Compare the physical development of the body through the life span.
- Describe the psychosocial development through the life span.
- Describe two models of change theory that may be applied to health care behavior.
- Describe each of the five stages of death acceptance (grief).

KEY TERMS

Addiction *(uh-DIK-shen)* Dependence on some habit; may be physical, psychological, or both

Anabolism *(ah-NAB-o-liz-uhm)* Any constructive process by which simple substances are converted by living cells into more complex compounds

KEY TERMS cont'd

Calorie *(KAL-o-ree)* Unit of heat

Carbohydrates *(kar-bo-HI-draytz)* Starches, sugars, cellulose, and gums

Catabolism *(kah-TAB-o-liz-uhm)* Breaking-down process by which complex substances are converted by living cells into simple compounds

Cholesterol *(ko-LES-ter-ol)* Pearly, fatlike steroid alcohol found in animal fats and oils; precursor of bile acids and hormones

Fat *(fat)* Adipose tissue; reserve supply of energy

Megadose *(MEG-uh-dos)* Overdose, 10 times the recommended dose

Metabolism *(mu-TAB-o-liz-uhm)* Sum of all the physical and chemical processes by which a living organized substance is produced, maintained, and transformed to produce energy

Mineral *(MIN-er-ul)* Nonorganic solid substance

Nutrients *(NOO-tree-ents)* Proteins, carbohydrates, fats, vitamins, and minerals necessary for growth, normal functioning, and maintaining life

Nutrition *(noo-TRISH-un)* Process of taking in nutrients and using them for body function

Protein *(PRO-teen)* Group of complex organic compounds that are the main part of cell protoplasm

Terminal *(TER-min-ul)* Illness or injury for which there is no reasonable expectation of recovery

Vitamins *(VIE-tuh-minz)* Organic compounds needed by the body for metabolism, growth, and development

Wellness

Wellness may be defined as a state of health on a continuum from a level of high energy and feeling of well-being to illness or death. Optimal wellness reflects a balanced relationship among the individual's physical, mental, and social health. Wellness is determined by the lifestyle choices a person makes. These choices include the amount of sleep, type of diet, exercise plan, personal habits, social relationships with others, and so forth. Many models have been designed to describe the type of lifestyle and personal habits that promote wellness, interrelating the body, mind, and spirit (Fig. 8-1). The body refers to physical health and development. The mind refers to intellectual and emotional development. The spirit includes inner and personal reflection.

Fitness may be evaluated by considering muscle strength and endurance, cardiorespiratory endurance, body composition, and flexibility. Some indicators that may be measured to evaluate optimal physical fitness include the following:

- Percentage of body fat (20% to 23% for women and 13% to 16% for men)
- Muscle strength
- Joint flexibility
- Balance and coordination
- Oxygen uptake
- Vital capacity

Some of the laboratory blood tests that may be used to indicate levels of wellness include the following:

- Cholesterol level
- Glucose level

An optimal state of wellness emphasizes self-care, personal responsibility, prevention of illness, and management of health through lifestyle choices. Concepts that may improve wellness include nutrition, stress reduction, counseling, habit cessation, and exercise.

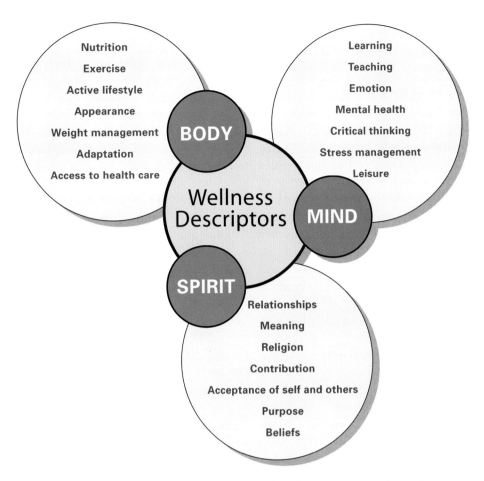

FIGURE 8-1 This model details different descriptors necessary for wellness.

Prevention

Preventative medicine includes the methods used to prevent disease in people instead of curing it. It can be classified into three categories, including primary, secondary, and tertiary prevention.

Primary prevention includes methods that are specifically directed toward a particular disease, such as immunizations or general interventions such as education. It is intended to protect the whole population. Primary prevention may be called health promotion. An example of health promotion would be regular exercise.

Secondary prevention is directed toward individuals who have risk factors for disease but have not yet developed it. It is intended to detect disease as early as possible. Examples of secondary prevention would be having regular mammograms to detect breast cancer and treatment of injuries to prevent infection.

Tertiary prevention includes the steps taken to minimize the disease when primary and secondary prevention have failed. It is designed to limit disability and rehabilitate the individual with disease. An example of tertiary prevention is the monitoring of medication and therapy in someone who has suffered a heart attack (Box 8-1).

BOX 8-1

Heart Health Prevention Categories

Primary Prevention: Screening for risk factors; avoiding disease by behavior modification such as losing weight, increasing exercise, and stopping smoking

Secondary Prevention: Identifying people at high risk for developing and those who have heart disease; cardiac rehabilitation

Tertiary Prevention: Limit complications and disabilities for person after myocardial infarction; cardiac rehabilitation

Nutrition

Nutrients

Metabolism refers to the physical and chemical processes that produce energy. The energy used by the body for growth and activity comes from the food that is eaten. Body cells metabolize or process food in two ways. **Anabolism** is the process of building tissues from small compounds, and it requires energy to occur. **Catabolism** is the breaking down of tissues into materials that may be reused or excreted. Catabolism releases energy that may be used for other activities of the cell.

Nutrition is the study of the food that is eaten and how it is used in the body. **Nutrients** are chemical materials in food and are vital to the body functions. Good nutrition is important in maintaining the best health possible.

Five nutrients have been identified as being essential to the maintenance of good health. They are carbohydrates, proteins, fats, vitamins, and minerals. Additionally, the body's cells need sufficient water to metabolize these nutrients. Effective use of one nutrient depends on the presence of all of the other nutrients in the body.

Since May 1994 all producers of processed foods have been required to comply with the Nutrition Labeling and Education Act. Labels on foods must be consistent and meet guidelines set by the U.S. Food and Drug Administration (FDA). Figure 8-2 lists the contents of processed food that must appear on the label. Additionally, foods that make health claims such as "low in ... ," "good source of ... ," or "lean" must meet specific guidelines for these statements, and claims can be made in only seven categories.

The FDA developed the reference daily intake (RDI), which indicates the nutrient value of processed foods and supplements. It replaced the term *recommended daily allowance* (RDA), which was previously used for labeling.

RDI (RDA) now indicates the amount of nutrients that should be consumed daily to meet the nutritional needs of almost all healthy people. The National Research Council committee establishes the RDI (RDA) guidelines. The committee, made up of nutritional scientists, has been providing these estimates

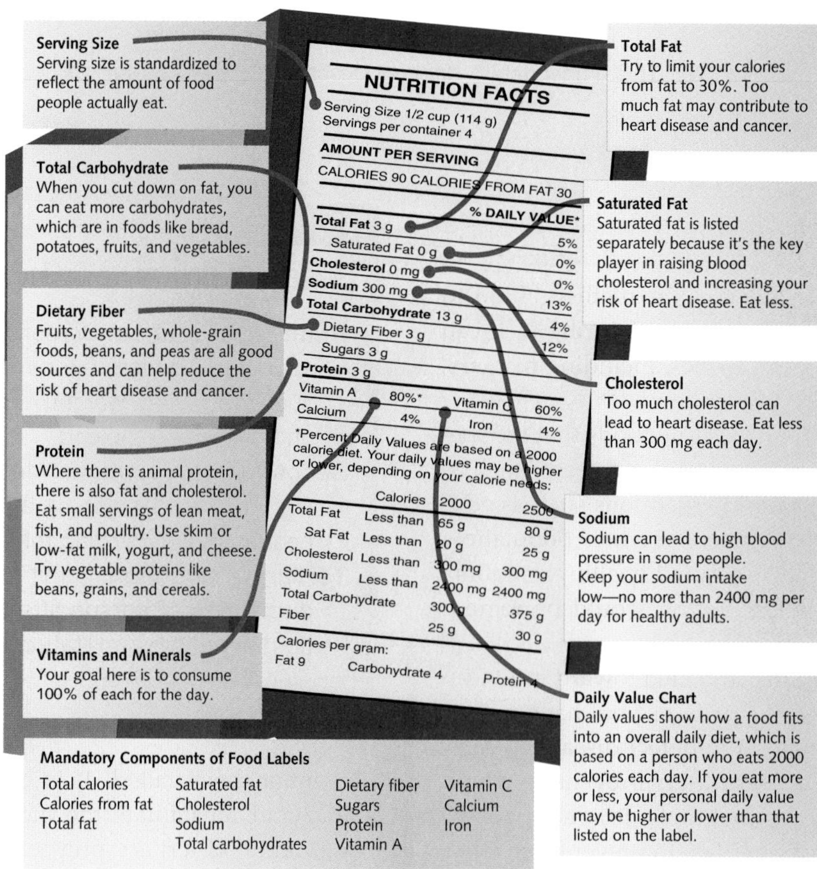

Serving Size
Serving size is standardized to reflect the amount of food people actually eat.
Total Carbohydrate
When you cut down on fat, you can eat more carbohydrates, which are in foods like bread, potatoes, fruits, and vegetables.
Dietary Fiber
Fruits, vegetables, whole-grain foods, beans, and peas are all good sources and can help reduce the risk of heart disease and cancer.
Protein
Where there is animal protein, there is also fat and cholesterol. Eat small servings of lean meat, fish, and poultry. Use skim or low-fat milk, yogurt, and cheese. Try vegetable proteins like beans, grains, and cereals.
Vitamins and Minerals
Your goal here is to consume 100% of each for the day.
NUTRITION FACTS
Serving Size 1/2 cup (114 g)
Servings per container 4
AMOUNT PER SERVING
CALORIES 90 CALORIES FROM FAT 30
% DAILY VALUE*
Total Fat 3 g 5%
Saturated Fat 0 g 0%
Cholesterol 0 mg 0%
Sodium 300 mg 13%
Total Carbohydrate 13 g 4%
Dietary Fiber 3 g 12%
Sugars 3 g
Protein 3 g
Vitamin A 80%* Vitamin C 60%
Calcium 4% Iron 4%
*Percent Daily Values are based on a 2000 calorie diet. Your daily values may be higher or lower, depending on your calorie needs:
Calories 2000 2500
Total Fat Less than 65 g 80 g
Sat Fat Less than 20 g 25 g
Cholesterol Less than 300 mg 300 mg
Sodium Less than 2400 mg 2400 mg
Total Carbohydrate 300 g 375 g
Fiber 25 g 30 g
Calories per gram:
Fat 9 Carbohydrate 4 Protein 4
Total Fat
Try to limit your calories from fat to 30%. Too much fat may contribute to heart disease and cancer.
Saturated Fat
Saturated fat is listed separately because it's the key player in raising blood cholesterol and increasing your risk of heart disease. Eat less.
Cholesterol
Too much cholesterol can lead to heart disease. Eat less than 300 mg each day.
Sodium
Sodium can lead to high blood pressure in some people. Keep your sodium intake low—no more than 2400 mg per day for healthy adults.
Daily Value Chart
Daily values show how a food fits into an overall daily diet, which is based on a person who eats 2000 calories each day. If you eat more or less, your personal daily value may be higher or lower than that listed on the label.
Mandatory Components of Food Labels
Total calories
Calories from fat
Total fat
Saturated fat
Cholesterol
Sodium
Total carbohydrates
Dietary fiber
Sugars
Protein
Vitamin A
Vitamin C
Calcium
Iron

FIGURE 8-2 Food labels provide nutritional information that reflects the content of the food.

since 1934 and revises its recommendations every 5 years.

Carbohydrates are found in all plants that are used as food sources. Carbohydrates are the main source of quick or immediate energy used by the body. Sugar and starch are the two main forms of carbohydrate. Foods that provide carbohydrates include cereal, potatoes, dried beans, corn, bread, and sugar. Carbohydrates found in fruit and vegetables also provide fiber or bulk to help with elimination of wastes. Carbohydrates also are necessary to use fat. If carbohydrates are not present in the diet, proteins are used as the alternate energy source.

Proteins are found in food from animal sources such as eggs, milk, meat, fish, and poultry. Additionally, dried beans, peas, and cheese provide this nutrient. Protein contains the compounds (amino acids) necessary to build muscle, bone, blood, and antibodies. Strict vegetarians who do not eat eggs or milk may combine legumes and whole grain products such as red beans and rice to obtain the nine essential amino acids. Amino acids that are called *essential* cannot be synthesized from other food sources.

Fats are found in the marbling or white part of meat, cooking oils, salad dressings, and in some milk products such as butter. Fat provides the most concentrated form of energy. Fat is necessary to repair cells and make hormones. Fats also supply essential fatty acids and fat-soluble vitamins. Fats are classified as saturated or unsaturated. Saturated fats are found in animal products and are solid at room temperature. Unsaturated fats are found primarily in vegetables and contain less cholesterol than saturated fats. **Cholesterol** is a waxy compound found in fats and is produced by the body. It is used by the brain to transmit nerve impulses and forms part of cell membranes. Cholesterol is necessary in the skin to produce vitamin D and is used in formation of bile acids and reproductive hormones. Cholesterol is sticky and may be deposited in the walls of blood vessels when too high a level accumulates in the blood. Because high cholesterol levels are linked to heart disease, unsaturated fats are believed to produce fewer health risks than saturated fats.

Vitamins are organic compounds that regulate cell metabolism. Each vitamin has specific functions (see Appendix: Vitamins and Minerals on Evolve). Vitamins are divided into two groups depending on whether they dissolve in water or fat. Vitamin supplements are not necessary if a varied and balanced diet, which contains all the nutrients, is eaten. Vitamins, especially vitamin C, may be destroyed when overcooked.

Minerals are simple compounds that regulate body processes. Nineteen minerals are used by the body. Seventeen are considered to be essential (see Appendix: Vitamins and Minerals on Evolve). Minerals are found in many food sources. Ten times the recommended daily allowance of vitamins and minerals is considered to be an overdose, or **megadose** (Table 8-1).

Food Groups

In June 2005 the USDA replaced the food group pyramid designed to help plan meals that provide all of the nutrients needed in a daily diet (Fig. 8-3). The new pyramid, called *MyPyramid,* provides an

TABLE 8-1
Effects of Vitamin and Mineral Megadosing

Vitamin or Mineral	Effect of Megadose
Vitamin A	Blurred vision, hearing loss, liver damage, headache
Vitamin B_6	Physiological dependency*
Vitamin C	Physiological dependency, kidney stones
Calcium	Drowsiness, impaired absorption of other minerals and vitamins
Iron	Toxic buildup in liver, pancreas, and heart
Zinc	Nausea, vomiting, premature birth, stillbirth

*Physiological dependency has occurred when the dosage is reduced to normal levels and symptoms of deficiency appear.

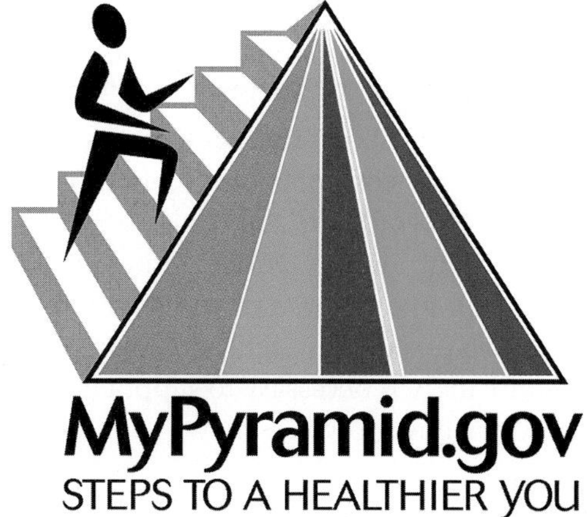

FIGURE 8-3 The food pyramid is used as a guide to provide a balanced diet. (From http://www.mypyramid.gov.)

TABLE 8-2
"MyPyramid" Sample Plans

Category	Individual 1	Individual 2	Individual 3
Age	16	16	16
Gender	Female	Female	Male
Physical activity*	<30 min daily	30-60 min daily	30-60 min daily
Grains	6 oz	6 oz	10 oz
Vegetables	2.5 cups	2.5 cups	3.5 cups
Fruits	1.5 cups	2 cups	2.5 cups
Milk	3 cups	3 cups	3 cups
Meat and beans	5 oz	5.5 oz	7 oz
Oils and discretionary calories	5 tsp (limit fats and sugars to 195 calories)	6 tsp (limit fats and sugars to 265 calories)	8 tsp (limit fats and sugars to 425 calories)

*Physical activity in addition to normal daily routine.

opportunity to personalize the plan for healthy eating and exercise. A healthy diet includes all of the recommended food groups to provide all of the required nutrients. The food groups include milk, meats and beans, vegetables, fruits, and grains. Servings of oils are not considered a food group because they contain calories but no nutrients. Additionally, they are found in a natural form in many other foods.

The new pyramid uses a symbol that includes all of the parts of healthy eating and physical activity. It includes activity, moderation, personalization, proportionality, variety, and gradual improvement. The pyramid calculates dietary information on the basis of age, gender, and levels of activity (Table 8-2). The plan includes tips to improve nutrition such as including calcium-rich foods, choosing lean proteins, varying vegetable selections, choosing whole grains, and focusing on fruits and physical activity. The flexibility of the plan provides alternatives to meet dietary needs due to religious, cultural, or health preferences.

The average person in the United States consumes 493 cans of soft drinks and 56 kg (123 lb) of sugar a year. Although the recommended daily allowance of salt is 2200 mg, or about 1 teaspoon, most people in the United States consume two to four times that amount. Most people in the United States could improve their nutrition by reducing their intake of fat, sugar, and salt. The amount of fruits and vegetables should be increased. Through adolescence, about 1 quart of milk daily is necessary to supply the minerals necessary for bone growth.

Calories

Another method used to measure the amount of food necessary to perform the body functions is counting calories. A **calorie** is the measurement of the amount of energy needed to raise 1 g of water 1° C. The amount of calories necessary daily depends on gender, age, size, general condition, and daily activity. In general, the caloric need can be estimated by multiplying the desired weight in pounds by 15 calories per pound per day (Box 8-2). A balanced diet provides 15% of the calories from protein sources. Fat sources should provide 30% of the daily calories, with the remaining 55% provided by carbohydrates.

BOX 8-2

Estimating Caloric Needs

Desired weight in pounds × 15 calories/lb per day = Necessary calories to maintain weight

Example: 150 lbs × 15 calories/lb per day = 2250 calories per day

To lose 1 lb each week, subtract 500 calories each day.

Example: 500 calories per day × 7 days = 3500 calories (1 lb)

Body mass index (BMI) is a number that is calculated using a person's weight and height. It indicates the amount of body fat and is used to screen for health problems. Although it does not measure the amount of fat directly, the results have been shown to correlate with measurements made using techniques like measuring skinfold thickness with callipers and hydrostatic (underwater) weighing. The BMI for adults (20 years or older) is calculated using a standard formula for men and women (Box 8-3).

For children and teens under 20 years of age, the BMI is specific for age and gender. This is because the

BOX 8-3

Body Mass Index Status*

Below 18.5	Underweight
18.5-24.9	Normal
25.0-29.9	Overweight
30.0 and greater	Obese

*Formula: weight (lb) / [height (in)]^2 × 703.

amount of fat changes with age and differs between girls and boys during growth years. The BMI status in children and teens is considered a screening tool, not a diagnostic tool. The CDC provides BMI-for-age growth or status charts for use with children and teens (Box 8-4).

BRAIN BYTE

According to the CDC, more than a third of adults and 16% to 33% of children in the United States are obese.

Weight can be regulated by counting calories. One pound (0.45 kg) of fat tissue is the equivalent of 3500 calories. Carbohydrates and protein provide 4 calories per gram. Fat provides 9 calories per gram. Vitamins and minerals do not contain any calories. Fad diets that limit the variety of foods eaten usually do not work on a permanent basis. One reason that quick weight loss is unsuccessful is that the body, when deprived of the essential nutrients, stores additional energy in the form of fat. Controlling weight results from balancing the number of calories taken in and the number of calories used as energy. The most successful method of weight loss is a gradual increase in caloric output by additional exercise and a decrease in the caloric intake of food. Weight loss of 1 to 2 pounds per week is considered safe and effective (Fig. 8-4).

Diet Therapy

Special diets are used to treat specific health conditions (Table 8-3). In addition to providing a balanced diet with adequate calories, the needs of special populations must be considered. Food habits are influenced by nationality, race, culture, religious beliefs, and personal preferences. Special diets must consider these factors, as well as nutrient requirements. The Dietary Guidelines for Americans (USDA, 2005) provide guidelines for older adults. A list of

BOX 8-4

Body Mass Index Weight Status Percentile Range for Children and Teens*

Underweight	Less than the 5th percentile
Healthy weight	5th percentile to less than the 85th percentile
Overweight	85th to less than the 95th percentile
Obese	Equal to or greater than the 95th percentile

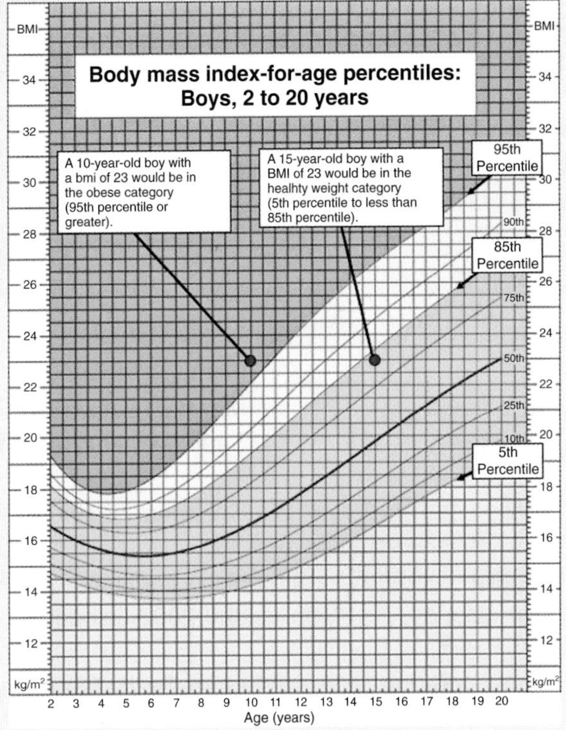

*From the Centers for Disease Control (CDC), available at: http://www.cdc.gov/healthyweight/assessing/bmi/childrens_BMI/about_childrens_BMI.html.

BRAIN BYTE

Eating 500 calories less each day results in 1 lb of weight loss each week.

CASE STUDY 8-1 You are helping admit a patient by measuring her weight and height. You find that she is 28 years old, 5′4″ tall and weighs 120 pounds. She tells you that she is embarrassed and depressed because she is so overweight. What should you do?

Answers to Case Studies are available on the Evolve website: ***http://evolve.elsevier.com/Gerdin***

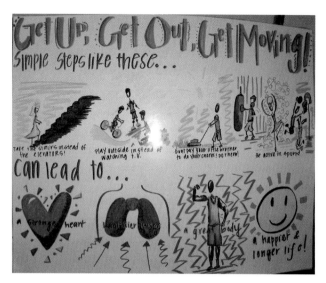

FIGURE 8-4 Simple changes in daily activities can increase exercise and the number of calories used. (Photo courtesy of National Health Occupations Students of America, Flower Mound, Tex.)

warning signs has been developed as a nutritional health checklist using the word *DETERMINE* (Box 8-5).

Stress Reduction

Identifying Stress

Stress is the body's nonspecific reaction to demands of everyday life. It affects a person physically and psychologically (Table 8-4). Stress is not the result of events that occur but rather the attitudes that are formed about the events. Individual responses to the same event may differ, and stress may result from a perceived threat that is not a real event. Some people do not take responsibility for the effects of stress in their own life, because they believe that others control it.

TABLE 8-3
Therapeutic Diets

Diet	Description	Use
Clear liquid	Minimal residue, dissolved sugar	Postsurgical, replace lost fluid
Full liquid	Strained, semiliquid, clear liquid	Progression to regular diet, digestive system upset
Soft	Chopped, strained, pureed, little fiber	Inability to chew, difficulty swallowing
Regular	No restrictions	
Low calorie	800-2000 calories	Overweight, arthritis, cardiac condition
High calorie	More than 2000 calories	Anorexia nervosa, hyperthyroidism, underweight
Bland	No highly seasoned foods, low fiber	Ulcer, colitis
Low sodium	No salt added on tray	Kidney disease, cardiovascular disorder, edema, hypertension
Restricted residue	Low in bulk, low fiber	Rectal disease, colitis, ileitis
Low carbohydrate	Sweets not allowed	Diabetes
Low cholesterol	Restricted saturated fat	Coronary disease, atherosclerosis
Low fat	High carbohydrates, low protein	Gallbladder disease, obesity, heart condition, liver disease
Lactose free	Lactose-free milk products, nondairy creamer, soy milk	Alactasia
High protein	Low carbohydrate, high protein	Pregnancy, postsurgical, children in growing years, burn victims
Diet substitutes	IV therapy, tube feeding	Dehydration, anorexia, poor nutrition, unconsciousness
Force fluids	Offer 8 oz of liquid every hour	Elderly, dehydration
Kosher	Separate utensils for meat and milk products	Observation of Jewish tradition

BOX 8-5

Nutritional Health Checklist

D—Disease
E—Eating poorly
T—Tooth loss or mouth pain
E—Economic hardship
R—Reduced social contact
M—Multiple medications
I—Involuntary weight loss/gain
N—Need of assistance in self-care
E—Elder years (older than age 80)

TABLE 8-4
Stress-Related Illness

Body Process	Effect of Stress
Cardiovascular system	Heart attack (myocardial infarction)
	High blood pressure (hypertension)
	Heart pain (angina)
	Migraine headache
	Stroke (cerebrovascular accident)
Digestive system	Ulcer
	Colitis
	Constipation
	Diarrhea
Skeletal system	Arthritis
Muscular system	Headache
	Backache
Respiratory system	Asthma
Endocrine system	Diabetes (type 2)
Nervous system	Accident proneness (decreased attention)
Immune process	Increased rate of infection
	Allergies
	Autoimmune disorders
Psychosocial process	Fighting
	Conflicts
	Alcoholism
	Drug abuse

Everyday stresses include pressures of urban life such as traffic, major life changes like birth and death, and management of a family and career. Social isolation may lead to stress when a person does not have an opportunity to express feelings or share in relationships with others. Financial concerns may also lead to the feelings of tension, frustration, and anxiety associated with stress.

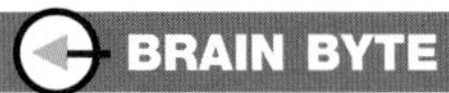

Stress does not decrease as you grow older, the cause just changes form.

Some of the common signs and symptoms of stress include the following:

- Increased heart rate
- Floating feeling of anxiety
- Trembling
- Indigestion
- Pain in the neck or back

Stress experienced for long periods has been linked to physical disorders, including the following:

- Hypertension
- Headache
- Atherosclerosis
- Back pain
- Ulcers
- Colitis
- Substance abuse
- Weight change
- Insomnia
- Accident proneness
- Skin disorder
- Rheumatoid arthritis
- Decrease in immune system efficiency

Stress Theory

In the 1950s Franz Alexander proposed that some specific illnesses resulted from the stress of life events. His theory introduced the concept of psychosomatic disorders or illness that result from actions of the emotions on the body. Also called psychophysiological disorders, psychogenic disease, or organ neuroses, this condition does not mean that the person is not ill, rather that the illness is caused by the person's own mind. Alexander proposed that certain specific personality traits combined with certain life events cause specific disorders of the body. Alexander's theory is now generally considered too rigid, but the idea that many illnesses are caused at least in part by emotional factors is well accepted. For example, the action of tightening muscles of the neck and back when under stress can lead to a headache.

One of many theories on personality types was developed by two cardiologists, Meyer Friedman and Ray Rosenman in 1959 (Table 8-5). They proposed that people with type A personalities were more

TABLE 8-5
Personality Types*

Description	Type A Personality	Type B Personality
Movement	Walks, eats, and talks rapidly	Lacks sense of urgency, enjoys relaxing without guilt
Action	Does two or more things at a time	Does one thing at a time
Temperament	Competitive, impatient, aggressive, achievement oriented, hostile, status conscious, focus on quantity more than quality, approval seeking	Patient, easygoing, passive, noncompetitive, little need for advancement, focus on quality, self-reflecting

*These descriptors are extremes of the characteristics.

prone to cardiovascular disorders and sudden death. Their theory has been supported by research that followed the health of men who were evaluated for behavior patterns. After 8½ years, the type A personalities in the study group had twice the incidence of coronary heart disease as the type B personalities. It has been shown that when the "fight or flight" response is triggered repeatedly, a resulting abnormal level of adrenaline and cortisol increases the level of cholesterol and fat in the bloodstream. A type C personality has been described as a person who can use the characteristics and behaviors of the type A personality without triggering a stress response.

Stress Management

Some methods used to manage stress include proper nutrition, exercise, relaxation techniques, and personal behavior changes. Another stress management technique includes methods of time management (Box 8-6). Because stress builds, intervention to decrease stress should be practiced regularly. The goal of stress management is lower rates for blood pressure, pulse, and respiration, as well as a refreshed feeling of peacefulness or calm.

Methods to help manage stress include the following:

- Identify the cause of stress.
- Make conscious choices to control stress.
- Develop coping and relaxation techniques.
- Practice good health habits.
- Plan ahead.
- Laugh.
- Use energy (adrenaline) in another manner (exercise).
- Relax.
- Seek emotional support.
- Maintain good nutrition.
- Avoid caffeine.
- Practice meditation, biofeedback, guided imagery, prayer, or hypnosis.
- Decrease alcohol or drug intake.
- Sleep.
- Take a warm bath.
- Walk.
- Decrease sugar intake.
- Play games or enjoy hobbies.
- Perform yoga.

BOX 8-6

Stress Management Techniques

- Plan and organize your workload.
- When possible, do things one at a time to completion.
- Occasionally plan to escape and have fun.
- Be positive about things and avoid criticizing others.
- Avoid unnecessary competition.
- Learn to negotiate.
- Get regular exercise.
- Tolerate, forgive, and learn to accept others.
- Talk to someone about things that are troubling you.
- Relax with methods such as biofeedback, yoga, and meditation.
- Use time-management techniques.
- Take mini-breaks during the day to relax and breathe.
- Practice acceptance of things that cannot be changed.
- Take responsibility for your own actions.
- Set realistic goals and expectations for yourself and others.
- Eat sensibly.

CASE STUDY 8-2 You notice that you are very tense and have a headache at the end of your shift every day. What should you do?

Answers to Case Studies are available on the Evolve website: ***http://evolve.elsevier.com/Gerdin***

Counseling

Guidance or counseling may be given by professionals for emotional concerns and for career decisions. As society has become more complex, the need for more specific types of counseling has emerged. Some of the signs and symptoms of a disorder of mental health include sadness, violent or erratic moods, an inability to make decisions, sleep disturbances, self-destructive behavior, physical disorders, fear, anger, anxiety, or a sense of hopelessness. Although friends can provide emotional support by listening, professional counselors including psychologists, psychiatrists, and others use specific techniques to help people cope with and solve their own problems (Table 8-6).

Habit Cessation

Addiction may be physical, psychological, or both. In a chemical addiction, the substance produces a feeling of pleasure similar to that produced by the brain's own endorphins and enkephalins. The regular use of narcotics can change the ability of the brain to produce these chemicals, leading to increased dependence on

TABLE 8-6
Family Counseling Techniques

Technique	Description
Patient control	The individual is taught to control the problem with specific directives of actions to be taken when situations occur.
Communication skill-building	The focus is on improvement of communication techniques such as listening, brainstorming, and relating in a nonjudgmental manner.
Family floor plan	Participant draws a floor plan of the generational or nuclear family information. Space and territory allotted to family members are evaluated.
Family photos	Discussion and observation of family members viewing family photos may be used to diagnose family relationships, rituals, communication, and roles.
Empty chair	An empty chair may be used to express feelings and thoughts to a family member. The role of the family member may also be played by the one expressing feelings.
Family choreography	Family members are asked to arrange the family as they believe it relates and then rearrange members in a manner that would be preferred.
Family counsel meeting	Rules are outlined and specific times are set for the family to meet and interact to provide structure for participation and communication.
Family sculpting	Family members represent their perceptions of the others to communicate in a nonverbal manner.
Genogram	This informational and diagnostic tool is developed by the therapist to show the family structure.
Prescribing indecision	A directive is given to the family member who usually makes decisions to let another member make decisions or to take a specified amount of time before a decision is made.
Reframing	An action that is perceived as negative is framed into a positive category.
Special days	Mini-vacations may be used to assist families to communicate or appreciate others.
Strategic alliance	One member of the family is given the role of helping another to implement behavioral change.
Tracking	The therapist listens to, records, and stores family events to identify possible interventions.

the narcotic. However, many other common habits or addictions can affect a person's level of wellness in a negative manner. For example, according to the *New England Journal of Medicine*, the lifetime medical cost for smokers is one third higher than nonsmokers, even though smokers have a shorter life span.

Many methods or treatments have been developed to treat addiction problems. No single method is considered effective in all cases. Some examples of treatment methods include the use of aversion therapy, support groups, and acupuncture. Experts generally accept that a long-term recovery program is necessary for any treatment to succeed. Many programs also use behavioral training and coping techniques in addition to the specific habit cessation method.

Exercise

The benefits of exercise are both emotional and physical (Fig. 8-5). A regular exercise program reduces the risk of cardiovascular disease and improves emotional outlook. Some specific physical benefits of exercise include increased bone density, decreased blood levels of cholesterol, improved ability to use glucose, and improved cardiac performance. The result of these effects is a decrease in the risk of developing heart disease, osteoporosis, diabetes, hypertension, and obesity. Exercise also causes the release of the brain's endorphins, leading to a feeling of well-being. It has been associated with an improvement in self-image and a reduction of depression, stress, and anxiety. Even a person with a sedentary lifestyle or limited mobility must maintain a certain amount of activity so that the body is able to function. Without some activity, the body begins to dysfunction or become disabled. For example, when a cast is applied to allow a fracture to heal, the muscles begin to atrophy and must be rebuilt to establish normal activity after the cast is removed.

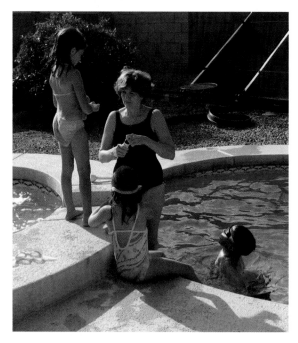

FIGURE 8-5 Exercise has both emotional and physical benefits.

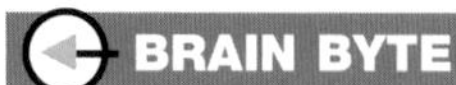

BRAIN BYTE

The CDC recommends that children and adolescents should have at least 60 minutes of physical activity every day, most of which should be moderate to intense aerobic activities.

Aerobic exercise programs are designed to improve cardiac performance. To achieve aerobic benefits, it is recommended to raise the heart rate, or pulse, to approximately 70% of the individual's maximum heart rate and maintain the elevated rate for 30 minutes at least three times each week. To calculate the maximum heart rate, the person subtracts his or her age from 220 and then multiplies the remainder by 70% (Box 8-7). Any exercise program should be started gradually to allow the body to adjust to the new stresses resulting from it.

CASE STUDY 8-3 You are caring for a patient that has an order to force fluids. What should you do?

Answers to Case Studies are available on the Evolve website: ***http://evolve.elsevier.com/Gerdin***

Growth and Development

The physical and psychological stage of a person changes rapidly from the moment of birth. Growth

BOX 8-7

Calculation of Heart Rate for Cardiovascular Exercise

Formula:	(220 − Age) × 0.7 = Maximum heart rate
Example:	(220 − 20) × 0.7 = 140*

*For a 20-year-old person, the recommended heart rate to maintain for 30 minutes at least three times a week is 140. The 70% is an average and may be adjusted to 60% for a less athletic person or to 80% for a more athletic person.

refers to the changes that can be measured in height and weight and in body proportions. Development describes the stages of change in psychological and social functioning (Fig. 8-6).

Physical Growth and Development

Physical changes occur in spurts throughout the life span (Table 8-8). At birth the baby, or neonate, is about 19 to 21 inches long and weighs 7 to 8 lb. The head is one fourth the length of the body compared with the adult ratio of one eighth. For the first 4 weeks, the baby is referred to as a neonate. As the person grows, the body proportions change and develop into an adult appearance.

The study of aging is called *gerontology*. Geriatrics refers to the care of the elderly. Aging is a normal process that occurs gradually through the life span. Elderly persons have specific needs resulting from the changes in body function and structure (Table 8-9).

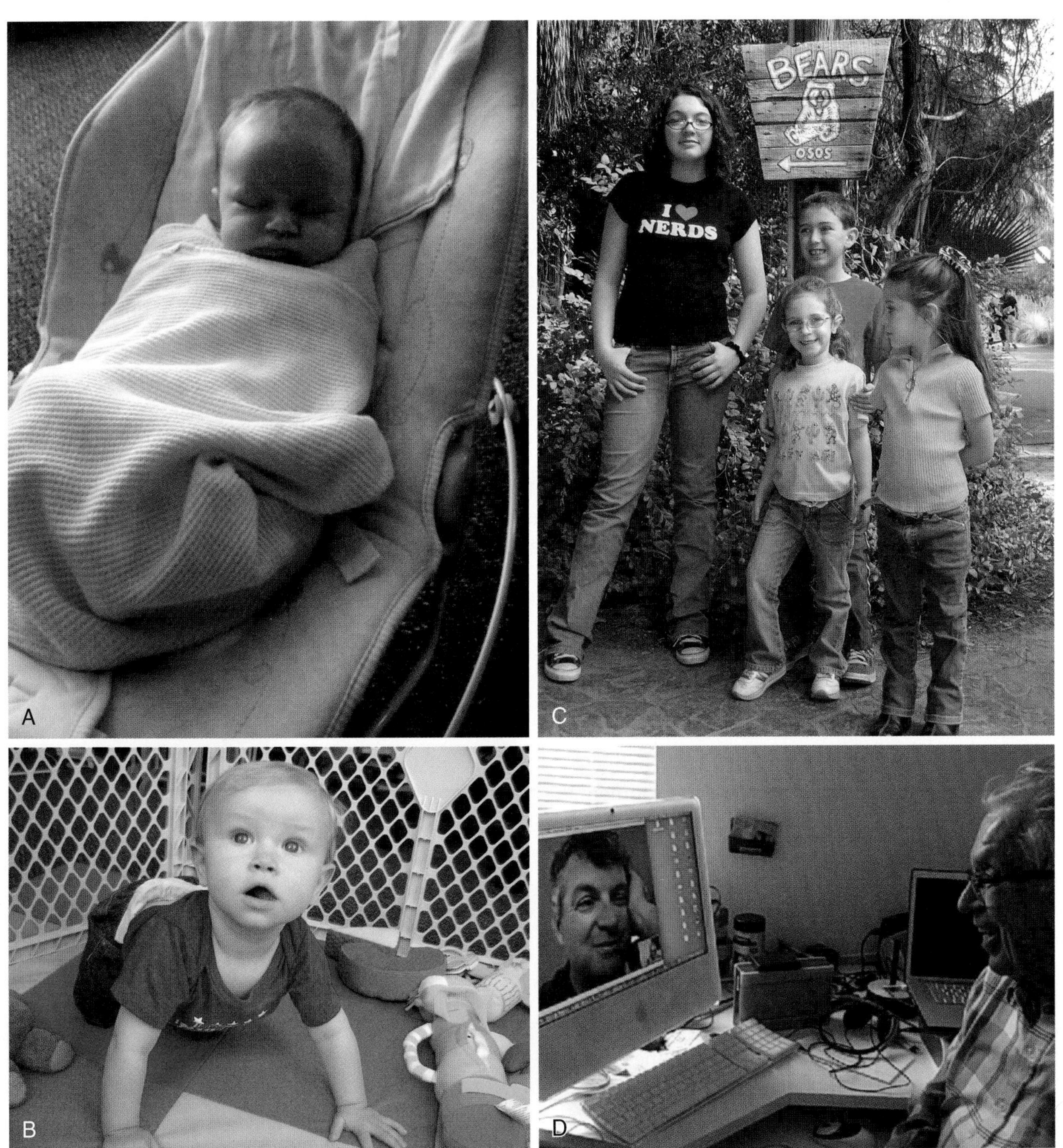

FIGURE 8-6 Psychosocial needs of an individual change from infancy to adulthood.

TABLE 8-7
Developmental Steps through the Life Span

Stage of Life	Developmental Changes
Infant (birth to 1 year)	Growth occurs in spurts, needs constant care, learns the differences in sensory input, sleeps in short periods, motor responses are uncontrolled, plays with own hands and feet, vital signs not stable, may experience separation anxiety at 8 mo
Toddler (1-2 years)	Takes first steps, mood changes quickly, begins to sense own energy and independence, learns to speak, coordination improves, suffers separation anxiety when away from family, self-loving, uninhibited, accidents and respiratory illness main threats to death
Preschooler (3-5 years)	Becomes a social being, recognizes peers, growth slows, has an excess of energy, needs clear-cut rules, can organize experiences into concepts, develops own self-concept and body image
School-age child (6-12 years)	Learns to channel energy, acquires knowledge and new skills quickly, peers become more important, growth is slow and steady, begins to reason about experiences, learns to compromise and cooperate
Adolescent (13-18 years)	Reaches puberty and sexual maturation, hormone levels increase, growth slows and stops, peers may assume primary importance, may rebel against family and society, forms own identity, needs limits, drug abuse and suicide may result from conflicts
Young adult (19 to 45 years)	Demonstrates place in society, establishes independence from family, may marry and start own family, plans for economic security, chooses lifestyle options
Middle-age adult (46-65 years)	Earns most of the money and makes most of the decisions for society, may question own life choices in self-assessment, decrease in hormone secretion leads to changes in body, metabolic rate decreases, eyesight may decline, skin thins and loses elasticity, learns to use leisure time
Older adult (66 years and older)	Must learn to reconcile life experiences with value system, slower neurologic responses lead to slower interpretation of sensory input, may suffer hearing loss, restriction in mobility, decreased ability to respond well to stress

Psychosocial Growth and Development

The psychosocial needs of the individual change as life progresses from birth to death. Developmental changes and abilities determine the type of care that is given (Table 8-7). Characteristic behaviors for each stage of development have been identified (Table 8-10). As a result of psychosocial development, children may not understand the confinement and pain resulting from illness and hospitalization (Fig. 8-7). In addition, a person who is ill or dying reacts psychologically. Coping strategies may include using defense mechanisms to deal with illness (Box 8-8). Defense mechanisms are unconscious psychological strategies used to cope and maintain self-image. In giving the care to the patient who is

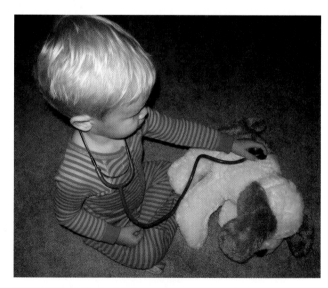

FIGURE 8-7 A child's understanding of treatments and tests can be improved through play.

TABLE 8-8
Physical Growth through the Life Span

Stage of Life	Milestones of Development
Infancy (birth to 1 year)	Head large in proportion to body; movement uncoordinated; vision unclear; good hearing, smell, and taste senses; teeth begin to erupt at 6 mo; physical growth is rapid; decline in amount of "baby fat"; lumbar curvature develops Learns to walk, communicate (talk), and understand some words; eats solid foods; forms relationships; sleeps and eats regularly
Toddler (1-2 years)	Muscles and nervous system become more coordinated, especially hands; physical growth continues less rapidly Learns to communicate with words; becomes less dependent and tolerates separation from person giving primary care; controls bowels and bladder; able to move by crawling, climbing, and running; plays in parallel (not together)
Early childhood (3-5 years)	Grows taller; gains little weight; increases coordination; begins to draw and write Ability to communicate increases; learns gender difference and modesty; learns right from wrong; plays with others; develops sense of family; provides some care of self
Middle childhood (6-8 years)	Grows in height and weight slowly; primary teeth are lost; hand coordination increases, allowing cursive writing; permanent teeth erupt Develops skills to play games; gets along with others of same age; learns basic skills of language and math; develops self-image of gender and self-esteem
Late childhood (9-12 years)	Muscles increase in strength, coordination, and balance; develops physical skills; grows in height (girls taller than boys); permanent teeth appear; secondary sexual characteristics appear Becomes independent; develops peer relationships; develops interest in sexual information
Adolescence (13-18 years)	Rapid physical growth; changes of puberty begin; growth uneven (clumsiness); "wisdom" teeth appear Rapid psychosocial development; relationships with peers and dating experiences develop
Young adulthood (19-45 years)	Little physical growth; bone growth plates close Chooses occupation; develops family unit with marriage, children, or others
Middle adulthood (46-65 years)	Gradual slowing of metabolism; changes of aging occur Lives on own or with adjusted family as children leave and parents age or die; develops leisure activities
Late adulthood (66 years and older)	Declines in physical strength, endurance, and overall health condition Adjusts to retirement, reduced income, and death of spouse; accepts own death

dying, at any age, it is important to consider psychosocial development.

The natural changes in physical, psychological, and social functioning with aging may lead to a change in role for the person and family (Box 8-9). A social role or identity is the expected or typical behavior expected by a person who fills a position in a group such as a family. For example, a person might fill the role of the mother, the child, student, and so forth. As a person becomes older, he or she might not be able to fill the roles that were previously held. New roles such as widowhood and retirement are

TABLE 8-9
Changes of Aging

System or Aspect	Change
Skeletal	Decrease in size; decalcification; bones more porous
Integumentary	Dry, thin, inelastic, pigment changes; hair thins; decrease in ability to make Vitamin D
Urinary	Number of nephrons decreases; bladder wall and meatus muscle tone lost
Respiratory	Costals harden; decrease in efficiency of system
Cardiovascular	Fatty deposits in vessels; hardening of vessels
Sensory	Decrease in muscle tone of eyes; hardening of lens; clouding of lens; increased pressure in eye; decrease in number of hair cells in ear; eardrum less flexible; decrease in number of taste buds; presbyopia decreases ability to focus
Reproductive	Menopause; decrease in amount of lubricant secretion and muscle tone of reproductive organs
Neurologic	Decrease in response time
Digestive	Decrease of water in body; less saliva; less absorption of nutrients; decrease in stomach acids, slowing digestion
Endocrine	Decrease in hormones, especially thyroid and sex hormones
Sociologic loss	Family, friends, and contemporaries die
Metabolic slowing	Drugs processed more slowly; weight gained more easily; less sleep needed; more sleeping difficulties

TABLE 8-10
Psychosocial Development through the Life Span

Stage of Life	Typical Behavior
Infant (birth to 1 year)	Responds reflexively; completely self-centered; detects changes; remembers responses and their results
Toddler (1-2 years)	Quickly changing moods; forming sense of independence; jealous when not center of attention; attached to mother and senses separation anxiety
Preschooler (3-5 years)	Speaks meaningfully; asks many questions, controls impulses, interacts with others of own age; forms theories about experiences
School-age child (6 to 12 years)	Learns quickly; curious; realistic; likes to associate with others of own age
Adolescent (13-18 years)	Reaches sexual maturity; seeks independence; able to learn quickly; develops concepts about life; develops slang and behaviors of peer groups
Young adult (19-45 years)	Expects physical health; continues to learn quickly; chooses career, family, or alternate lifestyle
Middle-age adult (46-65 years)	Makes decision for family, business, and society; seeks security for later years; questions meaning of life; finds ability to learn changing; memorization more difficult and spoken presentation less effective
Older adult (66 years and older)	Memory loss of recent events occurs; thinking process slows but is not impaired; learns best when focusing on one thing at a time; vision and mobility impaired; reviews life experiences

developed. The older person may fill the role of being dependent either physically, financially, or emotionally on others in the family. As roles change, the individual's dignity and worth must be reinforced and reestablished.

Change Theory

Methods of adaptation to change vary as a person ages. Many theories and models exist for describing behavior change as it relates to a person's health.

BOX 8-8

Emotional Reactions to Medical Illness

Emotions
- Anger
- Anxiety
- Conflict
- Depression
- Fear
- Helplessness
- Hostility
- Regression
- Stress

Defense Mechanisms*
- Denial
- Displacement
- Intellectualization
- Projection
- Rationalization
- Reaction formation
- Regression
- Repression
- Sublimation
- Suppression

*Sigmund Freud described 10 defense mechanisms used to deal with anxiety.

BOX 8-9

Characteristics of Successful Aging*

- Sense of worth and having a place in the world
- Sense of being competent and capable
- Economic security
- Ability to function independently
- Ability to make own decisions
- Good physical health
- Positive attitude
- Dignity and respect
- Leisure and meaningful activities
- Ability to contribute
- Meaningful relationships

*Adaptations may be necessary during aging to maintain these characteristics.

Change may be considered a linear process that occurs in one direction in a sequential manner. Complex changes are nonlinear and result from multiple interactions. Nonlinear approaches to change adaptation are found in learning, organization, and social cognitive theories.

Learning theories divide complex behaviors into small changes toward a larger goal. The habitual, older, and undesired behaviors are replaced by new ones. Reinforcement and rewards for the desired behaviors help the person maintain the behavioral change.

One of the first behavioral models applied to health care was the psychological Health Belief Model. It was developed in the 1950s to explain the lack of participation by the public in a program designed to screen for tuberculosis. The key variables are the perceived threat or susceptibility and severity, benefit, barriers, actions, and cues to action. Other variables in this model include demographics and the belief that the behavior will produce the desired outcome (self-efficacy).

The Transtheoretical Model of Change was developed in the 1980s. It is a model of intentional change focusing on individual decision making. The Transtheoretical Model is a process involving five stages. The five stages include precontemplation, contemplation, preparation, action, and maintenance.

Social cognitive theory and the theory of planned behavior are both social science theories as opposed to behavioral theories of change. They both state that change is influenced by behavioral, environmental, and personal factors. These theories emphasize the importance of the influence of other people in implementing behavioral change.

Another approach that has been developed to describe change is called the ecological approach. It assumes that environmental factors such as family, culture, and economics affect behavior. This model states that a change in the environmental factors leads to a change in the behavior.

Death and Dying

Death is a natural part of life. It is the end of life functions and results in the destruction of the body's cells. Biological death is the loss of cell function resulting in the absence of breathing and heartbeat. Clinical death, also called *brain death,* is the loss of function of the brainstem or the capacity for consciousness. Clinical death is defined legally as loss of brain activity for a specified amount of time. The study of death

BOX 8-10

Bill of Rights for the Terminally Ill

I have the right to say what I feel about my death and express my own philosophy or religious beliefs about it.

I have the right to health care to provide comfort and lessen pain provided by caring and knowledgeable professionals.

I have the right to help in making decisions about my care and to have my questions answered honestly.

I have the right to maintain hope to meet the goals I set regarding my death.

I have the right to maintain dignity and individuality as a person and be treated as a living person until I die.

I have the right to die with my family or someone caring present and to die in peace with dignity.

I have the right to expect that my body will be treated with respect after my death.

BOX 8-11

The Living Will

To My Family, My Physician, My Lawyer, and All Others Whom It May Concern,

Death is as much a reality as birth, growth, maturity, and old age—it is the one certainty of life. If the time comes that I can no longer take part in decisions for my future, let this statement stand as an expression of my wishes and direction, while I am still of sound mind.

If at such a time the situation should arise in which there is no reasonable expectation of my recovery from extreme physical or mental disability, I direct that I be allowed to die and not be kept alive by medications, artificial means, or "heroic measures." I do, however, ask that medication be mercifully administered to me to alleviate suffering even though this may shorten my remaining life.

This statement is made after careful consideration and is in accordance with my strong convictions and beliefs. I want the wishes and directions here expressed carried out to the extent permitted by law. Insofar as they are not legally enforceable, I hope that those to whom this Will is addressed will regard themselves as morally bound by these provisions.

(thanatology) became an area of research in the twentieth century. Legal and ethical controversy surrounds the definition of death and the rights of the **terminally** ill to refuse life-prolonging treatments (Box 8-10).

Most people die in hospitals, long-term care facilities, or hospices. In some cases the dying person may stay home until death with occasional visits from hospice personnel. Death may occur suddenly or may be expected as a result of injury or terminal illness. Dying patients often represent failure to the health care professional. The attitude of the health care worker directly affects the dying patient and family. Personal experience, religion, culture, and the ability to reason determine a person's attitude about death (Box 8-11). Grief is the process that gradually resolves the sense of loss resulting from death.

Attitudes about death often change with circumstances and increased age. Before 5 years of age, most children do not view death as final. However, children between 8 and 11 years of age understand that death is personal and inevitable. Because the arrangements for the rituals after death are often made by a funeral director, the family is isolated from direct contact with the dead. This isolation may result in a sense of mystery or fright because of unknown elements about death.

One theory to explain the acceptance of death was developed by psychiatrist Dr. Elisabeth Kübler-Ross. She identified five stages of grief. These stages are denial, anger, bargaining, depression, and acceptance. During denial, the individual refuses to believe that the death will occur or has occurred. Anger results as the person blames others or fate for the death or the prognosis. Bargaining with a higher power may occur to reconcile differences with a spiritual figure. Depression may occur when the person realizes the finality of the loss. The final stage is acceptance of the death or inevitability of dying.

Terminally ill individuals and their families do not always progress through all stages to acceptance. Psychological disorders may result as a failure to resolve this conflict. Dying people continue to have psychological, social, and spiritual needs. People usually need to communicate and resolve conflicts when death is expected. The health care worker provides quality care by allowing the patient to express his or her thoughts and feelings without judgment.

Some physical signs that indicate death is approaching include loss of muscle control, slowing of gastrointestinal functions, rise in body temperature, respiratory irregularities, and decrease in pain. The pulse rate is rapid, weak, and irregular. The patient may complain of feeling cold and have pale, cool skin caused by a decrease in circulation.

Signs that death has occurred include absence of pulse, respiration, and blood pressure. The "death rattle," caused by mucus collecting in the throat and bronchial tubes, may be heard. Only a physician can legally pronounce a person dead.

CASE STUDY 8-4 You are providing care for a patient who has been told of a terminal illness. The patient is very rude to you and throws the food tray to the floor when you enter the room. What should you do?

Answers to Case Studies are available on the Evolve website: ***http://evolve.elsevier.com/Gerdin***

Summary

- Three factors that may be used to determine level of wellness are mind, body, and spirit.
- Three categories of disease prevention are primary, secondary, and tertiary prevention.
- The function of carbohydrates is to provide a source for quick, immediate energy. Proteins are used to build tissues such as muscles. Fats are used to repair cells and make hormones. Vitamins regulate cell metabolism. Minerals regulate body processes.
- Weight control is a balance between the number of calories taken in and the number of calories used as energy.
- Therapeutic diets are used to treat specific health conditions. For example, a clear liquid diet is used after surgery and contains minimal residue.
- Five events that may result in a feeling of stress include traffic, birth, death, career, and family management.
- Five illnesses that may result from stress include a heart attack, high blood pressure, migraine headache, ulcer, and colitis.
- Methods used to manage stress include relaxation techniques, walking, taking a warm bath, and sleeping.
- Changes in physical development occur through the life span.
- Psychosocial development through the life span results in varied behaviors.
- Models of change theory that may be applied to health care include the Human Belief Model and the Transtheoretical Model of Change.
- The five stages of death acceptance (grief) described by Elisabeth Kübler-Ross are denial, anger, bargaining, depression, and acceptance.

Review Questions

1. List three factors that may be used to determine a level of wellness.
2. Describe the three categories of prevention of disease.
3. Describe the function of each of the five nutrients. Explain why water may also be considered a nutrient.
4. Draw a personalized USDA food pyramid that includes the groups and number of servings recommended for each. Design a daily meal plan that meets the recommended servings.
5. Explain the relationship of calories to weight loss and gain.
6. List five therapeutic diets and the conditions for which each might be required.
7. Describe five body reactions resulting from stress.
8. Describe four methods that may be used to manage stress.
9. Compare physical development of a 1-year-old, 10-year-old, and an adult.
10. Compare the psychosocial development of a 1-year-old, 10-year-old, and an adult.
11. Describe the five stages of death acceptance.
12. Use each of the following terms in one or more sentences that correctly relate their meaning: anabolism, calorie, catabolism, metabolism.

Critical Thinking

1. Investigate the chemical differences between and uses of the following forms of sugar:
   Brown
   Corn syrup
   Dextrose
   Fructose
   Honey
   Lactose
   Mannitol
   Raw
   Sorbitol
   Sucrose
   Xylitol

2. Investigate the interaction of common drugs and foods.
3. Investigate, compare, and contrast the USDA food pyramid to the Harvard Healthy Eating Pyramid and Oldways Preservation and Exchange Trust's Asian, Latin, Mediterranean, and vegetarian pyramids. Write an essay that compares the models and supports one of them.
4. Investigate the requirements for health claims on labeling, such as the percentage of fat that can be contained in a food labeled "low fat."
5. Keep a diary of daily food consumption and activity. Calculate the calories for each and determine whether weight will be lost or gained.
6. Investigate the diet of special populations found in the geographic area. Hypothesize about the success of several of the therapeutic diets with the local population.
7. Investigate and compare the developmental stages described by Levinson, Erickson, and Piaget.
8. Investigate how health care workers have used the Health Belief Model in treatment and prevention of sexually transmitted diseases.
9. Design a plan for change in a health-related behavior using the Transtheoretical or Health Belief Model of change.
10. Write an essay describing the meaning of death, including any personal experiences that may help determine its meaning.
11. Use the Internet to investigate what "cardiac rehabilitation" might include. Design a patient brochure that describes what it is, why it is used, and what is included in it.
12. Use the Internet to research and describe the defense mechanisms described by Freud and how they apply to medical illness.

Explore the Web

Nutrition

USDA

http://mypyramid.gov

http://www.myfoodapedia.gov/

WebMD

http://www.webmd.com/diet/food-fitness-planner

Medline

http://www.nlm.nih.gov/medlineplus/diets.html

Harvard Healthy Eating

http://www.hsph.harvard.edu/nutritionsource/what-should-you-eat/pyramid/

Oldways

http://www.oldwayspt.org/

Cardiac Rehabilitation

AHA

http://americanheart.org

Mayo Clinic

http://www.mayoclinic.com/health/cardiac-rehabilitation/MY00771

Development Stages

Search Key Terms: "Erickson" "Piaget" "Levinson" "compare"

BMI Calculators

CDC Child and Teen

http://apps.nccd.cdc.gov/dnpabmi/Calculator.aspx

CDC Adult

http://www.cdc.gov/healthyweight/assessing/bmi/adult_bmi/english_bmi_calculator/bmi_calculator.html

STANDARDS AND ACCOUNTABILITY*

Foundation Standard 9: Health Maintenance Practices

Health care professionals will understand the fundamentals of wellness and the prevention of disease processes. They will practice preventive health behaviors among the clients.

Accountability Criteria

9.1 Healthy Behaviors

9.11 Apply behaviors that promote health and wellness.

9.12 Describe strategies for the prevention of diseases including health screenings and examinations.

9.13 Discuss complementary (alternative) health practices as they relate to wellness and disease prevention.

*From the National Consortium for Health Science Education (2009). National Health Care Standards and Accountability Criteria. Available at: http://www.healthscienceconsortium.org.

UNIT TWO

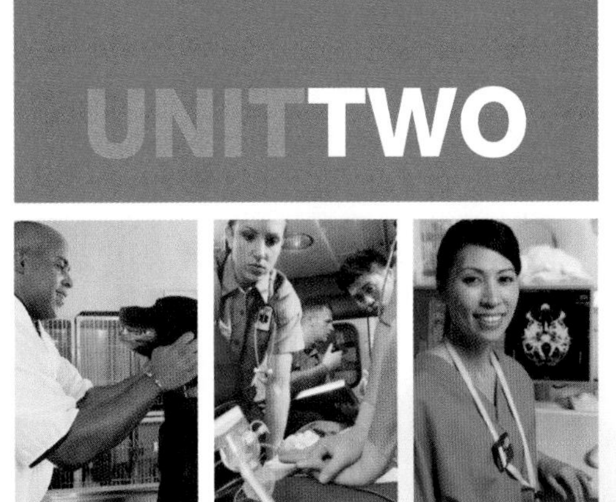

Anatomy and Physiology

CHAPTER 9

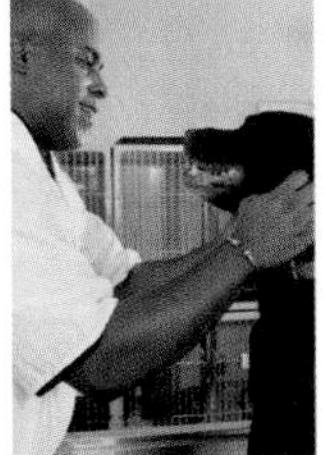
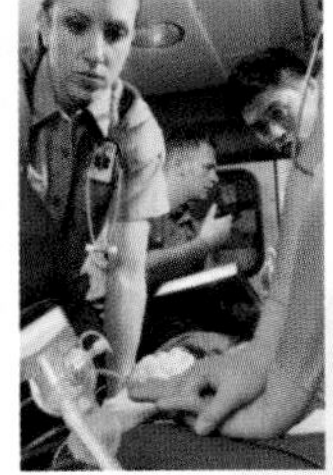
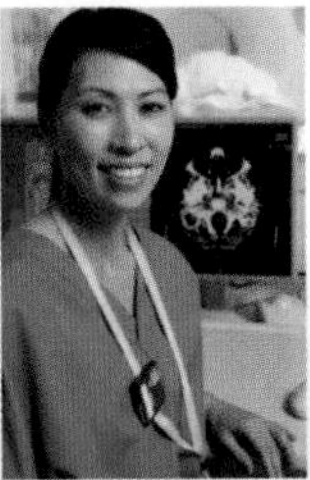

Body Organization

LEARNING OBJECTIVES

- Identify the meaning of 10 or more terms relating to the organization of the body.
- Describe the properties of life.
- Label the structures of the cell, and describe the function of each.
- Describe the organization of the body from the smallest unit to the largest.
- Describe organs of the body in relation to the plane, region, or cavity of location.
- Describe five or more disorders resulting from variations or defects in cell organization.

KEY TERMS

Autosome *(AW-toe-zome)* Any chromosome except the X or Y

Benign *(bi-NINE)* Self-limiting, not malignant

Condition *(kun-DISH-un)* Change from normal function that cannot be cured

Congenital *(kon-JEN-i-tal)* Referring to conditions that exist at birth regardless of cause

Disease *(di-ZEEZ)* Interruption of normal function of the body, usually caused by microorganisms; can be treated

Dominant *(DOM-i-nant)* Gene trait that appears when carried by only one in the pair of chromosomes

Electrolyte *(e-LEK-tro-lite)* Substance that separates into ions in solution and is capable of conducting electricity

Genotype *(JEEN-o-tipe)* Genetic pattern of an individual

Heredity *(he-RED-i-tee)* Genetic transmission of trait or particular quality from parent to offspring

Homeostasis *(ho-me-o-STAY-sis)* Tendency of an organism to maintain the "status quo" or the same internal environment

Malignant *(muh-LIG-nuh-nt)* Characterized by uncontrolled growth, invasive, tending to produce death

Mutation *(myoo-TAY-shun)* Permanent change in a gene or chromosome

KEY TERMS cont'd

Organism *(OR-gah-nizm)* Individual living thing, plant, or animal

Phenotype *(FEE-no-tipe)* Physical, biochemical, and physiological configuration of an individual determined by genes

Recessive *(re-SESS-iv)* Gene trait that does not appear unless carried by both members of a pair of chromosomes

Syndrome *(SIN-drome)* Set of symptoms that occur together

Body Organization Terminology*

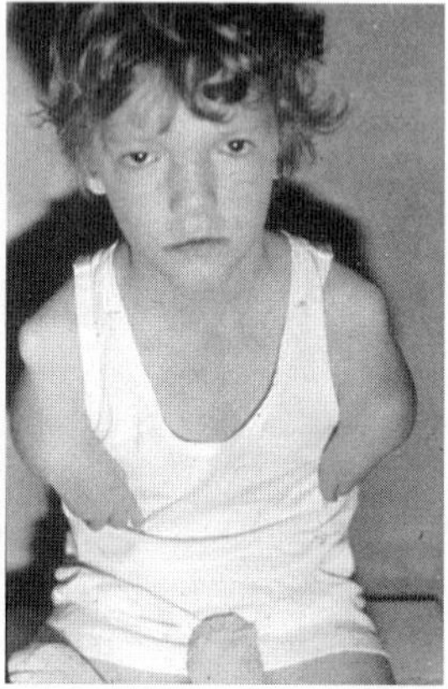

Thalidomide was a sleeping pill prescribed in the 1950s that caused more than 3000 children to be born with congenital birth defects. (Photograph courtesy of Dr. Olav Hilmar Iversen. In Damjanov I: *Pathology for the Health Professions*, ed 3, St. Louis, 2006, Saunders.)

Term	Definition	Prefix	Root	Suffix
Abduct	Draw away from the center	ab	duct	
Adduct	Draw toward the center	ad	duct	
Congenital	Born with	con	gen/it	al
Chemotherapy	Treatment by a chemical agent	chem/o*	therapy	
Cytoplasm	Nonorganelle material contained in cells	cyt/o	plasm	
Dysfunction	Impairment of function	dys	function	
Genetic	Pertaining to genes		gen/et	ic
Genotype	Genetic makeup of an organism		gen/o	type
Physiology	Study of function		physi	ology
Semipermeable	Allowing only some materials to enter and exit	semi	permeable	

*A short transition syllable or vowel may be added to or deleted from the word parts to make the combining form.

Abbreviations of Body Organization

Abbreviation	Meaning
A&P	Anatomy and physiology
ant	Anterior
CA^{+2}	Calcium ion
Cl^-	Chlorine ion
CVS	Chorionic villus sampling
DNA	Deoxyribonucleic acid
LUQ	Left upper quadrant
Na^+	Sodium ion
Post	Posterior
RLQ	Right lower quadrant

Anatomy and Physiology

The human body, like all living **organisms**, has four basic properties of life:

- Reception is the ability of the organism to control its actions and respond to changes in the environment.
- Metabolism is the process of taking in and using nutrients to produce energy and growth.
- Reproduction is the ability to reproduce offspring to continue the species.
- Organization divides the organism into distinct parts to perform these functions.

The two major types of study of the human body are called *anatomy* and *physiology*. Anatomy is the study of body structures and their location. Body structures are organized on five levels:

- Cells are the smallest unit of life.
- Tissues are combinations of similar cells.
- Organs are collections of tissues working together to perform a function.
- Body systems consist of organs that work together to provide a major body function.
- Organisms are the beings that result when the body systems work together to maintain life.

BRAIN BYTE

The median age of all Americans in 2000 was 35.3 years of age. The number of Americans 65 and older was 35 million, or one in eight.

Cell Structure

The major structures, called *organelles*, of the cell are shown in Fig. 9-1. These structures include:

- The nucleus controls the activity of the cell and directs reproduction.
- The cytoplasm is a semifluid material that surrounds the cell parts and transports chemicals and nutrients within the cell.
- Mitochondria produce the energy used for cellular processes.
- The cell membrane surrounds the cell and controls which substances enter and leave the cell.
- Lysosomes help to break down, or digest, molecules.
- Ribosomes attached to the rough endoplasmic reticulum work to make protein for the cell structures.

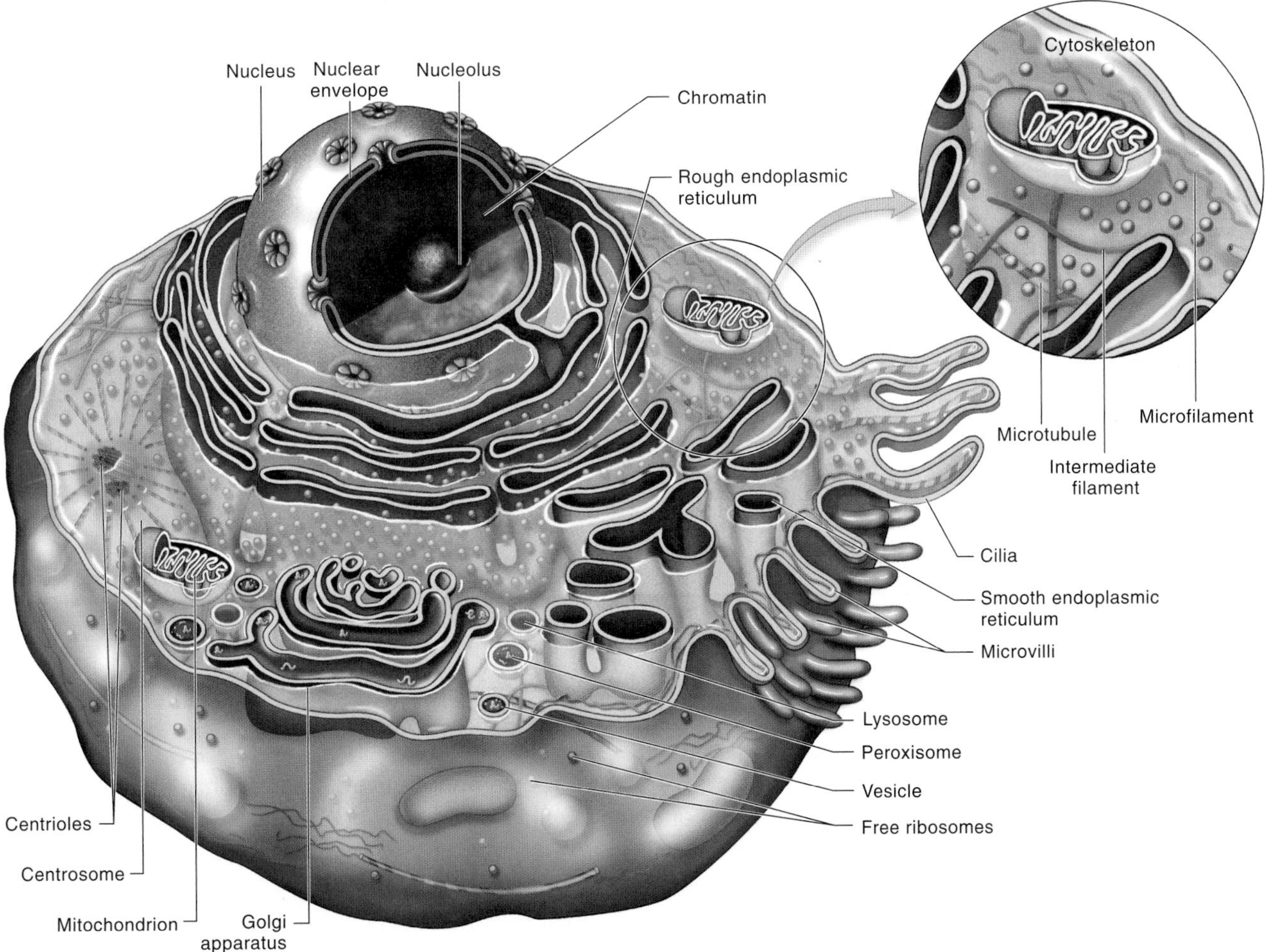

FIGURE 9-1 The structures of the cell. (From Patton KT, Thibodeau GA: *Anatomy & physiology*, ed 7, St. Louis, 2010, Mosby.)

- The Golgi apparatus helps to transport proteins made by the ribosomes out of the cell by making glycoproteins.
- The smooth endoplasmic reticulum makes fats (lipids), steroid hormones, and some carbohydrates.

Homeostasis is the tendency of a cell or the whole organism to maintain a state of balance. Homeostasis generally refers to maintaining constancy of the "internal milieu," or fluid surrounding the cells of the organisms. The composition of the tissue fluid that makes up this internal environment is kept constant despite changes in the external environment. Molecules pass into and out of the cell to maintain this balance. Some of the physiologic components of this state of balance include body temperature, gas exchange, pH values, water and ion balance, volume and pressure of fluids, waste removal, and nutrient intake (Table 9-1).

Electrolytes are compounds made of charged particles called ions. These ions can conduct electrical current in water or in the cytoplasm of the cell. A positive charge, or cation, creates an acid. A negative charge, or anion, creates a base. The pH of a fluid is a measurement of how much acid or base is present. Each body tissue has a normal pH. The cells do not function properly if the normal pH is not maintained for the area of the body (Fig. 9-2). Different electrolytes also have specific functions, as shown in Table 9-2.

Tissue Types

The body includes four main groups of tissue (Fig. 9-3).

- Epithelial tissue covers the body, forms glands, and lines the surfaces of cavities and organs.
- Connective tissue, formed by a protein, includes soft tissue such as fat and blood cells and hard tissues such as bones, ligaments, and cartilage.
- Muscle tissue, made of protein fibers, has the unique property of shortening in length to produce movement.
- Nervous tissue, composed largely of specialized cells called *neurons*, is found in the eyes, ears, brain, spinal cord, and peripheral nerves. Nervous tissue transmits communications.

Body Systems

The study of the functions of the body is called *physiology*. Functions are studied according to body systems. A body system is a group of related organs

TABLE 9-1
Homeostasis and Body Systems

Body System	Homeostasis Mechanism
Integumentary	Perspiration helps regulate body temperature.
Cardiovascular	Regulates blood pressure.
Circulatory	Red blood cells transport oxygen and carbon dioxide, as well as hydrogen ions. White blood cells fight infection. Platelets help to clot blood when needed. Nutrients needed by cells and the waste they produce are carried in plasma. Plasma proteins buffer blood to maintain pH. They also create osmotic pressure to remove excess fluid to the heart through lymph vessels.
Respiratory	Oxygen and carbon dioxide are exchanged in the lungs, blood vessels, and cells. Helps regulate pH of blood.
Skeletal	Level of calcium is regulated by parathyroid hormones.
Muscular	Shivering helps regulate body temperature.
Digestive	Digestive enzymes and bile break food down into nutrients. The liver breaks down toxic substances, stores glucose, and destroys old blood cells.
Urinary	Filters the blood to excrete waste products and regulate the amount of water in the body. Blood pressure is affected by fluid balance. Helps regulate pH of blood.
Endocrine	Hormones regulate action of glands that control metabolism, water retention, calcium blood levels, blood sugar, and many other body functions.
Nervous	Receives nutrients from blood. Regulates body temperature, breathing, blood pressure, and autonomic responses.
Sensory	Identifies hunger, pain, and other signs of homeostatic changes.
Reproductive	Oxytocin regulates the strength and frequency of contractions.

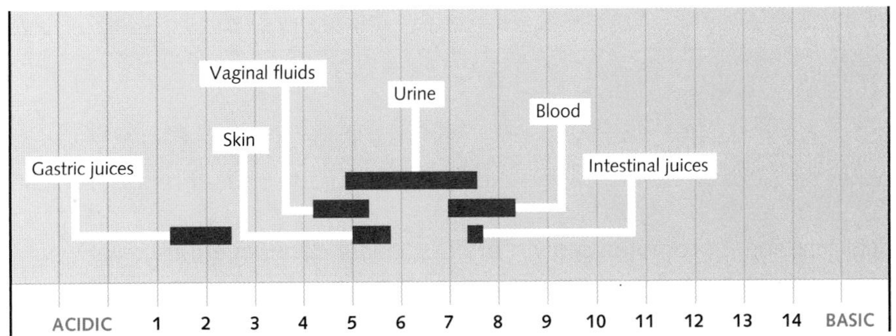

FIGURE 9-2 The body's pH. The body must maintain normal pH levels to function properly.

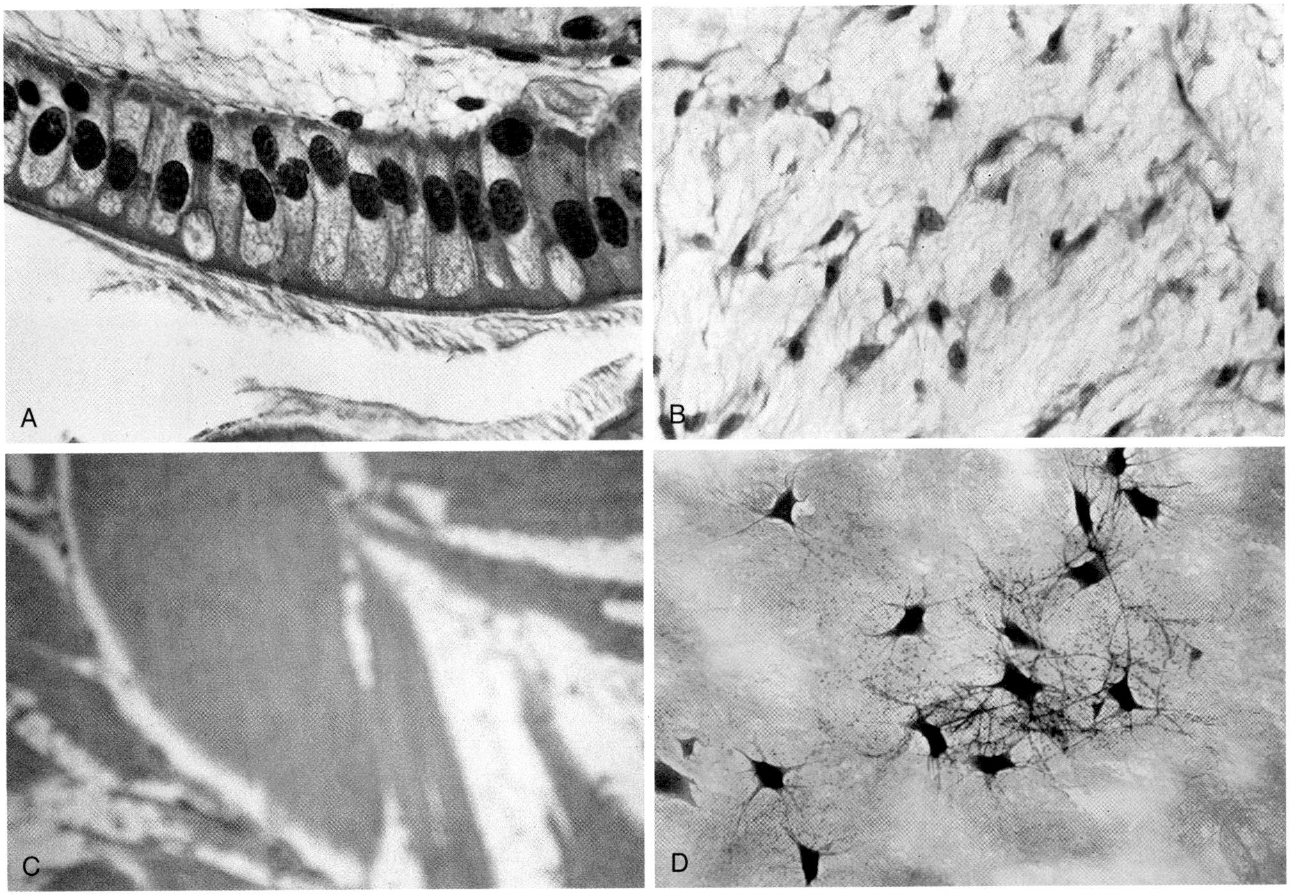

FIGURE 9-3 Tissues of the body. **A,** Epithelial. **B,** Connective. **C,** Muscle. **D,** Nervous. (A, B, and D, Courtesy Ward's Natural Science Establishment, Rochester, N.Y.)

that together accomplish functions necessary to maintain and support life. The 12 body systems are as follows:

- The integumentary system covers the body and protects other body systems.
- The cardiovascular system transports oxygen and nutrients to all body parts and removes waste products.
- The circulatory system includes the blood and lymph that move throughout the body.
- The respiratory system exchanges gases between the air and blood.
- The muscular system allows the body to move and controls movements within the body.
- The skeletal system provides body support and protection.
- The digestive system processes food and eliminates food waste.
- The urinary system filters the blood and removes liquid wastes.

TABLE 9-2
Electrolytes of the Body

Ion	Function
Cations (+)	
Sodium (Na^+)	Controls water distribution by increasing the ability of fluid to pass through the cell membrane
Potassium (K)	Maintains fluid balance, promotes growth of cells, nerve conduction, muscle contraction, and heart activity
Calcium (Ca^{+2})	Controls neuromuscular irritability, muscle contraction, and blood clotting; used to build bones and teeth
Magnesium (Mg^{+2})	Maintains neuromuscular system, activates enzymes, regulates level of phosphorus
Hydrogen (H^+)	Needed for cell and enzyme functions, binding of oxygen to hemoglobin
Anions (-)	
Bicarbonate (HCO_3^-)	Maintains acid-base balance
Phosphate (HPO_4^-)	Maintains fluid and acid-base balance
Chloride (Cl^-)	Maintains fluid balance
Sulfate (SO_4^-)	Maintains fluid balance

- The endocrine system coordinates body activities through hormones.
- The nervous system regulates the environment and directs the activities of other body systems.
- The sensory system perceives the environment and sends messages to and from the brain.
- The reproductive system provides for human reproduction.

The following 12 chapters discuss the body systems in more detail.

Describing the Body

The anatomical position is the standard position of the body used to describe the location of its anatomy. The person is in an erect standing position with mouth closed and eyes and head facing forward. The feet are slightly apart with the toes facing forward. The arms are close to the body, and the palms are facing forward with the fingers extended (Fig. 9-4). From this position, the parts of body may be described in relation to each other.

Body Planes

Structures of the body can be located and described in relation to planes that divide the body (Fig. 9-5). Three planes are used to describe the body:

- The coronal or frontal plane separates the front and back of the body.
- The transverse plane divides the upper and lower body.
- The sagittal plane divides the body into right and left sides.

The location of organs is described in relation to these planes. For example, an organ or growth may be below (inferior) or above (superior) the transverse plane. It may be close to (medial) or away from (lateral) the sagittal plane. It may be in front of (anterior or ventral) or behind (posterior or dorsal) the coronal plane. Other terms for location include close to (proximal) or away from (distal) a point where one organ attaches to another.

Body Cavities

The human body has five cavities (Fig. 9-6):

- The thoracic cavity contains the lungs, heart, esophagus, trachea, and major blood vessels.
- The abdominal cavity contains the stomach, gallbladder, pancreas, intestines, liver, spleen, adrenal glands, and kidneys.
- The pelvic cavity contains the reproductive organs, bladder, and rectum.
- The cranial cavity contains the brain, ventricles, and some glands.
- The spinal cavity houses the spinal cord and nerves.

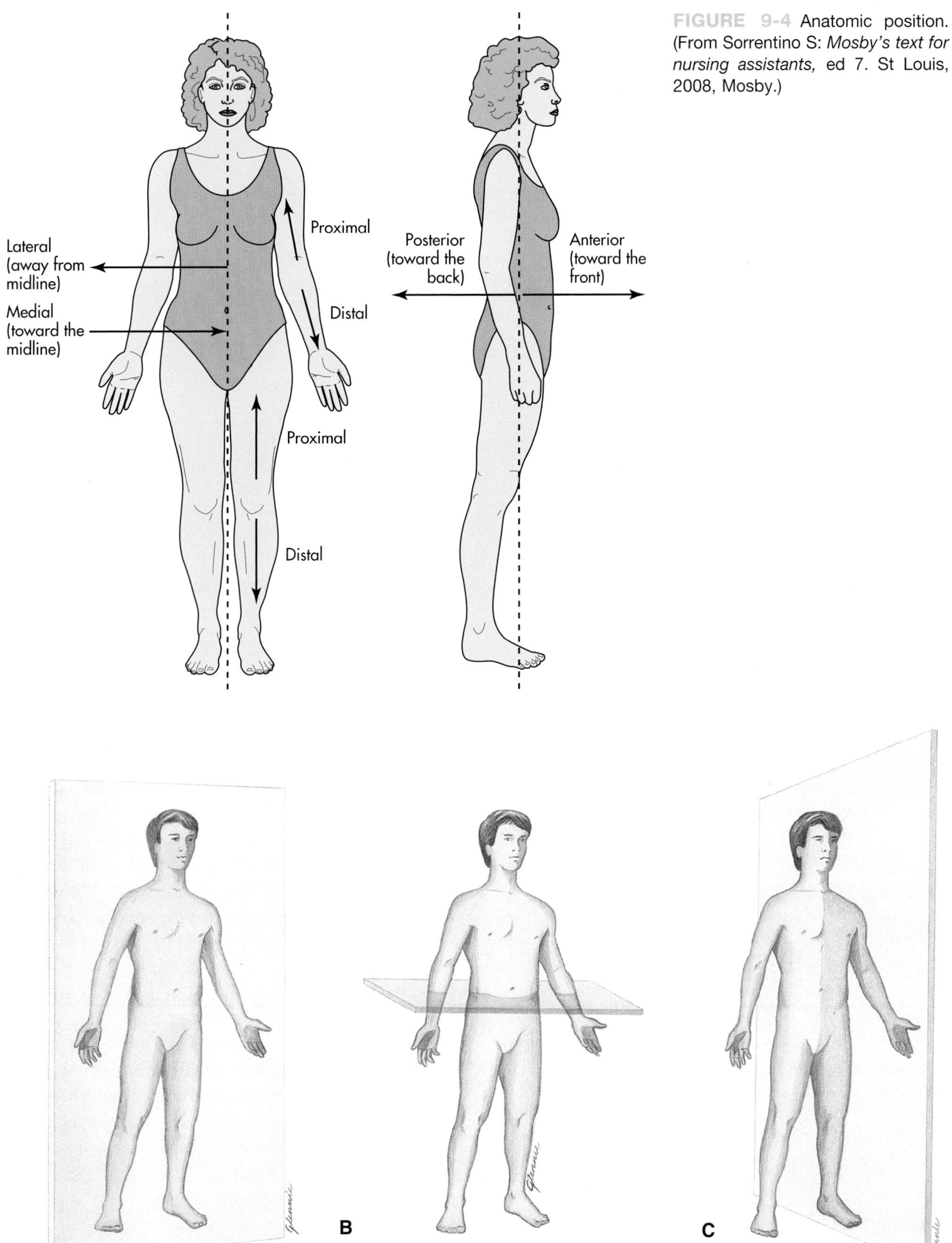

FIGURE 9-4 Anatomic position. (From Sorrentino S: *Mosby's text for nursing assistants,* ed 7. St Louis, 2008, Mosby.)

FIGURE 9-5 Body planes. **A,** Coronal. **B,** Transverse. **C,** Sagittal.

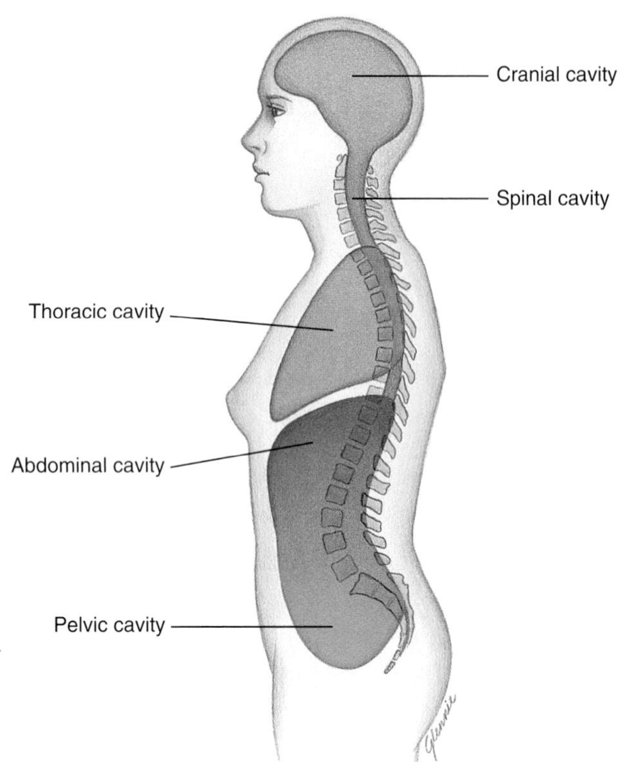

FIGURE 9-6 Cavities of the body.

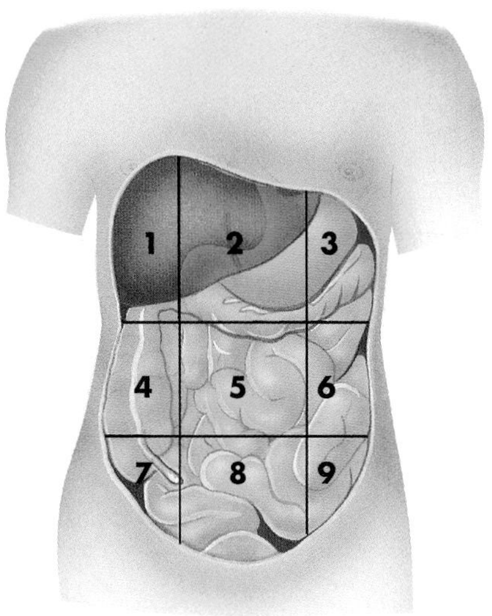

FIGURE 9-7 Body regions. *1,* Right hypochondriac. *2,* Epigastric. *3,* Left hypochondriac. *4,* Right lumbar. *5,* Umbilical. *6,* Left lumbar. *7,* Right inguinal. *8,* Hypogastric. *9,* Left inguinal. (From Patton KT, Thibodeau GA: *Anatomy & physiology,* ed 7, St Louis, 2010, Mosby.)

Body Regions

Locations within the abdominal and pelvic cavities are described in terms of nine regions (Fig. 9-7). The abdomen is also sometimes sectioned into four quadrants: the right upper, right lower, left upper, and left lower quadrants (Fig. 9-8).

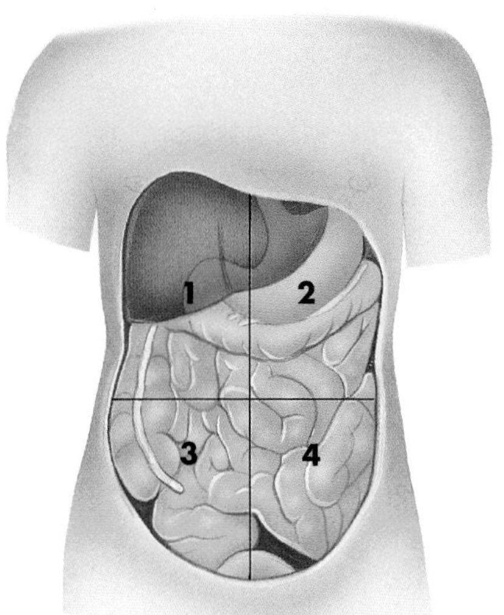

FIGURE 9-8 Division of the abdomen into four quadrants. Diagram shows relationship of internal organs to the four abdominopelvic quadrants: *1,* right upper quadrant (RUQ); *2,* left upper quadrant (LUQ); *3,* right lower quadrant (RLQ); *4,* left lower quadrant (LLQ). (From Patton KT, Thibodeau GA: *Anatomy & physiology,* ed 7, St Louis, 2010, Mosby.)

Cell Function

Cell Reproduction

Mitosis is the process by which a cell divides to reproduce, creating an identical copy with the same chromosomes. Each cell of an organism carries all of the genetic information of the organism. Humans have 46 chromosomes in each cell except the gametes (sperm and egg). With the exception of the sex chromosomes (X and Y), all of the chromosomes are paired and called homologous **autosomes**.

In the process of meiosis, the cell divides into two parts, each with only one half of the chromosomes. Meiotic cell division is part of the reproduction process and results in the formation of sex cells (gametes). The combination of two gametes with chromosomes from different parents into one cell is called fertilization. The offspring inherits any abnormal gene found on

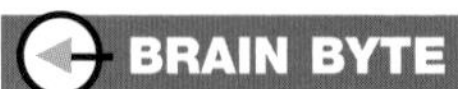

Sickle cell anemia is recognized as the first disorder with a known genetic cause. In 1956, V.M. Ingram determined that a substitution of amino acids in hemoglobin was the cause.

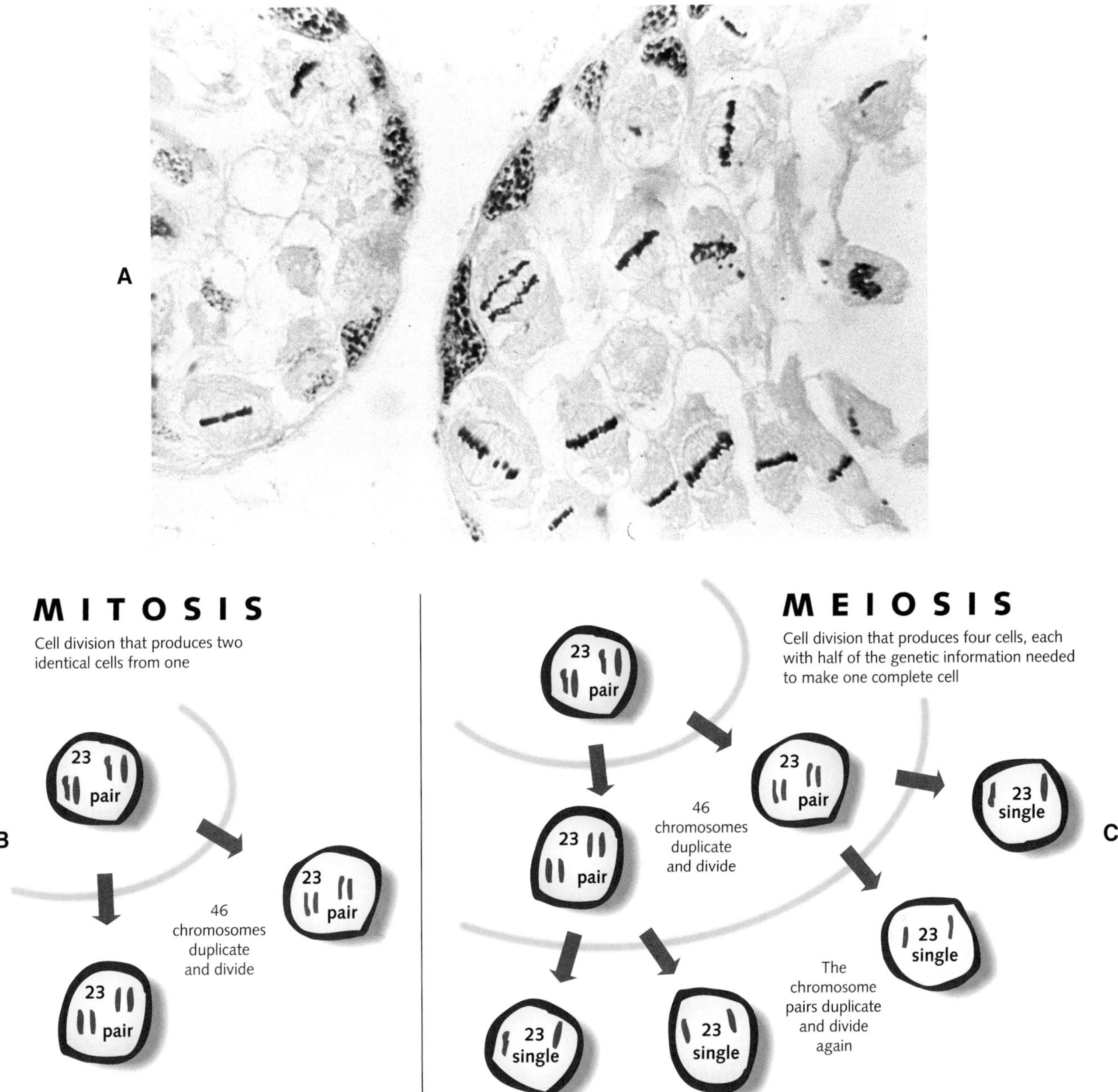

FIGURE 9-9 **A and B,** Mitosis produces two cells that are identical and complete. **C,** Meiosis results in four cells, each with one half of the genetic material of the cell.

the chromosome of either parent. Fig. 9-9 compares the processes of mitosis and meiosis.

Heredity

Heredity is the passing on of genetic information that determines the characteristics of an individual person. The arrangement of genetic material determines many characteristics, such as blood type, physical appearance, and gender. The hereditary information in the cell is found in the genes.

Genes are made up of chains of a molecule called *deoxyribonucleic acid* (DNA). The human genetic or DNA sequence (genome) has been completely "mapped" or identified, but the function of all of the genes has not yet been determined. There are almost three billion base pairs of DNA in the human genome on 46 chromosomes. Chromosomes are threadlike strands of DNA. The human genome or DNA sequence contains between 30,000 and 40,000 protein-coding genes that determine the person's general human and individual traits. A microscopic

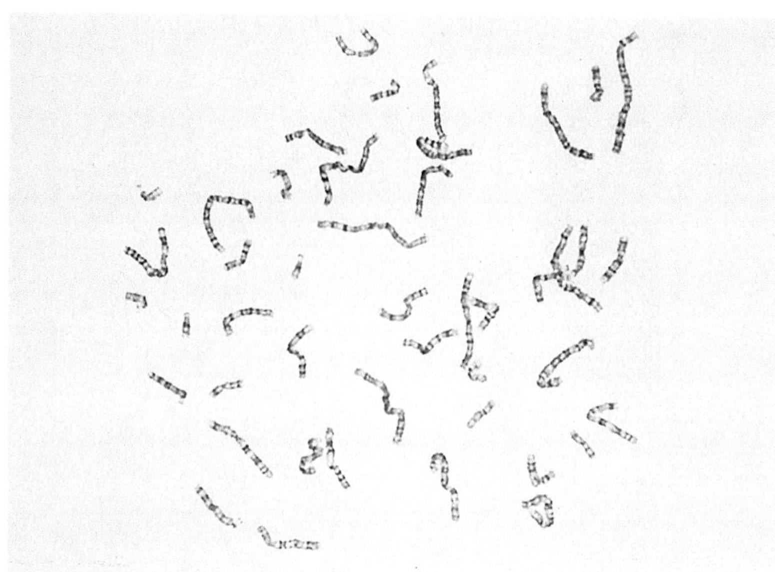

FIGURE 9-10 The karyotype is an organized picture of the chromosomes. (Courtesy Ward's Natural Science Establishment, Rochester, N.Y.)

TABLE 9-3
Causes of Genetic Disorders

Variation	Description	Examples
Single gene disorder	Mutation in a single gene (on one or both paired chromosomes)	Sickle cell anemia, cystic fibrosis, Tay-Sachs disease
Chromosomal disorder	Structural changes in chromosomes or excess/deficiency in number of genes	Down syndrome, Patau syndrome, Klinefelter syndrome
Multifactorial inheritance or polygenic disorder	Combination of genetic and environmental factors	Heart disease, breast cancer, diabetes, Alzheimer disease

photograph (karyotype) of the 46 chromosomes in the cell shows the chromosome composition (Fig. 9-10).

The configuration of genetic information in the chromosome is called the **genotype**. The trait or appearance that results from the genotype is called the **phenotype**. The characteristic of a **dominant** gene appears even when only one gene is inherited. Traits caused by **recessive** genes appear only when the gene is inherited from both parents and is present on both paired chromosomes. When two genes are alike on the chromosome pair, the combination is called homozygous. When they differ, they are called heterozygous.

The genetic information carried by the chromosomes is responsible for the development of all body cells and the formation of tissues, organs, and body systems. Chapter 35 provides more information regarding biotechnology, the study of genetic manipulation.

CASE STUDY 9-1 Your friend tells you that he is afraid that he inherited diabetes from his father who has the disorder. What should you say?

Answers to Case Studies are available on the Evolve website: ***http://evolve.elsevier.com/Gerdin***

Genetic Disorders

Abnormal genes or chromosomes cause many disorders, which are therefore called *inherited, hereditary,* or *genetic* disorders. Abnormalities may result when there is a **mutation** of one or more genes (Table 9-3). Researchers have identified more than 4000 disorders caused by gene variation. Not all people with the gene variant will develop the disorder. Most genetic disorders are multifactorial or caused by more than one factor or a combination of gene variations and environment. The National Center for Biotechnology Information has summarized more than 80 genetic disorders.

The terms **congenital** and **condition** are used to describe these disorders as opposed to the terms *contagious* and **disease**. An organism such as a virus or bacteria causes contagious diseases. Some genetic disorders affect only one body part or system, but others cause defects or symptoms in two or more body systems. When symptoms of a genetic disorder appear, the condition may be called a **syndrome**.

Common genetic disorders are included in the following body system chapters, according to the system primarily affected. The following are some of the most common genetic disorders:

- Cleft lip or palate (Chapter 10)
- Clubfoot (Chapter 14)
- Cystic fibrosis (Chapter 13)
- Down syndrome (Chapter 19)
- Huntington disease (Chapter 19)
- Klinefelter syndrome (Chapter 21)
- Neural tube defect (Chapter 19)
- Neurofibromatosis (Chapter 19)
- Phenylketonuria (Chapter 16)
- Sickle cell anemia (Chapter 12)
- Spina bifida (Chapter 19)
- Tay-Sachs disease (Chapter 16)
- Thalassemia (Chapter 12)

CASE STUDY 9-2 A husband and wife ask you what the chances would be that they might have a child with cystic fibrosis. They each have a sibling with the disorder, so they know it runs in their family. What should you say?

Answers to Case Studies are available on the Evolve website: ***http://evolve.elsevier.com/Gerdin***

CASE STUDY 9-3 A friend tells you that she is not going to have children because she does not want to have a baby with Down syndrome. She tells you she knows that Down syndrome runs in her family because she has a cousin with it. What should you say?

Answers to Case Studies are available on the Evolve website: ***http://evolve.elsevier.com/Gerdin***

Cancer

Cancer is the uncontrolled growth of abnormal cells that tend to spread (metastasize) and invade the tissue around them. Cancer is classified into five groups.

BOX 9-1

Warning Signs of Cancer*

- C—Change in bowel or bladder habits
- A—A sore that does not heal
- U—Unusual bleeding or discharge from any place
- T—Thickening or lump in the breast or other parts of the body
- I—Indigestion or difficulty in swallowing
- O—Obvious changes in a wart or mole
- N—Nagging coughing or hoarseness

*American Cancer Society.

Carcinomas have cells that cover internal and external parts of the body. Leukemia is found in the blood but starts in the bone marrow. Sarcomas are found in connective tissue like bones, muscle, fat, and cartilage. Lymphomas start in lymph nodes and immune system tissues. Adenomas affect the thyroid, pituitary gland, adrenal gland, and other glandular tissues.

A new growth of cells or neoplasm may be benign or malignant. **Malignant** growths spread and destroy body tissue. **Benign** growths are not cancerous and do not spread. Cancer cells are able to grow rapidly because they create their own blood vessels to take the oxygen and nutrients from the body. Common sites for development of cancer include the lungs, breast, colon, uterus, oral cavity, and bone marrow. Many malignancies are curable if detected early. Warning signs of cancer vary with the area affected (Box 9-1).

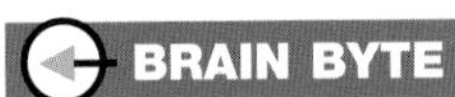

According to the American Cancer Society, most of the one million cases of nonmelanoma skin cancer are related to sun exposure.

Although the specific cause of cancer is not known, it results from a mistake or **mutation** in one single cell's division (Box 9-2). Cancer cells have properties similar to embryonic cells during fetal division. The DNA message that directs embryo cells to divide rapidly is chemically repressed when the fetal development is complete. In cancer this uncontrolled cell division begins again. It is theorized that this change is brought on by exposure to something that induces or starts it (carcinogen). More than 80% of the cancer cases are related to smoking or exposure to chemicals, radiation, and ultraviolet light such as the sun. Some

BOX 9-2

Factors Associated with Cancer

- Age
- Bacterial infection
- Carcinogens
- Diet
- Environmental factors
- Genetic mutations
- Immune system problems
- Physical activity
- Viruses
- Weight

BOX 9-3

Inherited Cancers*

- Breast
- Colorectal
- Cowden syndrome
- Melanoma
- Ovarian
- Prostate
- Retinoblastoma
- Von-Hippel-Lindau disease
- Wilms tumor
- Xeroderma pigmentosum

*Inheriting a gene mutation does not necessarily mean that the person will develop cancer in all types listed.

cancers are related to viral infections such as hepatitis B and Epstein-Barr virus. Genetic susceptibility in certain cancers is a factor in breast and basal cell skin cancer. More than 12 cancers are believed to be inherited directly from one or both parents. Genes that cause cancer are called oncogenes (Box 9-3).

In 2005 the National Institutes of Health started a pilot project using genetic sequencing to understand cancer on a molecular level. The Cancer Genome Atlas will develop and test technology to identify genetic mutation and changes associated with cancer.

In 1999 scientists at Emory University discovered enzymes that generate abnormal cell growth in both cancer and some forms of cardiovascular disease. The enzymes appear to change oxygen into a reactive form that has been theorized to cause damage to DNA and lead to an acceleration of the aging process. The reactive oxygen has been proven to cause cells to divide more rapidly. The scientists hypothesize that reactive oxygen may be a cause rather than a by-product of cancer.

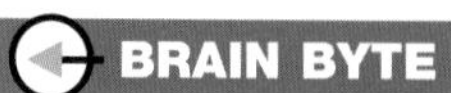

According to the World Health Organization, cancer is the leading cause of death worldwide. In the United States, it is the second leading cause of death.

New approaches to cancer treatment resulting from this research may include agents that block the enzymes or that destroy the reactive oxygen in cancer cells. The body fights cancer by forming antibodies against the abnormal cells. It is believed that small groups of cancer cells develop in the body continually without detection. These "silent cancers" are successfully removed by the body's immune processes.

CASE STUDY 9-4 Your friend tells you that he has been having aching abdominal pain that seems to be on the right side. He says it is sharper and hurts to touch the area. What should you do?

Answers to Case Studies are available on the Evolve website: ***http://evolve.elsevier.com/Gerdin***

Issues and Innovations

Genetic Engineering

At least 4000 disorders are known to result from single gene abnormalities. Research now shows that other disorders with no known cause, including some forms of retardation and cancer (Table 9-4), may also be genetically linked. Chromosomes also can be damaged by drugs, radiation, toxins, viruses, and other environmental agents. In all, approximately 1 of every 150 to 200 births involves a serious chromosomal defect.

Using advanced techniques, new procedures can now identify abnormal genes in the unborn fetus. Chorionic villus sampling (CVS) is a method of examining the chromosomes using a small sample of placental tissue at about the seventh to eighth week of pregnancy. Amniocentesis, a procedure that examines the fluid that surrounds the fetus in the uterus, can detect genetic defects in the 16th or 17th week of pregnancy. More than 200 disorders can be identified by amniocentesis. Some researchers are developing techniques to identify fetal disorders by using maternal blood samples that contain fetal cells. These fetal cells are present in the mother's blood after they have leaked through the placenta.

TABLE 9-4
Mapped Genetic Disorders*

Gene	Chromosome	Description
AD3	X	Alzheimer disease, type 3
AD4	1	Alzheimer disease, type 4
SOD1	21	Amyotrophic lateral sclerosis
APOE	19	Apolipoprotein E
BRCA1	17	Breast cancer, type 1
BRCA2	13	Breast cancer, type 2
CFTR	7	Cystic fibrosis
DMD	X	Duchenne muscular dystrophy
HD	4	Huntington disease
IDDM1	6	Type 1 diabetes
CDKN2	9	Malignant melanoma
NF2	22	Neurofibromatosis
OBS	7	Obesity
PAH	12	Phenylketonuria
DPC4	18	Suppressor of pancreatic carcinoma
FMR1	X	S-linked mental retardation

*In some cases the presence of the gene for a disorder does not guarantee that it will occur.

Preimplantation diagnosis combines the biotechnology of in vitro fertilization and genetic testing. In this procedure, embryos are created outside of the body in Petri dishes. A single cell sample is taken from the embryo when it has grown to eight cells in a process called embryo biopsy. The single cell is then examined for genetic defects. Only the embryos that are free from genetic error are then implanted.

Research teams are now investigating the possibility of correcting defective genes in humans. Gene splicing, the transplanting of genes, has been conducted successfully in "test-tube" animal embryos. Procedures are also being developed to implant a normal gene in a defective one by using a retrovirus to carry the normal gene into the cells of the affected individual after birth.

Genetic screening of potential parents can help determine the risk of a genetic disorder occurring. About 900 tests are available to find genetic disorders. Special counseling provides parents with information about their options before and after conception if a defect is expected or found. The couple's family medical and genetic histories are charted to determine the potential for chromosomal defects. All states test infants for phenylketonuria and congenital hypothyroidism.

Ethical decisions resulting from increased knowledge about genetics are a growing concern of health care workers now and in the future. Hospitals have ethics committees to decide what type of care should be given to infants born with genetic defects. Genetic research has raised ethical questions never before faced. Emergent techniques of genetic engineering will create new challenges and new ethical decisions. Chapter 35 provides more information regarding genetic engineering and biotechnology.

BOX 9-4

Types of Cancer Treatment

- Chemotherapy
- Gene therapy
- Hormone therapy
- Immunotherapy
- Radiation
- Surgery

Cancer Treatments

Using the theory that the body's immune system can treat cancer, scientists are developing cancer vaccines. The Food and Drug Administration (FDA) has approved two types of cancer-prevention vaccines. These are vaccines against the hepatitis B and human papillomavirus types 16 and 18. The FDA has not approved any cancer treatment vaccine.

Immunotherapy involves using chemicals that are isolated from bacteria infected with the cancer, killed suspensions of bacteria, and some biological substances that harm tumors (Box 9-4). The biological substances include interferon, interleukin, tumor necrosis factors, and growth factors. Other scientists are researching the possibility of replacing the genetic message of cancerous cells that causes the rapid cell division to occur.

In some cases lasers are used to destroy cancerous cells. Fiberoptic technology, called *photodynamic therapy,* is used to place a destructive wavelength of laser directly into the tumor. Hyperthermia, or an increase in temperature, is being used in combination with radiation to treat some tumors. The cells of the tumor can be raised to temperatures high enough to kill them without killing the surrounding body cells.

Summary

- The properties of life are reception, metabolism, reproduction, and organization.
- The structures of the cell include the nucleus, cytoplasm, and cell membrane.
- The organization of the body consists of cells that, when combined, make tissues. Tissues combine to make organs. Organs combine to make a body system. The combined body systems make an organism.
- The brain is located superior to the heart, which is anterior to the spinal cord.
- Five disorders resulting from defects in cell organization are cleft lip, clubfoot, cystic fibrosis, Down syndrome, and Huntington disease.

Review Questions

1. Describe four properties of living organisms.
2. List the four units of organization of the body from the smallest to the largest.
3. Describe the structure and location of the four types of tissue of the body.
4. Complete the following phrases using directional terms to describe the location of each body part. List the plane that is used to section the location.
   The eyes are located _________ to the nose.
   Plane: _________
   The head is located _________ to the neck.
   Plane: _________
   The spine is located _________ to the sternum.
   Plane: _________
   The stomach is located _________ to the heart.
   Plane: _________
   The fingers are located _________ to the hand.
   Plane: _________
5. List one body organ or structure located in each of the following sections of the body:

right upper quadrant	epigastric region
thoracic cavity	spinal cavity
left upper quadrant	abdominal cavity
hypogastric region	right inguinal region
umbilical region	left lumbar region

6. Differentiate between the genotype and phenotype of an individual.
7. Identify three tests used to detect genetic abnormalities of a fetus.
8. Describe two areas of research dealing with correcting genetic defects.
9. Use the following terms in one or more sentences that correctly relate their meaning: autosome, dominant, genotype, phenotype, recessive.

Critical Thinking

1. Investigate and compare the cost of at least three tests used to diagnose disorders relating to body organization.
2. Investigate at least five common medications used in treatment of body organization disorders.
3. List at least five health care occupations involved in the care of disorders of the body organization.
4. Investigate advanced techniques used in genetic engineering.
5. Investigate and write an essay about one type of cancer, its cause, signs and symptoms, and treatment.
6. Use the Internet to investigate and give an example of each of the following types of genetic disorders: point mutation, gene deletion, chromosomal aberration (missing or extra), trinucleotide repeat disorder.
7. Research and write a paragraph describing the origin of the name (eponym) of one genetic disorder.

Explore the Web

Genetic Disorders

National Center for Biotechnology Information (NCBI)
http://www.ncbi.nlm.nih.gov/bookshelf/br.fcgi?book=gnd&part=gnd_book_info

Genetic and Rare Diseases Information Center (GARD)
http://rarediseases.info.nih.gov/GARD/Default.aspx?PageID=4

National Institutes of Health
http://ghr.nlm.nih.gov/BrowseConditions

Genomic Science Project
http://www.ornl.gov/sci/techresources/Human_Genome/posters/chromosome/diseaseindex.shtml#top

Test and Treatment Costs

National Cancer Institute
http://www.cancer.gov/aboutnci/servingpeople/costofcancer

National Institutes of Health
http://ghr.nlm.nih.gov/handbook/testing/costresults

STANDARDS AND ACCOUNTABILITY*

Foundation Standard 1: Academic Foundation

Health care professionals will know the academic subject matter required for proficiency within their area. They will use this knowledge as needed in their role. The following accountability criteria are considered essential for students in a health science program of study.

Accountability Criteria

1.1 Human Structure and Function

1.11 Classify the basic structural and functional organization of the human body (tissue, organ, and system).

1.12 Recognize body planes, directional terms, quadrants, and cavities.

1.13 Analyze the basic structure and function of the human body.

1.2 Diseases and Disorders

1.21 Describe common diseases and disorders of each body system (prevention, pathology, diagnosis, and treatment).

1.22 Recognize emerging diseases and disorders.

1.23 Investigate biomedical therapies as they relate to the prevention, pathology, and treatment of disease.

1.3 Medical Mathematics

1.31 Apply mathematical computations related to health care procedures (metric and household, conversions and measurements).

1.32 Analyze diagrams, charts, graphs, and tables to interpret health care results.

1.33 Record time using the 24-hour clock.

*From the National Consortium for Health Science Education (2009). National Health Care Standards and Accountability Criteria. Available at: http://www.healthscienceconsortium.org.

CHAPTER 10

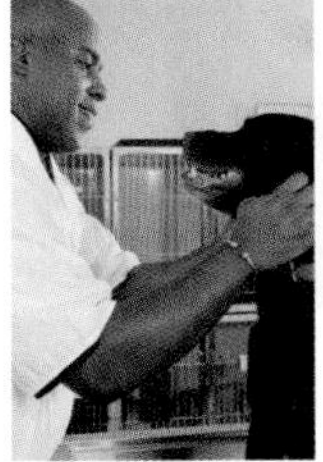
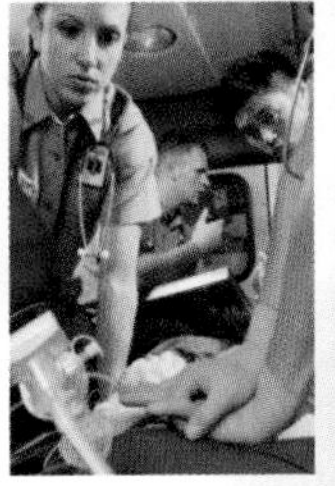
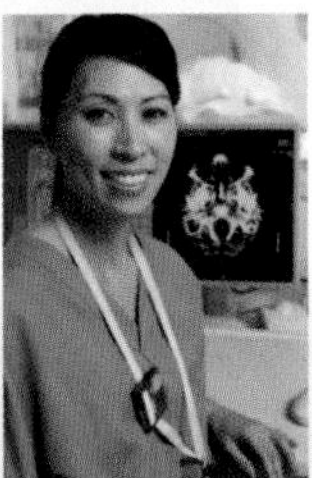

Integumentary System

LEARNING OBJECTIVES

- Define at least 10 terms relating to the integumentary system.
- Describe the function of the integumentary system.
- Identify at least five integumentary system structures and the function of each.
- Identify at least three methods used to assess the function of the integumentary system.
- Describe at least five disorders of the integumentary system.
- Describe three methods that can be used to maintain healthy skin.
- Identify three types of skin cancer and at least five methods for prevention.

KEY TERMS

Adipose *(AD-i-pose)* Of a fatty nature, fat

Biopsy *(BI-op-see)* Removal and examination of living tissue

Ceruminous *(se-ROO-min-us)* Pertaining to earwax

Dermatitis *(der-muh-TI-tis)* Inflammation of the skin

Dermis *(DER-mis)* Corium, or layer of skin beneath the epidermis

Epidermis *(ep-i-DER-mis)* Outermost and nonvascular layer of skin

Follicle *(FOL-ik-ul)* Sac or pouchlike depression or cavity

Lunula *(LOO-nuh-lah)* General term for a small crescent- or moon-shaped area of fingernail

Melanin *(MEL-uh-nin)* Dark, shapeless pigment of the skin

Papilla *(puh-PIL-uh)* Small, nipple-shaped projection or elevation

Pilus *(PIE-lus)* Hair

Sebaceous *(se-BAY-shus)* Pertaining to sebum or a greasy lubricating substance

Subcutaneous *(sub-kyoo-TAY-nee-us)* Beneath the skin

Sudoriferous *(soo-do-RIF-er-us)* Conveying sweat

Integumentary System Terminology*

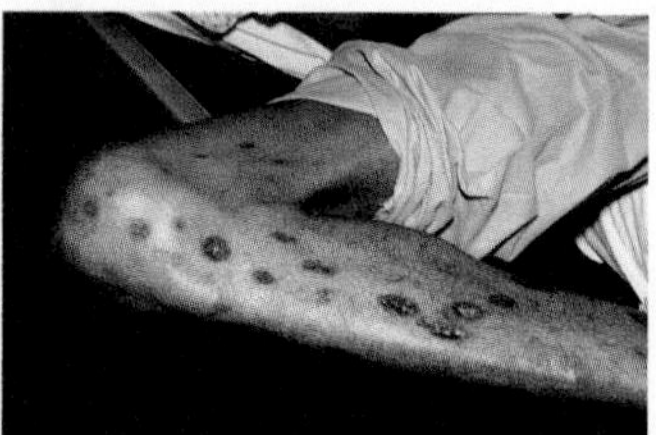

Kaposi sarcoma is the most common type of cancerous lesions in people with acquired immunodeficiency disease (AIDS). (From Damjanov I: *Pathology for the health professions*, ed 3, St. Louis, 2006, Saunders.)

Term	Definition	Prefix	Root	Suffix
Cheilorrhaphy	Suture of the lip		cheil/o	rrhaphy
Cutaneous	Pertaining to the skin		cutan	eous
Cyanoderm	Blue skin	cyan/o	derm	
Dermatitis	Inflammation of the skin		derm/at	itis
Melanoma	Tumor that is black		melan	oma
Psoriasis	Condition of the skin characterized by itching		psor	iasis
Rhinoplasty	Plastic repair of the nose		rhin/o	plasty
Sarcoma	Tumor of the flesh		sarc	oma
Sebaceous	Pertaining to oil		seb/ac	eous
Stomatitis	Inflammation of the mouth		stoma/t	itis

*A short transition syllable or vowel may be added to or deleted from the word parts to make the combining form.

Abbreviations of the Integumentary System

Abbreviation	Meaning
Bx	Biopsy
CA	Cancer
C&S	Culture and sensitivity
Etiol	Etiology
LE	Lupus erythematosus
mm	Millimeter
Oint	Ointment
PABA	Para-aminobenzoic acid
sc	Subcutaneous
SLE	Systemic lupus erythematosus

Structure and Function

The integumentary system is composed of the skin and accessory structures (Fig. 10-1). Accessory structures of the system include the hair, nails, specialized glands, and nerves. The main function of the integumentary system is to protect the other body systems from injury and infection. A second function is to help the body maintain homeostasis by regulating temperature, retaining body fluids, and eliminating wastes. The skin also helps to perceive the environment with sensory receptors. The skin stores energy and vitamins and produces vitamin D from sunlight. Some hormones, fat-soluble vitamins, and drugs may be absorbed through the skin.

Skin

The skin, covering 17 to 20 square feet (1.6 to 1.9 m^2), is the largest organ in the body. It varies in thickness from $\frac{1}{50}$ inch (0.5 mm) in the eyelids to $\frac{1}{4}$ inch (6.3 mm) in the soles of the feet. Changes in the skin often indicate the presence of other body system disorders, including anemia, respiratory disorders, liver disorders, cancer, and shock (Fig. 10-2).

BRAIN BYTE

The skin plays a major role in maintaining homeostasis by regulating body temperature.

The **epidermis**, or cuticle, is the outermost layer of the skin and is composed of a surface of dead cells with an underlying layer of living cells. Water-repellent cells made of protein (keratinocytes) make up 90% of the epidermis. Oil (**sebaceous**) and sweat (**sudoriferous**) glands and hair follicles lie in the epidermis. Melanocytes, which produce melanin, are located in this layer. **Melanin** is the pigment that

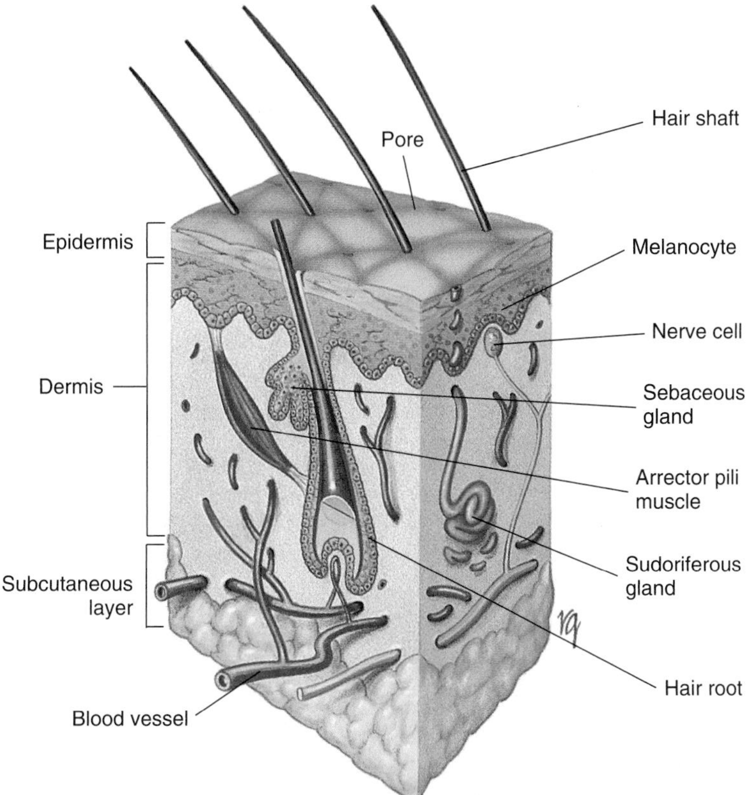

FIGURE 10-1 Structures of the skin.

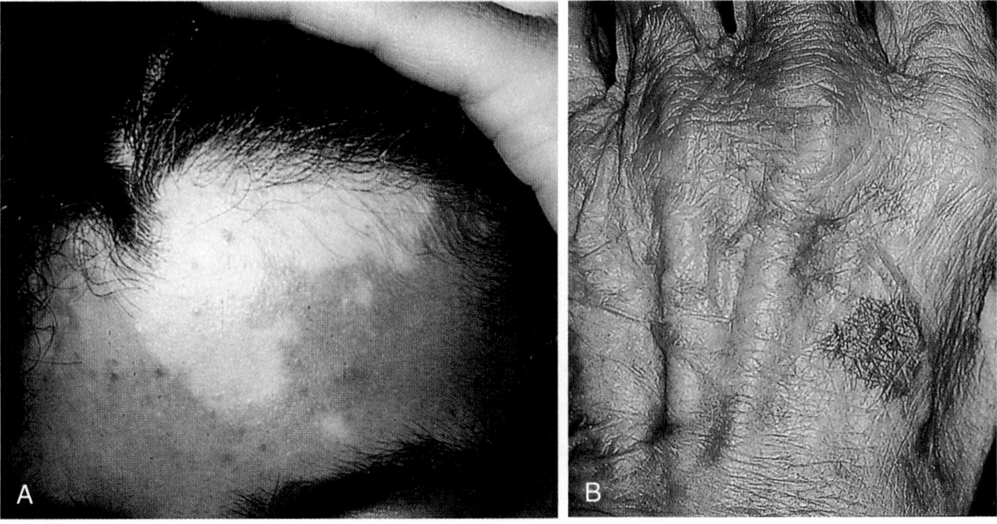

FIGURE 10-2 **A,** Vitiligo, a pigmentation disorder, has no known cause. **B,** Lentigo, a form of melanoma, is often found in people with extensive sun exposure. (**A,** Courtesy Jamie Tschen, MD; **B,** From *Mosby's medical, nursing, and allied health dictionary,* ed 6, St Louis, 2002, Mosby.)

gives skin its color (Fig. 10-3). The surface of the epidermis is covered with a film composed of sweat, oil, and epithelial cells that lubricates, hydrates, provides antibacterial protection, and blocks toxic agents from entering the body.

The **dermis**, or corium, is called the "true" skin. The dermis contains the blood vessels and nerves. Each inch of skin contains 15 square feet of blood vessels. The innermost layer of the skin is called the **subcutaneous** layer. Fatty (**adipose**) tissue of the subcutaneous layer cushions and insulates the body's organs. The nerve endings in the skin allow it to be sensitive to environmental stimuli. Skin senses pain, pressure, touch, and changes in temperature.

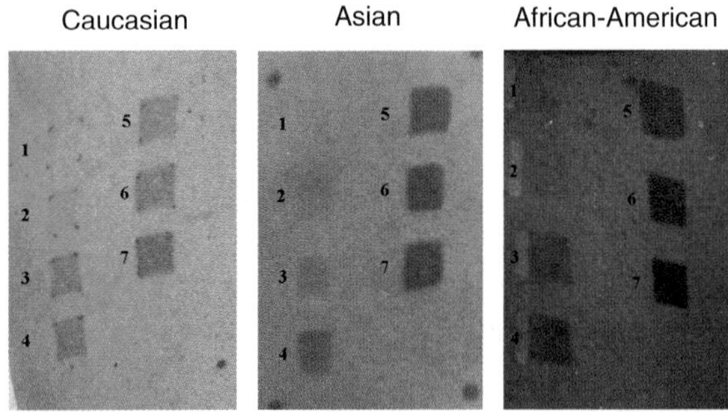

FIGURE 10-3 All skin types are affected by ultraviolet radiation, although white and lighter skins may become reddened and damaged more quickly after exposure. (From Patton KT, Thibodeau GA: *Anatomy & physiology,* ed 7, St. Louis, 2010, Mosby.)

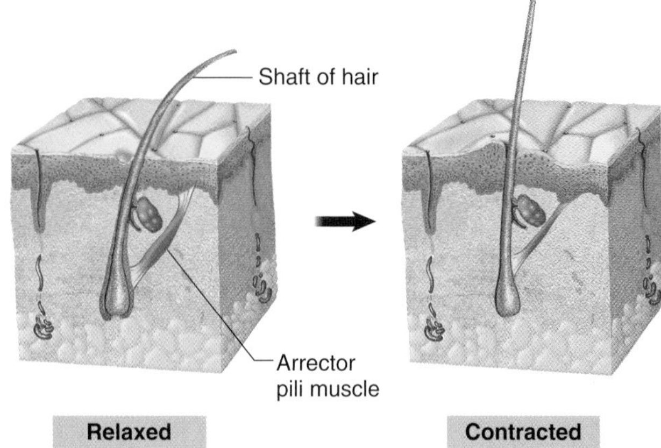

FIGURE 10-4 When the arrector pili muscle contracts, the hair and follicle are pulled up forming a "goose bump." (From Patton KT, Thibodeau GA: *Anatomy & physiology,* ed 7, St. Louis, 2010, Mosby.)

Hair and Hair Follicles

Skin normally has hair (**pilus**) in all areas except the soles of the feet and palms of the hands. Some hair blocks foreign particles from entering the body through structures such as the nose and eyes.

Each hair root originates in the dermis. The visible portion is called the shaft. The hair **follicle** is the root with its covering. One or two oil (sebaceous) glands are attached to each hair follicle. A tiny muscle (arrector pili) is attached to the hair shaft and causes "goose bumps" or the hair to "stand on end" in response to cold or fear (Fig. 10-4). Hair color and texture are inherited. The color depends on the amount of melanin in the cells.

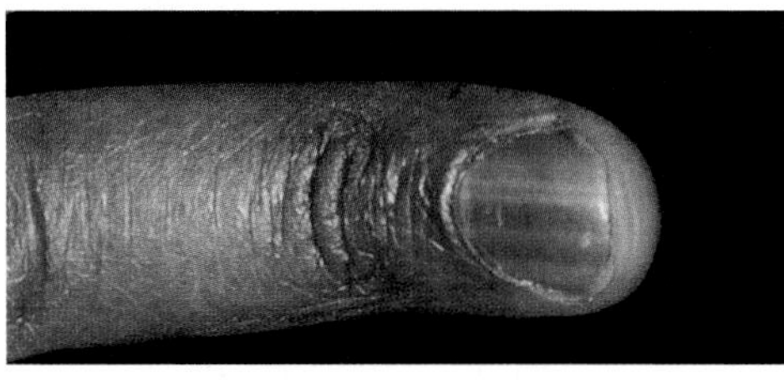

FIGURE 10-5 Although the nail bed is not usually pigmented in light-skinned individuals, yellowish or brown pigmented bands are common in individuals with darker skin. (From Patton KT, Thibodeau GA: *Anatomy & physiology,* ed 7, St. Louis, 2010, Mosby.)

Glands

The three types of glands in the skin are the sebaceous glands (oil), sudoriferous glands (sweat), and the ceruminous glands of the ear canal.

Sebaceous glands are located everywhere in the skin except the palms of the hands and the soles of the feet. Each square inch of skin has about 2000 sebaceous glands. Sebum, or oil, causes the skin to be soft and waterproof.

Sudoriferous glands originate in the subcutaneous layer of the skin. Some of these glands (apocrine) are attached to hair follicles, and others (eccrine) empty directly onto the skin. Apocrine glands are located in areas such as under the arms (axilla), the breasts, and pubic area. In some areas of the skin, each square inch contains about two million sudoriferous glands. Sudoriferous glands help regulate body temperature and excrete body wastes. The skin loses at least 500 mL of water each day; more water is lost through sweating caused by exercise or heat.

Ceruminous glands are located only in the auditory canal of the ear. These glands secrete wax that helps to protect the ear from infection and prevents entry of foreign bodies.

Nails

The function of the nails is to protect fingers and toes from injury. Fingernails and toenails are formed from dead, keratinized epidermal cells. The root or area of nail growth is covered by skin at the area of attachment to finger or toe. The crescent-shaped white area near the root is the **lunula** (Fig. 10-5).

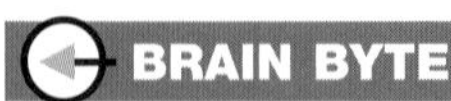

BRAIN BYTE

After compression, a return of normal color to the tissue under the nail bed within 2 seconds indicates good circulation.

Assessment Techniques

Dermatology is the study of skin. **Dermatitis** is the general term for inflammation of the skin. Skin disorders are usually uncomfortable and unattractive but not life threatening.

Assessment of the skin, hair, and nails includes palpation, olfactory (smell), and visual inspection. The color, temperature, texture, turgor (fullness or tension), and any moisture should be noted. The color of skin is genetically determined. Any change—such as paleness (pallor), redness (erythema), yellowishness (jaundice), or blueness (cyanosis)—may indicate a problem. Normal skin is warm, dry, and without open sores (intact). When a pinch or fold of skin on the forearm is lifted, it should rise easily and return to place quickly when released.

Skin lesions can usually be seen with visual inspection. The size, shape, texture, and color of a lesion often help reveal its cause. A **biopsy** or culture may be used to identify the causative organism.

The uppermost part of the dermis is composed of **papillae**, or ridges. The papillae form regular patterns in the fingers, palms of the hands, and soles of the feet, where the skin is thick. Fingertip and toe prints are unique to each person. In addition to forming a surface that permits gripping, the fingerprints allow the identification of each individual. The patterns of ridges in fingerprints and toe prints may also be linked to disorders such as Down syndrome.

DISORDERS OF THE Integumentary System

Acne vulgaris (AK-nee vul-GAYR-is) usually appears in adolescence and may continue into adulthood. Acne is often caused by the increased secretion of oil (sebum) related to increased hormones during puberty. Bacterial growth and blockage of the hair follicles cause papules, pustules, and blackheads. Acne primarily affects the face, chest, and back. Acne tends to run in families. Contrary to popular belief, diet does not cause or affect the severity of acne. Treatment may include exposure to ultraviolet light, oral or topical antibiotics, or removal of the top layers of skin that has scarred (dermabrasion).

Albinism (AL-bin-izm) is a rare inherited disorder in which the melanocytes do not produce enough or any melanin. Lack of melanin leads to pale skin, white hair, and pink eyes. People with albinism are prone to severe sunburn, and light may damage unprotected structures of the eyes. Although no cure for albinism exists, wearing sunglasses, applying sunscreen, and avoiding exposure to the sun may help avoid skin cancer and eye damage.

Alopecia (al-o-PEE-shee-uh), or baldness, is the inherited tendency to lose hair from the head. Production of androgenic (an-dro-JEN-ik) hormones beginning at puberty initiates the loss. Baldness is more common in men, but it may occur in women and may begin at any age. Drugs, radiation, pregnancy, high fever, anorexia, and cosmetics may cause temporary hair loss.

Athlete's foot, or *epidermophytosis* (ep-i-DER-mo-fi-TOE-sis) is a common fungal infection. The skin may itch, blister, and crack, especially between the toes. Athlete's foot most often occurs during warm weather and is contagious. It can be transmitted on wet floors, such as in gym showers. Treatment includes application of antifungal medication and keeping the area clean, ventilated, and dry. More serious infections may be treated with an oral antifungal medication.

Cellulitis (sel-yoo-LIE-tis) is a bacterial infection of the dermis and subcutaneous layer of the skin. Cellulitis may be caused by many different bacteria but is commonly caused by *Streptococcus* organisms. It occurs in people with low resistance to infection, such as older patients, children, and chronically ill patients. The infected person may experience fever, chills, and vesicles (VES-i-kulz) on a reddened, warm area of the skin. It most commonly occurs on legs and may cause impaired circulation and permanent lymphedema (lim-feh-DEE-muh). Treatment includes rest, immobilization and elevation of the infected area, and antibiotics.

Chloasma (klo-AZ-muh), or melasma, is a patchy discoloration of the face caused by high hormone levels that occur during pregnancy and by prolonged use of oral contraceptives. It may disappear at the end of the pregnancy or with stopping birth control pills. Chloasma may also be a sign of liver problems. Treatment is often unnecessary, but nonprescription cosmetic products can minimize the discoloration.

Cleft lip or *cleft palate* (kleft PAL-ut) occurs in 1 of 1000 (cleft lip) and 1 in 2000 (cleft palate) infants. In this condition the upper lip has a cleft or space where the nasal processes or palate does not meet properly. Heredity appears to be the direct cause in 25% of the cases, and environmental factors and premature birth may also cause the condition. Treatment includes surgical and dental correction, speech therapy, and psychological counseling.

Contact dermatitis is an allergic reaction that may occur after initial contact or as an acquired response. Some substances that commonly cause acquired dermatitis include poison ivy, nickel in jewelry, and preservatives in cosmetics. Latex in gloves may be an allergen for some health care workers. Redness, itching, swelling, and blisters may result from contact with the irritating substance. Treatment may include washing the affected area, applying anti-inflammatory creams, and avoiding exposure to the irritating substance.

Dandruff (DAN-druf), characterized by itching of the scalp, produces white flakes of dead skin cells. Massaging the scalp and brushing and shampooing the hair can control dandruff. Medicated shampoos designed to control dandruff often help.

Decubitus ulcers (de-KYOO-bit-us UL-serz), or decubiti, are sores or areas of inflammation that occur over bony prominences of the body as a result of prolonged pressure and hypoxia to the affected tissues. These "bedsores" are seen most often in older patients and in patients who cannot move themselves (immobilized). Frequent changes in position, good nutrition, and massage to the area help to prevent decubiti. Prevention of decubiti is easier than treatment. Decubiti are described in four stages by their severity and can be life threatening. Decubiti are often resistant to treatment, which may include application of antibiotics, removal of necrotic tissue, and frequent cleaning of open sores. Larvae (maggots) of blowflies, which feed only on dead tissue, have been used in some severe cases to clean sores. In addition to removing the dead tissue, the maggot larvae provide stimulation of the affected area with their movement and produce compounds that are lethal to bacteria that cause gangrene and similar infections. Deep pressure sores may require skin grafting. Negative pressure wound therapy (vacuum-assisted closure), as well as hyperbaric chamber therapy, may be used in some cases.

Eczema (EK-ze-muh), a form of dermatitis, is a group of disorders caused by allergic or irritant reactions. Eczema is characterized by swelling; redness; and itching, weeping, crusted skin lesions. Although it is not contagious, it seems to run in families. Eczema is chronic but may disappear as affected children become older. Treatment of eczema includes removing the irritant and keeping the affected skin clean and well moisturized. It is also helpful to avoid sudden changes in temperature and overheating. Outbreaks may disappear by avoiding harsh soaps and environmental factors or food that trigger outbreaks, as well as reducing stress.

Fungal (FUN-gul) skin infections live only on the dead, outer surface or epidermis. Some may cause no symptoms. Others may produce irritation, scaling, redness, swelling, or blisters. Most fungal infections occur in areas of the body that provide moisture and are named by the area in which they appear. Examples include athlete's foot (see earlier); jock itch; and scalp, nail, body, and beard ringworm. Fungal infections of the scalp or beard can cause hair loss. Treatment by the use of antifungal creams usually cures these skin conditions. In severe cases, oral antifungal medication may be necessary. Fungal infections of the skin may be prevented by keeping the skin dry; wearing loose, clean clothing; and avoiding shared use of towels, combs, and hairbrushes.

Furuncle (FER-ung-kl), commonly called a boil, is a bacterial infection of a hair follicle. Although it is usually caused by *Staphylococcus aureus (S. aureus)*, it may result from other bacteria or fungi. A carbuncle is several boils that join together. Recurring boils may indicate diabetes or an immune disorder. Boils are infectious, but the spread can be controlled with careful cleanliness and handwashing. Treatment includes hot compresses, antibiotics, and sometimes drainage by lancing. Boils may also be caused by methicillin-resistant *S. aureus* (MRSA). More information about MSRA is found in Chapter 3.

Hirsutism (HER-soot-izm), or *hypertrichosis* (hy-per-tri-KO-sis), is an abnormal amount of hair growth in unusual places. In women hair may appear on the face, back, and chest. Hirsutism may be caused by hormone supplements or may be a hereditary condition. Unwanted hair may be removed temporarily by shaving, waxing, or using depilatories, or it may be removed permanently by electrolysis. The disorder causing the hair growth, if any, should be treated when possible.

Impetigo (im-puh-TI-go) is a contagious bacterial skin infection that occurs most often in children. Impetigo is most often caused by *S. aureus*. It begins with small vesicles, which become pustules and form a crust. Itching and burning may occur. Ecthyma is a form of impetigo that creates open sores (ulcers) on the skin. Impetigo may lead to kidney infection, but lesions usually clear without causing lasting damage. It can be fatal in infants. Treatment includes antibiotics and isolation to prevent spread of the infection.

Kaposi sarcoma (KS) (kuh-POH-see sahr-KOH-muh) (Fig. 10-6) is a form of cancer that originates in blood vessels and spreads to the skin. KS appears as a round or oval spot on the skin that may be red, purplish, or brown in color. It has two forms. One

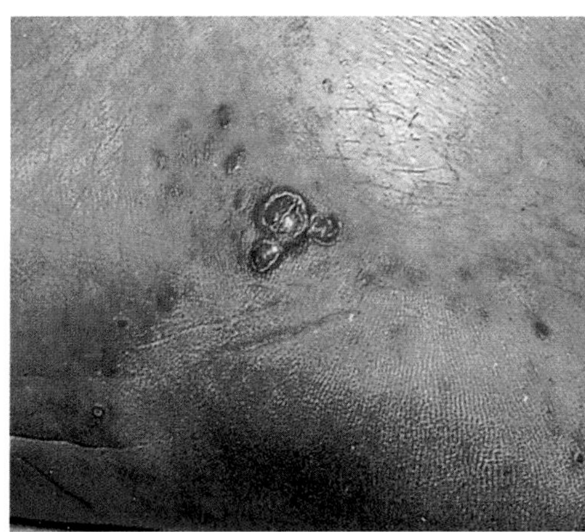

FIGURE 10-6 Kaposi sarcoma. (From Thibodeau GA, Patton KT: *Anatomy & physiology*, ed 5, St. Louis, 2003, Mosby.)

form affects older people and rarely spreads to other parts of the body. The second form is associated with diabetes, lymphoma, and AIDS. It grows more quickly and may spread to the lungs, liver, and intestines. Treatment for KS may include local treatment, systemic chemotherapy, or interferon.

Lupus erythematosus (LE) (LOO-pus air-ith-uh-mah-TOE-sis) may be a benign dermatitis or a chronic, relapsing systemic disorder. Its cause is usually unknown. In some cases, drugs used to treat heart conditions and tuberculosis may cause lupus, which disappears when the drug therapy ends. As dermatitis, it appears as a scaly rash and may lead to baldness. When systemic, lupus affects the vascular and connective tissues and also appears as a rash on the skin. Headaches, seizures, and mental disorders may be the first symptoms. Treatment includes protection from exposure to the sun and anti-inflammatory drugs.

Morgellons (mor-GEL-ens) may have been described for the first time 300 years ago. It is an unexplained skin condition characterized by blue and white fiber-like strands and black granules coming out of lesions on the skin. It causes a sensation of insects crawling, stinging, and biting the skin. The affected person may also have trouble concentrating, insomnia, and joint pain. In the past, Morgellons cases have often been diagnosed as psychosomatic illness. Another cause of Morgellons has not been determined, although some research indicates a link to Lyme disease. Treatment for Morgellons may include antibiotics and antidepressants. The CDC along with Kaiser Permanente's Northern California Division of Research, is conducting a study to determine who may be affected, the symptoms, and factors that contribute to the development of unexplained dermopathy (Morgellons).

Psoriasis (so-RY-uh-sis) is a common chronic skin disorder in which too many epidermal cells are produced. Psoriasis appears as red, thick areas, or plaques (plaks), covered with scales, which may be gray or silver. Although the cause is unknown, psoriasis may be triggered by stress and other factors. The disorder seems to run in families and appears in adolescence or early adulthood. Treatment includes topical medication, removal of the scales, and application of ultraviolet light.

Rashes may result from viral infection, especially in children (Table 10-1). Treatment is usually symptomatic, designed to prevent scratching that may result in scars. Complications from diseases that cause childhood rashes are possible but unlikely.

Scleroderma (skle-ro-DER-muh) is a rare autoimmune disorder that affects the blood vessels and connective tissues of the skin and other epithelial tissues. The first symptom is usually swelling. Hard, yellowish lesions are formed. Scleroderma usually remains localized but may become systemic. Treatment may include use of anti-inflammatory medication and physical therapy to prevent muscle contracture and deformity.

Skin cancer is the most common type of cancer and the most treatable, if diagnosed early. Usually it can be treated successfully by burning, freezing, or surgically removing the lesions. Radiation may be required. Skin cancer usually results from exposure to the sun. It has three basic forms: basal (BAY-zuhl) cell, which is the most common; squamous (SKWAY-mus) cell; and melanoma (mel-uh-NO-ma) (Fig. 10-10). Early signs of skin cancer include a spot or growth that does not heal or a mole or birthmark that changes size, color, thickness, or texture (Box 10-1). New treatment methods for squamous and basal cell carcinoma include medication to increase the action of the immune system, laser surgery, and drugs related to vitamin A. Vaccination and gene therapy are being tested to treat melanoma.

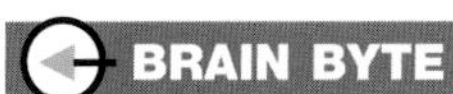

BRAIN BYTE

Basal and squamous cell carcinoma make up more than 95% of skin cancers.

Skin lesions differ in texture, color, location, and rate of growth. Skin lesions are uncomfortable but are not usually life threatening. They may result from irritation or infection. They may also indicate a condition of the body as a whole (Table 10-2).

TABLE 10-1
Viral Infections That Can Cause a Rash

Infection	Period of Incubation (days)	Contagious Period	Site of Rash	Nature of Rash
Measles (rubeola) (Fig. 10-7)	7-14 days	2-4 days before rash appears, plus 5 days	Ears, neck, face, trunk, arms, legs	Irregular, flat, red rash lasts 4-7 days
German measles (rubella) (Fig. 10-8)	14-21 days	Shortly before onset of symptoms until rash disappears	Face, neck, trunk, arms, legs	Pinkish, flat, begins 1-2 days after symptoms appear, lasts 1-3 days
Chickenpox (Fig. 10-9)	14-21 days	Before onset of symptoms until all vesicles have crusted	Trunk, face, neck, arms, legs, infrequently palms and soles	Small, flat, red spots from fluid-filled blisters followed by crusting, lasting a few days to 2 weeks

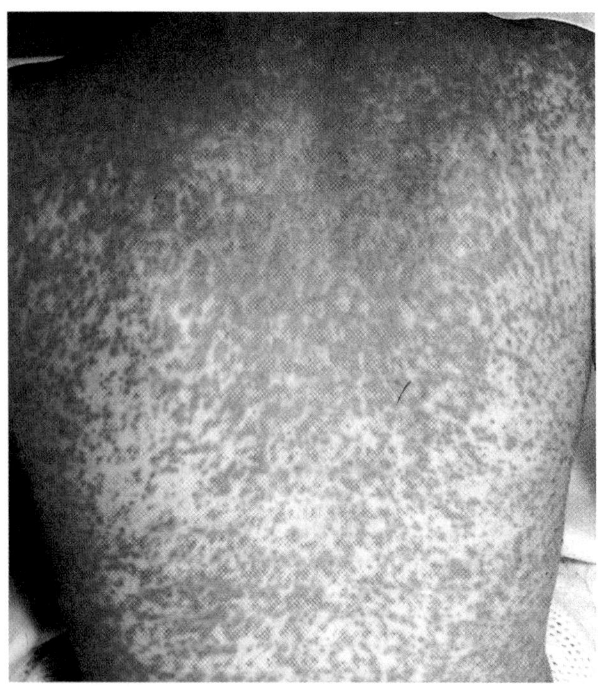

FIGURE 10-7 Measles (rubeola). (From Baren JM, et al: *Pediatric emergency medicine,* Philadelphia, 2008, Saunders.)

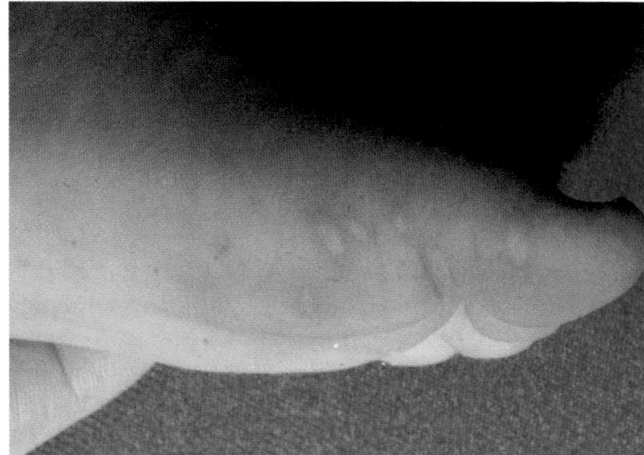

FIGURE 10-8 German measles (rubella). (From Lebwohl MG, Heyman WR, Berth-Jones J, et al: Treatment of skin disease. In *Comprehensive therapeutic strategies,* ed 3, London, 2010, Saunders.)

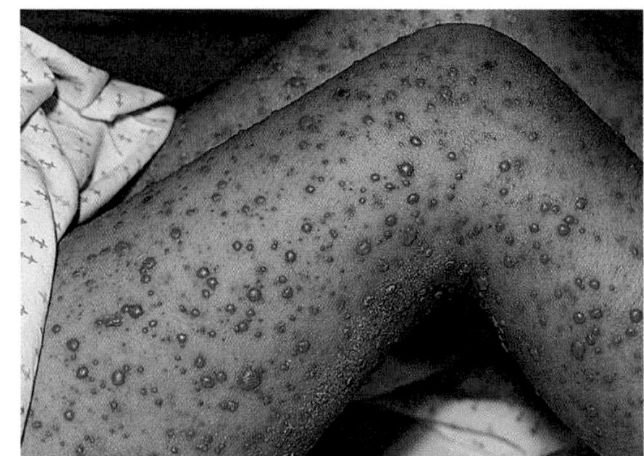

FIGURE 10-9 Chickenpox. (From Swartz MH: *Textbook of physical diagnosis*, ed 6, Philadelphia, 2010, Saunders.)

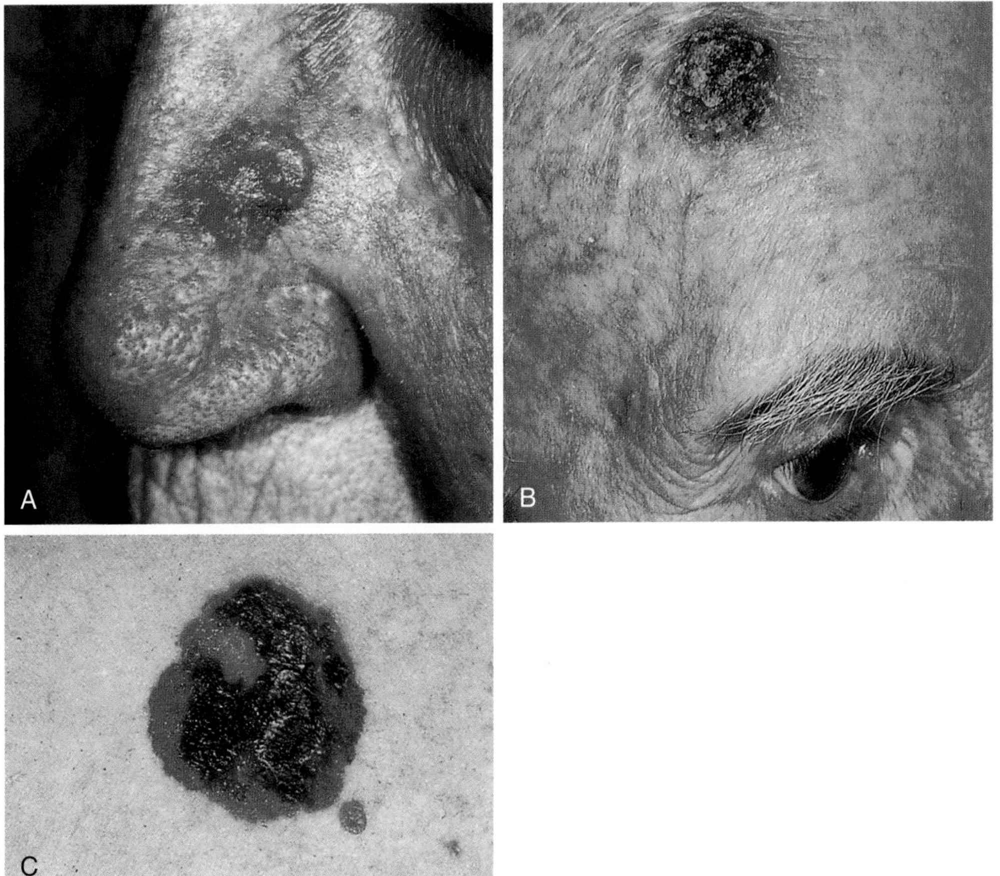

FIGURE 10-10 The three most common forms of skin cancer. **A,** Squamous cell. **B,** Basal cell. **C,** Malignant melanoma. (From Patton KT, Thibodeau GA: *Anatomy & physiology,* ed 7, St. Louis, 2010, Mosby.)

BOX 10-1

Warning Signs of Melanoma

- Change in size of a pigmented spot or mole
- Change in color of an existing mole (white, red, or blue pigmentation of the surrounding skin)
- Change in consistency or shape of the skin over a pigmented spot
- Inflammation of the skin around an existing mole

Streptococcus (strep-to-KOK-us) species are non-moving bacteria that affect many parts of the body. Each year 500 to 1500 cases of group A streptococcal infections appear as a skin disorder. Streptococci infections may become "flesh eating" in nature, destroying up to 1 cm^2 of skin each hour. If treated within 3 days, this bacterial infection can be cured easily with antibiotics. The condition may be fatal if not treated promptly.

Vitiligo (vit-il-EYE-go) is a condition that causes loss of pigment of the skin that results in irregular, smooth white patches. The condition may appear at any time and has an increased incidence in some families. The cause of vitiligo is unknown but may be the result of an autoimmune response. Most vitiligo goes untreated. Phototherapy and application of steroid creams may help replace color. Although some areas may repigment without any treatment, new patches may appear.

CASE STUDY 10-1 You have a patient with patches of skin that are white rather than flesh colored. The patient tells you that the areas are increasing in number and size and has been told it is vitiligo. He tells you it was caused by exposure to second-hand smoke from his parents. What should you say?

Answers to Case Studies are available on the Evolve website: ***http://evolve.elsevier.com/Gerdin***

A *wart* is a *papule* (PAP-yool) caused by a contagious viral infection of the skin. Plantar, common, and

TABLE 10-2
Skin Lesions

Lesion	Description	Possible Cause
Crust	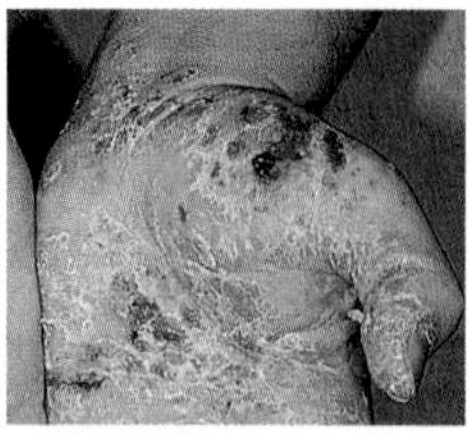 Dry pus, lymph, or blood covering injury, secondary skin lesion	Scab on abrasion; eczema
Cyst	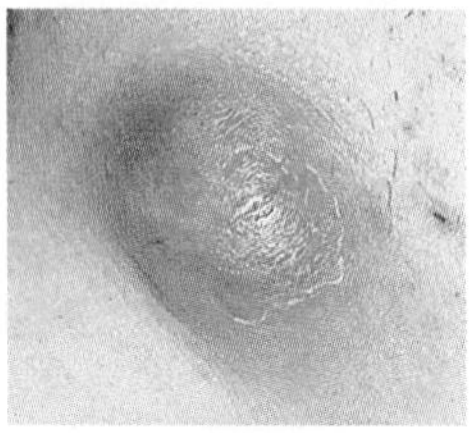 Sac of fluid or dead cells, solid to the touch	Plugged oil gland
Fissure	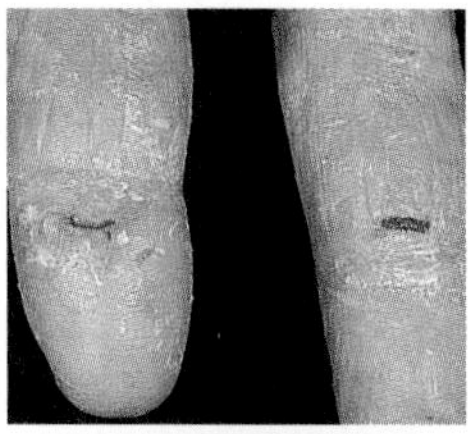 Deep groove in skin, crack	Athlete's foot
Keloid	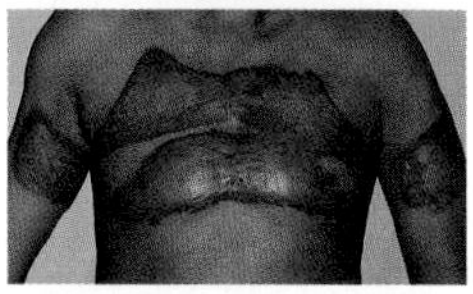 Progressively enlarging scar	Burn
Macule	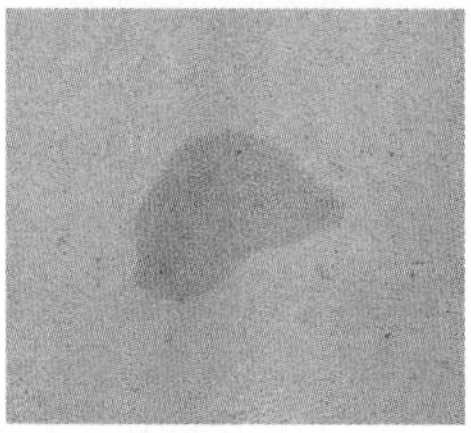 Discolored spot on skin; not raised or depressed	Measles, mononucleosis, freckles
Papule	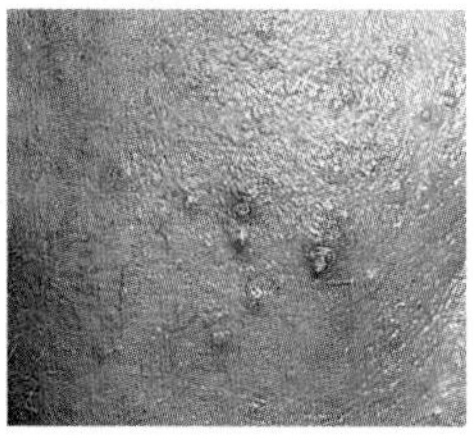 Raised, solid area, <1 cm in diameter	Warts, moles, pimples
Pustule	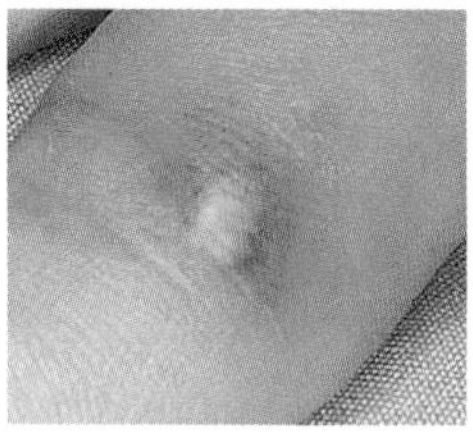 Pus-filled, raised area, white, yellow, greenish yellow	Pimples, acne

TABLE 10-2
Skin Lesions—cont'd

Lesion		Description	Possible Cause
Ulcer		Open sore, may bleed or have discharge	Bedsore
Varicose veins		Bluish, spiderweb-like veins	Pressure in peripheral veins
Vesicle		Raised fluid-filled pouch, specific location	Burns, scabies, shingles, chickenpox

(Varicose veins photo from Forbes CD, Jackson WF: *Color atlas and text of clinical medicine,* ed 3, London, 2003, Mosby Ltd. All other photos are from Callen JP, et al: *Color atlas of dermatology*, ed 2, Philadelphia, 2000, Saunders.)

flat warts are typical, and they may disappear after a few weeks or may last for years. Chemicals, freezing with liquid nitrogen, or burning can usually permanently remove warts. Chapter 21 provides information about the effect of warts on the reproductive system.

Issues and Innovations

Skin and Hair Care

People in the United States spend approximately $6 billion on skin and hair products each year. The major contribution to a clear complexion and attractive hair is good overall health. Cleanliness, nutritious meals, and exercise reduce the risk of skin disorders. With conditions such as acne, some commercial products lead to additional skin problems rather than solutions.

Regular washing is the best way to prevent skin eruptions caused by excessive oil. A drying agent (astringent) applied after washing can remove excess oil from the skin. Products such as cleansing creams, which contain oil, do not help individuals with excessive oil but may help people with dry skin.

Cosmetics manufacturers use many advertising techniques (gimmicks) to sell their products. Products are promoted as "imported," "scent free," "organic," "never rinse," "smell away," and "industrial strength," but none of these properties is beneficial to the cleanliness and health of skin. Creams that "reduce wrinkles" often contain alpha-hydroxy acids, which cause sloughing (loss) of dead cells and thickening of underlying tissues. A chemical peel or application of a strong exfoliant contains a greater percentage of this acid compound. The FDA has no record of serious injury from use of dewrinkling creams, although some reports of rashes and burns have been made. The FDA does not test cosmetics for effectiveness but establishes that the creams are safe in the doses currently being sold.

All soaps work by emulsification; they surround and bind to the dirt so that it can be rinsed off. The soap must be completely rinsed off to remove the dirt from the skin. Acne soaps may include antibacterial ingredients or abrasive materials to remove dead skin. One of the most effective antibacterial compounds is benzoyl peroxide. Antibacterial compounds are most effective when applied before a blemish appears. Hypoallergenic soaps contain no chemicals or fragrances that may irritate sensitive skin.

Many products are available to remove unwanted hair or add desired hair. Some of the more common ways to remove unwanted hair are shaving, waxing, and depilatory creams. Depilatory creams work by chemically destroying the hair above the surface of the skin. No evidence indicates that removal by shaving or with creams changes the pattern of growth or the texture of the hair. Hair can be removed permanently by electrolysis, which is the electrical destruction of each undesired hair follicle. No reliable evidence indicates that any cosmetic product stimulates hair regrowth. Minoxidil is a drug being used by some physicians to treat hair loss conditions. Hair transplants and hairpieces are effective ways to add desired hair.

Although the pigments in ink used for tattoos and permanent makeup (micropigmentation) are regulated by the FDA, the practice of tattooing is not. No color additives are approved for injection into the skin. Some states have established guidelines for tattooing ranging from age limitation to outlawing. The risks involved in tattoos include infection, dissatisfaction, allergic reaction, granulomas, keloid formation, and complications during magnetic resonance imaging. The American Association of Blood Banks requires blood donors to wait 1 year after being tattooed before donating blood because of the risk of acquiring hepatitis B and C and other infectious diseases from tattoo needles. The most common problem with tattoos is dissatisfaction with the result. Tattoos may be removed by dermabrasion, scarification (using acid to replace the tattoo with a scar), skin grafting, and laser treatment. Laser tattoo removal is painful, may take six to eight visits, and costs several thousand dollars.

BRAIN BYTE

It is estimated that 36% of Americans aged 18 to 29 have at least one tattoo.

CASE STUDY 10-2 Your friend got a tattoo on her ankle a week ago. You notice that the skin around it is red and swollen. What should you say?

Answers to Case Studies are available on the Evolve website: ***http://evolve.elsevier.com/Gerdin***

Sun and Skin Cancer

The skin defends against the damaging ultraviolet (UV) radiation of the sun by producing melanin. Melanin accumulates in the cells of the skin and causes a tan, but the skin is easily damaged by excessive sunlight. UV light of the sun causes damage to cells of the dermis and loss of moisture that result in wrinkled, dry, tough skin. Mild sunburn is actually a first-degree burn. A more serious second-degree burn with blister formation can also result. Newer skin products contain PABA (para-aminobenzoic acid), which is effective in blocking the UV rays of the sun. A broad-spectrum sunscreen with a sun protection factor of 15 may block 93% of the sun's UV type B rays for up to 2 hours following application.

UV rays in sunlight may change the DNA structure in skin cells. Such changes lead to mutations in the cells, or skin cancer. UV radiation is considered the main cause of skin cancer. Family history is also considered a risk factor for developing skin cancer. According to the American Cancer Society, more than 1 million cases of nonmalignant skin cancers occurred in 2009 in the United States, with more than 68,720 cases of melanoma; 8650 cases of melanoma resulted in death. Damage to the skin from the sun is cumulative, or adds up over the years, increasing the risk of developing skin cancers with each sun exposure.

Basal cell carcinoma is the most common type of skin cancer. It starts in the lowest layer of the epidermis and appears as waxy, pearly growths or red, scaly patches and is most often found on the face, arms, and hands. The cancer lesions may alternate bleeding and healing. Four standard treatment methods for skin cancer include surgery, radiation therapy, chemotherapy, and photodynamic therapy, which involves injecting an inactive drug into blood vessels surrounding cancer cells. When a laser light is shined on the skin above the area, the drug becomes active and kills the cancer cells with little damage to the healthy tissue. The *Journal of the American Medical Association* reported that incidence of basal cell carcinoma more than doubled in women younger than 40 years of age from 1976 to 2003. Only a small rate of increase occurred in men during this time period. Some skin cancer experts consider tanning beds to be a major cause of this increase. In 2009 the *Lancet* journal reported that the risk of developing skin cancer is increase by 75% if tanning bed use begins before age 30.

Squamous cell carcinoma is the second most common type and originates in the middle layer of the epidermis. It spreads more quickly than basal cell

CASE STUDY 10-3 You have a friend who goes to a tanning salon regularly to have a tan all year. You mention the risk of tanning salons and cancer. Your friend replies that she uses a spray-on tanning product to protect her when she goes to the tanning salon. What should you say?

Answers to Case Studies are available on the Evolve website: ***http://evolve.elsevier.com/Gerdin***

CASE STUDY 10-4 You have a friend who is often depressed during the winter. He tells you that he has seasonal affective disorder and may start going to a tanning booth to raise his spirits. What should you say?

Answers to Case Studies are available on the Evolve website: ***http://evolve.elsevier.com/Gerdin***

carcinoma and also appears on areas of skin most often exposed to the sun. This cancer looks like red, scaly patches that do not heal. Eventually, the cancer grows into the underlying tissues if not treated. Squamous cell carcinoma is removed with the same techniques used to treat basal cell carcinoma. Often Mohs microscopic surgery is used to treat basal and squamous cell cancer. This method removes affected tissue by layers. The location of the cancer cells is mapped to pinpoint the affected area. This method is considered to have the best cosmetic result.

Melanoma is the third and most serious form of skin cancer. It originates in the pigment-producing or melanin cells of the skin and is most often caused by exposure to the sun. The National Cancer Institute reports that women who use tanning beds more than once a month are 55% more likely to develop malignant melanoma that those who do not. It appears as a brown or black molelike growth on the back, legs, or torso. One half of the cases develop from existing pigmented moles. When treated early, cure rates are close to 100%. If not treated early, melanoma may be fatal. Melanoma is treated by removal of the growth. If the melanoma cells have spread, cure rates are low.

Malignant melanoma has been treated with some success by using gene therapy. A marked gene is inserted into the tumor and can be recognized for attack by the body's immune system. Another treatment, called extracorporeal photo chemotherapy (photopheresis), separates and irradiates white blood cells, which are then washed and reinserted. These cells act as a vaccine against the existing cancer.

Summary

- The function of the integumentary system is to protect the other body systems from infection and injury.
- Five integumentary structures include the hair, epidermis, dermis, sebaceous gland, and melanocytes.
- Three methods used to assess the integumentary system are visual inspections, biopsy, and culture.
- Five disorders of the integumentary system are acne, albinism, alopecia, athlete's foot, and dandruff.
- Three methods used to maintain healthy skin are cleanliness, nutritious meals, and exercise.
- Three types of skin cancer are squamous cell carcinoma, basal cell carcinoma, and melanoma. Methods to prevent skin cancer include wearing sunblock, avoiding sun exposure, and wearing protective clothing.

Review Questions

1. Describe five functions of the integumentary system.
2. Describe the location and function of each of the following parts of the integumentary system.

Ceruminous glands	Nerves
Dermis	Sebaceous gland
Epidermis	Shaft
Hair follicle	Subcutaneous gland
Nails	Sudoriferous gland

3. List three disorders of the integumentary system that are caused by a pathogen.
4. List three signs that may indicate a cancerous growth.
5. List three precautions that help to avoid skin cancer.
6. List five diseases or conditions in other body systems that might be detected by changes in the skin.
7. Use the following terms in one or more sentences that correctly relate their meaning: adipose, dermis, epidermis, subcutaneous

Critical Thinking

1. Research and compare the cost of at least three tests used to diagnose disorders of the integumentary system.

2. Investigate the function of at least five common medications used to treat the integumentary system.
3. List at least five occupations involved in the health care of integumentary system disorders.
4. Describe three commercials that are used to sell skin and hair products. Identify the technique or claim in each that is used to sell the product.
5. Write an essay about pressure sores. Research and report the incidence of pressure sores (decubitus ulcers) in long-term care facilities. Describe the daily care of an immobilized patient that would reduce the risk for development of a pressure sore. Research and report the treatment methods used for pressure sores.
6. Investigate the incidence of tattooing and state regulations or guidelines. Compare the positive and negative aspects of tattoos.
7. Use the Internet to investigate and prepare a pamphlet that tells readers about good skin care.
8. Use the Internet to investigate and prepare a report on a skin disorder. Include the incidence, cause, signs, symptoms, treatment, and method of prevention if any is known.

Explore the Web

Skin Care

Kid's Health

http://kidshealth.org/kid/stay_healthy/body/skin_care.html

Mayo Clinic

http://www.mayoclinic.com/health/skin-care/SN00003

Skin Disorders

Merck

http://www.merck.com/mmhe/sec18.html

Web MD

http://www.webmd.com/skin-problems-and-treatments/default.htm

Skin Cancer

Skin Care Physicians

http://www.skincarephysicians.com/skincancernet/whatis.html

CHAPTER 11

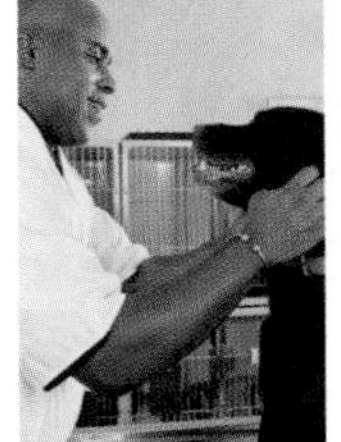
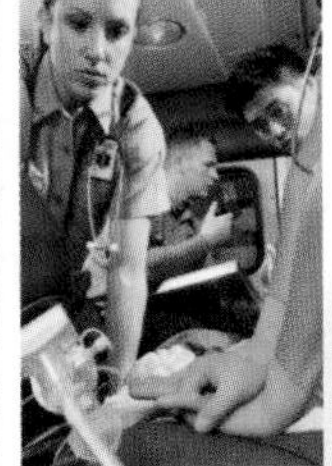
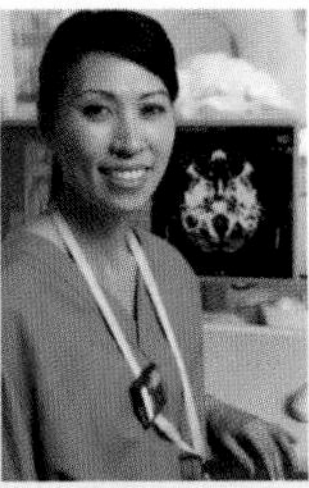

Cardiovascular System

LEARNING OBJECTIVES

- Define at least 10 terms relating to the cardiovascular system.
- Describe the function of the cardiovascular system.
- Identify at least 10 cardiovascular system structures and the function of each.
- Identify at least three methods of assessment used to evaluate the cardiovascular system.
- Describe at least five disorders of the cardiovascular system.

KEY TERMS

Cardioversion *(kar-dee-o-VER-zhun)* Restoration of normal heart rhythm by electrical shock

Contract *(kon-TRAKT)* Shorten, reduce in size

Coronary *(KOR-uh-nay-ree)* Pertaining to the heart; coronary arteries supply blood to the heart muscle

Diastole *(di-AS-to-lee)* Dilation of the heart; resting phase or filling of the ventricles, alternating with systole

Infarction *(in-FARK-shun)* An area of tissue death (necrosis) caused by loss of oxygen (ischemia) as a result of obstruction of circulation to the area

Pulmonary circulation *(PUL-muh-nayr-ee ser-kyuh-LAY-shun)* Carrying venous blood from the right ventricle to the lungs and returning oxygenated blood to the left atrium of the heart

Rate *(rayt)* Expression of speed or frequency of an event in relation to a specified amount of time; number of contractions of the heart per minute

Rhythm *(RITH-um)* Measured movement; recurrence of an action or function at regular intervals; interval of heart contractions

Stenosis *(ste-NO-sis)* Narrowing or stricture of a duct or canal

Stethoscope *(STETH-o-skohp)* Instrument used to listen to body sounds (auscultation), such as the heartbeat

KEY TERMS cont'd

Systemic circulation *(sis-TEM-ik ser-kyuh-LAY-shun)* General circulation; carrying oxygenated blood from the left ventricle to tissues of the body and returning the venous blood to the right atrium of the heart

Systole *(SIS-toe-lee)* Filling of the atria and contraction of the ventricles of the heart, alternating with diastole

Vessel *(VES-el)* Any one of many tubules in the body that carry fluid

Cardiovascular System Terminology*

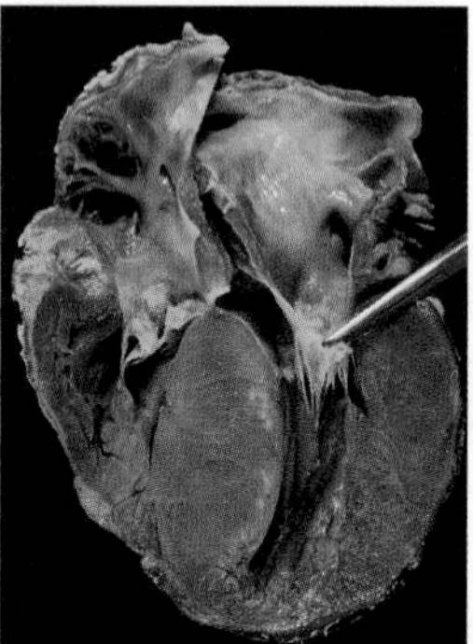

Hypertrophic cardiomyopathy is a congenital or genetic condition that may cause heart failure without symptoms. (From Patton KT, Thibodeau GA: *Anatomy & physiology,* ed 7, St. Louis, 2010, Mosby.)

Term	Definition	Prefix	Root	Suffix
Atherosclerosis	Condition of hardening of the arteries		ather/o	sclerosis
Cardiology	Study of the heart		cardi/o	ology
Congenital	Born with	con	gen	ital
Electrocardiography	Recording of the electrical activity of the heart	electro	cardi/o	graphy
Hypertension	High blood pressure	hyper	tension	
Myocardial	Pertaining to the muscle of the heart	myo	card	ial
Pericardial	Around the heart	peri	card	ial
Phlebitis	Inflammation of the veins		phleb	itis
Subclavian	Below the clavicle	sub	clav	ian
Thrombitis	Inflammation of a clot		thromb	itis

*A transition syllable or vowel may be added to or deleted from the word parts to make the combining form.

Abbreviations of the Cardiovascular System

Abbreviation	Meaning
AP	Apical
BP	Blood pressure
CHF	Congestive heart failure
chol	Cholesterol
ECG	Electrocardiogram
HB	Heartbeat
HDL	High-density lipoprotein
LDL	Low-density lipoprotein
MI	Myocardial infarction
PVC	Premature ventricular contraction

Structure and Function of the Cardiovascular System

The structures of the cardiovascular system are the heart and blood **vessels**. The heart beats more than 100,000 times a day, circulating about 5 L of blood. The functions of the cardiovascular system are the following:

- Transport nutrients and oxygen to the body
- Transport waste products from the cells to the kidneys for excretion

- Distribute hormones and antibodies throughout the body
- Help control body temperature and maintain electrolyte balance (homeostasis)

Heart

The heart is a two-sided, double pump. It weighs less than a pound and is slightly larger than a fist. The heart is located between the lungs in the thoracic cavity, positioned partially to the left of the sternum. The base or topmost (superior) part of the heart has a flatter shape than the tapered apex or lower (inferior) portion.

The right side of the heart pumps oxygen-poor (deoxygenated) blood to the lungs, where carbon dioxide is exchanged for oxygen. This is referred to as **pulmonary circulation**. The left side pumps the oxygen-rich (oxygenated) blood to the rest of the body. This is referred to as **systemic circulation**. The blood returns to the right side of the heart from the body to complete the cycle (Fig. 11-1).

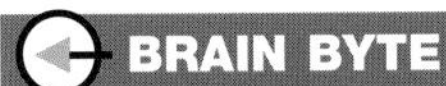

BRAIN BYTE

The heart pumps 5 quarts of blood a minute or about 2000 quarts each day.

Hepatic circulation refers to the path of the blood from the intestines, gallbladder, pancreas, stomach, and spleen through the liver. The liver stores and modifies nutrients in the blood for use by the body. It also removes or alters toxic substances so that they can be eliminated by the urinary system. The nutrient-rich blood, which has been filtered by the liver, is returned to the heart through the inferior vena cava for use throughout the body.

The heart has four chambers (Fig. 11-2). The top chambers are called *atria*. The lower chambers are called *ventricles*. The blood enters the heart through the atria and leaves the heart from the ventricles. The septum divides the right and left sides of the heart. Four valves prevent the blood from flowing backward through the system. Two of these valves are called atrioventricular (AV) valves. They separate the atria and ventricles on each side of the heart. The semilunar

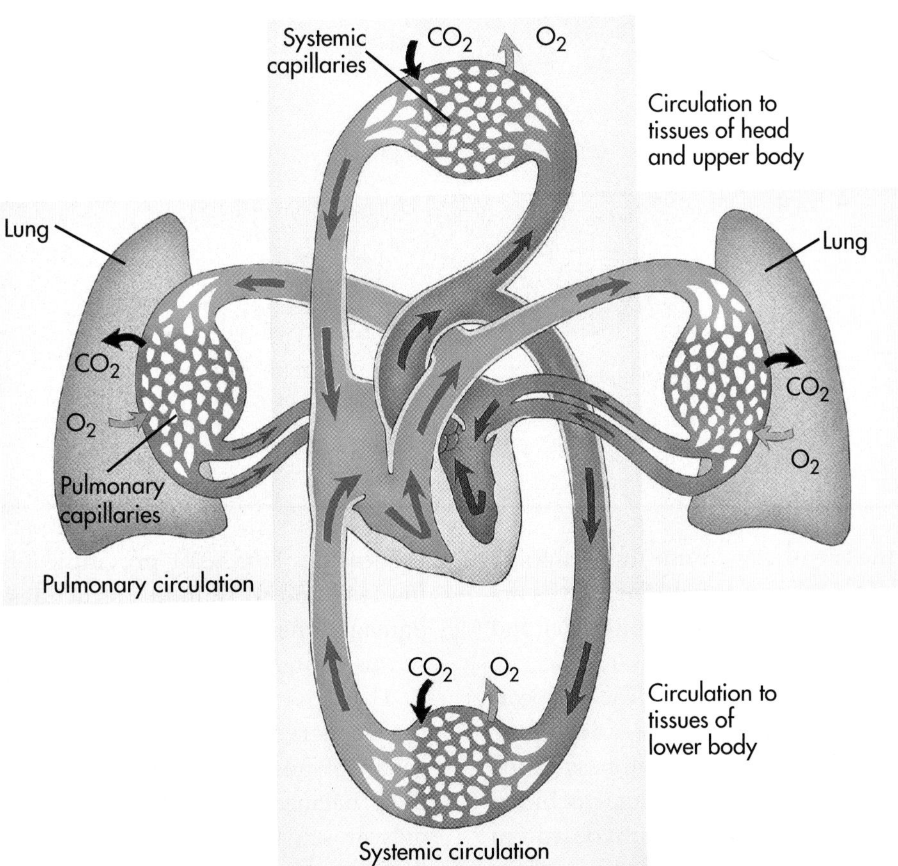

FIGURE 11-1 Blood flow through the cardiovascular system. (From Patton KT, Thibodeau GA: *Anatomy & physiology,* ed 7, St. Louis, 2010, Mosby.)

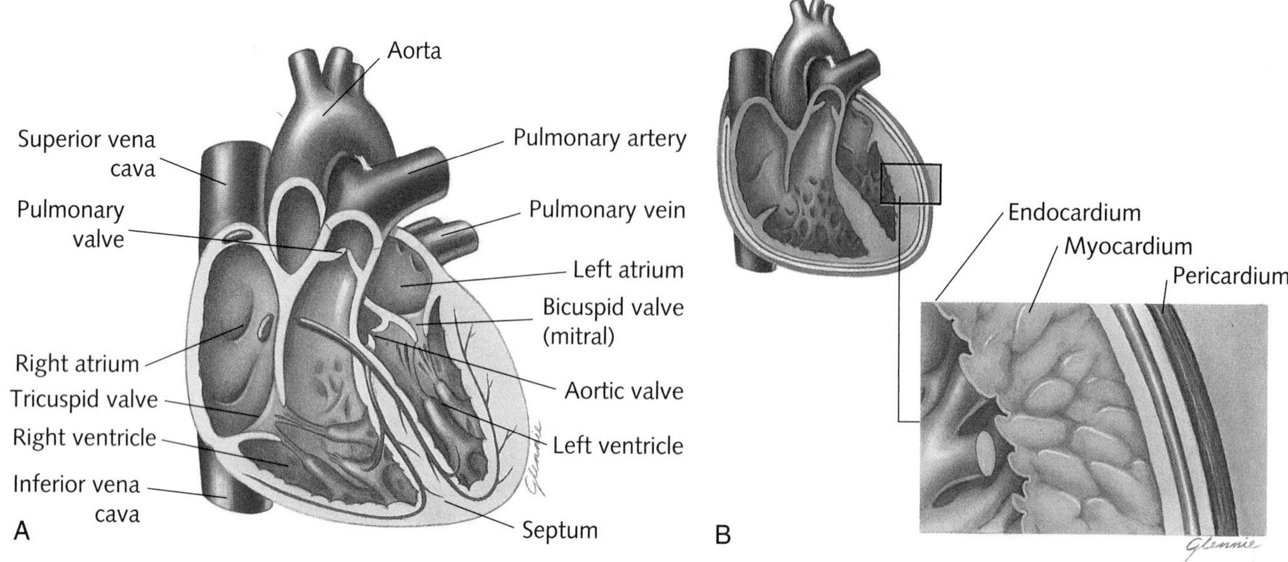

FIGURE 11-2 **A,** Structures of the heart. **B,** Layers of the heart.

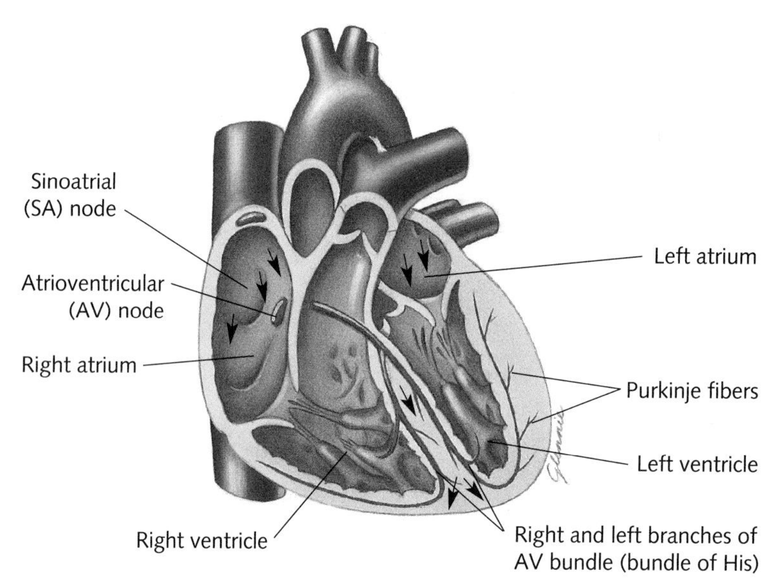

FIGURE 11-3 Path of electrical conduction in the heart.

valves separate the ventricles from the outgoing vessels (pulmonary artery and aorta). The valves are named according to their structure (semilunar) and location (pulmonary or aortic).

The heart has three layers of tissue. The endocardium is a smooth layer of cells lining the inside of the heart and forming the valves. The smoothness of the endocardial tissue helps prevent damage to blood cells circulating through the system. The myocardium is the thickest layer, consisting of muscle tissue. This part of the heart pumps blood through the system. The pericardium is a double membrane that covers the outside of the heart, providing lubrication between the heart and surrounding structures to prevent tissue damage. The pericardial sac is made up of the inner serous (watery) and outer fibrous layers.

The activity of the heart muscle is controlled largely by the nervous system but is affected also by the action of hormones and other mechanisms such as fluid balance. Additionally, the heart contains the only muscle tissue that can stimulate its own contractions. Specialized sinoatrial (SA) cells in the right atrium (SA node) act as a pacemaker to start a heart contraction (Fig. 11-3). The change in the electrical

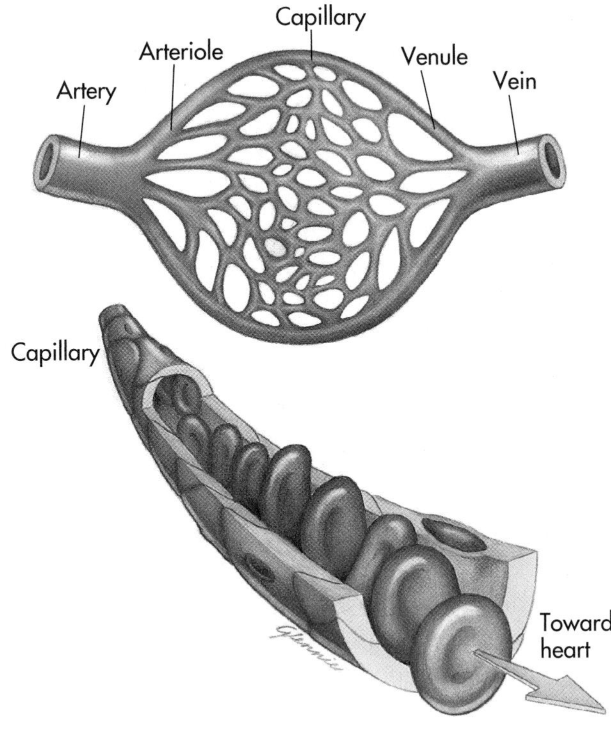

FIGURE 11-4 Blood vessels.

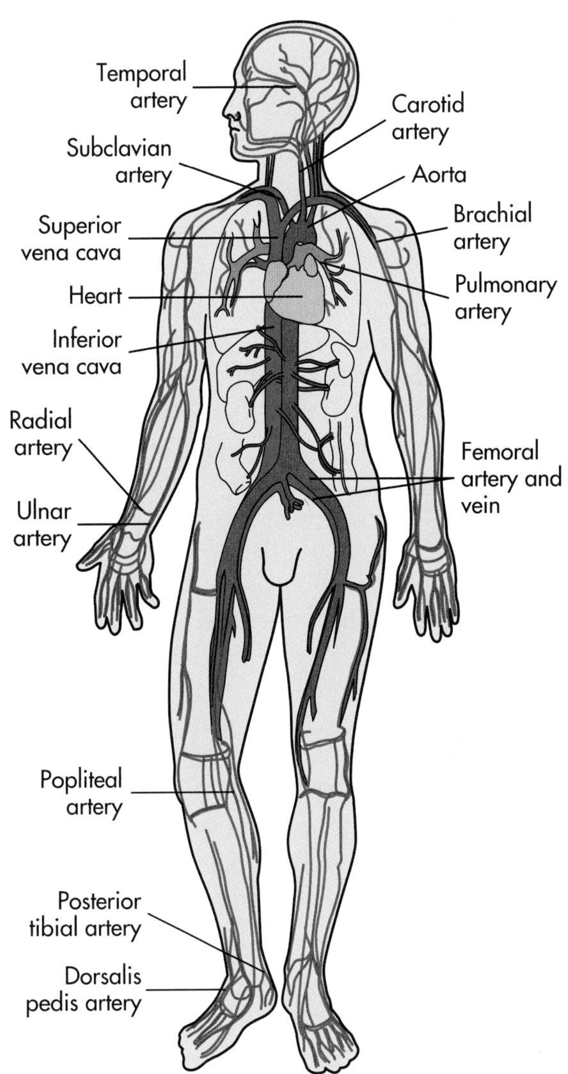

FIGURE 11-5 Principal arteries and veins. (From Sorrentino SA: *Mosby's textbook for nursing assistants*, ed 7, St. Louis, 2008, Mosby.)

potential of these cells stimulates another group of cells, called the atrioventricular node (AV node), to send the impulse into the lower portions of the heart. The impulse of the AV node stimulates specialized bundles of muscle called the *AV bundle* or *bundle of His*. These fibers then stimulate the Purkinje fibers, which surround the lower portions of the ventricles. The Purkinje fibers cause the ventricles to contract. Another unique property of the heart is the ability to adjust the strength of the contractions on the basis of the amount of blood in its chambers. Without the influence of the nervous system and other controls, the heart would contract only 40 times each minute instead of the normal 60 to 90 times. The adult heart beats 10,000 times a day.

Blood Vessels

The body has three main types of blood vessels (Fig. 11-4):

- Arteries carry blood away from the heart.
- Veins carry blood back to the heart.
- Capillaries are microscopic vessels that carry blood between the arterial and venous vessels.

Blood is pumped from the heart to the body by the largest artery in the body, the aorta. Fig. 11-5 shows the principal arteries of the body. The aorta branches into other arteries, which in turn branch into smaller vessels called *arterioles*. The blood moves from arterioles to microscopic capillaries. Gases, nutrients, and wastes are exchanged through the thin walls of the capillaries. The blood, which has now given up its oxygen, flows from the capillaries into tiny veins called *venules*. Venules branch together to form larger veins (Fig. 11-5). The blood is returned to the heart in the body's largest veins, the superior vena cava and inferior vena cava. With the exception of the pulmonary artery, blood in the arteries is oxygenated. Except for the pulmonary vein, blood in veins is deoxygenated.

Arteries have a muscular layer of tissue that helps pump blood out to the body. Veins have a much thinner muscular layer. Gravity and the movement of the muscles surrounding the veins help deliver blood back to the heart. Veins also have valves that prevent blood from flowing back, away from the heart, once it has moved forward.

Path of the Blood Through the Heart

Tracing the path of a blood cell through the heart is one way to learn the heart's structures and understand its functions (Table 11-1). Although the heart is considered a two-sided pump to differentiate the systemic and pulmonary circulation, the two atria contract at the same time, then the ventricles contract. Deoxygenated blood enters the right atrium of the heart from the body through the inferior and superior vena cavae. Additionally, blood from the heart muscle itself returns through a structure called the coronary sinus. The blood then passes through the tricuspid valve into the right ventricle. This valve closes as the pulmonary valve opens, allowing the passage of blood from the right ventricle to the pulmonary arteries. The pulmonary valve closes as the blood enters the lungs for the diffusion of oxygen and carbon dioxide. The oxygenated blood then travels through the pulmonary veins to the left atrium. From the left atrium the blood travels through the bicuspid or mitral valve to the left ventricle. The mitral valve closes as the blood leaves the left ventricle through the aortic valve. The blood then travels through the aorta to the rest of the body. As the ascending aorta leaves the heart, it branches in three directions to supply blood to the head and upper limbs. Two coronary arteries, which supply blood to the heart, branch off of the ascending aorta. The descending portion of the aorta supplies blood to the abdominal area and lower extremities. Deoxygenated blood is returned to the heart through the inferior and superior vena cavae from the body to complete the path.

TABLE 11-1
Path of the Blood through the Heart

Structure	Oxygen Content
Body	Exchange of carbon dioxide and oxygen
Superior and inferior vena cavae	Deoxygenated
Right atrium	Deoxygenated
Tricuspid valve	Deoxygenated
Right ventricle	Deoxygenated
Pulmonary valve	Deoxygenated
Pulmonary artery	Deoxygenated
Lungs	Exchange of carbon dioxide and oxygen
Pulmonary vein	Oxygenated
Left atrium	Oxygenated
Mitral valve	Oxygenated
Left ventricle	Oxygenated
Aortic valve	Oxygenated
Aorta	Oxygenated
Body	Exchange of carbon dioxide and oxygen

Assessment Techniques

Health care workers assess the activity of the heart as an indicator of overall body condition. Methods to assess the heart's condition include the following:

- Measuring pulse and blood pressure
- Listening to heart sounds
- Determining cardiac output
- Measuring muscle activity with electrocardiography
- Inserting a cardiac catheter
- Using echocardiography
- Radionuclide imaging

Pulse

With each heartbeat, blood surges against the walls of arteries. That surge, called a *pulse*, can be felt and counted in arteries close to the skin. The pulse can be counted in eight body locations (Fig. 11-6). The most commonly used site is the radial artery of the wrist. The large carotid artery in the throat is used in emergency situations. The brachial artery is used to measure the blood pressure. Other locations include the temporal, femoral, popliteal, posterior tibial, and pedal arteries. The normal pulse range for adults is 60 to 90 beats per minute, depending on the person's age, weight, fitness level, and emotional state. A pulse rate outside the normal range may indicate a disorder.

CASE STUDY 11-1 Your friend says her heart rate is usually about 60. She wonders whether she has something wrong with her heart. What should you say?

Answers to Case Studies are available on the Evolve website: ***http://evolve.elsevier.com/Gerdin***

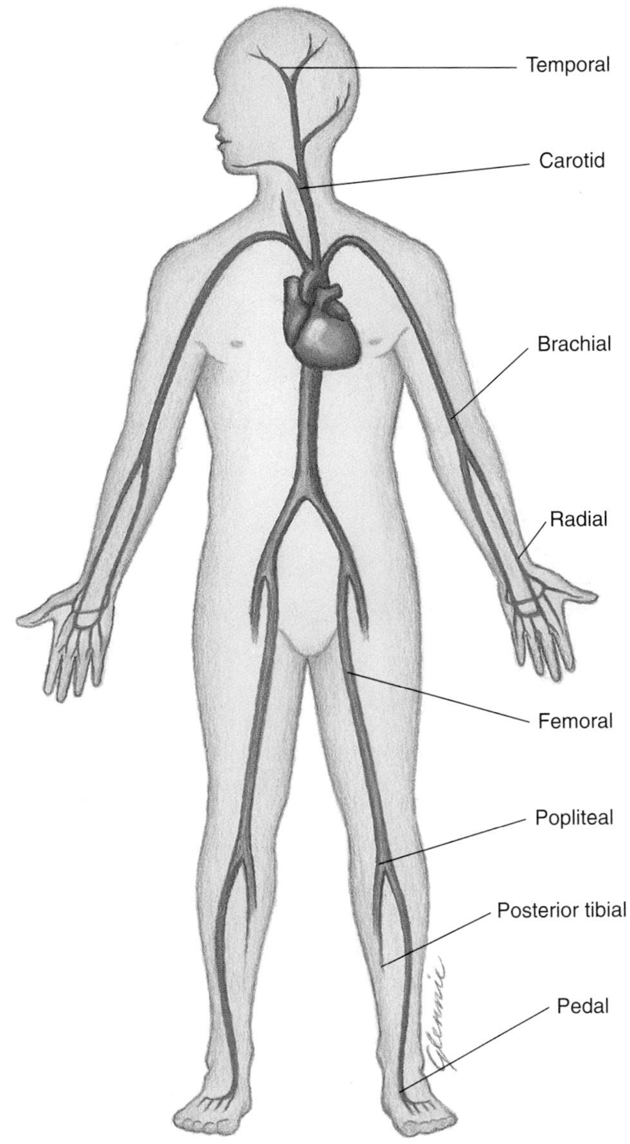

FIGURE 11-6 Peripheral pulse points.

Blood Pressure

Blood pressure is the force of the blood against the walls of the arteries. The systolic blood pressure, or systole, occurs when the ventricles of the heart contract, pushing blood through the arteries. The diastolic pressure, or diastole, occurs when the ventricles relax. Normal blood pressure is written as 120/80 (systolic/diastolic). However, blood pressure varies greatly among people. A healthy systolic pressure is usually less than 120. The diastolic pressure should be less than 90. A blood pressure outside this range may indicate a disorder such as hypertension or renal failure.

Heart Sounds

The "lub-dup" sound of the heart can be heard with a stethoscope. This characteristic sound results from the opening and closing of the valves in the heart as the blood is pumped from the atria to the ventricles and then to the lungs and then throughout the body. Abnormal or extra sounds are called murmurs. Murmurs are classified by the timing, intensity, location, pitch, and quality of the sound. Some heart murmurs are benign (causing no ill effect), but other murmurs indicate a disorder. A vibration caused by an abnormal flow of blood can sometimes be felt by touching over an artery and is called a "thrill."

Cardiac Output

The heart regulates the rate at which the blood circulates to the tissues. This measurement is called the *heart rate*. The stroke volume is the amount of blood contained in the ventricles. This blood is pumped into the arteries with each heartbeat. The volume of blood that is pumped from the heart by each contraction, multiplied by the heart rate, is called cardiac output:

$$\text{Stroke volume (mL/beat)} \times \text{Heart rate (beats/min)} = \text{Cardiac output (mL/min)}$$

For example, the cardiac output of an individual with a heart rate of 70 beats/min and a stroke volume of 70 mL/beat is 4.9 L. The normal cardiac output ranges from 4 to 8 L of blood per minute. The cardiac output affects the blood pressure. An abnormally high or low cardiac output may indicate a disorder of the cardiovascular system.

CASE STUDY 11-2 Your patient is monitoring his pulse rate because he worries about high blood pressure. You notice that he is counting his pulse for 6 seconds and multiplying by 10. What should you do?

Answers to Case Studies are available on the Evolve website: ***http://evolve.elsevier.com/Gerdin***

Electrocardiography

The pattern of electrical activity in heart contractions can be measured graphically using an electrocardiogram (Fig. 11-7). Electrodes attached to different sites on the body measure electrical changes occurring during heart contractions. Each section of the electrocardiogram pattern indicates a specific part of the heart's electrical activity (Fig. 11-8). Normal and abnormal heart activities have characteristic wave patterns (Fig. 11-9).

Some heart problems appear only during strenuous or specific activities. These can be diagnosed by using stress testing with electrocardiography or by wearing a portable electrocardiograph to compare heart activity with a log of activities during a specified time period.

Cardiac Catheterization

Cardiac catheterization is a procedure in which a tube is inserted through a blood vessel into the heart. A dye is then released through the catheter and traced by using radiography. This procedure is called *contrast coronary angiography*. Cardiac catheterization is used to measure the pressure in the chambers of the heart, take blood samples, and view obstructions in the vessels. Ultrasound transducers also have been inserted into the tip of catheter to allow viewing of an image of the inside of the arteries.

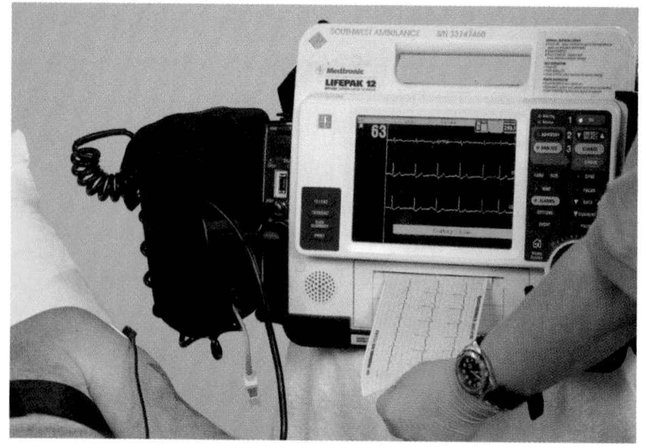

FIGURE 11-7 Electrical activity of the heart is measured with electrocardiography. (From Aehlert BJ: *Paramedic practice today*, St. Louis, 2010, Mosby.)

Echocardiography

Echocardiography is a procedure using ultrasonic waves that show the structures and motion of the heart. This procedure sends high-pitched sounds, which cannot be heard by the human ear, into the body. A special instrument called a *transducer* plots the echoes of these sounds to produce a graphic picture of the heart and valves. Echocardiography is used to detect conditions such as mitral valve defects and atrial tumors. If the image is unclear, a transesophageal echocardiogram may be used. After the back of the throat is numbed, a scope with an ultrasonic device is lowered into the esophagus to complete the echocardiogram.

Radionuclide Imaging

Radionuclide imaging, also called *radioisotope scanning*, uses a gamma camera to create an image after injection of a radioactive material such as thallium-201. Single-photon emission CT takes a series of pictures around that chest that are used to generate a three-dimensional computerized image. Myocardial perfusion produces images after the heart muscle absorbs radionuclides. Radiolabeled markers that group in areas of damaged heart tissue are shown in infarct avid imaging.

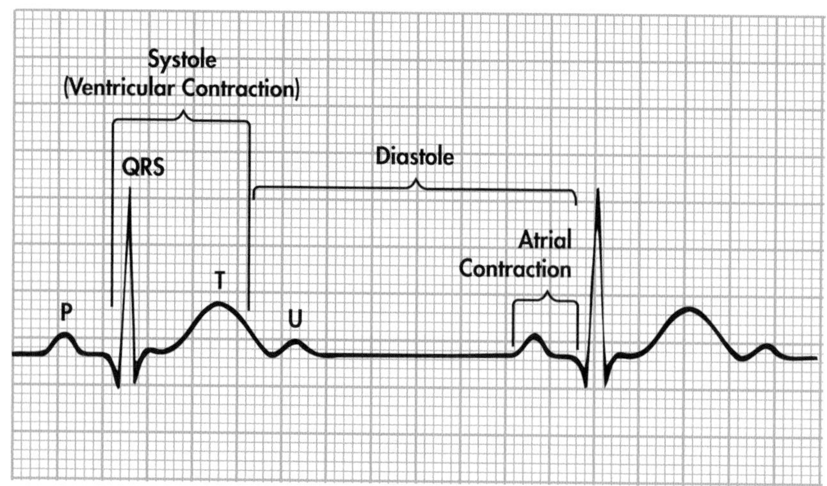

FIGURE 11-8 A normal electrocardiogram pattern with descriptions. (From Grauer K: *A practical guide to ECG interpretation*, ed 2, St. Louis, 1998, Mosby.)

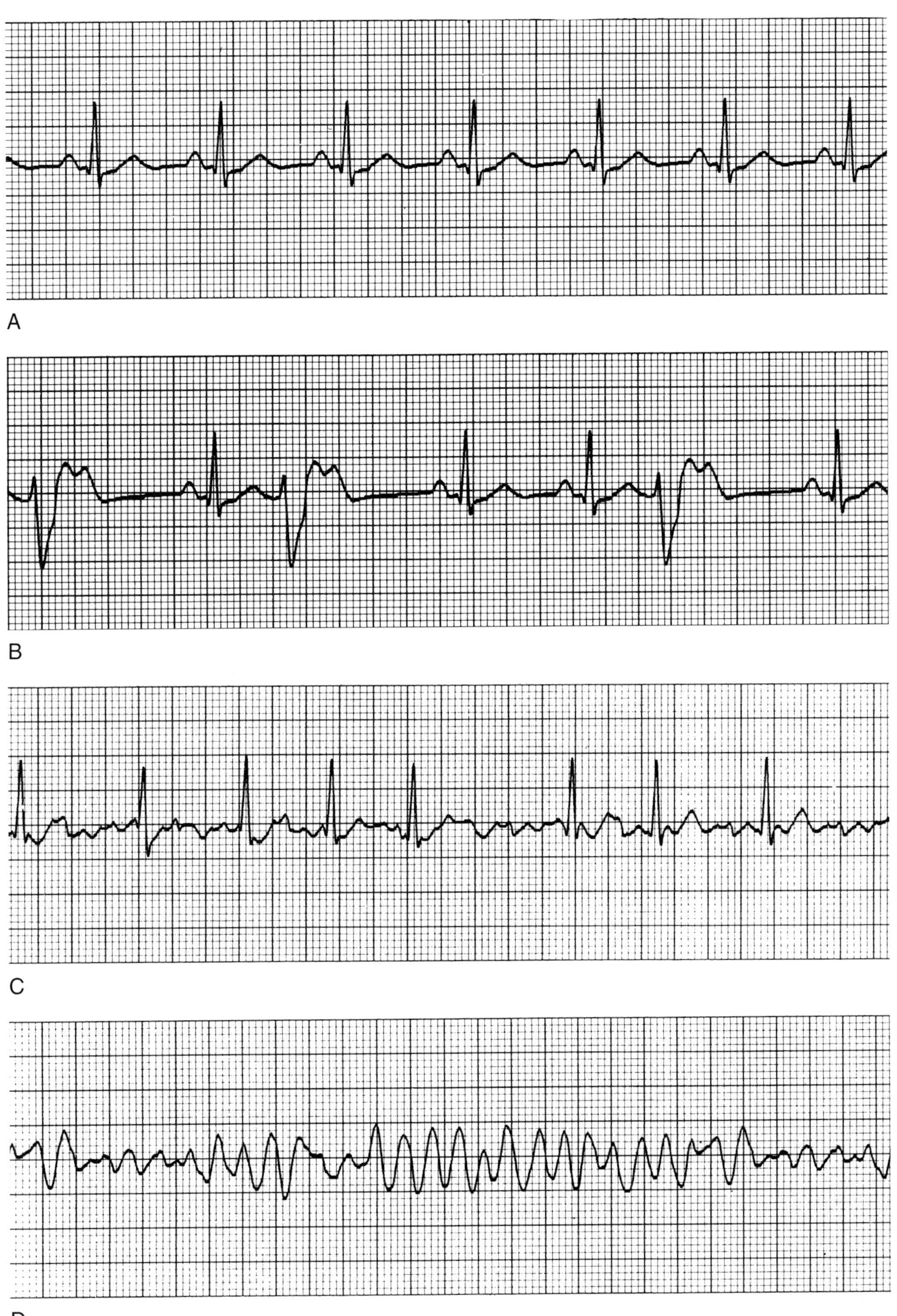

FIGURE 11-9 Electrocardiogram patterns. **A,** Normal sinus rhythm. **B,** Unifocal premature ventricular contractions. **C,** Atrial fibrillation. **D,** Ventricular fibrillation. (From Tait C: *EZ ECGs booklet,* ed 2, St. Louis, 2001, Mosby.)

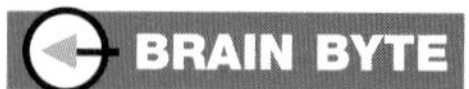

Molecules released from damaged cells are used as markers to confirm a heart attack has occurred.

DISORDERS OF THE Cardiovascular System

An *aneurysm* (AN-yoo-rizm) is an area of a blood vessel that bulges because of a weakness in the wall. Most aneurysms occur in the aorta, but they can occur in other vessels. The condition can be congenital and may cause no symptoms, but if an aneurysm ruptures, the person may have a life-threatening drop in blood pressure because blood is released into the body cavities. An aneurysm may be diagnosed if it displaces other body structures. Abnormal blood flow caused by an aneurysm sometimes can be heard with a stethoscope over the area. The sound of this abnormal blood flow is called a *bruit*. Aneurysms often can be corrected surgically by replacing the weak section of vessel.

Atherosclerosis (ath-er-o-skle-RO-sis) is a narrowing of blood vessels caused by deposits of fatty material containing calcium and cholesterol. This condition is sometimes called "hardening of the arteries" because the vessels lose their elasticity. When this narrowing occurs, the tissue that is deprived of blood will die. The exact cause of atherosclerosis is not known, but poor diet and lack of exercise increase the risk of developing it. Atherosclerosis can occur in any area of the body, but often it is found in the coronary arteries of the heart or in the arteries of the brain. Tissue death in the brain caused by atherosclerosis is called a *stroke*. Blockage of the blood vessels of the heart results in a heart attack (see following section on myocardial infarction). A person with atherosclerosis may experience chest pain, shortness of breath, fainting, and other indications of insufficient blood supply. Controlling risk factors, such as diet and exercise, may be used to treat atherosclerosis. Surgical removal of fatty deposits is possible in some vessels. Other treatments include drug therapy and surgery to lessen symptoms of the condition.

Cardiac arrhythmia (uh-RITH-mee-uh) is a disturbance of the heart's **rhythm** caused by a defect in the heart's pacemaker cells or by damage to heart tissue. The rhythm may be too fast, too slow, or irregular. The person with cardiac arrhythmia may experience dizziness, changes in heart rate, and poor blood circulation. Treatment, if necessary, may include insertion of an artificial pacemaker or implanted cardioverter-defibrillator, the procedure of **cardioversion**, or medication.

Cardiovascular disease is a general term for the combined effects of arteriosclerosis, atherosclerosis, and several related conditions, which are collectively called *coronary artery disease* **(CAD)**. It is responsible for more than 40% of all deaths in the United States and is three times more common than cancer. CAD might appear as a heart attack, peripheral artery disease, angina, or stroke. According to the CDC, heart attack is the leading cause of death of both men and women in the United States. Stroke is the third leading cause. Health care for cardiovascular disease is directed toward prevention, including a healthy diet, exercise, and avoidance of tobacco products. Treatments for CAD may include medication and are numerous (Table 11-2).

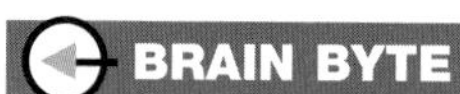

Cardiovascular disease (heart disease and stroke) is the leading cause of death for Americans age 35 and older.

Congenital (kon-JEN-i-tal) **heart disease** is a group of disorders that affect about one in eight newborns each year in the United States. Although the exact causes of many abnormalities in fetal heart development are not known, genetic or chromosome and maternal infections such as rubella during pregnancy may be causes. Use of some medication, alcohol, or drug abuse during pregnancy may also result in congenital diseases. Common defects include narrowing, or **stenosis**, of vessels to the heart and atrial or ventricular septal defects. Coarctation (ko-ark-TAY-shun) of the aorta and patent ductus arteriosus (PA-tent DUK-tus ar-tee-ree-O-sus), a condition in which the opening between the pulmonary artery and aorta does not close at birth, may also occur. Individuals with a heart defect often experience shortness of breath and bluish discoloration of the skin, called *cyanosis* (si-uh-NO-sis). This is caused by inadequate perfusion of oxygen to the tissues. Some mild heart defects may not need any treatment or can be treated with medication. Heart defects often can be corrected surgically.

Congestive (kon-JES-tiv) *heart failure* **(CHF)**, usually caused by disease in another body system, is the inability of the heart to pump blood adequately to meet the body's needs. CHF may occur suddenly or

TABLE 11-2
Treatment of Coronary Artery Disease and Angina*

Procedure	Description	Characteristics
Coronary artery bypass graft (CABG)	A blood vessel from another part of the body (often the leg) is grafted in front of and beyond the artery blockage to provide a new route for blood flow.	Preferred if there are three or more blocked arteries, when the main artery is blocked more than 50%, and in diabetics
Percutaneous transluminal coronary angioplasty (PTCA)	A camera is used to guide a catheter into the blocked artery. The artery is opened by inflating a balloon. A mesh tube may be inserted (stent) to reinforce the opening.	Less invasive than CABG; narrowing or reclosing of the artery occurs in about 50% of the patients, requiring reopening
Enhanced external counterpulsation (EECP)	An air pump inflates and deflates cuffs around the legs, causing blood to be pushed to the heart.	Used in China and in clinical trials in the United States; will not replace CABG or PTCA
Ultrasound thrombolysis	High-frequency sound waves are used to dislodge and dissolve fatty plaques in coronary arteries.	Experimental; initial cases have a low incidence of restenosis
Endoscopic transthoracic sympathicectomy	Nerves that cause chest pain are blocked to relieve angina.	Experimental; blocks symptoms of heart attack if it occurs
Angiogenesis	A gene is injected into heart to cause growth of new blood vessels.	Experimental; genetic therapy

*No surgical procedure cures coronary artery disease. A healthy lifestyle and possible medication will still be necessary after surgery.

develop over time. It leads to inadequate respiratory and kidney function. The person with CHF usually experiences shortness of breath; rapid heartbeat called *tachycardia* (tak-ee-KAR-dee-uh); and fluid retention. Treatment includes medication to lessen the symptoms and lifestyle changes to reduce risk factors.

Hypertension (hy-per-TEN-shun), also called *high blood pressure*, affects about one in five people in the United States. The cause of most cases of high blood pressure is not known. When the cause is not known, it is called essential or primary hypertension. Some cases result from other conditions, such as kidney disease and adrenal gland disorders. These cases are called secondary hypertension. A tendency toward high blood pressure may be inherited. High blood pressure is one of the major risk factors for development of a heart attack, stroke, heart failure, and kidney failure (Box 11-1). The rate of high blood pressure in children and adolescents is increasing. Because most people with high blood pressure have no symptoms at all, hypertension is sometimes called "the silent killer." The person may sometimes experience headaches, dizziness, and shortness of breath. Treatments for hypertension may include exercise, diet modification, avoiding tobacco products, and regular use of medication.

CASE STUDY 11-3 You are trying to lower your blood pressure. While you are attending a party, you want to have a snack. Your choices are cheese dip with crackers, shrimp dip with crackers, and fresh vegetables with onion dip. Which should you eat?

Answers to Case Studies are available on the Evolve website: ***http://evolve.elsevier.com/Gerdin***

Myocardial (my-o-KAR-dee-al) **infarction**, known as heart attack, can begin with a buildup of fatty deposits in the lining of the coronary arteries that feed the heart muscle. If the delivery of oxygen is obstructed, a heart attack occurs. It can also result from blockage of the blood vessels to the heart by a clot called an *embolus*. The area of the heart that is deprived of oxygen quickly dies. The victim of a heart

BOX 11-1

Effects of High Blood Pressure*

Damage to Arteries
- Atherosclerosis
- Arteriosclerosis
- Aneurysm

Damage to the Heart
- Coronary artery disease
- Enlarged left heart (hypertrophy)
- Heart failure

Damage to the Brain
- Transient ischemic attack
- Stroke
- Dementia
- Mild cognitive impairment

Damage to the Kidneys
- Kidney failure
- Kidney scarring (glomerulosclerosis)
- Kidney artery aneurysm

Damage to the Eyes
- Blood vessel damage (retinopathy)
- Fluid buildup under retina (choroidopathy)
- Nerve damage (optic neuropathy)

*http://www.mayoclinic.com

attack usually experiences chest pain called *angina pectoris*. The person may also experience dizziness, sweating, nausea, shortness of breath, or a combination of these effects. In some cases there are no symptoms at all. The damaged areas of the heart form scar tissue, making the heart less efficient in delivering blood to the body. If a large area of the heart is affected, it may stop functioning entirely. This situation is called *cardiac arrest* (Fig. 11-10). Treatment begins with reestablishing a pulse and then immediate and complete rest to minimize the damage to the heart muscle. In addition, drugs may be given to dissolve or prevent clotting of blood or to increase the heart's ability to work. This treatment is followed by rehabilitation and lifestyle changes to reduce the risks (Box 11-2). These may include control of blood pressure, a diet low in cholesterol and saturated fats, avoidance of tobacco products, weight reduction, and regular exercise.

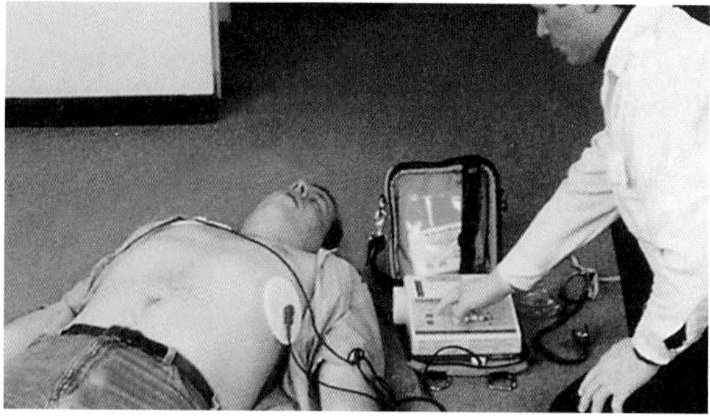

FIGURE 11-10 Many lives can be saved using the automatic external defibrillator (AED) device. (From Patton KT, Thibodeau GA: *Anatomy & physiology*, ed 7, St. Louis, 2010, Mosby.)

BOX 11-2

ABCs of Preventing Heart Disease, Stroke, and Heart Attack*

A—Avoid tobacco
B—Become more active
C—Choose good nutrition

*American Heart Association, http://www.americanheart.org/

BRAIN BYTE

People who smoke or lack physical activity have twice the risk of having a heart attack than nonsmokers and the physically active.

CASE STUDY 11-4 Your friend's mother is overweight. She is complaining of her arm hurting, shortness of breath, and is perspiring. What should you do?

Answers to Case Studies are available on the Evolve website: ***http://evolve.elsevier.com/Gerdin***

Phlebitis (fle-BY-tis) is inflammation of a vein, often with formation of a clot (thrombus). If the thrombus breaks free, then it is called an *embolus* (EM-bo-lus), and it may lodge in a smaller artery and cause tissue damage or sudden death. Phlebitis often results from damage to the vessel wall or prolonged sitting or standing. The person may experience swelling, stiffness, and pain in the affected part. Treatment of phlebitis includes administration of blood-thinning medications (anticoagulants), compression stockings, and elevation of the affected limb. Treatment may also include surgical removal of the clotted vein or injection of dissolving drugs to remove the clots.

Rheumatic (roo-MAT-ik) *heart disease* is a condition in which the heart muscle and valves are damaged by a recurrent bacterial infection that usually begins in the throat. The bacteria produce a toxin that causes inflammation and damage to the heart valves. Rheumatic fever is most common in children 5 to 15 years of age. The person experiences swelling of the joints, fever, shortness of breath, and chest pain (angina). The damaged heart valves may harden (sclerosis) and not close completely, allowing blood to leak through the valves. If the damage is great, affected valves may be replaced surgically. Treatment of strep throat with antibiotics such as penicillin can usually stop rheumatic fever from developing.

Varicose (VAYR-ih-kos) *veins* is a common condition in which veins become enlarged and ineffective. This commonly occurs in the leg veins of people who stand for long periods. Congenitally malformed valves, pregnancy, or obesity may also cause varicose veins. The person may experience swelling, visible bluish veins, redness, and pain. Treatment includes increased exercise and elevation of the affected part. Support hosiery is often helpful. If the condition warrants, surgery can be performed to remove the veins.

Issues and Innovations

Heart Replacement

The first heart transplant was performed in 1967. Each year, about 2300 heart transplants are performed in the United States. Dr. William DeVries implanted the first artificial heart in a human being in 1982. The Jarvik-7 was connected to an external power source and pump. Along with newer versions of this type of device, the Jarvik-7 is considered a temporary bridge to stabilize a person waiting for a donor heart. Currently it takes more than 6 months to obtain a heart for transplant once the recommendation has been made for the procedure. Most transplant recipients live for more than a year and can return to work.

In May 1991 the Texas Heart Institute in Houston began using a portable heart-assist device to decrease the workload of the heart. Another development is the use of an implantable defibrillator that senses an abnormal electrical activity in the heart and delivers an immediate shock to resume a normal rhythm or prevent sudden death.

In July 2001 the AbioCor self-contained artificial heart was used for the first time by developer Dr. O. H. Frazier (Fig. 11-11). The first recipient, Mr. Robert Tools, lived 151 days with the heart. Five people were recipients of this heart by December 2001. The AbioCor clinical trial that Mr. Tools and the other recipients participated in was designed to test whether

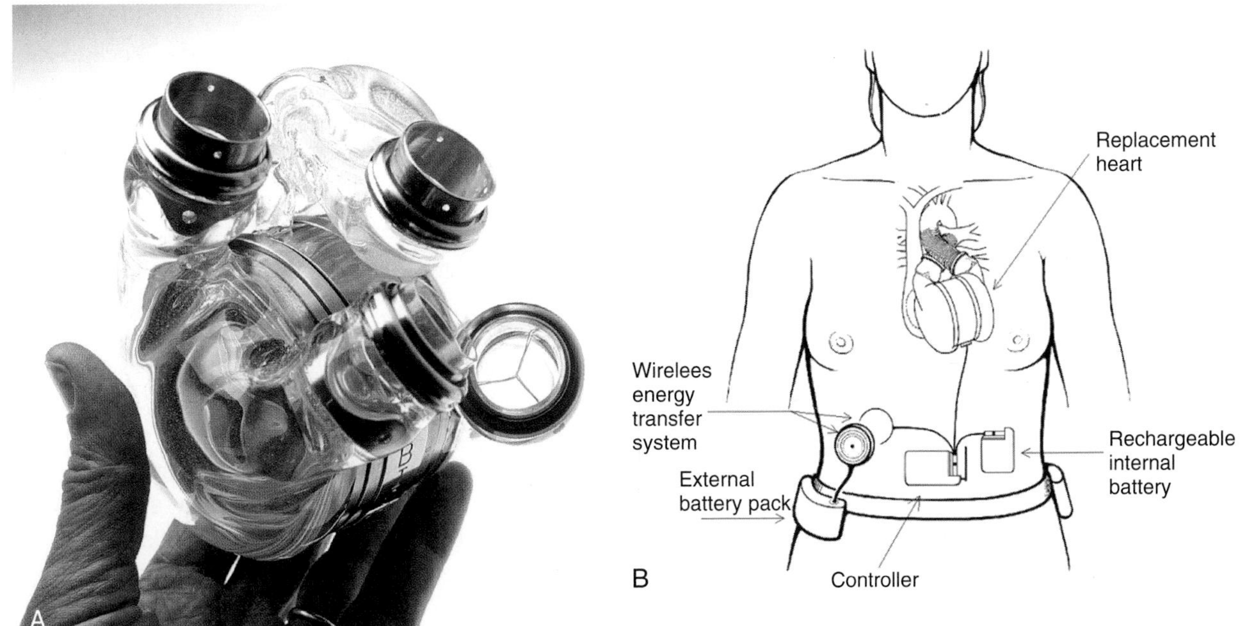

FIGURE 11-11 **A,** AbioCor heart. **B,** Placement of AbioCor heart in the body. (Courtesy ABIOMED, Inc., Danvers, Mass.)

the AbioCor Implantable Replacement Heart could extend life for people with end-stage heart failure who have no other clinical option and provide them with a good quality of life. To be accepted into the trial, the patient had to be ineligible for heart transplantation and have a high probability of dying within 30 days.

In 2005 the U.S. Food and Drug Administration (FDA) approved the use of a total artificial heart designed to support life functions until a transplant becomes available. The SynCardia CardioWest Temporary Total Artificial Heart (TAH) may be used in patients with irreversible failure of the ventricles. The CardioWest TAH-t is the only FDA–approved artificial heart that can provide full circulation restoration in patients with this condition. The goal of the company is to develop smaller, more portable devices.

According to the Organ Procurement Transplantation Network, in 2006 more than 3000 people were on a waiting list for a heart transplant. The American Heart Association reports that a new name is added to the national organ transplant list every 16 minutes.

Cholesterol Controversy

Cholesterol, which is found in all animal cells, is a waxlike substance used in the body to make cell membranes, hormones, and vitamin D. The liver makes enough cholesterol for all these needs. Cholesterol does not mix in water, so it is carried in the blood in proteins (lipoprotein). Cholesterol is found in both low-density lipoprotein (LDL) and high-density lipoprotein (HDL) forms. The HDL form takes cholesterol to the liver, whereas the LDL form blocks the arteries. Elevated blood cholesterol is one of the major risk factors for development of heart disease. Triglycerides or fats carried in the blood from food are also measured. The World Health Organization estimates that more than 50% of heart attacks and almost 20% of strokes are linked to high cholesterol.

Guidelines given to the public for the recommended types and amount of cholesterol have been confusing and disputed in the past. In 2004 the National Cholesterol Education Program updated guidelines on cholesterol management. Currently for adults older than 20 years, the emphasis is placed on the ratio of LDL to HDL in the blood as well as an overall value of less than 200 mg/dL (milligrams of cholesterol per deciliter of blood). The HDL portion should be greater than 40 mg/dL. The LDL levels should be less than 100 mg/dL. Triglycerides should be less than 150 mg/dL. A lipoprotein profile every 5 years or more often is recommended.

Harvard researchers have studied the link between fat in the diet and cholesterol blood levels over the past 20 years. They concluded that the type of fat in the diet, not the amount, changes the cholesterol level. Fats that were determined to lower LDL and raise HDL were monounsaturated and polyunsaturated fats such as olives, canola oil, avocados, fish, and most nuts. These fats are usually liquid at room temperature. Fats that raise both LDL and HDL are saturated fats, including whole milk, butter, cheese, red meat, chocolate, and coconut oil. These fats are generally solid at room temperature. Trans-fats, which are solid or semisolid at room temperature, raise the LDL and lower the HDL. They are considered the worst kind of fat. Foods containing trans-fat include most margarines, vegetable oils, shortening, deep-fried, and most fast foods. The Harvard researchers concluded that the amount of unsaturated fat in the diet does not necessarily raise blood cholesterol. In fact, replacing other calories with unsaturated fats such as fish may lower the risk for heart disease. They recommend limiting intake of saturated fats and eliminating transfats completely.

Losing excess weight, exercising, and not smoking will increase the overall HDL value. A diet with low-cholesterol foods such as fruits and vegetables is the best method for reducing the values. Some medications are used to reduce the level of cholesterol in the blood. Recently claims have been made that vitamins that prevent the oxidation (chemical breakdown) of cholesterol help prevent heart disease. However, this type of treatment is not recommended because of the harmful effects of large doses of these vitamins. Some research done in England has indicated that smaller, more frequent meals lower the amount of LDL produced.

Summary

- The function of the cardiovascular system is to transport oxygen, nutrients, waste products, hormones, and antibodies, as well as to control body temperature and maintain homeostasis.
- Structures of the cardiovascular system include parts of the heart and blood vessels.
- Methods of assessment used to evaluate the cardiovascular system include measuring blood pressure and pulse, listening to heart sounds, and determining cardiac output.

- Disorders of the cardiovascular system include aneurysms, atherosclerosis, CHF, phlebitis, and varicose veins.

Review Questions

1. Describe the four functions of the cardiovascular system.
2. Explain the differences in structure of the arteries, veins, and capillaries.
3. Identify the location of the following parts of the Cardiovascular system:

Carotid artery	Radial artery
Mitral valve	Inferior vena cava
Endocardium	Sinoatrial node
Pericardium	Left ventricle
Femoral artery	Tricuspid valve

4. Explain the action of the heart during systolic and diastolic contraction.
5. Which disorder of the cardiovascular system is called the "silent killer"?
6. Describe the location of eight pulse points that can be used to assess the rate of the heart.
7. Draw and identify a normal and three abnormal electrocardiogram patterns. Note the heart activity that is indicated by each peak of the normal graph.
8. Use the following terms in one or more sentences that relate their meaning: cardioversion, infarction, rhythm, vessel.

Critical Thinking

1. Investigate and compare the cost of at least three tests used in diagnosing disorders of the cardiovascular system.
2. Investigate the function of at least five common medications used in treatment of the cardiovascular system.
3. List at least five occupations involved in the health care of cardiovascular system disorders.
4. Investigate the way candidates are chosen for heart transplant surgery and its benefits and drawbacks.
5. Investigate the types of foods that contain trans-fats. Create a chart that identifies foods that contain trans-fat and foods with no trans-fats that would fill the same place in a menu.
6. Use the Internet to design a brochure to teach patients about cardiac disease rehabilitation.
7. Use the Internet to design a brochure to teach patients about cardiac disease prevention.
8. Use the Internet to investigate the increase in hypertension in children and adolescents. Write a paragraph with data that supports a possible reason.

Explore the Web

Cardiovascular Disease Rehabilitation

American Heart Association (AHA)

http://www.americanheart.org/presenter.jhtml?identifier=3035374

http://www.americanheart.org/presenter.jhtml?identifier=4490

Mayo Clinic

http://www.mayoclinic.com/health/heart-disease-prevention/W000041

Cardiac Disease Prevention

American Heart Association (AHA)

http://www.americanheart.org/presenter.jhtml?identifier=4723

Hypertension

About.com

http://highbloodpressure.about.com/od/quickfacts/f/pediatric_rate.htm

University of Chicago

http://www.funandeducation.org/Health/heathinfo/cvs/hypertension.htm

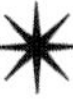

CHAPTER 12

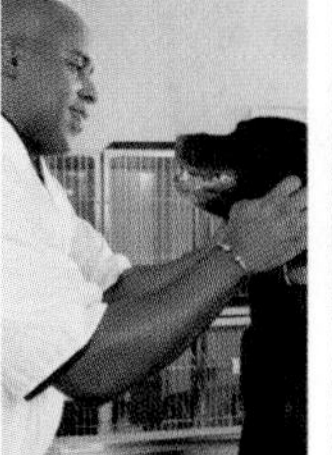
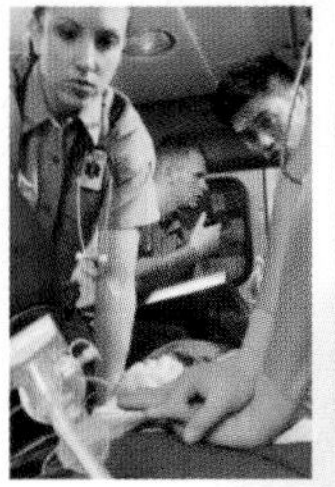
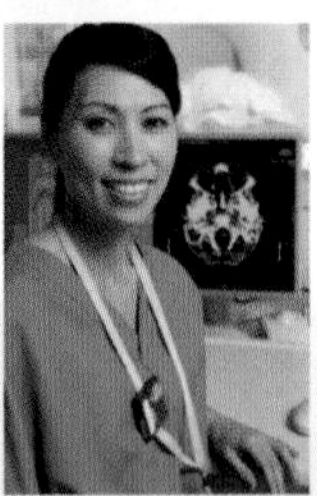

Circulatory System

LEARNING OBJECTIVES

- Define at least 10 terms relating to the circulatory system.
- Describe two functions of the circulatory system.
- List five functions of blood.
- Describe the function of lymph.
- Identify at least three methods of assessment of the circulatory system.
- Describe at least five disorders of the circulatory system.

KEY TERMS

Allergen *(AL-er-jen)* Substance capable of inducing specific hypersensitivity

Anemia *(uh-NEE-mee-uh)* Below normal number of red blood cells

Antibody *(AN-tih-bod-ee)* Molecule that interacts with specific antigen

Coagulation *(ko-ag-yoo-LAY-shun)* Process of clot formation

Erythrocyte *(e-RITH-ro-site)* Red blood cell or corpuscle

Immunity *(ih-MYOO-nih-tee)* Security against a particular disease

Inflammation *(in-fluh-MAY-shun)* Localized protective response to injury or destruction of tissue resulting in pain, heat, redness, swelling, and loss of function

Leukocyte *(LOO-ko-site)* White blood cell

Plasma *(PLAZ-muh)* Fluid portion of blood

Serum *(SEER-um)* Fluid portion of blood with clotting proteins removed

Spectrophotometry *(spek-tro-fo-TOM-uh-tree)* Measurement of quantity of matter in solution by passing light through spectrum

Thrombocyte *(THROM-bo-site)* Blood platelet

Circulatory System Terminology*

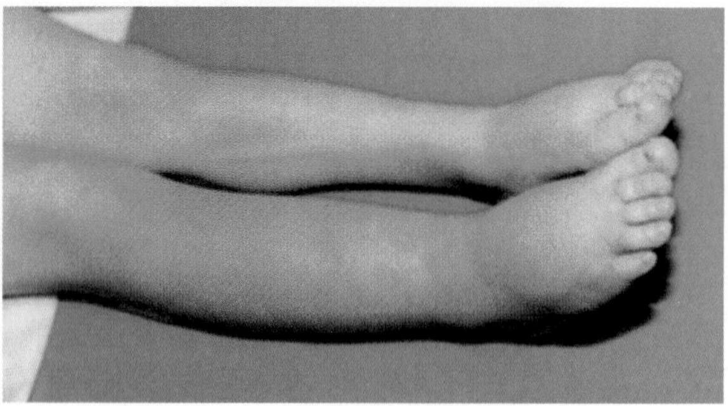

Lymphedema causes swelling in the tissues around the lymph vessels. (From Patton KT, Thibodeau GA: *Anatomy & physiology*, ed 7, St. Louis, 2010, Mosby.)

Term	Definition	Prefix	Root	Suffix
Anemia	Without blood	a/n	emia	
Erythrocyte	Red blood cell	erythro	cyte	
Hemogram	Record of blood	hemo	gram	
Leukocyte	White blood cell	leuk/o	cyte	
Lymphedema	Swelling due to lymph	lymph	edema	
Phagocyte	Eating cells	phag/o	cyte	
Polycythemia	Abnormal increase in the number of blood cells	poly	cyt/h	emia
Septicemia	Condition of poisoning of the blood		sept/ic	emia
Splenomegaly	Enlargement of the spleen		splen/o	megaly
Thrombocyte	Blood platelet	thromb/o	cyte	

*A transition syllable or vowel may be added to or deleted from the word parts to make the combining form.

Abbreviations of the Circulatory System

Abbreviation	Meaning
ABG	Arterial blood gas
AIDS	Acquired immuno-deficiency syndrome
Alb	Albumin
Bl	Blood
CBC	Complete blood cell count
FBS	Fasting blood sugar
Hct	Hematocrit
H&H	Hematocrit and hemoglobin
RBC	Red blood cell count
WBC	White blood cell count

Structure and Function of the Circulatory System

The circulatory system includes the blood and lymph that move through the body. Both blood and lymph are tissues that function to maintain homeostasis and give the body **immunity**.

Blood

Hematology is the study of blood. The body contains approximately 4 to 5 L of blood, making up about 8% of the body's weight. The functions of blood include the following:

- Transporting nutrients, oxygen, and hormones
- Removing metabolic wastes and carbon dioxide
- Providing immunity (resistance to disease) through antibodies
- Maintaining body temperature and electrolyte balance
- Clotting to prevent bleeding from a wound

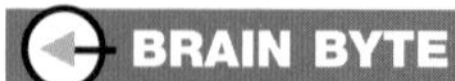

BRAIN BYTE

There are more than 60,000 miles of vessels that carry blood in the body.

Blood divides into solid and liquid portions when spun in a centrifuge (Fig. 12-1). The solid parts, called formed elements, are red blood cells (RBCs), white

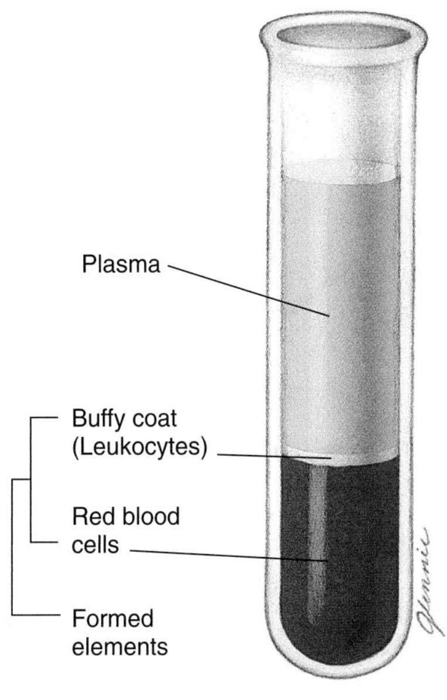

FIGURE 12-1 Hematocrit.

blood cells (WBCs), and platelets (**thrombocytes**). Table 12-1 shows the formed elements of blood. The remaining liquid portion is composed of the buffy coat and **plasma**. The buffy coat is a mixture of the WBCs and platelets.

Red Blood Cells

More than 25 trillion RBCs, also called **erythrocytes**, circulate in the body's 4 to 5 L of blood (Fig. 12-2). Erythrocytes contain a protein called hemoglobin that carries oxygen to all cells and removes carbon dioxide. Each RBC lives only 90 to 120 days. New cells are manufactured by the red marrow or myeloid tissue in bones (see Chapter 14). A few million new RBCs are made each second in a process called *hemopoiesis*. The liver and spleen remove dead RBCs and reuse the material.

TABLE 12-1
Formed Elements of Blood

Cell Type	Description	Function
Erythrocyte	Biconcave disk; no nucleus; 7-8 μm in diameter	Transports oxygen and carbon dioxide
Leukocyte		
Neutrophil	Spherical cell; nucleus with connected filaments; cytoplasmic granules stain light pink to reddish-purple; 12-15 μm in diameter	Phagocytizes microorganisms
Basophil	Spherical cell; nucleus with two indistinct lobes; cytoplasmic granules stain blue-purple; 10-12 μm in diameter	Releases histamine, which promotes inflammation, and heparin, which prevents clot formation
Eosinophil	Spherical cell; nucleus often with two lobes; cytoplasmic granules stain orange-red or bright red; 10-12 μm in diameter	Releases chemicals that reduce inflammation; attacks certain worm parasites
Lymphocyte	Spherical cell with round nucleus; cytoplasm forms a thin ring around the nucleus; 6-8 μm in diameter	Produces antibodies and other chemicals responsible for destroying microorganisms; responsible for allergic reactions, graft rejection, tumor control, and regulation of the immune system
Monocyte	Spherical cell; nucleus round, kidney, or horseshoe shaped; contains more cytoplasm than lymphocytes; 10-15 μm in diameter	Phagocytic cell in the blood leaves the blood and becomes a macrophage, which phagocytizes bacteria, dead cells, fragments, and debris within tissues
Platelet	Cell fragments surrounded by a cell membrane and containing granules; 2-5 μm in diameter	Forms platelet plugs; releases chemicals necessary to blood clotting

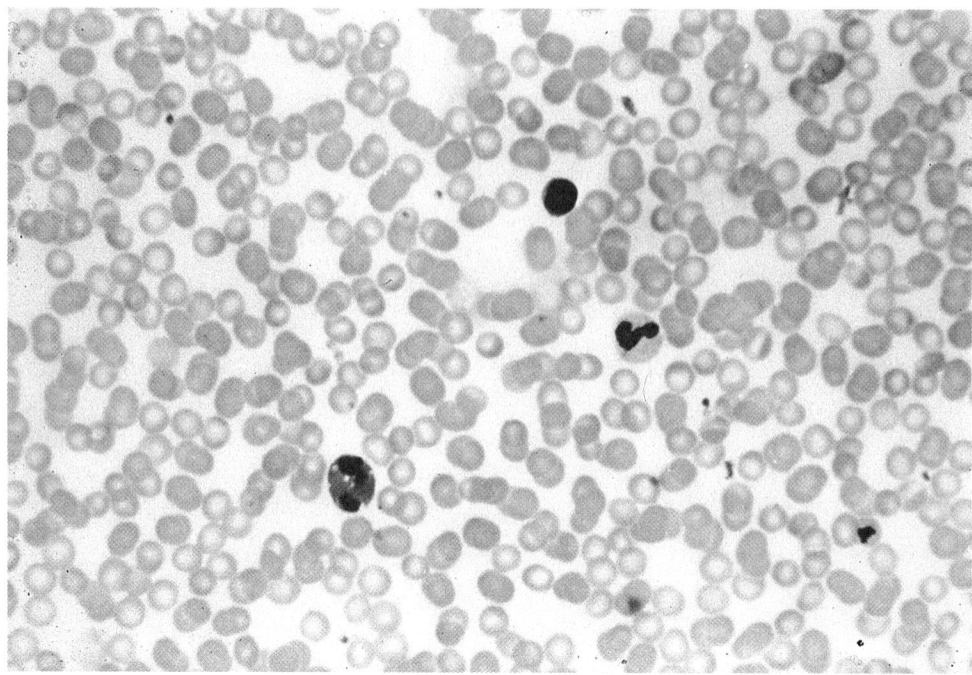

FIGURE 12-2 Erythrocytes circulating in the blood. (Courtesy Ward's Natural Science Establishment, Rochester, N.Y.)

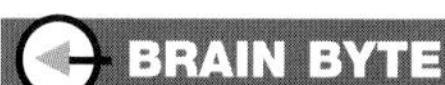

It takes 20 seconds for a red blood cell to circulate around the body.

White Blood Cells

WBCs, also called **leukocytes**, fight disease and infection. There are fewer WBCs than RBCs, and they are larger. Leukocytes live about 9 days and can move out of the blood vessels as part of the immune process. WBCs remove foreign particles, fight infection, and help prevent disease. Pus consists of WBCs mixed with bacteria.

The five types of WBCs are listed as follows (Table 12-1):

- Neutrophils (NOO-truh-filz) engulf and digest bacteria in a process called *phagocytosis.*
- Basophils (BAY-suh-filz) contain the anticoagulant substance heparin and participate in the inflammatory response of the body.
- Eosinophils (ee-uh-sin-uh-filz) defend the body from allergic reactions and parasitic infections and may help remove toxins from the blood.
- Lymphocytes (LIM-fuh-sites) participate in the production of antibody and plasma cells and help destroy foreign particles.
- Monocytes (MON-uh-sites) help remove foreign materials and bacteria in the process of phagocytosis.

Platelets

Platelets, also called *thrombocytes*, are the smallest blood cells. They promote clotting to prevent blood loss. As platelets pass over a rough spot in a vessel, they become sticky. They may form a plug to seal small vessels by themselves or start the clotting process. To form a clot, platelets combine with a protein, called *prothrombin*, and calcium to form thrombin. This mass combines with another protein called *fibrinogen* to form a gel-like substance called *fibrin*, which forms the clot. Thrombocytes are usually produced in red bone marrow and live for about 5 to 9 days.

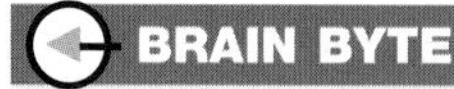

The heart pumps about 4000 gallons of blood each day.

Plasma

Plasma is a pale yellow liquid that is left when the formed elements are removed from blood. Whole blood is 55% plasma. Plasma is 90% water and approximately 10% proteins. It contains nutrients, electrolytes, oxygen, enzymes, hormones, and wastes. The proteins help fight infection and assist in the clotting (**coagulation**) of blood. **Serum** is plasma without the clotting proteins. Serum may be used for identification and research of antibodies.

TABLE 12-2
Blood Types and Blood Group Components

Group	Antigen Marker*	Antibody†	Compatible Donor
A	A	Anti-B	A, O
B	B	Anti-A	B, O
AB	A, B	None	A, B, AB, O
O	None	Anti-A, Anti-B	O

*Found on red blood cells.
†Found in plasma.

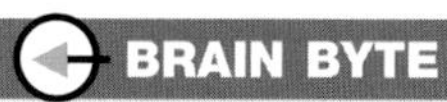

BRAIN BYTE

Each drop of blood contains five million RBCs, 10,000 WBCs, 250,000 platelets, and half a drop of plasma.

Blood Typing

A person's blood type is an inherited characteristic of the blood. Before a transfusion is given, many factors are checked to prevent an adverse reaction in the person receiving the blood. Blood type is determined by antigens located on the surface of the RBC. Clumping of the blood cells may occur when the antigens of donated blood react with antibodies in the plasma of the person receiving it. This clumping of incompatible cells blocks the blood vessels and may cause death.

The four major blood types are A, B, AB, and O (Table 12-2). Type AB blood is called the universal recipient because it has no antibodies in the plasma to react with other blood cells and can receive any type of blood safely. Type O blood is the universal donor because the blood cells have no antigens to react with the antibodies in the plasma of the other blood types. Therefore type O blood can be given safely to a person of any blood type.

CASE STUDY 12-1 A friend tells you that her biology class is going to do their own blood typing. She asks you if she could get AIDS or hepatitis from doing it. What should you say?

Answers to Case Studies are available on the Evolve website: ***http://evolve.elsevier.com/Gerdin***

Another important aspect of blood typing is the identification of the antigen known as the Rh factor. The Rh factor is found in the RBCs. About 85% of North Americans have this factor and are said to be Rh-positive (Table 12-3). If Rh-positive blood is given to someone with Rh-negative blood, that person's blood considers the Rh-positive blood a foreign particle and tries to combat it by forming antibodies. A second transfusion of Rh-positive blood can be fatal to an Rh-negative person. The Rh factor also becomes important in the Rh-negative mother having a second Rh-positive baby (Fig. 12-3).

TABLE 12-3
Approximate Distribution of Blood Types in the U.S. Population*

Blood Type	Prevalence (%)
O Rh-positive	38
O Rh-negative	7
A Rh-positive	34
A Rh-negative	6
B Rh-positive	9
B Rh-negative	2
AB Rh-positive	3
AB Rh-negative	1

Data from American Association of Blood Banks, 2002.
*Distribution may differ for specific racial and ethnic groups.

Lymph and Lymphatic Tissues

Lymph has two important functions. The first is maintaining the body's fluid balance. Lymph is a watery substance formed from fluid that filters into the body tissues or interstitially. This fluid is returned to the body through the lymph vessels, which operate independently from the circulatory vessels. Lymph capillaries are more porous than blood capillaries, allowing the fluid in the tissues to collect and be returned to the circulatory system. Fats, protein molecules, and some cancerous cells may also use this method of transportation in the body. Unlike blood, lymph flows in only one direction toward the heart. Lymph moves from the tissues into capillaries that drain into lymphatic ducts that lead into the blood. Unlike blood, lymph circulates slowly. Movement of the body muscles surrounding the lymph vessels keeps the lymph flowing.

The lymphatic tissues consist of the tonsils, thymus, spleen, nodes, and lymph vessels. The tonsils consist of three sets of lymphoid tissue: palatine, pharyngeal

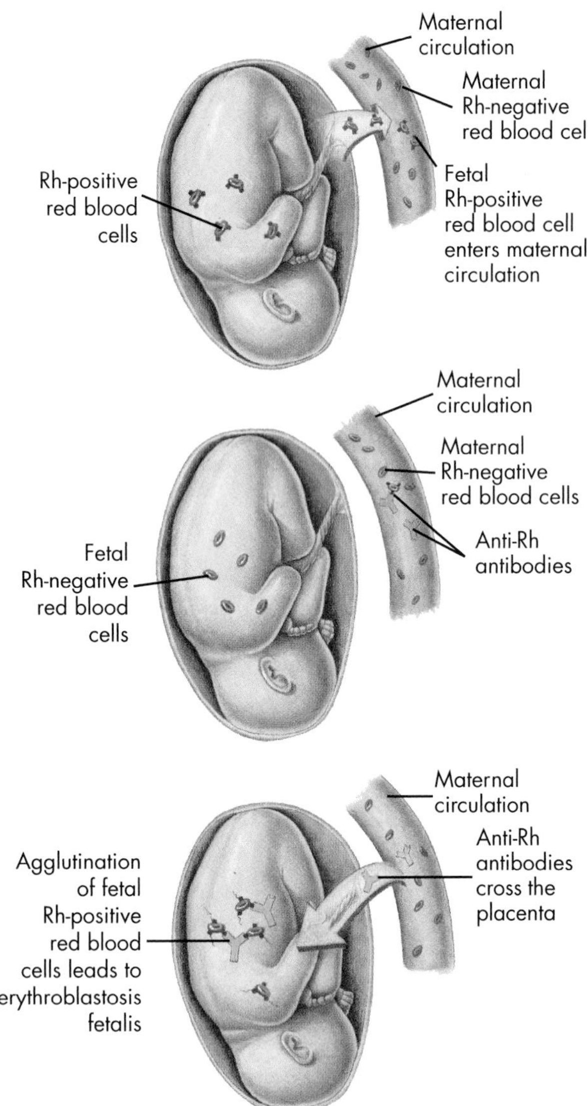

FIGURE 12-3 In erythroblastosis fetalis, an Rh- (Rh negative) mother may form antibodies against the Rh+ blood of a fetus. That infant is not harmed, but when a second Rh+ (Rh positive) fetus is formed, the mother's antibodies will attack the unborn baby's blood. (From Patton KT, Thibodeau GA: *Anatomy & physiology*, ed 7, St. Louis, 2010, Mosby.)

(adenoids), and lingual. The thymus, located in the chest, is a source of lymphocytes before birth and through puberty. At that time, this organ is gradually replaced by fat and connective tissue in a process called *involution*. The thymus is considered by some to be the "biological clock" that indicates the progress of the aging process. The thymus also has endocrine functions (see Chapter 18).

The spleen is the largest lymphoid mass in the body and an important part of the circulatory system. In addition to storing about 1 pint of blood, the spleen filters bacteria and foreign substances so that they can be destroyed by phagocytic leukocytes. The spleen also makes lymphocytes and monocytes. Worn RBCs are broken apart, and the iron is retrieved for further use by the spleen.

Lymph vessels are located in all body tissues except the brain and placenta (Fig. 12-4). Lymph nodes, located in clusters along the path of lymph vessels, are biological filters that remove bacteria and cancerous cells from the body. Nodes are small, about 0.5 to 1 cm in diameter, but they may swell during an infection as they filter bacteria and produce additional leukocytes.

Immunity

Lymph is also important in the process of immunity. The immune response takes two forms—specific and nonspecific. The nonspecific, or innate, reaction provides general protection. It includes the barrier of the skin, mucous membranes, tears, and the leukocytes. The leukocytes form antibodies in response to antigens or foreign materials that enter the body.

The inflammatory response, a type of nonspecific defense, may be a localized or systemic reaction. The usual progression of a localized response occurs following tissue damage by bacteria or infection. The response of the injured cells is the release of chemicals, which cause vascular dilation and an increase in blood flow. This vascular dilation allows other molecules to enter the area, walling off the injured tissue. The bacteria are then destroyed by phagocytic action of WBCs. The area appears reddened and is warm and painful. It often causes swelling and decreased function.

CASE STUDY 12-2 Your friend says her mother often has swelling in her arm since she had a mastectomy last year. She asks you if that could be the cancer returning. What should you say?

Answers to Case Studies are available on the Evolve website: ***http://evolve.elsevier.com/Gerdin***

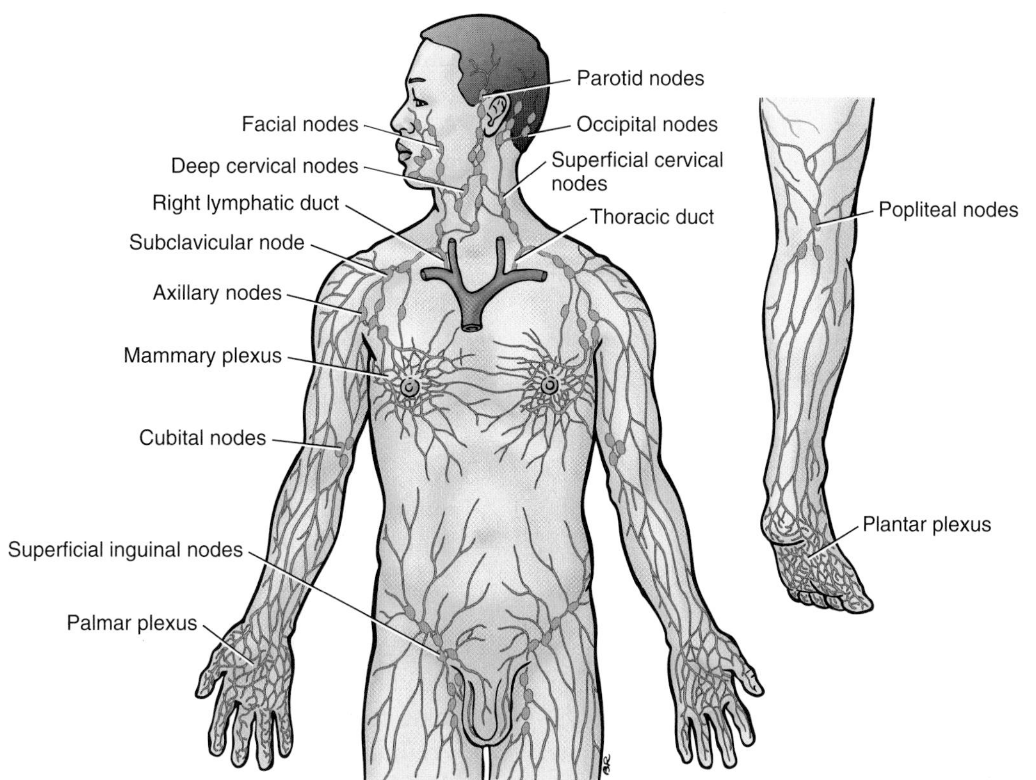

FIGURE 12-4 Lymph vessels and nodes. (From Fritz S: *Mosby's fundamentals of therapeutic massage*, ed 4, St. Louis, 2008, Mosby.)

Another nonspecific response is the systemic inflammatory response that affects the entire body. In addition to all the signs and symptoms of a localized response, it also includes an increase in neutrophil production, elevated temperature, and fluid loss into the tissues. This reaction may lead to shock and death if not stopped.

Two types of specific immunity protect the body at the cellular level. These are acquired and inherited immunity. Inherited immunity develops before birth and is a genetic trait. For example, humans are not susceptible to some diseases that affect dogs or cats.

Acquired immunity can be either natural or artificial, depending on how it is attained. Natural immunity is caused by exposure to the agent unintentionally. For example, the formation of antibodies to prevent the reoccurrence of measles is natural immunity. Immunity that is obtained by the fetus from the mother or in breast milk is an example of passive natural immunity.

Artificial acquired immunity is obtained intentionally. For example, vaccination against poliomyelitis is a form of active, artificial immunity. Injection of gamma globulin taken from one person and given to another is an example of passive artificial immunity.

An immune response resulting in tissue damage may be triggered by hypersensitivity to an antigen. Four main types of hypersensitivity exist. Type I occurs when plasma and memory cells are produced on first exposure to an **allergen**. On the second exposure, an immediate anaphylactic response occurs. A type II or cytotoxic response occurs when antibodies react with foreign or normal cells causing the destruction of cells. An example is the reaction of an incompatible blood transfusion or Rh incompatibility reaction. In type III hypersensitivity, phagocytes are released to remove antigen-**antibody** complexes that are deposited in the tissues. The by-products of the phagocytic action to remove these complexes damage the tissues. More than 12 hours after exposure to the antigen, a type IV, or delayed hypersensitivity, reaction occurs. It also results in tissue destruction as a result of both phagocytic and cytotoxic cells that are produced.

Assessment Techniques

Blood and lymph can be assessed by direct examination, chemical tests, and coagulation studies. Table 12-4 shows the normal values of some blood components. Some common tests for direct examination of the blood include the following:

- The hemoglobin test measures the amount of oxygen-carrying ability of the blood.
- The hematocrit test measures the volume of erythrocytes in the blood.
- Sedimentation rates or "sed rate" measure how long it takes for erythrocytes in the blood to settle to the bottom of a container.
- Reticulocyte studies measure the number of immature RBCs.
- RBC counts determine the number of circulating RBCs in 1 mm^3 of blood.
- Platelet or thrombocyte counts measure the number of platelets in 1 mm^3 of blood to determine clotting ability.
- Aspiration biopsy cytology studies examine bone marrow from the iliac crest of the hip.
- Serum iron, total iron-binding capacity, serum ferritin, and transferrin saturation evaluate iron metabolism.

Chemical tests use a process called **spectrophotometry** to measure the exact chemical makeup of a blood sample. Spectrophotometry calculates the concentration of substances in solution by measuring the amount of light it absorbs. Chemical tests measure proteins, glucose, uric acid, cholesterol, enzymes, and electrolyte ions. Two routine blood tests include several of these tests combined:

- Complete blood cell count (CBC) measures at least six tests including the number of RBCs and WBCs and the proportional difference between the number of RBCs and WBCs (differential).
- Sequential multiple analysis includes both the cell counts and the chemistry tests.

Two kinds of coagulation studies assess the ability of the blood to clot:

- Bleeding time is the amount of time an incision takes to clot.
- Prothrombin time uses an anticoagulant to measure the blood sample's clotting rate.

TABLE 12-4
Components of a Complete Blood Cell Count (CBC)*

Test	Name	Description
WBC	White blood cell	WBCs fight infection.
% Neutrophil	Neutrophil/band/seg/gran	Each type of WBC has a different function.
Lymphs	Lymphocyte	
% Mono	Monocyte	
% Eos	Eosinophil	
% Baso	Basophil	
Neutrophil	Neutrophil/ban/seg/gran	
Lymphs	Lymphocyte	
Mono	Monocyte	
Eos	Eosinophil	
Baso	Basophil	
RBC	Red blood cell	RBCs carry oxygen.
Hgb	Hemoglobin	Hgb is the oxygen-carrying protein in the blood.
Hct	Hematocrit	Hct indicates the proportion of RBCs to plasma in the blood.
MCV	Mean corpuscular volume	MCV is the average volume of RBCs.
MCH	Mean corpuscular hemoglobin	MCH is the average amount of Hgb per RBC.
MCHC	Mean corpuscular hemoglobin concentration	MCHC is the average amount of Hgb in cells.
RDW	RBC distribution width	RDW measures the variation in size in the RBCs.
Platelet	Platelet	Platelets help blood clotting.
MPV	Mean platelet volume	MPV measures the size of platelets.

*Reference values on factors such as patient age, gender, and test method. Different laboratories may have different numeric values for ranges.

DISORDERS OF THE Circulatory System

Acquired immunodeficiency syndrome (AIDS) is a dysfunction of the immune system caused by a virus. Since the first reported case in the United States in 1981, more than 900,000 cases of AIDS have been reported. In 2006 the Centers for Disease Control and Prevention (CDC) estimated that 1.1 million Americans may be infected with human immunodeficiency (HIV), and of that number 56,300 were diagnosed in that year. A person infected with HIV might not show any severe symptoms for up to 6 years. During this time, the person may experience fever, headache, fatigue, and enlarged lymph nodes. This condition is known as AIDS-related complex syndrome. The virus eventually uses the cell's own materials to make viral DNA, damaging the host cell. The damaged T-lymphocytes of affected WBCs allow disease to enter the body. Victims of AIDS generally die of sarcoma or protozoal pneumonia. HIV is transmitted by the exchange of body fluids such as blood and semen. No cure exists. Research is being conducted to develop a vaccine against HIV and to stop it from reproducing in the body. Treatment for HIV and opportunistic infections includes the use of antiviral and other medications. Cancers that occur are treated with radiation, chemotherapy, or injections or interferon. In 2008 a doctor in Berlin reported that a leukemia patient was cured of AIDS after receiving a bone marrow transplant. The transplanted cells had a gene mutation (delta-32 CCR5) that is resistant to HIV infection. Research is working to make naturally occurring proteins called *zinc fingers* cause this same mutation in the T cells of AIDS patients.

Allergy (AL-er-jee) is a hypersensitive response by the immune system to an outside substance. An otherwise harmless substance becomes an allergen in the body. Then antibodies are formed in the blood to combat the allergen. Common allergens include pollen, dander, feathers, and plant oils. Either a skin or blood test can be used to identify the allergen that is causing symptoms. The allergic person may experience **inflammation** of the respiratory, gastrointestinal, and integumentary systems. In severe cases the condition may be life threatening. Treatment may include desensitization to the allergen or administration of anti-inflammatory drugs.

Anemia (uh-NEE-mee-uh) is the most common blood disorder. An anemic patient's blood has an inadequate amount of hemoglobin, RBCs, or both. More than 400 types of anemia exist. Pernicious anemia involves inadequately developed RBCs. It results from poor absorption of vitamin B_{12}, which is necessary in the formation of RBCs. Iron-deficiency anemia involves an inadequate amount of hemoglobin caused by a shortage of iron. Aplastic anemia occurs when radiation, chemicals, or medications destroy bone marrow. This type of anemia is often the result of cancer treatment. Two types of hemolytic anemia include sickle cell and thalassemia (see pp. 213–214). A person with anemia may experience fatigue, shortness of breath, pallor, and rapid heart rate. The treatment of anemia may include dietary supplements or blood replacement.

Autoimmune (aw-toe-im-YOON) *diseases* are conditions in which the immune system of the body turns against itself (Table 12-5). Systemic lupus erythematosus (LOO-pus er-i-thuh-muh-TOE-sus) affects connective tissue. It may also affect the kidneys, lungs, and heart. Hashimoto disease results in destruction of the thyroid. Myasthenia gravis (my-as-THEE-nee-uh GRA-vis) affects the nerves and causes paralysis. The treatment of these disorders includes immunosuppressive drugs and steroids to relieve inflammation. Some conditions may be treated with enzymes or gene therapy.

Elephantiasis (el-uh-fun-TIE-uh-sis), a form of lymphedema, is a massive accumulation of lymphatic fluid in body tissues causing an abnormally large growth of tissue or hypertrophy (hy-PER-tro-fee). Elephantiasis is caused by obstruction of the lymph vessels by tiny worms (*filariae*) that are common in tropic and subtropic areas (Fig. 12-5). The larvae of

TABLE 12-5
Autoimmune or Autoimmune-Related Disorders

Disorder	Body System Affected
Addison disease	Endocrine
Dermatomyositis	Integumentary and muscular
Diabetes mellitus	Endocrine
Graves disease	Endocrine
Hashimoto thyroiditis	Endocrine
Multiple sclerosis	Nervous and muscular
Myasthenia gravis	Nervous and muscular
Pernicious anemia	Circulatory
Rheumatoid arthritis	Muscular and skeletal
Systemic lupus erythematosus	Multiple systems

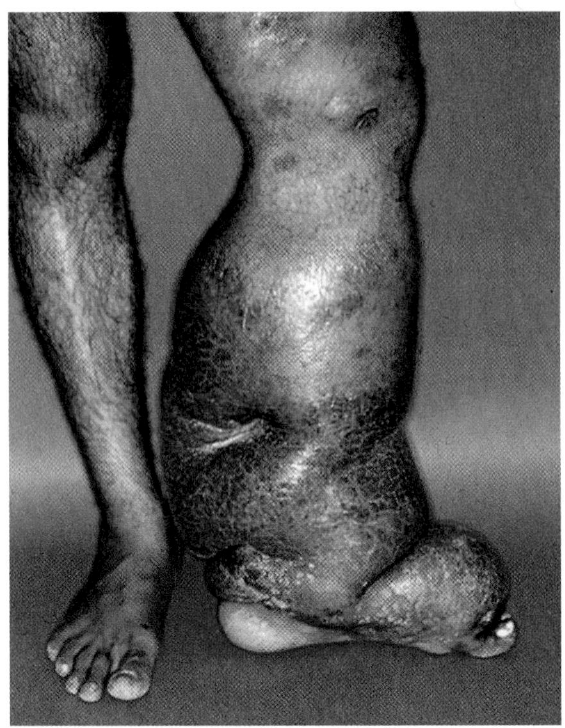

FIGURE 12-5 Swelling from *Filaria* worms in elephantiasis may require surgery to remove the extra tissue. (From Patton KT, Thibodeau GA: *Anatomy & physiology*, ed 7, St. Louis, 2010, Mosby.)

the worms enter the lymph system through an insect bite such as a mosquito. Early on, the infected person experiences fever, chills, and ulcer formation. Individuals with elephantiasis are more susceptible to infections. No cure is known for this condition. Control of carrier mosquitoes can prevent exposure. If necessary, medication can be taken to prevent the condition. Treatment includes the use of medication that kills the worms. Surgery may also be used to remove excess tissue and dead worms.

Erythroblastosis fetalis (e-rith-ro-blas-TOE-sis fuh-TAL-is) is a condition in an unborn infant in which the mother forms antibodies against the antigens in the baby's blood. This condition may result in an Rh-positive child of an Rh-negative mother and Rh-positive father or the mother and infant have different blood types. The condition may cause brain damage in the infant. Treatment includes monitoring of bilirubin levels during pregnancy and intrauterine blood transfusion if necessary (see Fig. 12-3). An exchange transfusion of blood may be required at the time of birth.

Hemophilia (hee-mo-FIL-ee-uh) is a rare sex-linked genetic blood disease in which the blood is missing a clotting factor. The person with hemophilia may have uncontrolled and prolonged internal and external bleeding. Bleeding under the skin may appear as extensive bruising. Two different clotting factors may be missing, resulting in hemophilia. Hemophilia appears in two forms. Hemophilia A is the classic and most common form. Hemophilia B is also called *Christmas disease*. According to Medscape, approximately 1 of every 5000 males born in the United States have hemophilia A. Treatment includes giving plasma that contains the missing clotting factor. No cure is known for this condition. Experimental gene therapy has been tested at Boston's Beth Israel Deaconess Medical Center, where researchers inserted the missing normal genes into skin cell samples of hemophiliacs. The cells were then reinjected into the fatty tissue of the abdomen with a modest increase in the production of blood-clotting proteins.

Hepatitis (hep-uh-TIE-tis) is a viral infection of the blood (Table 12-6). Two forms, hepatitis B (HBV) and hepatitis C virus (HCV), can be transmitted through body fluids including blood. Hepatitis A is transmitted when an object or food contaminated with infected feces enters another person's mouth. About 5% to 6% of Americans have hepatitis. Vaccines are available to prevent hepatitis A and B. According to the CDC there were 17,000 new cases of HCV in 2007, with 3.2 million people living with chronic cases. The official number is believed to be much higher because most people do not have symptoms. More than one method of treatment for HCV exists and may include α-interferon and ribavirin. The World Health Organization estimates that 3% of the world's population is infected with HCV. The CDC reports 12,000 deaths associated with viral hepatitis each year in the United States. Blood donations are routinely tested for hepatitis.

CASE STUDY 12-3 Your friend is training for a sports competition and asks you if you think blood doping will help. What should you say?

Answers to Case Studies are available on the Evolve website: ***http://evolve.elsevier.com/Gerdin***

Hodgkin (HODJ-kin) *disease* is a malignant cancer of the lymph system that usually appears in people between the ages of 15 and 30. The person with Hodgkin disease experiences a painless enlargement

TABLE 12-6
Hepatitis*

Type	Transmission	Symptoms	Prevention and Treatment
A	Ingestion of feces, contaminated object, food, or water	Flulike symptoms, jaundice	Vaccine available; immunoglobulin on exposure, bed rest
B	Direct blood contact with infected body fluids or contaminated objects such as needles. Neonates can be infected during birth.	Flulike symptoms, cirrhosis and cancer of the liver, jaundice	Vaccine available; interferon reduces chance of recurrence
C	Direct blood contact with infected body fluids or contaminated objects such as needles. Neonates may be infected during birth.	Chronic liver damage, cirrhosis and cancer of the liver; most people have no symptoms	No vaccine; interferon, ribavirin
D	Direct blood contact with infected body fluids or contaminated objects such as needles. Neonates may be infected during birth.	Flulike symptoms, cirrhosis and cancer of the liver, jaundice; more severe than hepatitis B	Hepatitis B vaccine; interferon
E	Ingestion of feces or contaminated water	Liver inflammation, flulike symptoms; many people have no symptoms	No vaccine; bed rest, fluids

*More information about hepatitis infections may be found in Chapter 16.

of the lymph nodes (lymphoma) along with itching, weight loss, fever, anemia, and difficulty swallowing. Hodgkin disease appears most often in men and is one of the most curable cancers. Treatment may include chemotherapy, radiation of the lymph nodes, or bone marrow transplant.

Leukemia (loo-KEE-mee-uh), also called blood cancer, is an abnormal malignant increase in the number and longevity of WBCs. The leukemia cells, which are immature and less effective in fighting disease, replace RBCs. Leukemia may be chronic or acute. In chronic leukemia the abnormal blood cells function until their number is large. Acute leukemia quickly gets worse. The person experiences anemia and bleeding gums, and the condition is often life threatening. Treatment may include radiation, chemotherapy, immunotherapy, or bone marrow transplantation. The patient with leukemia may also be isolated from others to prevent infection.

Non-Hodgkin's lymphoma (lim-FO-muh) is a group of malignant cancers of lymph tissues other than Hodgkin disease. Lymphoma may develop at any age but commonly appears in middle age. The affected person has a painless enlargement of the lymph nodes. The disease spreads to the bone marrow and causes anemia, weight loss, night sweats, skin itching, and red patches. The treatment of lymphoma may include chemotherapy and radiation.

Polycythemia vera (pol-ee-sie-THEE-mee-uh VEH-ruh), or myeloproliferative disorder, is an abnormal increase in the number of RBCs, making the blood thicker and slower flowing. The amount of WBCs and platelets may also increase. The person with polycythemia experiences increased blood pressure, dizziness, an enlarged spleen, and reddened skin. Polycythemia results from excessive development of the bone marrow, but the cause is unknown. It has no cure, but treatment may include removing blood or therapy to slow the production of blood cells. Anagrelide (Agrylin), an orphan drug, has been approved by FDA to control platelet level. It is effective in more than 90% of patients.

Septicemia (sep-tih-SEE-mee-uh), commonly called *blood poisoning*, is an infection that occurs when pathogens enter the blood. The infected person experiences nausea, vomiting, fever, chills, shortness of breath, and an increased leukocyte count. Treatment includes antibiotics, oxygen therapy, and plasma transfusion. Septicemia can lead to shock and death.

Sickle cell (SIK-el sel) *anemia* is a genetic condition that results in misshapen RBCs. The "sickled" cells are more fragile and cause pain as the vessels are blocked and less oxygen is delivered. Sickle cell anemia occurs in 1 of every 400 births of African Americans. The condition may result in no symptoms when only one gene (allele) is affected. The gene is found in one of every 600 African Americans and in one of every 1000 Hispanics. Sickle cell anemia can lead to death in severe cases. Treatment of sickle cell anemia may include antibiotics to prevent infection and other actions to maintain good health. Pain relievers and a prescription drug (hydroxyurea) may be used in severe cases. No cure for sickle cell anemia is known, but bone marrow transplant has been used with some success. Gene research may also lead to therapy to alter or block the defective gene.

Splenomegaly (splee-no-MEG-uh-lee) is an enlargement of the spleen caused by an acute infection such as mononucleosis or anemia. Some liver diseases and cancers may also cause it. The person with splenomegaly may experience no symptoms or those similar to anemia and leukemia. Treatment may require removal of the spleen (splenectomy).

CASE STUDY 12-4 Your friend tells you that his mother may have her spleen removed after a car accident. He asks you if that is very serious. What should you say?

Answers to Case Studies are available on the Evolve website: ***http://evolve.elsevier.com/Gerdin***

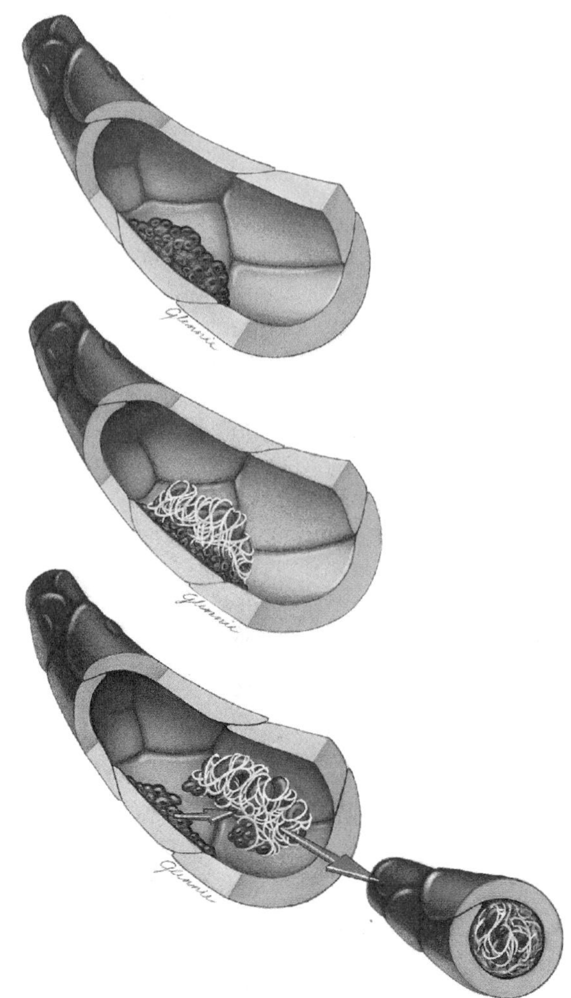

FIGURE 12-6 Development of an embolus.

Thalassemia (thal-ah-SEE-mee-uh) is one of the most common genetic blood disorders. It appears in two forms, called *alpha* and *beta*, which are identified by which gene is involved. Thalassemia affects the production of hemoglobin and may cause anemia. β thalassemia occurs most often in people of Mediterranean origin. In the most severe form, it is called *thalassemia* major or *Cooley anemia*. At age 1 or 2 years, a child with this form may experience listlessness, poor appetite, and infections. The condition leads to yellow skin (jaundice), enlarged spleen, and cardiac malfunction. Treatment includes blood transfusions to lessen the effects. New treatments include medication that affects RBC production. Gene manipulation and bone marrow transplants are also treatments.

Thrombocytopenia (throm-bo-sie-toe-PEE-nee-uh) is a decrease in the number of platelets in the blood. This condition can be caused by a drug reaction, radiation, chemotherapy, or an autoimmune disorder. The person with thrombocytopenia experiences symptoms similar to those of leukemia: skin rash, nosebleed, bleeding, and bruising. Treatment method chosen depends on the original cause of the platelet decrease.

Thrombosis (throm-BO-sis) is a condition in which a blood clot, called a *thrombus*, forms in the blood vessel (Fig. 12-6). The clot slows the flow of blood to the tissues. A deep vein thrombosis (DVT) is one that forms in veins that are deep in the body and usually occur in the lower leg or thigh. If the clot breaks away, it is called an *embolus*. Clots formed by DVT are more likely to form an embolus than those closer to the surface. The embolus may lodge in a blood vessel and cause tissue death in the area (Fig. 12-7). The person with thrombosis feels pain in the area of the clot because of a lack of oxygen in the tissues. Treatment includes elevation of the affected part and may include anticoagulants. In severe cases surgery may be necessary to remove the clot.

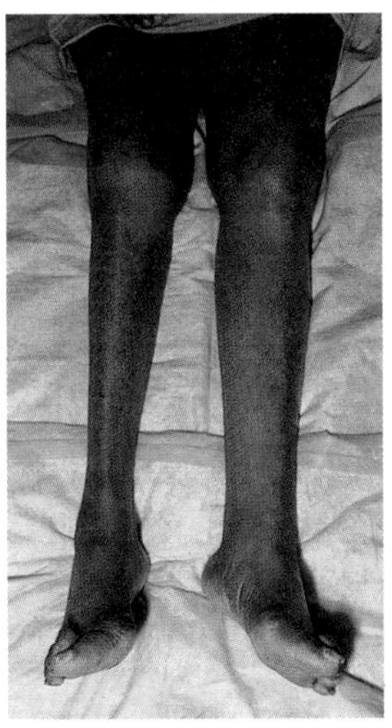

A

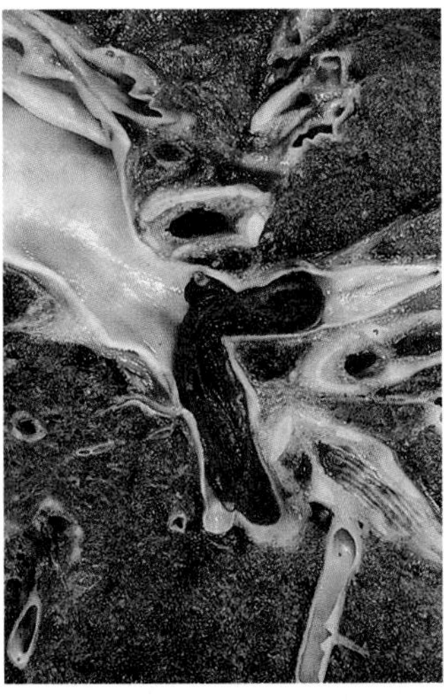

B

FIGURE 12-7 **A,** Deep vein thrombosis (DVT) causes swelling of the leg. **B,** An embolus from a DVT blocks blood flow in the pulmonary artery. (From Patton KT, Thibodeau GA: *Anatomy & physiology*, ed 7, St. Louis, 2010, Mosby.)

Issues and Innovations

Transfusion

According to the National Blood Data Resource Center, hospitals in the United States transfused 14.65 million units of whole blood and RBCs in 2006. Transfusions are given to improve the blood's ability to carry oxygen to the cells, increase blood volume, improve immunity, and correct clotting problems. New methods of transfusion have been developed to minimize the risk of this procedure. These methods, as well as improved methods for testing blood transfusions, have reduced the risk of an adverse reaction or infection by a blood-borne organism. As a result of blood screening and heat treatment, the risk of contracting HIV from a blood transfusion is small. Some facilities offer a service called *direct donation*. In this procedure, blood is donated to a specific person from family and friends. The FDA regulates the testing of the blood supply.

Autologous transfusion is the collection and transfusion of a person's own blood. For example, up to one unit of blood may be given each week for 6 weeks before an elective surgery is planned. Whole blood can be refrigerated safely for up to 35 days or frozen for several months before use. Hemodilution, or blood dilution, is the removal of one or more units just before surgery for transfusion at the end of surgery. Fluids are given to the person to dilute the remaining blood.

When a person is bleeding after an accident, his or her own blood may be collected and returned to the person in a process called *intraoperative salvage*. Autotransfusion prevents complications of blood transfusion such as mismatched blood types, the risk of disease transmission, and tissue rejection. PolyHeme, a temporary blood substitute, has been used in trauma and surgical settings on a trial basis and other oxygen therapeutics are under development.

Platelets can be donated through a process called *apheresis* to be used for patients undergoing bone marrow transplant, surgery, chemotherapy, radiation treatment, or organ transplant. Platelets have a 5-day storage life. Before apheresis, platelets for one transfusion required donations from 5 to 10 people. In apheresis the donated blood is separated into parts by using a centrifuge. The platelets are recovered separately, and the rest of the blood is returned to the donor. With this technique, a single donation provides a complete platelet transfusion.

Interferon

Interferon is a protein that prevents a virus from reproducing. It is made in the body by T-lymphocyte cells (WBCs). Synthetic interferon is now being manufactured by using gene-splicing techniques with bacteria. It is being used to fight viruses and some cancers. Interferon is being tested in prevention of many viral diseases, including AIDS and the common cold. It has also been used to treat leprosy and malaria. Interferon can also be used to diagnose tumors and hepatitis.

Interferon consists of three versions: alpha (α), beta (β), and gamma (γ). α-interferon is used to treat hairy cell leukemia, malignant melanoma, and Kaposi sarcoma, and β-interferon is used to treat relapsing multiple sclerosis and genital warts. γ-interferon is used to treat infections, including two rare conditions called *chronic granulomatosis* and *osteopetrosis*. The cause of granulomatosis is not known. It affects the lungs and bones. Osteopetrosis is an autosomal genetic bone disorder in which the bones are too dense. It is usually discovered within the first year of life. Initial symptoms include vision problems, anemia, and recurrent infection.

Monoclonal Antibodies

Monoclonal antibodies are proteins with unique abilities in the blood. Specific antibodies can be "harvested" and fused to new cells in laboratory tissue cultures. These "hybridomas" can be used to treat some cancers and some specific viruses. Monoclonal antibodies are being used in organ transplants to prevent rejection; slow the progress of autoimmune diseases; and help diagnose malignant tumors, leukemia, and some sexually transmitted infections. Monoclonal antibodies have also been used to treat breast cancer and lymphomas. Monoclonal antibodies are found in some over-the-counter products to test for pregnancy, ovulation, and blood in the stool. Research is now beginning to find other uses of these proteins for circulatory system disorders.

Entry Inhibitors

People infected with HIV have been able to live longer and healthier lives because of medications. Entry inhibitors, also called fusion inhibitors, include drugs that locate and attach to the virus before it enters the T cells that are affected by it. This type of entry inhibitor prevents infection from occurring and is called a *fusion inhibitor*. The first entry inhibitor, Fuzeon, was approved by the FDA in 2003.

Summary

- Two functions of the circulatory system are to maintain homeostasis and give the body immunity.
- Functions of the blood are to transport nutrients, gases, hormones, and wastes. It also functions to provide immunity, maintain body temperature and electrolyte balance, and prevent blood loss by clotting.
- The function of lymph is to maintain fluid balance and provide immunity.
- Methods used to assess the circulatory system include blood surveys such as hemoglobin, hematocrit, and sedimentation rates. Bone marrow may also be examined by using an aspiration biopsy.
- Disorders of the circulatory system include allergies, anemia, elephantiasis, hemophilia, and hepatitis.

Review Questions

1. Describe the two functions of the circulatory system.
2. Describe the five functions of the blood.
3. Describe the role of lymph in the circulatory system.
4. Describe the function of each of the WBCs.
5. Describe three tests used to assess the function of the circulatory system.
6. Describe two types of autotransfusion. List three benefits of autotransfusion.
7. Use the following terms in one or more sentences that correctly relate their meaning: allergen, antibody, immunity, and inflammation.

Critical Thinking

1. A test to detect HIV was introduced in blood banks in 1985. The first hepatitis C test was not used until 1990. Hepatitis C has infected four times as many people as HIV. Describe a plan that would not cause panic or discrimination against victims but could inform the public about the risks of contracting or not treating hepatitis C.
2. Investigate and compare the cost of at least four tests used in diagnosing circulatory system disorders.
3. Investigate the function of at least five medications used in treatment of circulatory system disorders.
4. List at least five occupations involved in the health care of circulatory system disorders.
5. Use the Internet to investigate the Orphan Drug Act and approval, use, and cost of orphan drugs such as anagrelide.
6. Use the Internet to investigate the use of blood substitutes.
7. Use the Internet to investigate gene therapy designed to replace defective sickle cell genes.
8. Use the Internet to investigate AIDS survival, including the number of people living with AIDS, current treatments, and research such as the use of zinc fingers to inhibit or stop HIV infection.

Explore the Web

HIV and AIDS

AIDS.gov
http://AIDS.gov
Search Key Terms: AIDS, cure, zinc fingers

Orphan Drugs

FDA

http://www.fda.gov/forindustry/developingproductsforrarediseasesconditions/overview/ucm119477.htm

National Institutes of Health

http://gateway.nlm.nih.gov/MeetingAbstracts/ma?f=102211500.html

About.com

http://biotech.about.com/od/faq/f/orphandrugs.htm

Sickle Cell

National Institutes of Health

http://www.nhlbi.nih.gov/new/press/01-12-13.htm

Sickle Cell Information Center

http://www.scinfo.org/bonemarr.htm

WebMD

http://www.webmd.com/cancer/news/20071206/stem-cells-ease-sickle-cell-anemia

CHAPTER 13

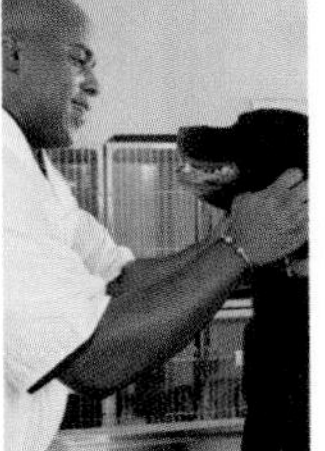
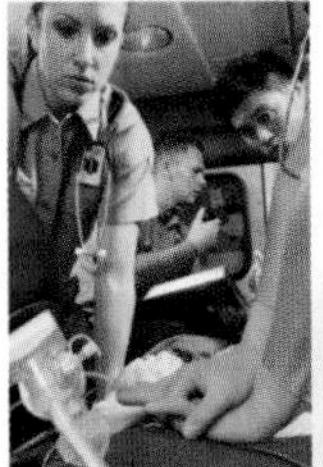
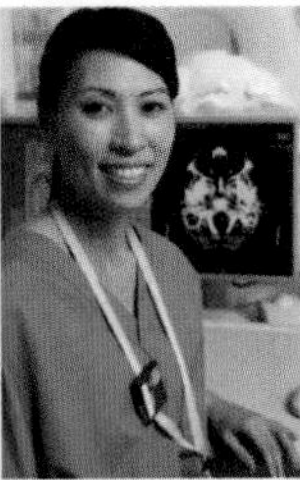

Respiratory System

LEARNING OBJECTIVES

- Define at least 10 terms referring to the respiratory system.
- Describe the three functions of the respiratory system.
- Identify at least 10 respiratory system structures and the function of each.
- Describe at least three methods of assessment of the respiratory system.
- Describe at least five disorders of the respiratory system.

KEY TERMS

Apnea *(AP-nee-uh)* Cessation of breathing

Bradypnea *(brayd-IP-nee-uh)* Abnormally slow rate of breathing

Chronic *(KRON-ik)* Persisting over a long period of time

Cilia *(SIL-ee-uh)* Hairlike projections from the surface of a cell

Dysphagia *(dis-FAY-jee-uh)* Difficulty swallowing

Dyspnea *(DISP-nee-uh)* Difficult or labored breathing

Eupnea *(YOOP-nee-uh)* Easy or normal breathing

Expiration *(ek-spih-RAY-shun)* Act of breathing out, exhalation

Inspiration *(in-spih-RAY-shun)* Act of drawing air into the lung, inhalation

Mediastinum *(mee-dee-uh-STI-num)* Thoracic space between the two lungs

Phlegm *(flem)* Thick mucus secreted by the tissues in the respiratory passages and usually discharged through the mouth

Pulmonary *(PUL-mo-nayr-ee)* Pertaining to the lungs

Respiration *(res-pih-RAY-shun)* Exchange of oxygen and carbon dioxide between the atmosphere and the cells of the body, also called ventilation

Tachypnea *(tak-IP-nee-ah)* Excessively fast respiration

Respiratory System Terminology*

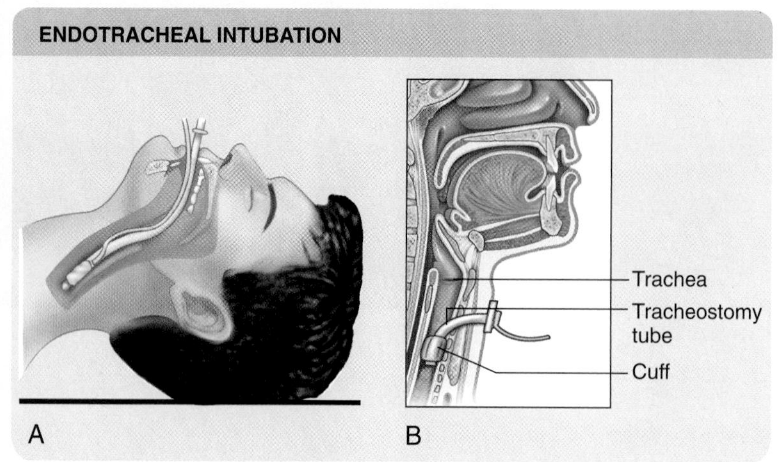

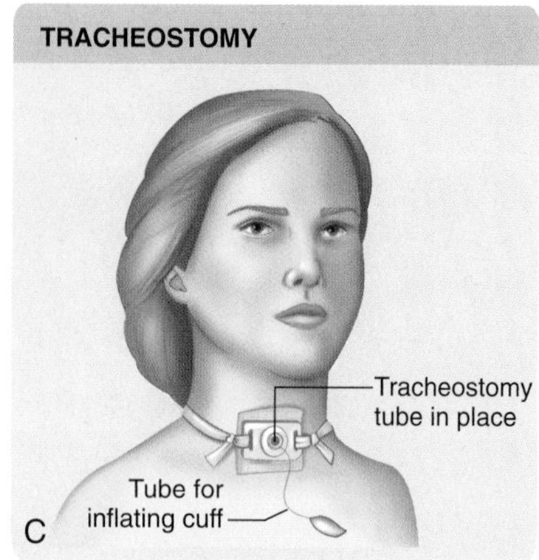

A tracheotomy and endotracheal tube may be used to temporarily open the airway, but a tracheostomy may be more permanent. (From Patton KT, Thibodeau GA: *Anatomy & physiology*, ed 7, St. Louis, 2010, Mosby.)

Term	Definition	Prefix	Root	Suffix
Apnea	Without breathing	a	pnea	
Bronchitis	Inflammation of the bronchus		bronch	itis
Dysphagia	Difficulty swallowing	dys	phag	ia
Eupnea	Normal breathing	eu	pnea	
Laryngitis	Inflammation of the voice box (larynx)		laryng	itis
Pleuritis	Inflammation of the lining of the lung		pleur	itis
Pneumonectomy	Removal of the lung		pneumon	ectomy
Tachypnea	Fast respiration	tachy	pnea	
Tonsillitis	Inflammation of the tonsils		tonsill	itis
Tracheotomy	Incision into the windpipe (trachea)		trache	otomy

*A transition syllable or vowel may be added to or deleted from the word parts to make the combining form.

Abbreviations of the Respiratory System

Abbreviation	Meaning
ABG	Arterial blood gases
BS	Breath sounds
CF	Cystic fibrosis
CO_2	Carbon dioxide
COPD	Chronic obstructive pulmonary disease
ENT	Ears, nose, and throat
TB	Tuberculosis
TCDB	Turn, cough, deep breath
Trach	Tracheotomy
URI	Upper respiratory infection

Structure and Function of the Respiratory System

The respiratory system brings oxygen into the body through the breathing process. With **inspiration**, or inhaling air, oxygen is brought into the lungs. With **expiration**, or exhalation, carbon dioxide is removed from the lungs.

The respiratory system functions in three ways:

- It exchanges gases between the blood and the lungs.
- It helps regulate body temperature by cooling or warming the blood.
- It helps maintain the blood's electrolyte balance.

TABLE 13-1
Breathing Reflex Actions

Reflex	Cause	Action
Cough	Irritation to the trachea or bronchi	Epiglottis and glottis close, muscles raise pressure in lungs, and then they open, releasing a burst of air to remove foreign matter
Diving	Submersion in cold water	Heart and breathing rate slow, blood diverted to the brain, heart, and lungs until breathing resumes
Gasp	Sudden sensation (cold, surprise, pain, sleep apnea)	Deep inhalation of air through mouth
Hiccup	Cause unknown, lack of sleep, overeating or drinking, stress, chronic hiccups may indicate tumor or laryngitis	Rib muscles and diaphragm contract, causing rapid inhalation
Sneeze	Irritation of nasal passages, respiratory illness, allergy, can be exposure to bright light (genetic)	Eyes and nasal passages secrete fluid, diaphragm causes large breath to be inhaled, followed by contraction of chest muscles to push air out of nose and mouth
Sniff	Identify smell, nasal congestion	Small audible inhalations with little exhalation
Yawn	Bored, tired, stress (hypotheses include low oxygen content in blood, regulation of brain temperature, muscle stretching)	Mouth opens wide to take in deep breath; air is released after lungs are expanded to capacity

There are three processes of **respiration**:

- External respiration, or ventilation, brings oxygen into the lungs.
- Internal respiration exchanges oxygen and carbon dioxide between blood and body cells.
- Cellular respiration changes acid produced during metabolism into harmless chemicals in the cells.

Both the voluntary and involuntary nervous systems control respiration. The body chemically regulates the rate (how fast the breaths are) and depth (how deep they are). If the concentration of gases in the blood changes, the brain adjusts respiratory rate and depth to counteract the changes to maintain homeostasis (Table 13-1).

Air enters the respiratory system (Fig. 13-1) through the nose (nasal cavity). The nasal cavity is lined with hairs called **cilia** to help filter out any foreign particles.

BRAIN BYTE

Nostrils take turns breathing. This can be demonstrated by breathing onto a mirror and observing the size of the condensation.

It also helps to warm and moisten the air. Air also enters through the mouth (oral cavity), when the nasal cavity is blocked. The tonsils and adenoids at the back of the throat help the body resist infection.

The sinuses are hollow spaces in the bones of the skull that open into the nasal cavity. Sinuses help regulate the temperature of air before it reaches the sensitive lungs. They also humidify and filter the air. The spaces act as chambers for vibration of the air producing "vocal resonance" or the sound quality of the voice.

The air from the nose or mouth is then funneled through the throat (pharynx) and into the windpipe (trachea). The pharynx is divided into three portions: nasopharynx (nose), oropharynx (mouth), and laryngopharynx (larynx).

The trachea or windpipe is lined with rigid cartilage to keep the passageway open. Sometimes an opening is made into the trachea as an alternative method for the exchange of gases (tracheotomy).

The voice box (larynx) is located below the pharynx. Voice sounds are made when air moves through it. A flap of tissue called the *epiglottis* covers the voice box or larynx during swallowing to prevent food and liquid from entering the bronchi and lungs. The pharynx also contains the opening for tubes through which air reaches the middle ear to adjust for pressure changes (eustachian tubes).

The trachea branches into two tubes called *bronchi*. Each bronchus enters one of the lungs and then

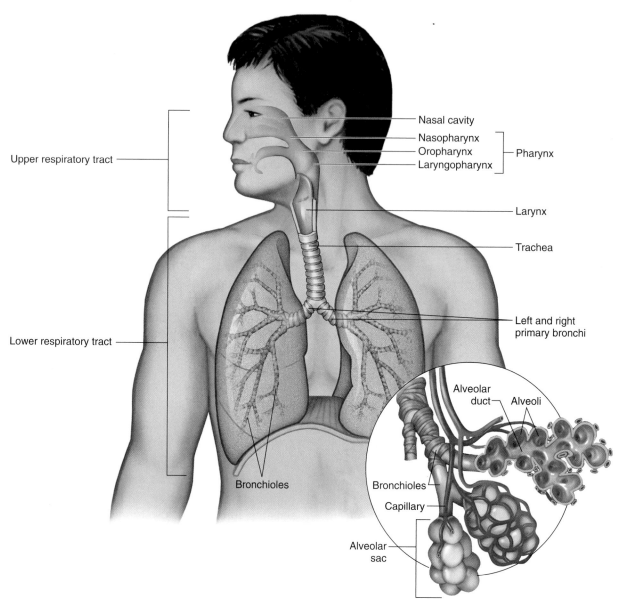

FIGURE 13-1 Structure of the respiratory system. (From Patton KT, Thibodeau GA: *Anatomy & physiology*, ed 7, St. Louis, 2010, Mosby.)

branches into smaller tubes called bronchioles. The bronchi and bronchioles are lined with tiny hairs called cilia and sticky mucus called **phlegm** to catch dust and germs. The respiratory system produces approximately 125 mL of mucus each day, which is removed by the movement of the cilia.

The bronchioles have small sacs at their ends called *alveoli*. Capillaries in the walls of the alveoli exchange oxygen and carbon dioxide by the process of diffusion. Each alveolus is lined with a liquid called surfactant through which the diffusion occurs.

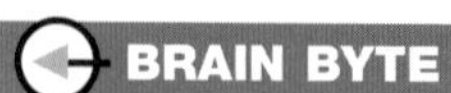

The lungs contain about 1500 miles of airways and over 300 million alveoli.

The large number of alveoli, nerves, lymph tissues, and capillaries give the lungs a spongelike texture. The lungs are divided into sections called *lobes*. The right lung has three lobes, and the left lung has two lobes. The space separating the lungs (**mediastinum**) contains the esophagus, heart, and bronchi.

Each lung is surrounded by a double membrane called *pleura*. The pleurae separate and lubricate the delicate lung tissues. The pleurae are slippery, allowing a gliding motion of the lungs during respiration. The ribs support and protect the chest cavity (thorax).

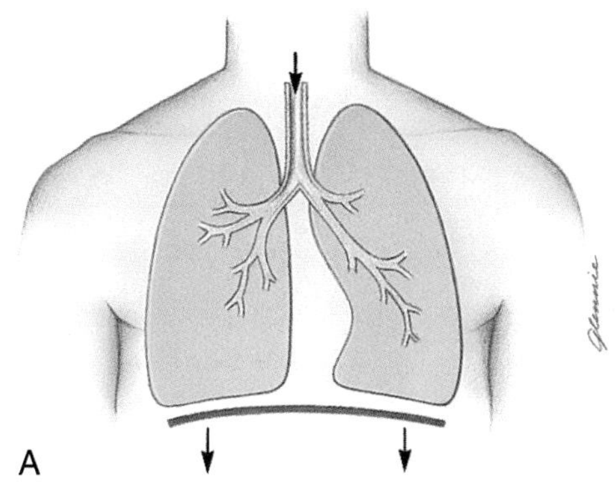

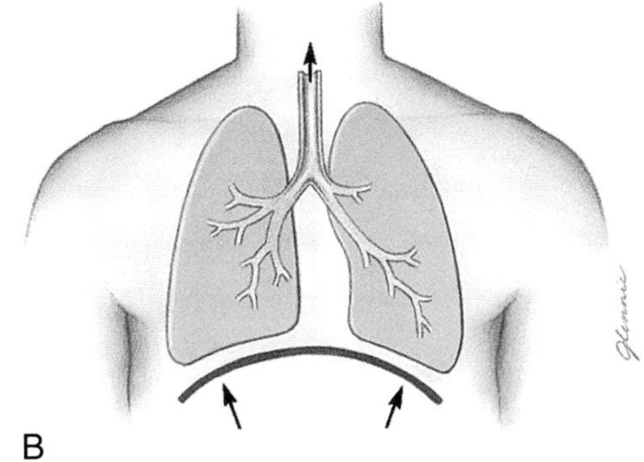

FIGURE 13-2 The mechanics of breathing. **A,** The diaphragm contracts to pull air into the lungs. **B,** As the diaphragm relaxes, the air is released.

During breathing, muscles lift and separate the ribs to help the lungs expand.

The diaphragm is a large, flat muscle that separates the thoracic cavity from the abdominal cavity. The diaphragm contracts and moves downward during inhalation. This creates suction, and air is pulled in from outside the body. Exhalation occurs when the diaphragm relaxes (Fig. 13-2).

Assessment Techniques

Different indicators of respiratory function can be assessed. These include the respiration rate, character, sounds, lung volume, and blood gases.

Rate

The normal rate of respiration varies with age, gender, posture, exercise, temperature, and other factors. Children breathe more than 20 times per minute, adults breathe 16 to 20 times per minute, and older adults often breathe fewer than 16 times per minute. Normal respiration is called **eupnea**. Painful or difficult respiration is **dyspnea**. **Tachypnea** is an abnormal respiratory rate greater than 24 per minute, and **bradypnea** is fewer than 10 per minute.

Character

Respirations should have a regular rhythm, occurring at regular intervals. Irregular rhythms of respirations may occur in different patterns, such as a rapid series followed by a pause or by no respiration, called **apnea**. Respirations may also be dry, which is normal, or wet. They can also be characterized as deep or shallow.

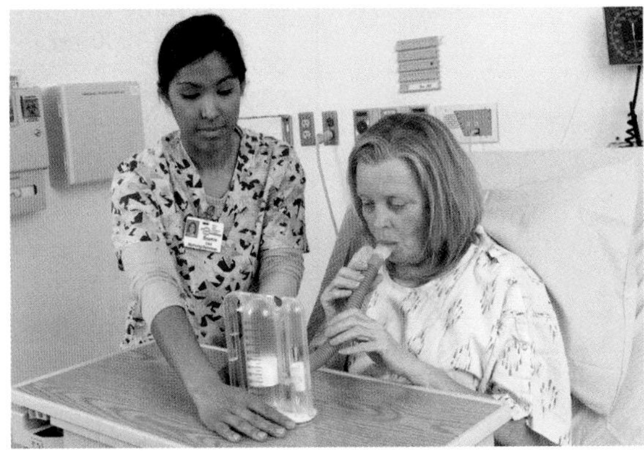

FIGURE 13-3 An incentive spirometer encourages the patient to breath deeply and measures the amount of air inhaled. (From Sorrentino SA: *Mosby's textbook for nursing assistants*, ed 7, St. Louis, 2008, Mosby.)

Sounds

Breath sounds can be heard by using a stethoscope. The quality of the sound varies with the location of the stethoscope over the bronchial tree but should be dry and clear. Wheezing or other abnormal or misplaced (adventitious) sounds in the upper respiratory tract may indicate an abnormal condition.

Lung Volume

The amount of air that can be brought into the lungs is called *respiratory capacity*. It is measured using a spirometer (Fig. 13-3). Lung capacity depends on age and physical condition. The measurement of respiratory capacity is called *lung volume* (Fig. 13-4). The vital capacity includes the tidal volume, inspiratory reserve, and expiratory reserve.

The tidal volume is the amount of air normally exchanged with each cycle of inspiration and expira-

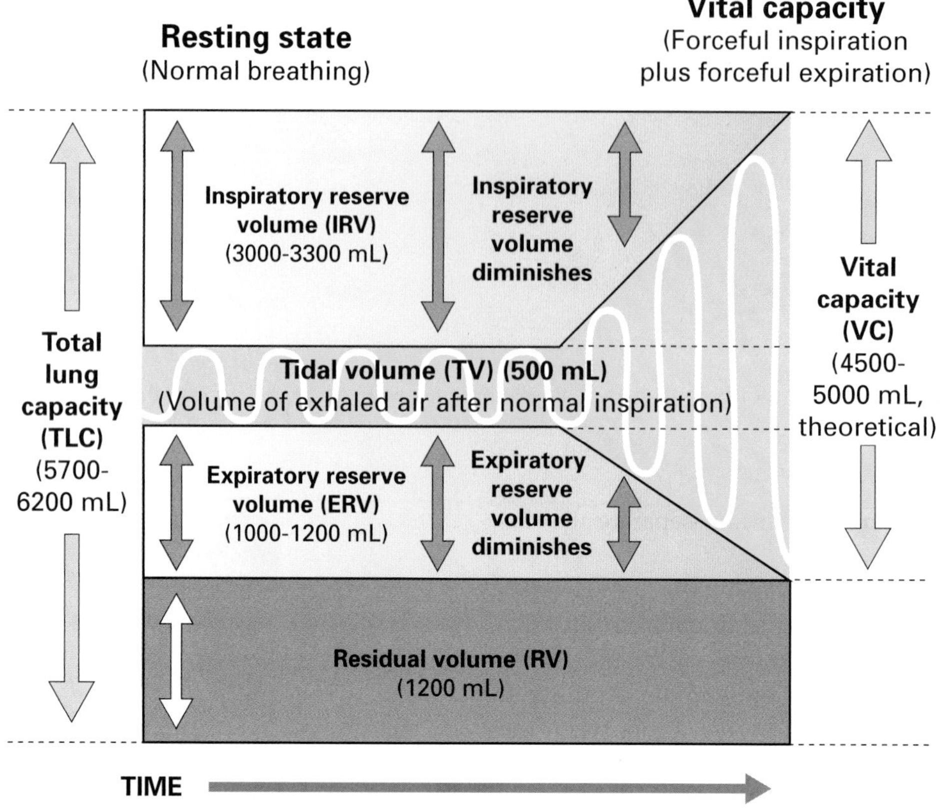

FIGURE 13-4 Respiratory capacity.

tion. Inspiratory reserve is an additional amount of air that can be inhaled with conscious effort. Expiratory reserve is the additional amount of air that a person can exhale beyond the normal amount with conscious effort.

The sum of these three values is called the *vital capacity*. This is the total amount of air that can be exchanged by that person. A certain amount of air is always in the lungs to maintain their shape. This is called the *residual volume*.

Blood Gases

Blood gas studies measure the amount of gases such as oxygen (O_2) and carbon dioxide (CO_2) in the blood and the blood's pH. These tests provide an accurate assessment of respiratory function (Table 13-2).

DISORDERS OF THE Respiratory System

Anthrax (AN-thraks) occurs naturally and is caused by spores of the bacteria *Bacillus anthracis*. The spores may be present in the soil for years and occasionally infect grazing animals. In humans, anthrax may appear as an infection of the skin, digestive system, or respiratory system. Inhalation anthrax has a death rate of more than 80%. In 2001 anthrax spores were sent through the U.S. postal system as a type of biological terrorism, which resulted in the death of five people. A vaccine for anthrax has been developed and is available to special military units and researchers. After exposure, early treatment with antibiotics may prevent infection.

Asthma (AZ-muh) is a chronic condition that can be life threatening. According to the American Academy of Allergy, Asthma, and Immunology, 10 million Americans have allergic asthma. Its cause is not completely understood, although an antibody produced by exposure to an allergen causes the symptoms. Therefore the conventional belief is that asthma is an allergic reaction. However, some studies indicate that cells in the airway may trigger the attack, not the immune system. Asthma attacks may result from exposure to an allergen, cold temperature, exercise, or emotion (Box 13-1). The bronchi narrow and contract in spasms, and the affected person may experience wheezing and difficulty exhaling. Treatment includes

TABLE 13-2
Blood Gas Analysis

Test	Normal Range*	Description
Arterial O_2 saturation (SaO_2)	93%-98%	Ratio of oxygen content and capacity
Arterial O_2 tension (PaO_2)	80-104 mm Hg	Partial pressure of oxygen
pH (arterial)	7.38-7.44	Hydrogen ion concentration
Arterial CO_2 tension ($PaCO_2$)	36-42 mm Hg	Partial pressure of carbon dioxide
Total CO_2 (venous)	26-30 mEq/L	Measurement from all compounds containing CO_2 in plasma
Bicarbonate HCO_2 (venous)	25-28 mEq/L	Concentration bicarbonate ion in plasma
Base excess (arterial)	−2.4 to +2.3 mEq/L	Excess of basic ions; value should be zero

*Value may vary with differing laboratories.
mm Hg, millimeters of mercury.

BOX 13-1

Triggering Agents of Asthma

- Air pollution
- Cockroaches
- Cold
- Dust mites
- Emotion
- Exercise
- Foods or food additives
- Humidity
- Mold
- Pets
- Secondhand smoke

relaxation and medication to clear air passages. If the cause is determined to be the airway cells, treatment might include inhalation of genes that stop the reaction. Although there is no known cure for asthma, half of all children with asthma outgrow the condition by their teens.

CASE STUDY 13-1 Your friend tells you that he always thinks he has asthma because he feels a burning pain in his head and chest when he has to shovel snow in cold weather. What should you say?

Answers to Case Studies are available on the Evolve website: ***http://evolve.elsevier.com/Gerdin***

Atelectasis (at-uh-LEK-tuh-sis) is collapse of part or all of a lung caused by a tumor in the thoracic cavity, pneumonia, or injury. The person feels severe pain and shortness of breath, or dyspnea. Treatment corrects the cause and reexpands the lung with pulmonary suction.

Bronchitis (bron-KIE-tis) is an infection of the bronchi. Inflammation causes the bronchial walls to thicken, and less air can be exchanged. Bronchitis often results in a heavy cough and much mucus eliminated as sputum. Treatment may include the use of expectorant medications and postural drainage.

Carbon monoxide poisoning usually occurs from breathing carbon monoxide from automobile exhaust fumes. Breathing too much carbon monoxide can be life threatening because the carbon monoxide takes the place of oxygen on hemoglobin molecules. With no place for oxygen on the hemoglobin, the body cells do not receive it. Carbon monoxide poisoning first causes nausea and drowsiness. The person should be removed from the area of the gas, and oxygen should be administered.

BRAIN BYTE

Carbon monoxide is the leading cause of accidental poisoning deaths in America.

Chronic obstructive pulmonary disease (COPD) is a group of chronic respiratory disorders that includes asthma, chronic bronchitis, and pulmonary emphysema. These conditions have similar symptoms and treatments. The symptoms include shortness of breath (dyspnea) and tissue overgrowth called *hyperplasia* (hi-per-PLAY-zhee-uh). Treatment includes giving oxygen; an antidiuretic (an-tie-die-uh-RET-ik), a medication used to increase the amount of fluids excreted by the body, and a bronchodilator (brong-ko-die-LAY-ter), a medication used to dilate the bronchi and bronchioles for easier breathing.

A *cold* is a respiratory infection caused by one of more than 200 viruses. It lasts from 1 to 2 weeks. It may cause a sore throat, sneezing, aches, pains, a runny nose, and fever. Cold medications may relieve the symptoms, but there is no cure.

CASE STUDY 13-2 Your friend tells you that he cannot catch your cold because he had one a few months ago. What should you say?

Answers to Case Studies are available on the Evolve website: *http://evolve.elsevier.com/Gerdin*

CASE STUDY 13-3 Your friend's baby is 1 year old and has a cold. Your friend asks you what over-the-counter medication you should give the baby. What should you say?

Answers to Case Studies are available on the Evolve website: *http://evolve.elsevier.com/Gerdin*

Cystic fibrosis (SIS-tik fie-BRO-sis) is a genetic disorder of the exocrine (EK-so-krin) glands, usually diagnosed before the age of 3. The mucus in the respiratory system becomes thicker (more viscous), and excess salt appears on the skin. Cystic fibrosis requires intensive pulmonary care to prevent chronic disorders. With consistent treatment, people with cystic fibrosis may live for 30 or more years.

Emphysema (em-fuh-SEE-ma) results when the alveoli lose elasticity, usually after 50 years of age. The alveoli become dilated and do not exchange gases well. Emphysema can result from smoking or several disorders of the respiratory system. Treatment includes use of "pursed lip breathing," the very slow exhalation of air to allow alveoli to respond.

Hanta virus (HAN-tuhvi-rus) is a respiratory condition spread by breathing in materials contaminated by urine or saliva of infected rodents such as deer, mice, and chipmunks. The symptoms appear like influenza and include fever; cough; muscle ache; and inflamed, reddened eyes. This virus has a rapid onset and is often fatal. Treatment is supportive to assist the infected person with respiratory function.

Hay fever is a respiratory inflammation caused by allergens such as plants, dust, and food. It may cause headache, nausea, and watery drainage from the eyes and nose. Treatment includes medication for the symptoms or desensitization therapy.

Lung cancer is directly linked to smoking and smoke products (Fig. 13-5). The American Cancer Society reports that lung cancer is the leading cause of cancer-related deaths in both men and women. The cancer is usually not detected until it is widespread. The cancer may spread to many parts of the body through the lymph nodes. Treatment may include surgical removal of lung segments, as well as chemotherapy and radiation.

Pleural effusion (PLER-uhl e-FYOO-zhun) is a condition in which air or fluid enters the pleural cavity. The space for respiration becomes limited. Pleural effusion is usually caused by cancer, infection, or congestive heart failure. The person with pleural effusion may feel shortness of breath and pain. Treatment may include thoracentesis (tho-ra-sen-TEE-sis), which removes the fluid with a needle or a suction drainage tube.

Pleurisy (PLOO-rih-see) is an inflammation of the membranes that line the lungs. It is usually a

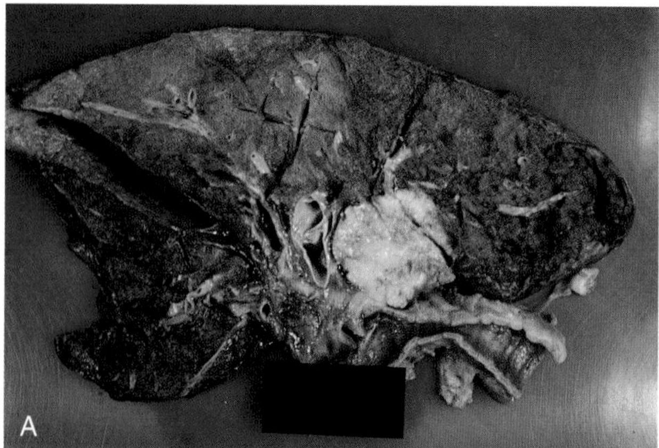

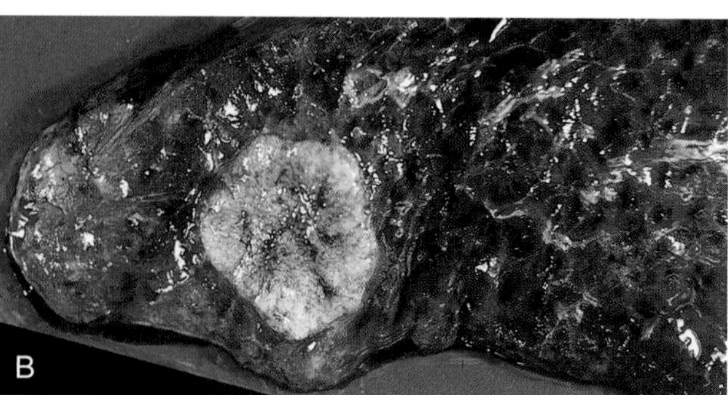

FIGURE 13-5 Normal lungs are bright red in color. **A and B,** Cancer causes blacking and loss of moisture in the tissues. (From Damjanov I: *Pathology for the health professions,* ed 3, St. Louis, 2006, Saunders.)

complication of a severe respiratory infection such as pneumonia. The person with pleurisy experiences difficulty breathing; pain; and grating breath sounds, also known as *crepitus* (KREP-ih-tus).

Pneumonia (noo-MO-nee-ah) is an inflammation of the lungs, in which a buildup of excessive moisture impairs breathing. Bacteria, viruses, or chemical irritants may be the causative agents of pneumonia. When a foreign substance, such as vomitus, causes it by entering the respiratory passage, it is called aspiration pneumonia. Treatment is directed at the original cause and includes medication to decrease the moisture.

Pneumoconiosis (noo-mo-ko-nee-O-sis) is an inflammation in the lungs caused by inhaled irritants. These may include dust, asbestos, sand, iron, and coal particles (Fig. 13-6). The lungs may have excessive fluid, and the person feels shortness of breath.

Respiratory acidosis (RES-per-uh-tore-ee as-ih-DO-sis) is a buildup of carbon dioxide in the blood, causing a lowered blood pH. The condition may result from COPD or drug overdose. The person with respiratory acidosis may experience decreased mental functioning or delusions (delirium); death may also result. Treatment may include giving oxygen or providing ventilation with a respirator.

Respiratory alkalosis (RES-pir-uh-tore-ee al-kah-LOH-sis) is a deficiency of carbon dioxide in the blood. It is most often caused by hyperventilation, or rapid breathing, resulting from anxiety or exercise at high elevations. The person with respiratory alkalosis experiences extreme nervousness, tingling in the extremities, and muscle spasms (tetany). It is rarely life threatening. Treatment involves breathing slowly or breathing into a paper bag. These techniques increase the carbon dioxide level in the blood.

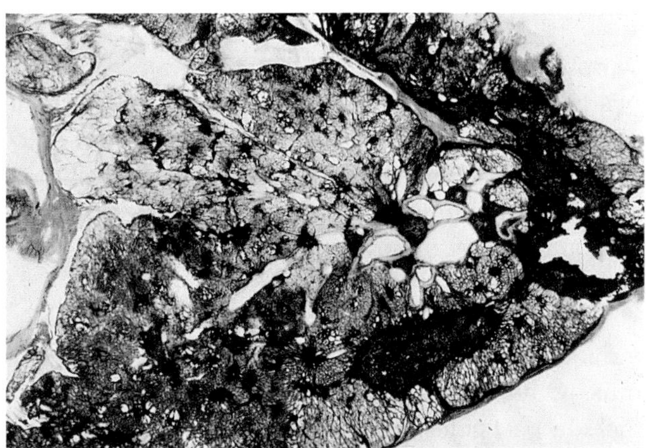

FIGURE 13-6 Deposits of carbon particles make the lungs appear black in coal-workers' lung disease. (Courtesy Dr. W. Thurlback, Vancouver, BC, Canada. In Damjanov I: *Pathology for the health professions*, ed 3, St. Louis, 2006, Saunders.)

CASE STUDY 13-4 Your friend tells you that he gets a 'stitch' or sharp pain in his side when he runs. He says he won't keep running because it hurts too much. What should you say?

Answers to Case Studies are available on the Evolve website: ***http://evolve.elsevier.com/Gerdin***

Respiratory distress syndrome is a condition that occurs when the alveoli do not inflate properly. Adult respiratory distress syndrome may result from inhaling foreign substances and swelling (edema) of respiratory tissues. Infant respiratory distress syndrome (IRDS) is one of the leading causes of death in premature births. According to the National Institutes of Health, IRDS affects 10% of premature infants. Treatment is the delivery of oxygen and in infants, application of surfactant through tubes into the lungs.

Sinusitis (sine-us-I-tus) is an inflammation of one or more of the paranasal sinuses. It can result as a complication of an upper respiratory or dental infection or changes in atmosphere, such as in swimming or air travel. Symptoms include pain, pressure, headache, fever, and increased secretions. Treatment includes nasal decongestants, steam inhalations, and antibiotics if infection is present.

BRAIN BYTE

Since 2005 the Patriot Act has required a signature and identification for purchase of over-the-counter nasal decongestant remedies that contain pseudoephedrine.

Sudden infant death syndrome (SIDS) is a respiratory disorder of newborns. More than 2500 infants in the United States die of SIDS each year. The SIDS diagnosis is given for the sudden death of an infant younger than 1 year of age that remains unexplained after a complete investigation. SIDS may be called crib death because it often occurs while the infant is sleeping. The cause of SIDS may be related to a defect in a part of the brain, but environmental and metabolic factors are also considered risk factors. Infants who are at high risk for SIDS may be monitored with heart and respiratory devices while sleeping. One new technique to prevent death is pajamas that have respiratory and heart monitors built into them.

Tuberculosis (tuh-ber-kyoo-LO-sis) (TB) caused by bacteria that are difficult to destroy, is transmitted through the air. It leads to excessive sputum production and coughing. Since 1991 more cases of tuberculosis have developed than in all previous time. The Centers for Disease Control and Prevention (CDC) reports that the reduction in rate in 2003 and 2004 was the lowest since national reporting began in 1953. It is the most common fatal infectious disease in the world today. Recently a strain of the bacteria that is resistant to the medications used previously has evolved, and the incidence of this strain of infection is currently increasing. Treatment includes medication for up to 2 years and may require surgical removal of the affected tissue to destroy the bacteria. Respiratory isolation may be necessary to prevent the spread of tuberculosis.

Upper respiratory infections (URI) are caused by a virus or bacteria in the nose, pharynx, or larynx. Pharyngitis (fare-in-JIE-tis) is a sore throat often accompanied by difficulty in swallowing (dysphagia). Laryngitis (lare-in-JIE-tis) may cause hoarseness or loss of voice. Tonsillitis (ton-sil-I-tis) is painful inflammation of the lymph nodes and may require surgical removal of the tonsils. Treatment for all types of upper respiratory infections includes rest and medication to relieve pain, reduce fever, and combat the cause of the infection.

Issues and Innovations

Tobacco Issues

Cigarette smoking has been linked to many illnesses, such as heart disease and cancer. Research shows that nonsmokers subjected to "passive," "secondhand," or "side-stream" smoke from the cigarettes of other people also face these risks. The CDC considers smoking to be the leading preventable cause of death in the United States. It estimates that more than 20% of adult Americans smoke cigarettes.

Studies have demonstrated that a person who works in a restaurant or bar where smoking is permitted has a 50% greater chance of developing lung cancer than someone who does not. The American Lung Association has reported that 20% of the U.S. population is at risk of developing lung disease from secondhand smoke. The U.S. Department of Health, Education, Welfare, and Public Health Services reports that secondhand smoke has higher levels of tar, nicotine, and carbon monoxide than that inhaled by the direct smoker.

The federal Environmental Protection Agency has classified secondhand smoke as a group A carcinogen, along with asbestos and radon. In many regions new laws restrict smoking to designated areas to protect nonsmokers from exposure to the smoke. Insurance companies often have higher rates for smokers because of the greater health risks and problems of safety. Smoking has been an issue used to determine custody in divorce settlements.

Some advertisements of "smokeless" tobacco, such as chew or tobacco powder, imply that it does not involve the same health risks; however, placing smokeless tobacco between the lower lip and teeth (dipping) is actually as dangerous as smoking and perhaps more so because the juice from tobacco causes a change in mouth tissue called *leukoplakia* (loo-ko-PLAY-kee-uh). These white, leathery patches become mouth cancer in 5% of cases (Fig. 13-7). Damage to the taste buds on the tongue affects a person's sense of taste. Tobacco and the sweeteners in the smokeless tobacco products also damage the gums, causing the teeth to decay and loosen.

Cancer may develop in the esophagus if the tobacco juices are swallowed. Ulcers may occur in the stomach from increased production of gastric acid. The nicotine habit develops with smokeless tobacco just as with cigarette smoking. Heart disease may result from an increase in blood pressure and heart rate. Cancer of the bladder, pancreas, and kidney has been shown to occur more often in those using smokeless tobacco.

Environmental Health Risks

Various inhaled inorganic substances can be hazardous to one's health. For example, miners who inhale coal dust develop black lung disease (pneumoconiosis) or silicosis. Inhalation of asbestos leads to chronic scarring of the lung tissue. Berylliosis can result from inhalation of beryllium used in fluorescent light bulbs and the aerospace industry.

Inhalation of biological contaminants such as bacteria, fungus, and dust mites can lead to allergic rhinitis. Other items of concern in the environment include pesticides, particulates in air pollution, and combustible gases. New environmental risks are continually being identified. The American Lung Association reports that occupational lung disease is the major reason for lost workdays and loss of productivity in the United States. It considers occupational

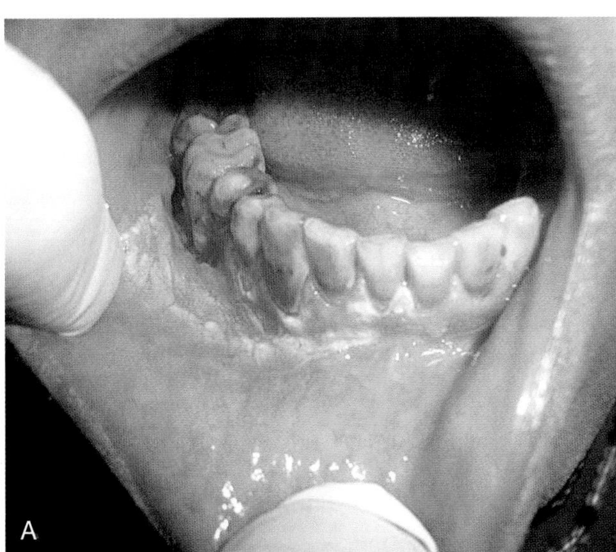

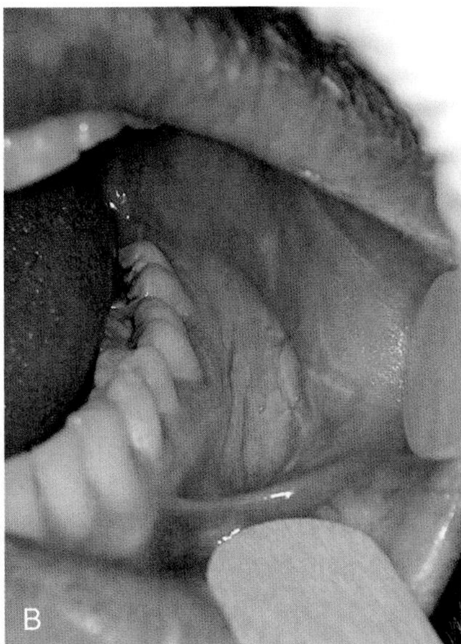

FIGURE 13-7 **A and B,** Leukoplakia is a precancerous tissue growth of the mucous membranes of the mouth. It is directly related to the use of smokeless tobacco products. (Copyright www.entusa.com. All rights reserved.)

asthma to be the most common form of occupational lung disease.

In a long-term study of 45 different neighborhoods, three areas in Pennsylvania were found to have three times the usual rate of lung cancer. In these areas a high level of sulfur dioxide was found in the air. These studies have implicated the power plants as the source of the sulfur dioxide. A study released by the Maryland Nurses Association in 2006 links 700 premature deaths, 30,000 asthma attacks, and 400 pediatric emergency department visits to the pollution from power plants yearly.

In the Silicon Valley area of California, hundreds of workers experienced symptoms apparently resulting from exposure to toxic chemicals used in the computer industry. The symptoms experienced include hypersensitivity to ordinary chemicals, memory loss, fatigue, impaired concentration, and violent mood swings.

Sick building syndrome includes several environmental conditions that can lead to sickness. Most often, sick buildings do not have windows that open to the outside, and their heating and cooling ducts start at a common source. An elevated level of carbon dioxide in the building causes sickness. Specific types of sick building syndrome include "air-conditioner lung" and "humidifier fever."

Exposure to "toxic mold" has been determined to be a health hazard for perhaps hundreds of thousands of affected people. Although the mold itself is not toxic, some molds such as *Stachybotrys* or *Chaetomium* produce mycotoxins that are poisonous. Exposure to molds may cause anything from a minor allergic reaction to more serious conditions including chronic bronchitis, heart problems, and learning disabilities.

Summary

- Functions of the respiratory system include exchanging gases between the blood and lungs, regulating body temperature, and maintaining electrolyte balance.
- Structures of the respiratory system include the nasal cavity, lungs, bronchi, alveoli, and diaphragm.
- Methods of assessment of the respiratory system include respiration rate, character, breath sounds, lung volume, and blood gases.
- Disorders of the respiratory system include asthma, atelectasis, bronchitis, chronic obstructive pulmonary disease, and cystic fibrosis.

Review Questions

1. Describe the three functions of the respiratory system.
2. Describe the function of each of the following structures of the respiratory system:

Epiglottis	Sinus
Pleura	Tonsil

3. Describe three tests used to assess the function of the respiratory system.
4. Describe five body systems that are affected by the use of tobacco in any form.
5. Describe two health hazards that have been attributed to inhalation of environmental materials.

Critical Thinking

1. Investigate the rate of tobacco use by adolescents. Design a brochure for middle school-age children about the hazards of using tobacco.
2. Investigate at least five common medications used in treatment of respiratory system disorders.
3. List at least five occupations involved in the health care of respiratory system disorders.
4. Investigate the current research being conducted about respiratory disorders that result from environmental factors.
5. Research and review an article regarding a recent development or treatment method relating to the respiratory system.
6. Use the Internet to investigate cystic fibrosis or another respiratory disorder. Create a poster that describes the condition including the cause, treatment, and outlook.

Explore the Web

Cystic Fibrosis

Cystic Fibrosis Foundation

http://www.cff.org/treatments/Therapies/

National Heart Lung and Blood Institute

http://www.nhlbi.nih.gov/health/dci/Diseases/cf/cf_what.html

Tobacco

KidsHealth

http://kidshealth.org/teen/drug_alcohol/tobacco/smokeless.html

CDC

http://www.cdc.gov/tobacco

CHAPTER 14

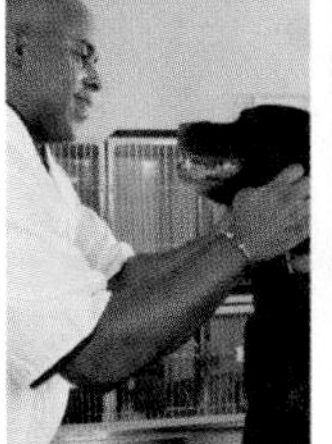
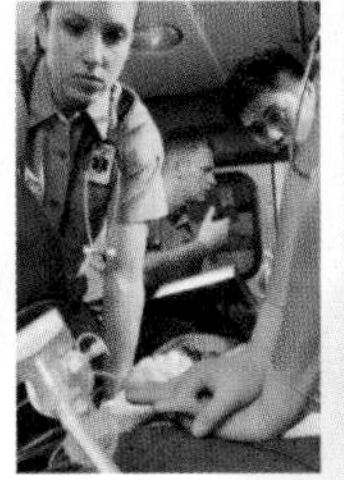
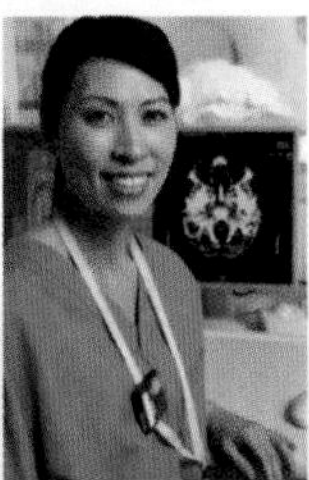

Skeletal System

LEARNING OBJECTIVES

- Define at least 10 terms relating to the skeletal system.
- Describe the five functions of the skeletal system.
- Identify at least 10 structures of the skeletal system.
- Identify at least three methods of assessment of the skeletal system.
- Describe at least five disorders of the skeletal system.

KEY TERMS

Articulation *(ar-tik-yoo-LAY-shun)* Joint; place of junction between two bones

Bursa *(BER-sah)* Saclike cavity filled with fluid to prevent friction

Cancellous *(KAN-seh-lus)* Spongy or latticelike structure

Cartilage *(KAR-tih-lij)* Specialized, fibrous connective tissue

Collagen *(KOL-uh-jen)* White protein fibers of the skin, tendons, bone, and cartilage (connective tissue)

Compact *(KOM-pakt)* Having a dense structure

Degenerative *(de-GEN-er-uh-tiv)* Having progressively less function

Extremities *(ek-STREM-ih-tees)* Arms or legs

Ligament *(LIG-uh-ment)* Band of fibrous tissue that connects bones and supports joints

Marrow *(MARE-o)* Soft organic material filling the cavities of bones

Orthopedic *(or-tho-PEE-dik)* Pertaining to the correction of deformities

Periosteum *(per-ee-OS-tee-um)* Specialized connective tissue covering all the bones of the body

Resorption *(re-SORP-shun)* Loss of bone tissue caused by the action of specialized cells (osteoclasts)

Synovial *(sin-O-vee-uhl)* Pertaining to transparent alkaline fluid contained in joints

Tendon *(TEN-dun)* Fibrous cord by which a muscle is attached to a bone

Skeletal System Terminology*

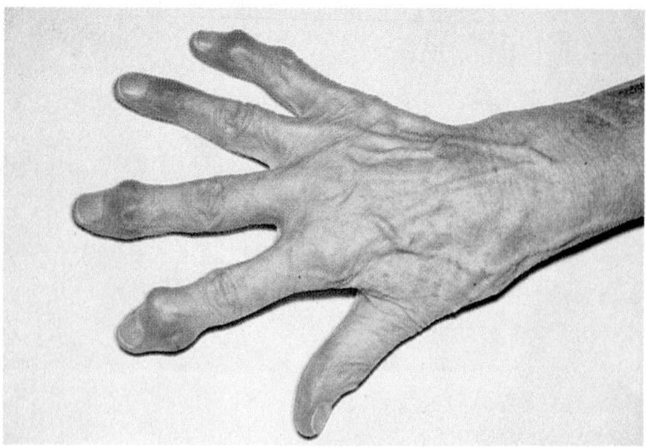

Osteoarthritis may cause Heberden's nodes to form around the knuckles. (From Kamal A, Brocklehurst JD: *A color atlas of geriatric medicine*, ed 2, St. Louis, 1991, Mosby.)

Term	Definition	Prefix	Root	Suffix
Arthritis	Inflammation of the joint		arthr	itis
Arthrodesis	Surgical union or fixation of the joint		arthr/o	desis
Arthroplasty	Plastic reconstruction of the joint		arthr/o	plasty
Cervical	Pertaining to the neck		cervic	al
Chondrectomy	Removal of the cartilage		chondr	ectomy
Intercostal	Between the ribs	inter	cost	al
Odontology	Study of the tooth		odont	ology
Orthopedics	Pertaining to correcting or straightening the bones	ortho	ped	ics
Osteoarthritis	Inflammation of the bones and joints	osteo	arthr	itis
Periodontal	Around the tooth	peri/o	dont	al

*A transition syllable or vowel may be added to or deleted from the word parts to make the combining form.

Abbreviations of the Skeletal System

Abbreviation	Meaning
AKA	Above knee amputation
Amb	Ambulatory
Bil	Bilateral
CAT	Computed axial tomography
CXR	Chest x-ray
Ext	Extremity
Fx	Fracture
Lat	Lateral
Lt	Left
Ortho	Orthopedics

Structure and Function of the Skeletal System

The human body has more than 200 bones (Table 14-1). The skeletal system works directly with the muscular system to perform many functions, including the following:

- Providing shape and support
- Protecting internal organs
- Storing minerals and fat
- Producing blood cells and platelets
- Assisting in movement

Bone tissue is composed of inorganic salts (particularly calcium phosphate), water, and organic material such as bone cells, blood vessels, nerves, and elastic material (**collagen**). Like other body cells, bone cells must continuously receive food and oxygen. However, bones and their adjoining structures, ligaments, and tendons have fewer nerves and blood vessels than other body structures.

Bones continue to grow for the first 18 to 20 years of life. Even after growth stops, bone cells die and are replaced by new cells throughout life. Osteoblasts are cells in the bone tissue that produce new cells. Osteoclasts are cells that break down bone cells (**resorption**).

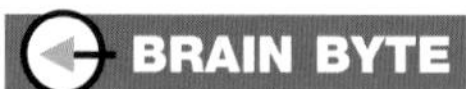

BRAIN BYTE

Most people reach peak bone density around age 20.

TABLE 14-1
Bones of the Body

Part of Skeleton	Body Part	Body Part Division	Names of Bones
Axial skeleton	Skull (28)	Cranium (8)	Frontal (1), parietal (2), temporal (2), occipital (1), sphenoid (1), ethmoid (1)
		Face (14)	Nasal (2), maxillary (2), zygomatic (2), mandible (1), lacrimal (2), palatine (2), inferior concha (2), vomer (1)
		Ear bones (6)	Malleus (2), incus (2), stapes (2)
	Hyoid (1)		
	Spinal column (26)		Cervical vertebrae (7), thoracic vertebrae (12), lumbar vertebrae (5), sacrum (1), coccyx (1)
	Sternum and ribs (25)		Sternum (1), true ribs (14), false ribs (10)
Appendicular skeleton	Upper extremities (64)		Clavicle (2), scapula (2), humerus (2), radius (2), ulna (2), carpals (16), metacarpals (10), phalanges (28)
	Lower extremities (62)		Coxal bones (2), femur (2), patella (2), tibia (2), fibula (2), tarsals (14), metatarsals (10), phalanges (28)

Bones may have **cartilage**, a fibrous connective tissue, on some surfaces to prevent friction. Bones are attached to other bones by **ligaments**. A sheet of fibrous tissue connecting bone to bone is called an *aponeurosis* (ap-o-noo-RO-sis). Bones are joined to muscles by **tendons**. Fascia (FASH-ee-uh) is a variable fibrous connective tissue that joins organs. Chapter 15 provides more information about the muscular system. The two major types of bone tissue are dense (**compact**) and loosely packed or spongy (**cancellous**).

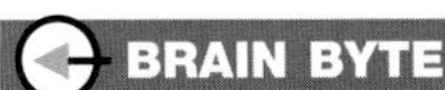

When a person is born, the body has more than 300 separate bones. After some fuse, there are only 206.

Types of Bones

The skeletal system consists of two major groups of bones (Fig. 14-1):

- The axial skeleton includes the 80 bones of the head and trunk.
- The appendicular skeleton includes the 126 bones of the pelvis, shoulders, arms, and legs (**extremities**).

Bones are also classified by shape (Table 14-2):

- Long bones are longer than they are wide.
- Short bones have similar length and width.
- Flat bones have two layers with space between them.
- Irregular bones are those that do not fit into the other categories.

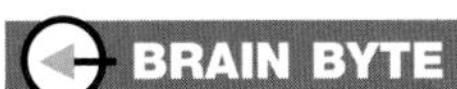

The longest bone is the femur of the leg, and the shortest is the stapes (stirrup) of the ear.

Skull

The skull includes the bones of the cranium, face, and ear. The cranium is made up of eight bones (Fig. 14-2). The sinus cavities make the skull lighter and the voice sound stronger. At birth, the bones of the cranium have two openings called *fontanels*. These close by 2 years of age. The face is made up of 13 bones (Fig. 14-3). The lower jaw (mandible) is the only movable bone of the skull.

Teeth

The adult has 32 teeth after the deciduous or primary teeth are replaced (Fig. 14-4). Each tooth has a number of parts (Fig. 14-5):

- The crown is the white section above the gum.
- The root is below the gum.

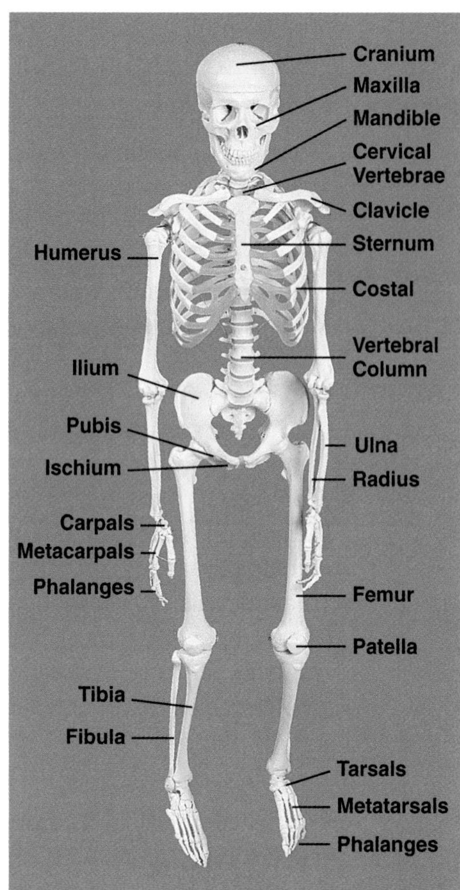

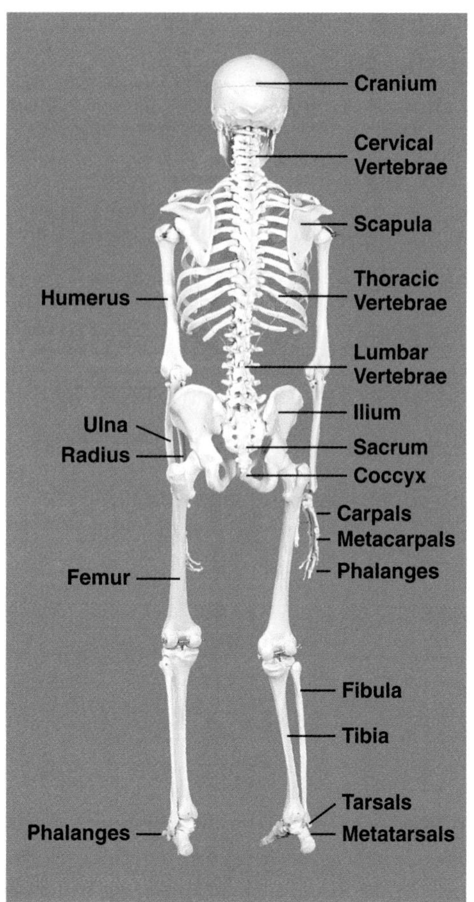

FIGURE 14-1 Common skeletal bones. **A,** Front view. **B,** Back view.

TABLE 14-2
Bones by Shape

Shape of Bone	Examples
Long	Femur, humerus, radius, ulna, tibia, fibula
Short	Tarsal, carpal, metatarsal, metacarpal
Flat	Cranium, costal, scapula, sternum
Irregular	Vertebrae, mandible, ilium, ossicle, patella

- Enamel, the hardest substance in the body, covers the crown.
- Cementum is the hard, bonelike substance covering the root.
- Dentin is located between the enamel and the pulp.
- The pulp is the soft living portion of the tooth, containing the nerves and blood vessels.

The four major types of teeth have different shapes and functions (Table 14-3).

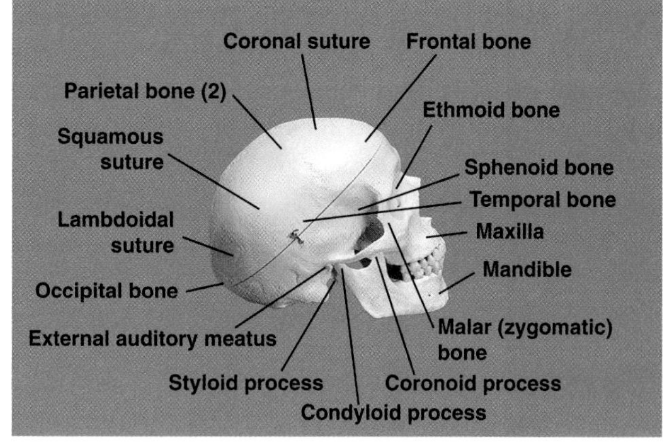

FIGURE 14-2 The bones of the skull include the cranium, face, and ears.

Thorax

The thorax is the part of the skeletal system that includes the ribs, sternum, and vertebral bones that protect the lungs and heart (Fig. 14-6). The first seven pairs of ribs are called "true" ribs and are attached to the sternum. The lower five pairs of ribs are called "false" ribs and are not attached directly to the sternum. The costal cartilage of each false rib attaches it to the rib above it. The bottom two pairs of false ribs are attached only to the spine and are called "floating" ribs. The area between the ribs is called *intercostal space*. It contains muscles, blood vessels, and nerves.

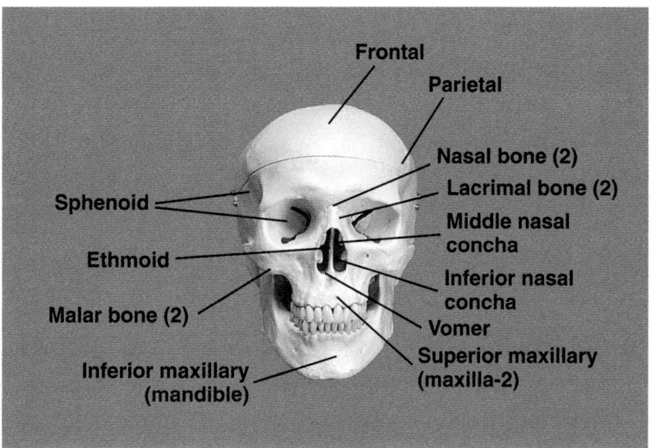

FIGURE 14-3 The skull includes the bones of the face. (The palate [2] and inferior turbinate [2] are not visible.)

Vertebral Column

The adult vertebral (spinal) column consists of 26 vertebrae and has five parts (Fig. 14-7). The curvature of the vertebral column gives it strength and flexibility. Between the vertebrae are disks of cartilage that cushion the bones and allow movement.

Long Bones of the Extremities

The long bones of the arms and legs contain marrow that makes blood cells for the body. Long bones grow and lengthen from a layer of cartilage called the *epiphyseal plate*. This area becomes completely ossified when the bones stop growing. The different parts of the long bone are shown in Fig. 14-8.

The diaphysis, or shaft, of the long bone contains fatty tissue and yellow marrow in its cavity. This fatty

Central incisor
Lateral incisor
Cuspid
First bicuspid
Second bicuspid
First molar
Second molar
Third molar

Central incisor
Lateral incisor
Cuspid
First molar
Second molar

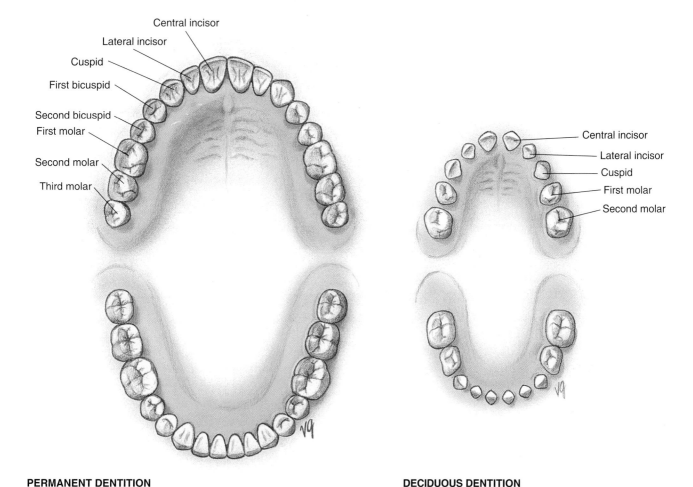

PERMANENT DENTITION

DECIDUOUS DENTITION

FIGURE 14-4 Tooth development.

TABLE 14-3
Teeth Types

Type of Tooth	Number	Function	Location	Description
Incisor	8	Cuts food	Front of mouth (central or lateral)	Broad, sharp edge
Cuspid (canines or eyeteeth)	4	Tears food	At angles of lips	Longest in mouth
Bicuspid (premolar)	8	Pulverizes or grinds food	Between cuspids and molars	Flat
Molar	12*	Grinds food	Back of mouth	Largest, strongest

*The third molar is called the "wisdom" tooth. It does not appear in all individuals.

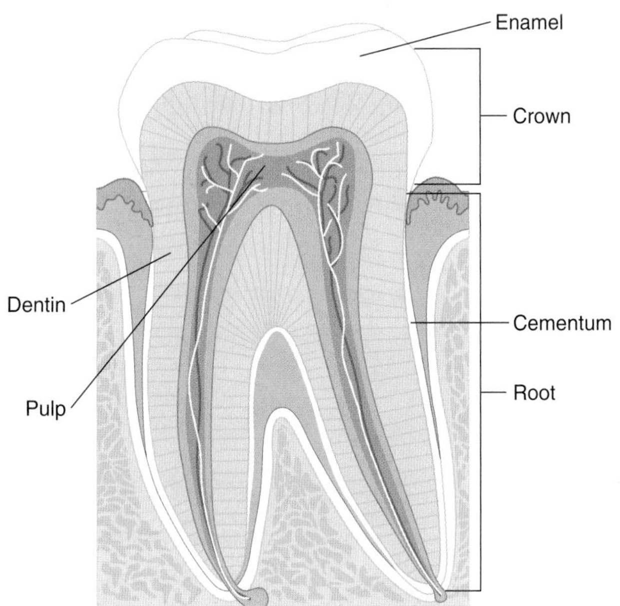

FIGURE 14-5 Parts of a tooth. (From Bird DL, Robinson DS: *Torres and Ehrich modern dental assisting*, ed 7, Philadelphia, 2003, Saunders.)

tissue provides stored energy. The epiphysis, or end of the long bone, contains the red marrow that produces red blood cells. The red marrow also destroys old red blood cells, forms all but one type of white blood cell, and produces platelets. Children have red marrow throughout the body. It is replaced by yellow marrow in all bones except the flat and long bones as they become adults.

The **periosteum**, or membrane that covers the bone, contains osteoblasts, special cells that form new bone tissue. In addition to arteries, nerves, and veins, the medullary cavity, or hollow inner tube of the diaphysis, also contains specialized cells called *osteoclasts*. Osteoclasts enlarge the diameter of the cavity by removing bone cells.

CASE STUDY 14-1 Your friend tells you that he has grown 6 inches this year and cramping pains in his legs from growing are hurting him at night. What should you say?

Answers to Case Studies are available on the Evolve website: ***http://evolve.elsevier.com/Gerdin***

Bone Markings

Bone markings are the shapes of different parts of bones (Table 14-4). There are four major types of bone markings:

- Projections bulge from a bone and attach to muscles, ligaments, and tendons.
- Openings are holes or spaces in bones.
- Depressions include openings and cavities in bone.
- Ridges are lines on a bone surface.

Joints

Two or more bones join together at a joint, also called an **articulation**. Joints are commonly named by the bones that are joined. For example, the sternoclavicular joint is between the sternum and clavicle. The following list describes the three types of joints:

- Immovable (synarthrosis)
- Slightly movable (amphiarthrosis)
- Freely movable (diarthrosis)

An example of an immovable joint is any one of the sutures of the cranium after they have ossified and closed. An example of a slightly movable joint is a pelvic bone.

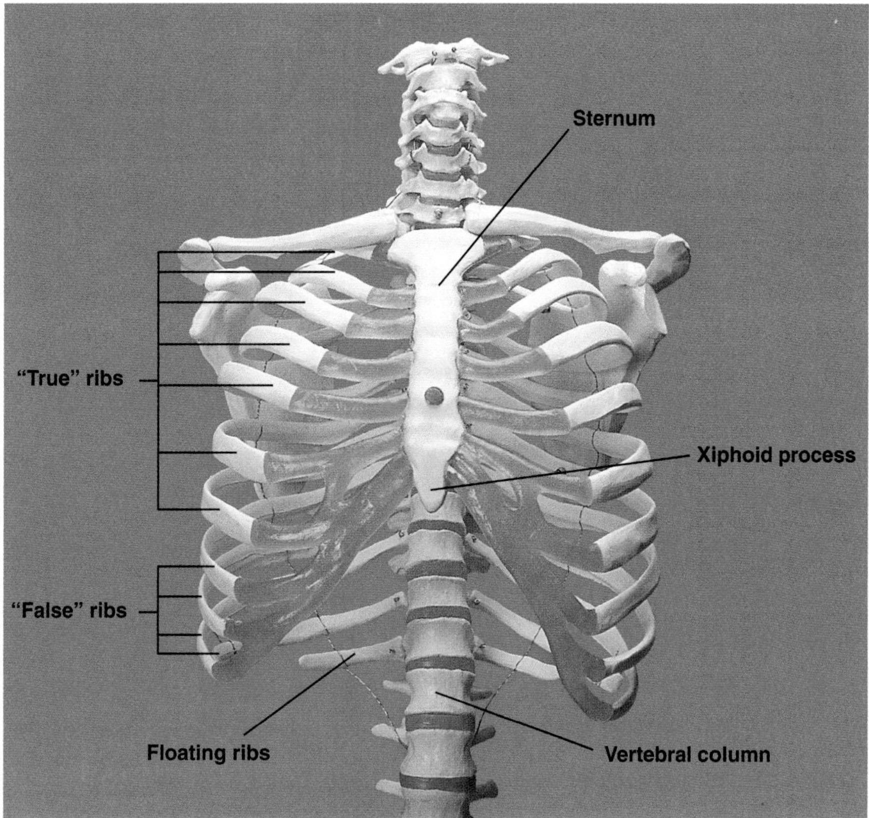

FIGURE 14-6 The thorax.

Movable joints are also called synovial joints. They contain a protective bursa, which is a sac filled with synovial fluid that cushions the moving parts. Bursae are found at the freely movable joints such as the elbows, knees, hips, shoulders, and ankles. The six types of diarthrosis joints are named according to how they move (Fig. 14-9):

- Ball and socket joints of the shoulders and hips
- Hinge joints of the elbow and knee
- Gliding joints of the wrists
- Pivot joint at the base of the skull
- Saddle joint of the thumb
- Gomphosis, such as the attachment of a tooth into its socket in the jaw

The ball and socket joint allows the movements of flexion, extension, abduction, adduction, and a limited rotation. Hinge joints have limited movement in only one direction, like a hinge. Gliding joints allow the bones to slide. The pivot joint at the base of the skull is unique, allowing rotation of the head. The saddle joint allows many movements, such as the thumb touching the fingertips. Gomphoses are specialized joints that allow slight movement and attach a peglike structure such as a tooth into a socket like the jaw.

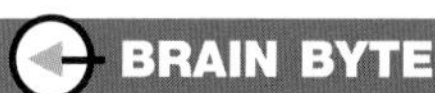

Humans have more than 230 joints that are movable or semimovable.

Assessment Techniques

Radiographic images (commonly referred to as *x-rays*) use electromagnetic energy that is absorbed by the body's tissues to produce images on photographic film. X-ray machines may be portable or stationary. They may be used to detect bone fractures, cancer, infection, arthritis, and deformities (Fig. 14-10). They may also be used to determine bone age, congenital skull deformities, and injuries resulting from abuse in children. Although having an x-ray taken has minimal risk and is painless, it is less sensitive than a bone scan in detecting bone destruction.

Bone marrow aspiration or sampling is accomplished by inserting a long needle into the spinal column to remove marrow. The sample is used to determine the cause of an abnormal blood test or unexplained blood disorders such as leukemia, sample for pathogens or chromosome abnormality, and evaluate a response to cancer treatment. It may be performed in the hospital or as an outpatient procedure.

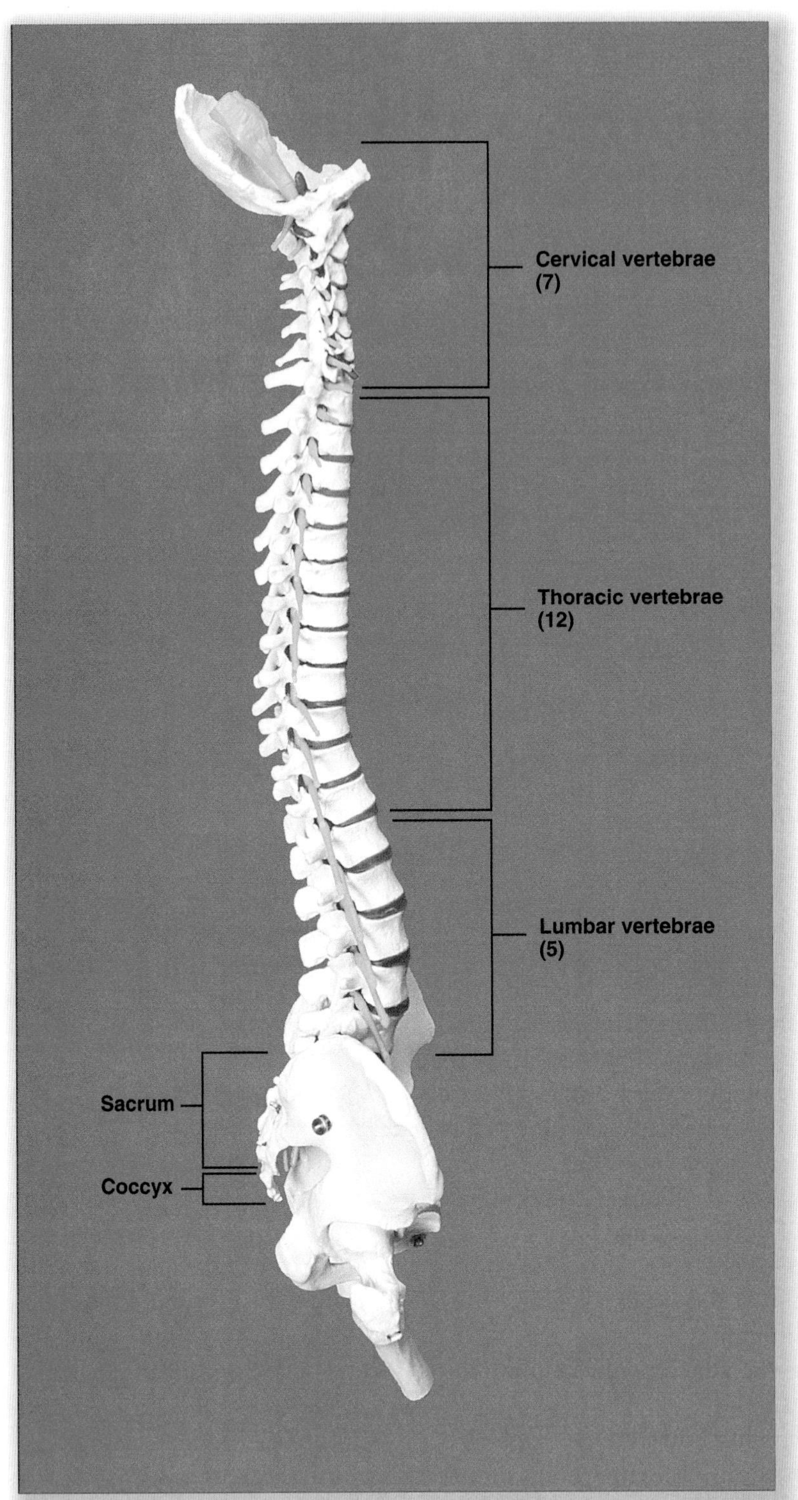

FIGURE 14-7 The lateral view of the vertebral column shows its five major parts. These five parts contain a total of 26 vertebrae.

CASE STUDY 14-2 You have a friend who has been diagnosed with leukemia. He is afraid he is going to die from it. What should you say?

Answers to Case Studies are available on the Evolve website: ***http://evolve.elsevier.com/Gerdin***

Although the procedure has relatively few complications, it may cause discomfort.

A bone marrow biopsy is used to obtain a piece of bone containing intact marrow to identify abnormalities such as thrombocythemia. It is also used to diagnose tumors, lymphoma, and the cause of an

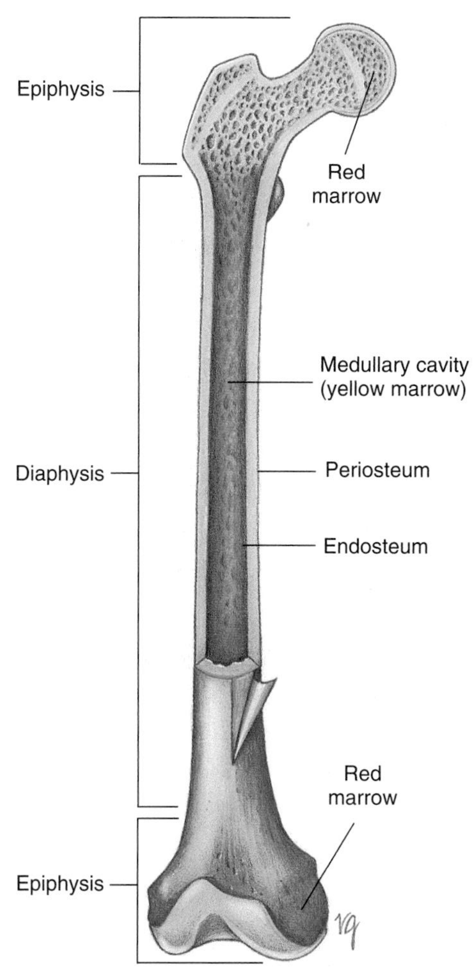

FIGURE 14-8 The anatomy of a long bone.

unexplained fever. It may also be used if bone marrow aspiration is unsuccessful. The procedure is similar to the bone marrow aspiration except that a core of bone is removed for examination.

A radionuclide bone scan or bone scintigraphy is used to detect bone cancer when x-rays do not show any abnormalities but a malignancy is suspected. It may also be used to locate a bone infection and other abnormalities. Stress fractures that do not show on x-rays may be seen by using a bone scan. The procedure involves injection of the radionuclide, which spreads through the bone. Increased concentration of the material indicates a diseased area.

A computed tomography (CT) scanner is a machine that sends several beams of x-rays simultaneously from different angles. A computer determines the relative density of the tissues examined by the strength of the beams. The technique of CT scanning was developed by Sir Geoffrey Hounsfield, who was awarded the Nobel Prize for his work. The CT scanner is used for taking pictures of every part of the body.

Magnetic resonance imaging (MRI) uses magnetic and radio waves to show computerized images of the body. No exposure to x-rays or any other damaging forms of radiation occurs with an MRI. Because the MRI scan shows detailed pictures, it is the best technique to identify tumors (benign or malignant) in the brain. The MRI scan can also show the heart and blood vessels. It is also used to examine the joints,

TABLE 14-4
Bone Markings

Type of Marking	Description	Example
Process		
Crest	Narrow ridge	Iliac crest
Condyle	Rounded process that articulates with another bone	Occipital condyle of skull
Tubercle	Small, rounded elevation that attaches muscles and ligaments	Proximal end of humerus
Tuberosity	Large, rounded elevation that attaches muscles and ligaments	Ischial tuberosity
Trochanter	Very large projection	Greater trochanter of femur
Head	Rounded projection from neck of bone, articulates with cavity	Head of humerus
Depression		
Sinus	Chamber or cavity in bone	Frontal sinus of skull
Foramen	Opening for nerves and blood vessels	Foramen magnum
Fissure	Narrow slit, cleft, or groove	Inferior orbital fissure of the eye
Fossa	Shallow concave depression on bone surface	Acetabular fossa

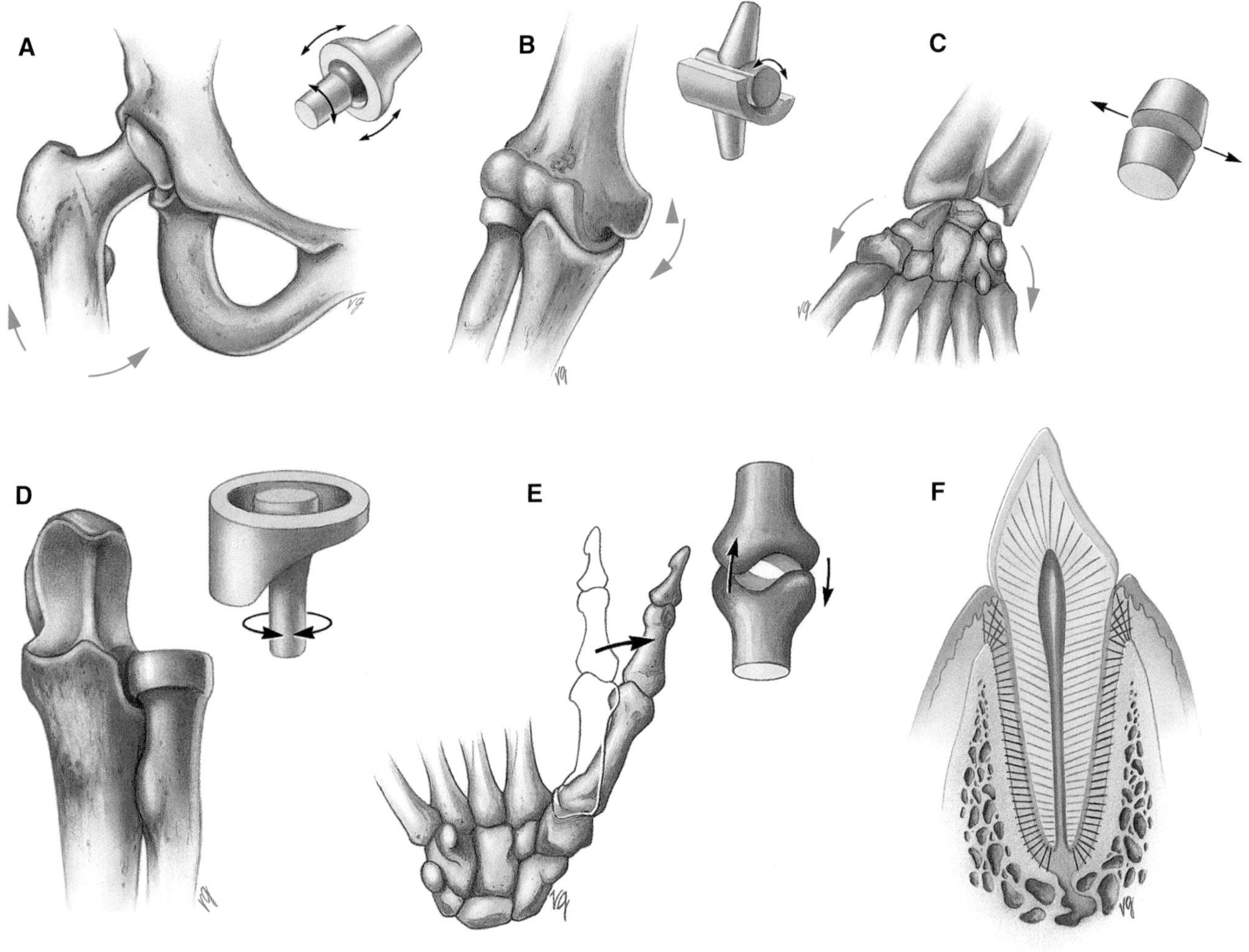

FIGURE 14-9 Types of joints. **A,** Ball and socket. **B,** Hinge. **C,** Gliding. **D,** Pivot. **E,** Saddle. **F,** Gomphosis.

spine, and sometimes the soft parts of the body, such as the liver, kidneys, and spleen.

The Centers for Disease Control and Prevention (CDC) reports that more than 10 million Americans older than 50 years of age have osteoporosis (Fig. 14-11). About 1.5 million fractures occurring each year are related to the condition. Bone densitometry or bone mineral density measures the amount of minerals such as calcium in bones to determine the extent of osteoporosis and fracture risk. Common techniques include dual-photon absorptiometry and dual-energy x-ray absorptiometry.

DISORDERS OF THE Skeletal System

Ankylosing spondylitis (ang-kil-O-sing spon-dih-LIE-tis) is a hereditary chronic spinal disease of unknown cause. Some or all of the bones and joints of the spine fuse together as a result of this condition. It results in stiffness, decreased mobility, and possible back deformity. Although no cure exists, treatment can slow the progression of the disease. Treatment includes a combination of rest, exercise, pain relievers, anti-inflammatory medication, and heat applications.

Arthritis (ar-THRIE-tis) includes a group of more than 100 disorders evidenced by inflammation of a joint, pain, and stiffness during movement. According to the CDC, one in five American adults has been diagnosed with some form of arthritis. Arthritis may be caused by joint disease, infection, gout, or trauma, but most cases are of unknown cause. Three forms of arthritis are ankylosing spondylitis, **degenerative** joint disease, and rheumatoid arthritis (each described separately here). Although no cure is available, treatment can relieve discomfort and promote movement in the joint. Controlled activity, rest, diet, application of heat and cold, and medication are all used for

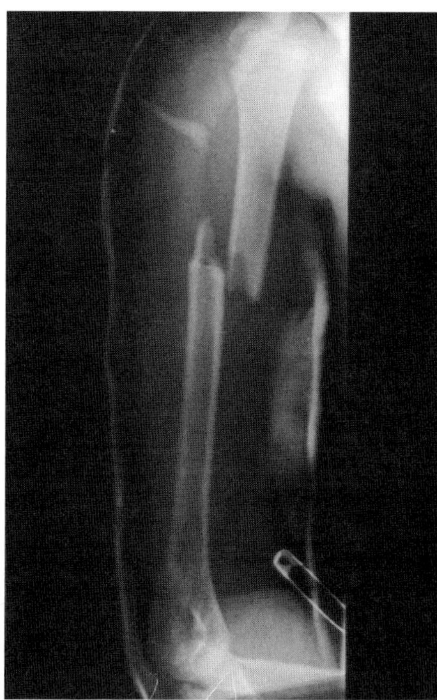

FIGURE 14-10 A fracture of the humerus. (Courtesy of Dr. Mercer Rang, The Hospital for Sick Children, Toronto, Ontario, Canada. In Gould BE, Dyer R: *Pathophysiology for the health professions*, ed 4, St. Louis, 2011, Saunders.)

treatment. Surgery to replace joints may be used in severe cases (Fig. 14-12).

Avulsion (uh-VUL-shen) fractures occur when a ligament or tendon pulls off part of a bone during an injury. This type of injury may occur in the ankles, legs, hip, and upper arms. Small fractures may not need treatment and may not cause pain or discomfort. Large avulsion fractures may require surgical reattachment.

Bursitis (bur-SIE-tis) is inflammation of the sac around a joint and is caused by trauma or irritation. Bursitis results in swelling and restricted movement. Treatment includes protection of the joint, rest, medications, and removal of excess fluid. The condition can become chronic if the joint is injured repeatedly.

Caries (KARE-eez), also called cavities, are a major cause of tooth loss in young people. Bacteria cause dental cavities. If the infection is extensive, the bone supporting the tooth can be damaged. Treatment may include "filling" the cavity with a restorative material such as amalgam or a composite resin. Air abrasion is a method used to remove tooth decay. A stream of particles such as silica, aluminum oxide, and baking soda are sprayed at the decayed portion of the tooth. In some cases the tooth may be removed.

Carpal (KAR-pul) *tunnel syndrome* (CTS) is a common disorder caused by pressure on the median nerve of the wrist resulting from repetitive use or trauma. The person with carpal tunnel syndrome may feel numbness, burning, tingling, pain, and weakness in the hand. Treatment may include resting the affected wrist, splinting, anti-inflammatory medication, or surgical correction.

Degenerative (de-GEN-er-ruh-tiv) *joint disease*, also called *osteoarthritis* (os-tee-o-ar-THRIE-tis), is usually associated with aging, but the cause is unknown. It is the most common form of arthritis. The condition has gradual onset as the cartilage in the joint softens. The person feels pain after exercise and stiffness after inactivity. Treatment for osteoarthritis includes medication to ease the pain and reduce inflammation. In severe cases the joint may be surgically replaced.

A *dislocation* (dis-lo-KAY-shun) occurs when bones move out of their proper location, usually in the shoulder or hip. Dislocation is either congenital or the result of trauma. The person feels pain and loss of mobility. The bones may relocate by themselves or require surgery. Ligaments may be damaged with dislocation injuries.

A *fracture* (FRAK-chur) is a broken bone caused by trauma. A fracture may be open (the skin is broken) or closed (skin is not broken). Swelling, bruising, and pain may occur. Treatment includes use of casts, traction, and electrical stimulation or ultrasound to increase the rate of healing (Fig. 14-13).

Gout is painful swelling of a joint that results from the buildup of uric acid crystals, most commonly in the great toe. Fever and chilling may also occur. The condition is usually due to an inability to adequately remove uric acid from the blood. Signs and symptoms of gout can result as a complication of another disorder. Treatment includes the use of medications, weight loss, and diet therapy that restricts the intake of purine.

A *herniated* (HER-nee-ate-ed) *disk* is a ruptured or "slipped" disk between vertebrae. It results in pain and reduced mobility. Treatment includes pain medication, bed rest, and possibly surgical correction.

Kyphosis (kie-FO-sis), also called "hunchback" or "humpback," is an abnormal curvature of the thoracic part of the spine (Fig. 14-14). The person with kyphosis may feel pain caused by affected nerves. The cause may be congenital or the effect of rheumatic arthritis, rickets, poor posture, or chronic respiratory diseases. Osteoporosis is the most common cause of kyphosis in adults. Treatment may include exercise to strengthen the back and bracing.

Lordosis (lore-DOE-sis), also called "swayback," is an abnormal curvature of the lumbar spine (see

FIGURE 14-11 "Widow's hump" or "dowager's hump" and fractures may result from osteoporosis. (From Damjanov I: *Pathology for the health professions*, ed 3, St. Louis, 2006, Saunders.)

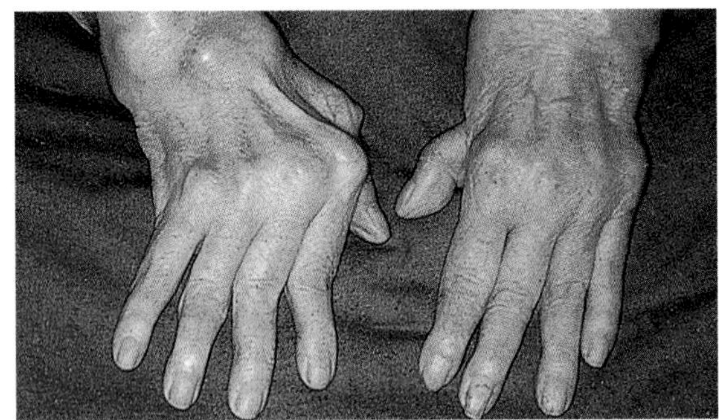

FIGURE 14-12 The hands may become deformed in rheumatoid arthritis as the joints soften. (From Stevens A, Lowe J: *Pathology: illustrated review in color*, ed 2, London, 2000, Mosby.)

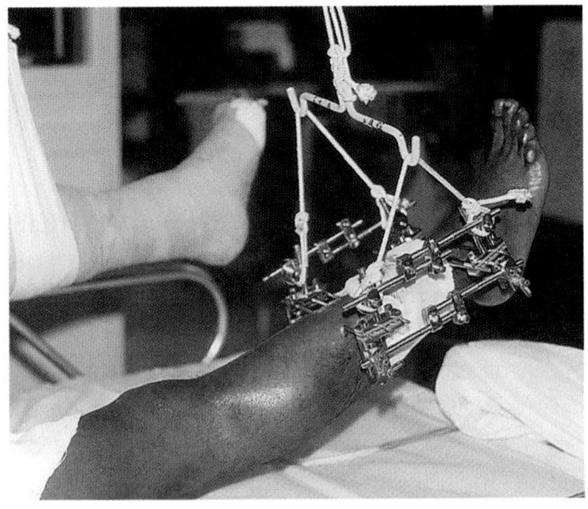

FIGURE 14-13 External fixator. (From McCance KL, Huether SE: *Pathophysiology: The biologic basis for disease in adults and children*, ed 6, St. Louis, 2010, Mosby.)

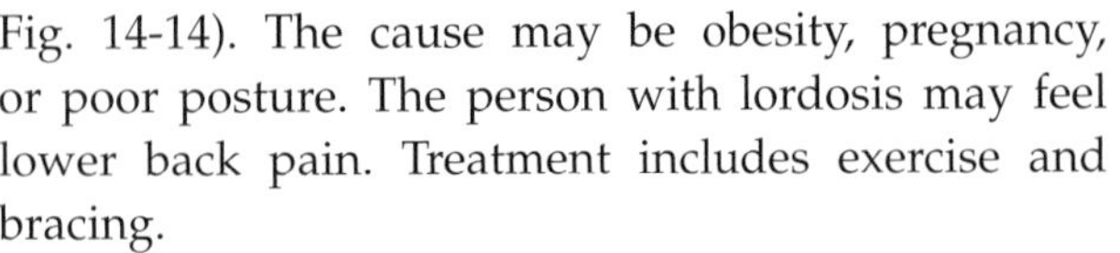

Fig. 14-14). The cause may be obesity, pregnancy, or poor posture. The person with lordosis may feel lower back pain. Treatment includes exercise and bracing.

Meningomyelocele (muh-ning-go-MIE-uh-lo-seel), also called *spina bifida* (SPY-na BIF-ih-da), is a

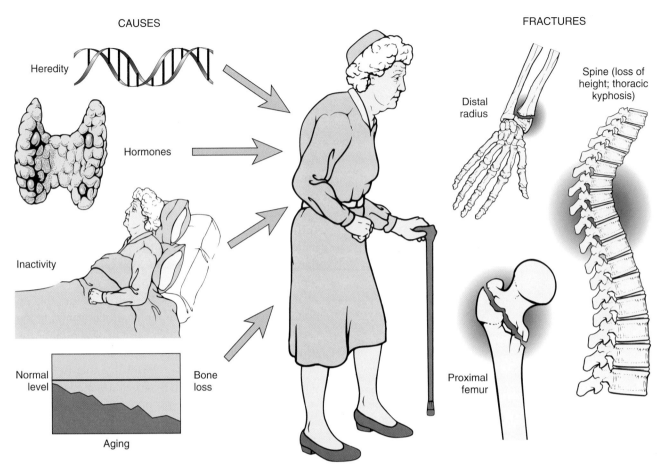

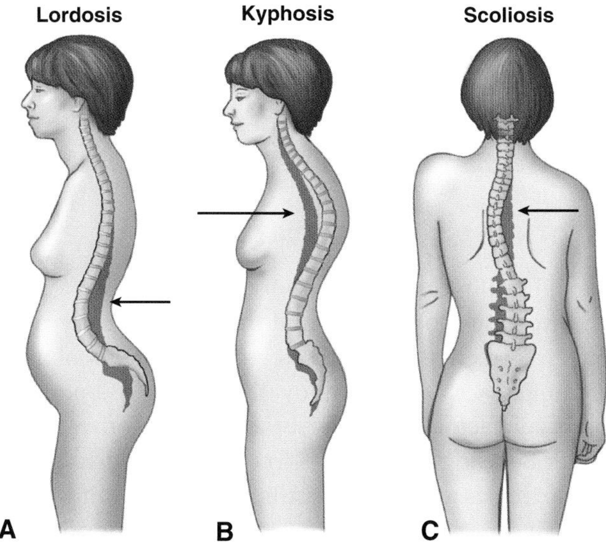

FIGURE 14-14 **A,** Lordosis. **B,** Kyphosis. **C,** Scoliosis. Arrows indicate abnormal curvature of the spine. (From Patton KT, Thibodeau GA: Anatomy & physiology, ed 7, St. Louis, 2010, Mosby.)

congenital condition of the spinal column. It can cause paralysis and nervous system disorders because of pressure on the spinal nerves. Most individuals with spina bifida do not have learning disabilities, although it may occur in some cases. Spina bifida is caused by genetic and environmental factors. Folic acid taken as a nutritional supplement before and during pregnancy reduces the risk of spina bifida. Treatment includes surgery and the prevention of infection. Surgical correction of the opening has been done while the fetus is still in the uterus in some cases.

An *osteoma* (os-tee-O-ma) is a bone tumor. It may be noncancerous (benign) or cancerous (malignant). Its symptoms depend on the location and size of the growth. A benign growth can be cured by surgical removal. Some malignant bone tumors may require chemotherapy or surgical removal.

Osteomalacia (os-tee-o-muh-LAY-she-a), also called *rickets* in children, is a softening of the bones caused by vitamin D and calcium deficiency. The person may experience pain, muscular weakness, anorexia, loss of weight, and deformity. Treatment includes adding nutrients to the diet.

Osteomyelitis (os-tee-o-my-uh-LIE-tis) is a bacterial infection of bone. Sudden fever and pain may occur. The bacteria enter the bone via the bloodstream or from tissues around the bone that are infected. Treatment includes immobilization of the part and antibiotics.

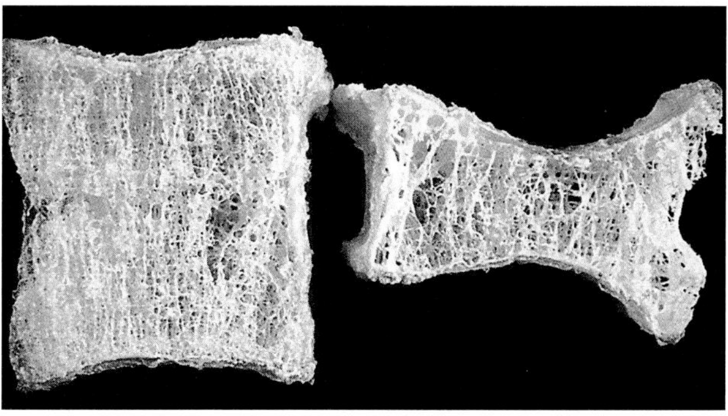
FIGURE 14-15 Normal vertebral body *(left)* and osteoporotic specimen *(right)*. (From Patton KT, Thibodeau GA: *Anatomy & physiology*, ed 7, St. Louis, 2010, Mosby.)

Osteoporosis (os-tee-o-po-RO-sis) is a weakening of the bones that affects more than 10 million people in the United States (Fig. 14-15). Another 34 million have osteopenia, or low bone mass, which may lead to osteoporosis. The bones become fragile and break usually in the hip, spine, and wrist. Women with small, thin builds are most likely to develop it, especially after menopause. Inadequate calcium in the diet, lack of exercise, and excessive use of caffeine and alcohol may also be associated with this condition. Lower back pain and abnormal curvature of the spine may result. No cure exists, but treatment to reduce symptoms includes dietary supplements of calcium and vitamin D. Estrogen and other hormone replacement therapies have been shown to improve bone density. In addition to pain medications and bracing, vertebroplasty may be used to control pain caused by compression fractures caused by osteoporosis. In this procedure, medical-grade cement is injected around the area of fracture to stabilize the bones. Kyphoplasty is a similar procedure but also expands the collapsed vertebra before injecting the cement. Bisphosphonates are a group of medications used to slow or repair the damage of osteoporosis.

CASE STUDY 14-3 Your friend tells you that her mother has shrunk more than 1 inch in height, and she thinks she is doing the same. What should you say?

Answers to Case Studies are available on the Evolve website: ***http://evolve.elsevier.com/Gerdin***

Paget (PAJ-et) *disease*, also called *osteitis deformans*, is a condition of unknown cause. It usually appears after the age of 35. Because of excessive destruction of bone cells, the long bones become bowed, and the flat bones are deformed. Although there may be no symptoms, bone pain, dizziness, headache, and deafness may result. Treatment, if necessary, includes medication, mild exercise, and a high-protein diet.

Periodontitis (pair-ee-o-don-TIE-tis) affects more than one in three people older than 30 years of age in the United States, according to the American Academy of Periodontology. It is the cause of most tooth loss in people older than the age of 35. Periodontitis is an inflammation of the tissues that keep teeth in place. It may start as sore, bleeding gums and may include persistent bad breath and tender, swollen, and receding gums. In advanced stages, pus may form and teeth may loosen. Treatment may include removing the tooth, scraping the gums, and performing root canal surgery to remove the infected area.

Rheumatoid arthritis (ROO-mah-toid ar-THRIE-tis) is a condition that affects many parts of the body and joints. Its cause is unknown. It may lead to crippling deformity and atrophy of the muscle tissue. In rheumatoid arthritis the synovial membrane thickens, causing pain and stiffness in the joints. Treatment includes physical therapy or orthopedic braces. Although there is no cure, antiinflammatory medications and rehabilitative care can slow the spread to other joints.

Rickets (RIK-ets) is a painless deformity at the epiphysis of the bones caused by insufficient vitamin D. In children the fontanels may close late and the arms and legs may be bowed. Treatment includes dietary supplements of vitamin D.

Scoliosis (sko-lee-O-sis) is an abnormal lateral spinal curvature (see Fig. 14-14). It may cause one shoulder to become higher than the other. It may be congenital, but it develops in the early teens during the growth spurt. It also may be caused by rickets, shortening of one leg, or other spinal disorders. The person with scoliosis may feel discomfort in walking and experience lower back pain. Treatment includes corrective exercise; braces; possibly casting; and in some cases, surgical correction.

Subluxation (sub-luk-SAY-shun) is partial dislocation of a joint, such as occurs in the neck in a "whiplash" injury. The person with subluxation may feel mild or severe pain in areas affected by the spinal cord nerves. Treatment includes manipulation of the spine and may include bracing or surgery.

Talipes (TAL-i-pez) is a congenital deformity involving the foot and ankle. Clubfoot is one type of talipes in which one or both feet are turned, usually inward, affecting mobility. Treatment may include surgery, corrective (orthopedic) shoes, or both.

Issues and Innovations

Progress in Dental Care

Dental health care includes more than repair of caries and treatment of periodontal disease. Dentistry now offers corrective measures for damaged, discolored, and misplaced teeth. Innovations include bonding, porcelain facing, bleaching, bracing, and tooth replacement. Bonding is a process to correct the surface of a tooth that is damaged or discolored. Bonding uses adhesive materials such as epoxy and ceramic powder. Porcelain veneers, another method of correcting surfaces, use composite resins. These last longer than bonding but are more costly. Sealants or plastic coatings are used to fill spaces to prevent formation of caries.

New methods of bleaching are also used to remove stains from tooth surfaces. Gas plasma or blue light, pastes, and chemical strips are being used to whiten the surface of teeth. Exact coloration may be difficult with bleaching, and the process may weaken the tooth. Metal brackets, also called *braces*, traditionally worn by children, are now used by people of all ages. Other new methods to move teeth include plastic braces, which are less visible, and electrical stimulation.

Osteointegration is the process of placing implants into the bone to replace missing teeth. This process takes several months and more than one surgical treatment to place hardware made of inert substances such as titanium into the jaw bone (endosseus). Although there is a greater risk of infection than in other replacement techniques, the implants are more stable and last longer.

A chemical has been developed that softens areas of decay in a tooth. The decay dissolves and can be painlessly removed, reducing the need for traditional drilling of cavities. About 3000 dentists in the United States are now using this method. The chemical treatment usually costs more than drilling, and it takes longer to remove the decayed area, but this new chemical method may provide a better surface for bonding to the metals used for fillings. Dentists may also use air abrasion or lasers to remove dental caries. Amalgam fillings may be replaced by a composite material for patients who have a concern about the release of mercury into the body from fillings.

CASE STUDY 14-4 Your friend tells you she has three wisdom teeth, but her dentist says they do not have to be removed. What should you say?

Answers to Case Studies are available on the Evolve website: ***http://evolve.elsevier.com/Gerdin***

Bone Substitutes and Repairs

Several materials have been found to replace missing or damaged bones. One type of material, called *organo-apatites*, consists of a mineral network that can mesh together with existing bone. This implant material has been shown to promote growth and repair of existing bone tissue.

Coral from the ocean has been used to repair bones by grafting (Fig. 14-16). This animal leaves a calcium deposit that is not rejected by the human body's immune system. Another advantage of using this material is its relative abundance. Coral is generally used for cranial grafts because it is not as rigid as bone or some other substitutes. Blocks of wood have been used as bone substitutes by researchers in Italy. In 2009 the researchers had implanted rattan wood as artificial bone in sheep. They estimate that human trials may start in 5 years.

Bone tissue engineering techniques include the use of bone marrow cells that are taken from a patient and then multiplied in culture. After shaping, the structures are implanted in the patient.

Medical researchers are using a process called *stereolithography* to make surgical implants for cranial and joint injuries. Stereolithography was adapted from the process used to make floor covering like linoleum. In the process, digital computer imaging is used to create an implant that is shaped with lasers and liquid plastic. The laser forms layer upon layer of the plastic until the implant matches the computer image.

Bone regeneration using the Ilizarov method was first introduced in the United States in 1987. The orthopedic surgical procedure involves making cuts in the affected bone surface without damaging the underlying nerves and blood vessels. Pins and a brace are placed around the bone, allowing it to be pulled apart gradually. Natural bone tissue is allowed to regrow in the split area. Bones can be lengthened approximately 1 mm every 24 hours, and reports have been made of lengthening up to 14 inches. The orthopedic surgery has been successful in treating bone deformities resulting from polio, trauma, and other degenerative conditions.

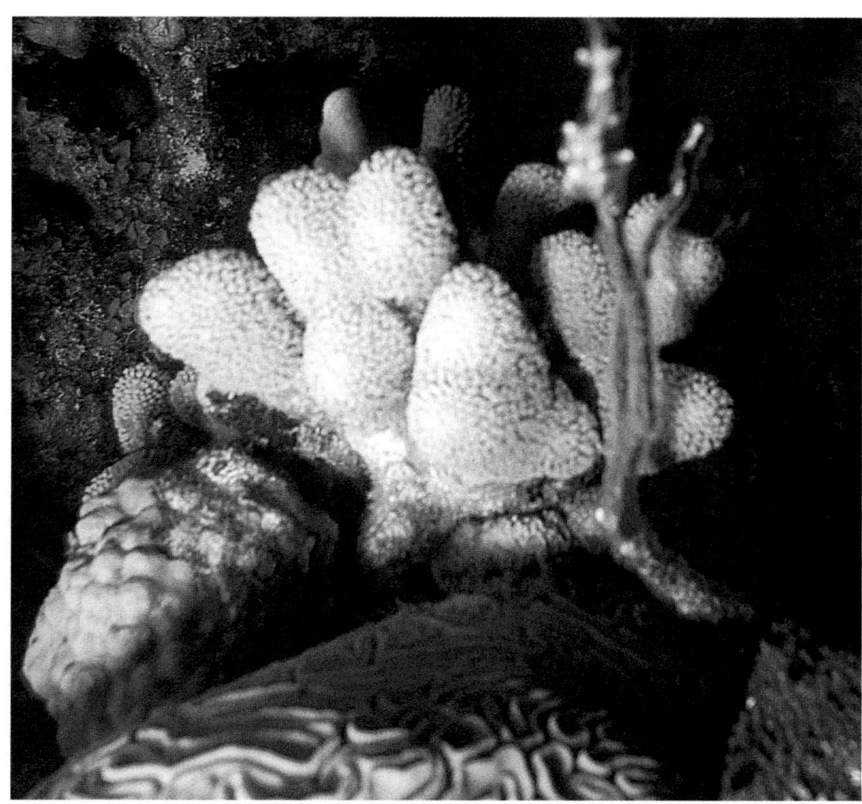

FIGURE 14-16 Coral has been used in grafting procedures to repair human bones.

Summary

- Functions of the skeletal system include protecting internal organs, storing minerals and fat, producing blood cells and platelets, and assisting in movement.
- Structures of the skeletal system are divided into the axial and appendicular skeleton and include bones such as the cranium, humerus, femur, and ulna.
- Methods of assessment of the skeletal system include x-rays, bone marrow aspiration, biopsy, CT, and MRI scans.
- Disorders of the skeletal system include avulsions, fractures, caries, carpel tunnel syndrome, and kyphosis.

Review Questions

1. Describe the five functions of the skeletal system.
2. In one or more sentences, identify the location of each of the following bones of the skeletal system and the characteristics these bones have in common: femur, fibula, humerus, radius, tibia, and ulna.
3. Identify a disorder of the skeletal system that has similar effects as kyphosis.
4. Describe the functions of red and yellow bone marrow.
5. Describe six types of joint movement.
6. Describe three methods of bone replacement or repair.
7. Use the following terms in one or more sentences that correctly relate their meaning: collagen, ligament, synovial, and tendon.

Critical Thinking

1. Investigate and compare the cost of at least three tests used to diagnose disorders of the skeletal system.
2. Investigate the function of at least five common medications used in treatment of skeletal system.
3. List at least five occupations involved in the health care of skeletal system disorders.
4. Use the Internet to investigate first-, second-, and third-class lever movement of joints.
5. Use the Internet to research the process and techniques used for bone repair after a fracture.
6. Use the Internet to make a poster or pamphlet showing the recommendations for healthy bones, including nutrition and exercise.
7. Use the Internet to investigate and make a poster or pamphlet that describes the methods for improving dental care and cosmetic appearance.

Explore the Web

Bone Health

WebMD

http://www.webmd.com/osteoporosis/bone-mineral-density

National Institute of Arthritis and Musculoskeletal and Skin Disease (NIAMS)

http://www.niams.nih.gov/Health_Info/Bone/Bone_Health/Exercise/default.asp

Bone Repair

Medscape

http://www.medscape.com/viewarticle/405699_6

Medline

http://www.nlm.nih.gov/medlineplus/ency/article/002966.htm

Dental Hygiene

Academy of General Dentistry

http://www.agd.org/public/oralhealth/Default.asp?IssID=290&Topic=B&ArtID=1123#body

American Dental Association (ADA)

http://www.ada.org/public/topics/whitening_faq.asp

CHAPTER 15

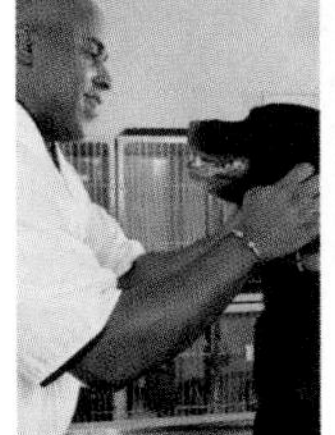
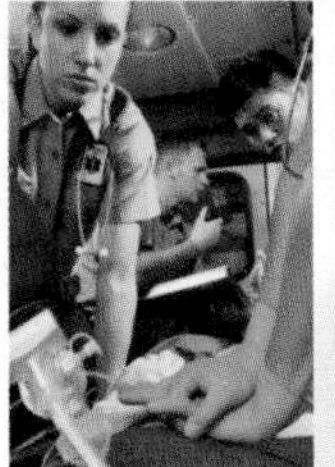
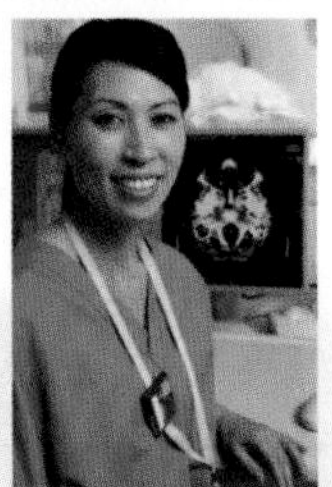

Muscular System

LEARNING OBJECTIVES

- Define at least 10 terms relating to the muscular system.
- Describe the six functions of the muscular system.
- Identify at least 10 structures of the muscular system and the function of each.
- Describe at least three methods of assessment of the muscular system.
- Describe at least five disorders of the muscular system.

KEY TERMS

Antagonist *(an-TAG-uh-nist)* Muscle that acts in opposition to the action of another muscle, which is its agonist

Atrophy *(AT-ro-fee)* Wasting away, decrease in size

Contraction *(kon-TRAK-shun)* Shortening or development of tension in muscle tissue

Contracture *(kon-TRAK-chur)* Permanent shortening of tendons and ligaments of a joint resulting from atrophy of muscle

Dystrophy *(DIS-tro-fee)* Muscle disorder resulting from defective or faulty nutrition, abnormal development, or infection

Myalgia *(my-AL-jee-uh)* Muscle pain

Paralysis *(puh-RAL-ih-sis)* Loss or impairment of motor function

Posture *(POS-chur)* Attitude or position of the body

Prime mover *(prime MOO-ver)* Muscle that acts directly to bring about a desired movement, agonist

Range of motion *(raynj uhv MO-shen)* Active or passive movement of muscle groups to full extent possible, used to prevent contracture

Sarcomere *(SAR-ko-meer)* Repeating units of muscle fibers with the ability to contract

Skeletal *(SKEL-e-tal)* Pertaining to the framework of the body

KEY TERMS cont'd

Stimulus *(STIM-yoo-lus)* Any agent, act, or influence that produces a change in the development or function of tissues

Tonus *(TO-nus)* Slight, continuous contraction of muscle

Visceral *(VIS-er-al)* Pertaining to any large interior organ in any one of the cavities of the body

Muscular System Terminology*

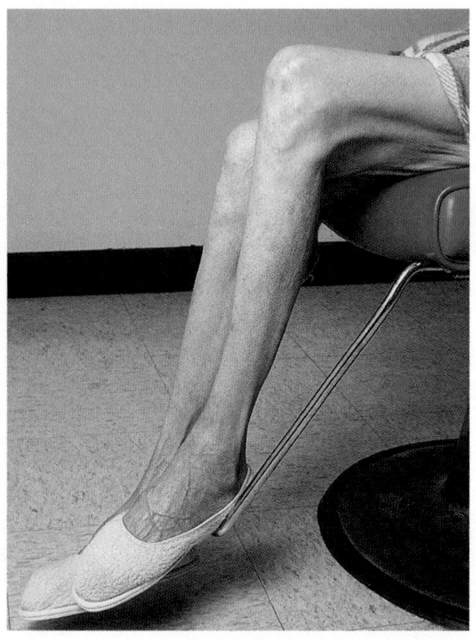

Atrophy or wasting of muscle tissue may result from immobility, such as bed rest. (From Sorrentino SA: *Mosby's textbook for nursing assistants,* ed 7, St. Louis, 2008, Mosby.)

Term	Definition	Prefix	Root	Suffix
Atrophy	Without growth, wasting away	a	troph	y
Biceps	Muscle with two heads	bi	ceps	
Blepharospasm	Uncontrolled muscle contraction of the eyelid		blepharo	spasm
Dystrophy	Faulty growth	dys	troph	y
Fibromyositis	Inflammation of the muscle tissues	fibro	my/os	itis
Myalgia	Muscle pain		my	algia
Myoma	Tumor of the muscle		my	oma
Myometrium	Muscle of the uterus	my/o	metrium	
Quadriceps	Muscle with four heads	quadr/i	ceps	
Visceral	Pertaining to the inside		viscer	al

*A transition syllable or vowel may be added to or deleted from the word parts to make the combining form.

Structure and Function of the Muscular System

The human body has more than 600 muscles. The three types of muscle tissue are skeletal, visceral, and cardiac (Table 15-1). Muscles do the following:

- Aid in movement
- Provide and maintain posture
- Protect internal organs
- Provide movement of blood, food, and waste products through the body
- Open and close body openings
- Produce heat (Fig. 15-1)

Muscle contraction is the movement of muscles when stimulated. Tonus is the muscle's ability to maintain

Abbreviations of the Muscular System

Abbreviation	Meaning
ATP	Adenosine triphosphate
Bx	Biopsy
Ca^{+2}	Calcium
EMG	Electromyogram
IM	Intramuscular
LP	Lumbar puncture
MD	Muscular dystrophy
MI	Myocardial infarction
OT	Occupational therapy
PT	Physical therapy

TABLE 15-1
Types of Muscle Tissue

Muscles	Appearance	Manner of Control
Skeletal	Striated	Voluntary
Visceral	Smooth	Involuntary
Cardiac	Indistinctly striated	Involuntary

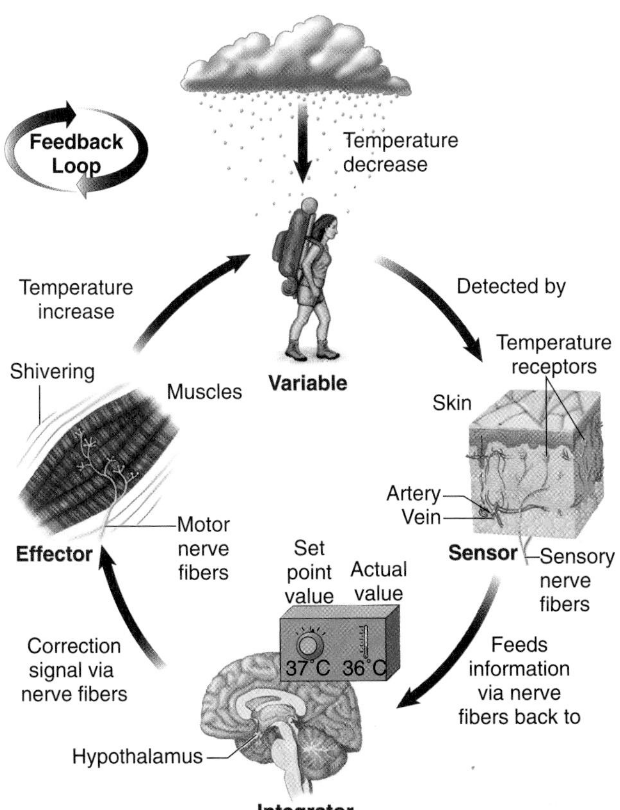

FIGURE 15-1 A drop in body temperature is corrected by muscle contraction (shivering) that produces heat. (From Patton KT, Thibodeau GA: *Anatomy & physiology*, ed 7, St. Louis, 2010, Mosby.)

slight, continuous contraction. Muscles can be stimulated electrically, mechanically, or chemically. Muscles are flaccid, or soft, when not contracted. Muscle tissue has several unique characteristics:

- Irritability or excitability is the muscle's ability to respond to a **stimulus** such as a nerve or hormone.
- Contractility is the muscle's ability to shorten forcefully when stimulated.
- Extensibility is the muscle's ability to stretch and lengthen.
- Elasticity is the muscle's ability to recoil to its resting length when relaxed.

BRAIN BYTE

The face has more than 30 muscles that create surprise, happiness, sadness, and frowning images. Fourteen muscles create a smile, whereas 43 create a frown.

Types of Muscle Tissue

Skeletal Muscle

Skeletal muscles make up more than 40% of a person's body weight. They increase in size and weight with exercise and decrease with inactivity. Muscle size and strength vary among people because of genetic differences and nutritional and exercise habits. Muscles are attached to bones by tendons, which are narrow strips of dense connective tissue. Muscles are named according to their location, related bones, shape, action, or size (Fig. 15-2).

Skeletal muscle tissue looks striated, or banded, under the microscope (Fig. 15-3). Striated muscle is made of bundles of fine fibers. The number of muscle fibers does not increase much after birth. Increase in muscle mass is due to an increase in the size of the fibers. Fascia is a layer of fibrous connective tissue that separates individual muscles.

The basic unit of muscle fibers that causes muscle contraction is called a **sarcomere**. Sarcomeres are organized units made up of actin and myosin myofibrils. Most skeletal muscles contract under a person's voluntary control.

Skeletal muscles have three parts (Fig. 15-4):

- The origin is one end of the muscle, attached to the less movable part of the bone.
- The insertion is the other end of the muscle, attached to the more movable part of the bone.
- The action, or body, is the thick, middle part of the muscle.

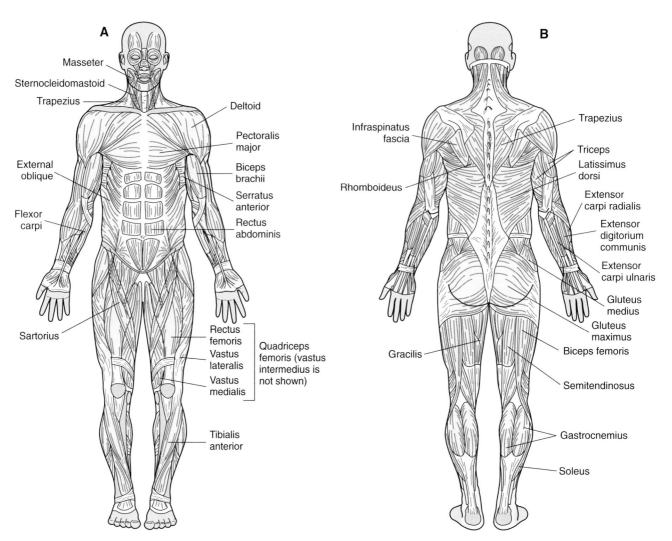

FIGURE 15-2 Common muscle groups. **A,** Front view. **B,** Back view. (From Sorrentino S: *Mosby's textbook for nursing assistants*, ed 7, St. Louis, 2008, Mosby.)

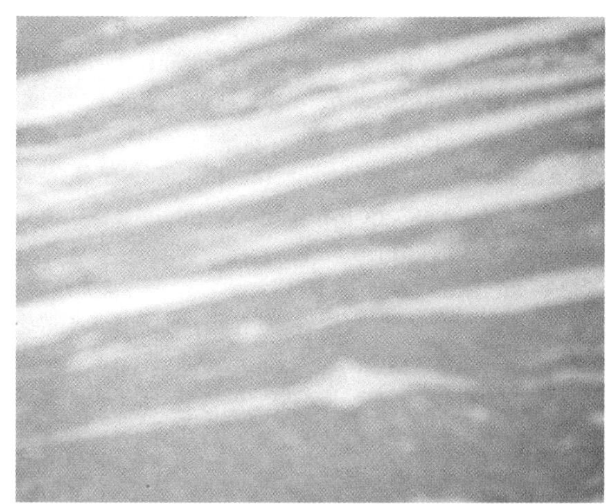

FIGURE 15-3 Skeletal muscle tissue.

- Skeletal muscles produce movement by pulling bones. Fig. 15-5 shows how skeletal muscles work in pairs; one contracts and pulls while its counteracting muscle relaxes.
- The **prime mover**, or agonist muscle, pulls to cause the movement.
- The **antagonist** muscle relaxes when the agonist contracts.
- Other muscles, called *synergists* and *fixators*, help keep the muscle and bone stable during movement.

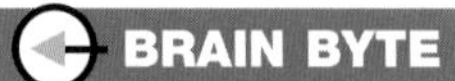

Muscles make up about 50% of your body weight.

Skeletal muscles can make seven basic types of body movements (Fig. 15-6). Flexion moves a bone closer to another bone, and extension moves a bone farther from another bone. Rotation is a circular or

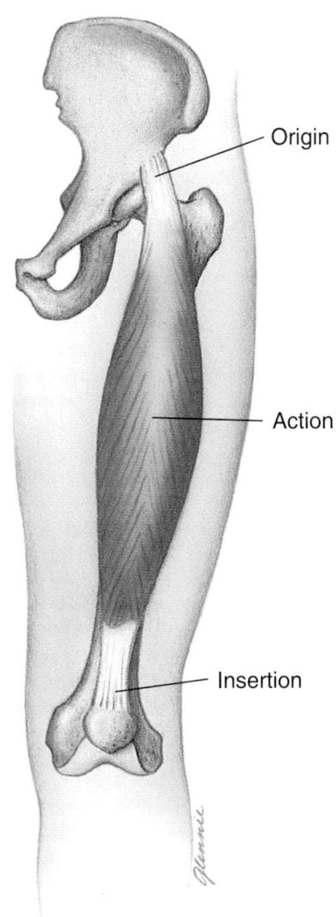

FIGURE 15-4 Parts of a muscle.

semicircular motion. Abduction is movement of a body part away from the midline, and adduction is movement toward the midline. Pronation is turning the hand or foot downward or backward, and supination is the opposite of pronation, turning the hand or foot upward or forward.

Visceral Muscle

Visceral muscle lines various hollow organs, makes up the walls of blood vessels, and is found in the tubes of the digestive system. Visceral muscle is smooth and has no striations like the bands of the skeletal muscle (Fig. 15-7). Like skeletal muscle, it contracts when stimulated. Visceral muscles are controlled by the autonomic nervous system. One example of a visceral muscle is the sphincter (circular) muscles, which open and close the pupil of the eye.

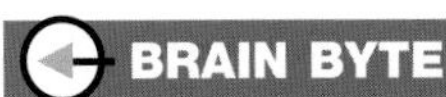

The largest muscle in the body is the gluteus maximus in the buttocks, and the smallest muscles are in the middle ear.

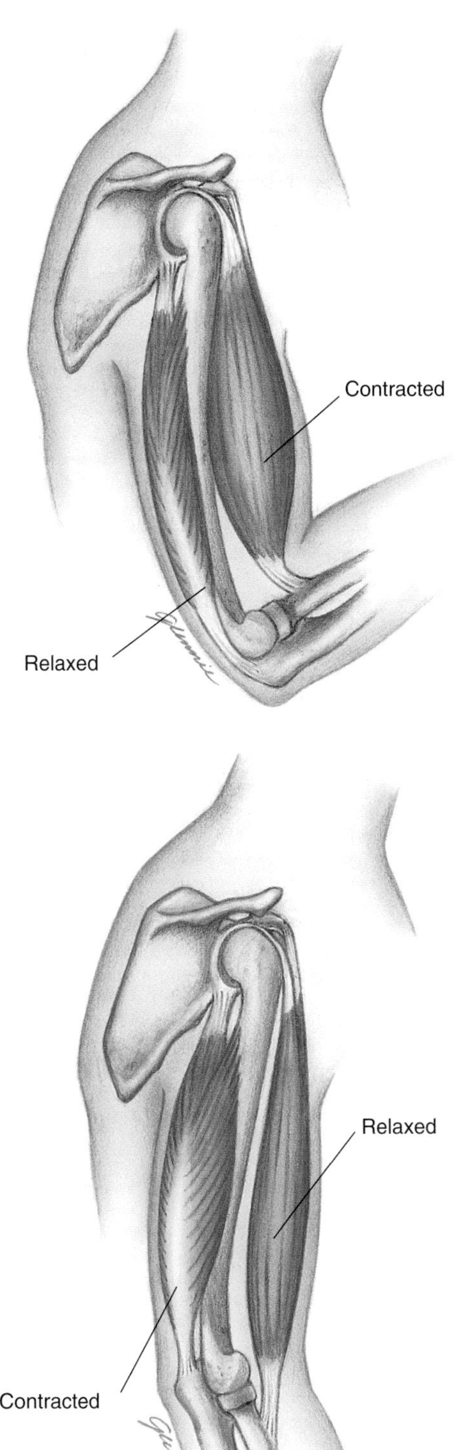

FIGURE 15-5 Skeletal muscle movement.

Cardiac Muscle

Cardiac muscle is found only in the heart. It is indistinctly striated muscle and is under involuntary control (Fig. 15-8). Cardiac muscle has specialized cells that provide a stimulus for contraction. Because of this

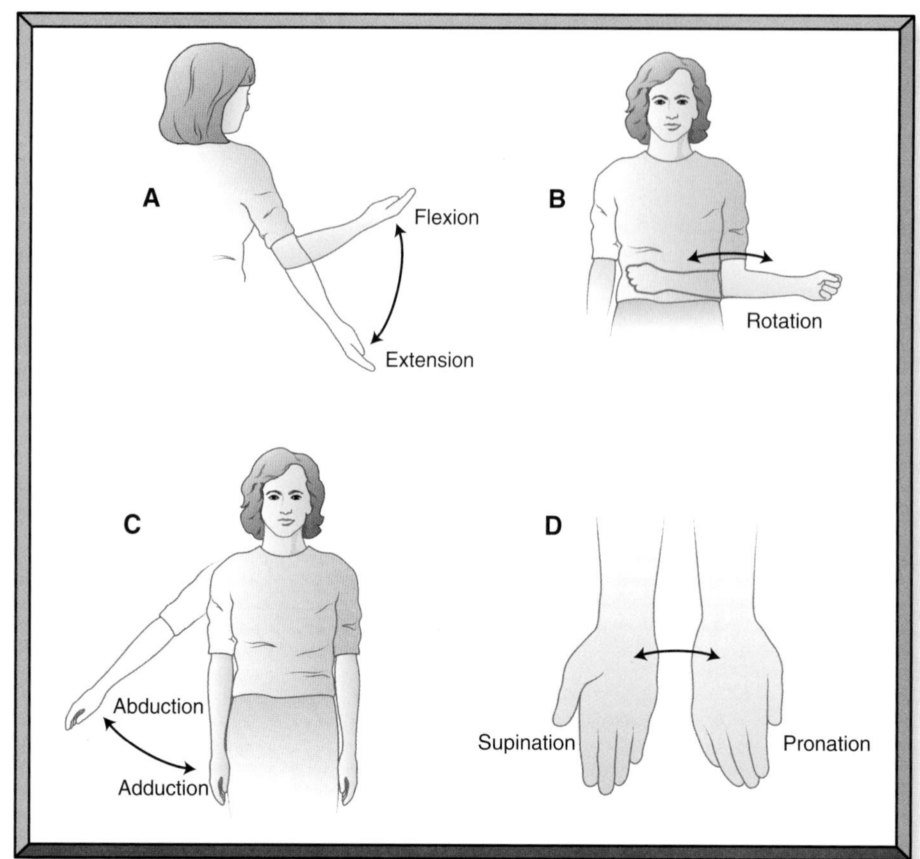

FIGURE 15-6 Types of muscle movement. **A,** Flexion and extension. **B,** Rotation. **C,** Abduction and adduction. **D,** Pronation and supination.

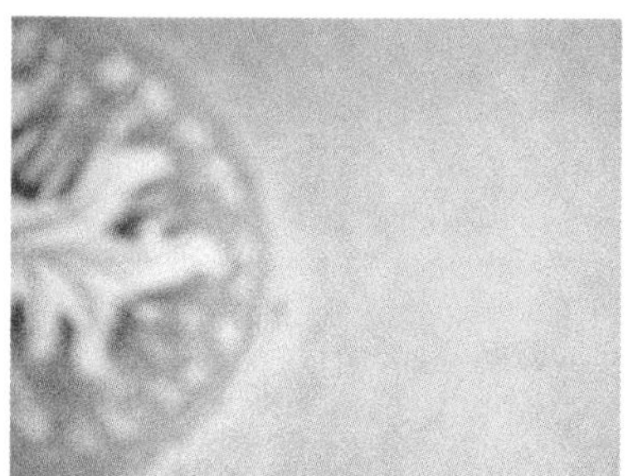

FIGURE 15-7 Visceral muscle tissue.

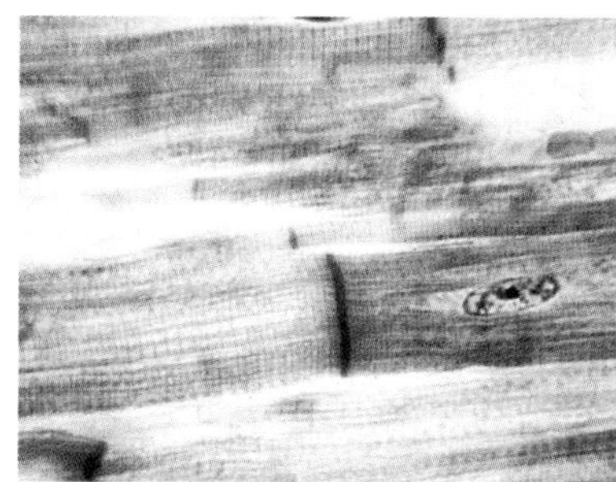

FIGURE 15-8 Cardiac muscle tissue. (Courtesy Ward's Natural Science Establishment, Rochester, N.Y.)

"pacemaker," the heart continues beating when not stimulated by neural impulses. Chapter 11 provides more information about the heart.

How Muscles Contract

When stimulated, a complex chain of molecular actions is responsible for muscle contraction. One theory used to explain this process is the sliding filament theory of muscle contraction. It states that proteins and other molecules in the muscle tissue interact when stimulated, and the resulting molecules are shorter than they were originally, thereby making the tissue contract.

Muscle cells use a form of glucose (glycogen) to provide the energy used for contraction. The glucose is used to fuel the adenosine diphosphate–adenosine triphosphate (ADP-ATP) cycle for energy production in the muscle cells. In the ADP-ATP cycle, ADP combines with a phosphate to store energy as ATP and breaks this bond to release energy for use by the muscle tissue. The ADP-ATP cycle provides the energy necessary to combine the proteins actin and myosin into actomyosin. Calcium is necessary for the reaction to occur. The lactic acid that is produced from the metabolism of glycogen is converted to water and carbon dioxide in the presence of oxygen. If oxygen is in short supply, lactic acid, a by-product of this process, can build up in the muscle and cause soreness. Heat is produced by this action as another by-product.

Types of Muscle Contraction

The strength of a muscle contraction depends on the strength of nerve impulses received in the muscle from the brain. Each muscle fiber contracts either completely or not at all. The stimulus must be strong enough to cause the contraction. This is the "all-or-none" law of skeletal muscle contraction. Not all muscle contractions are the same.

- Isotonic contraction is muscle shortening that produces movement such as skeletal muscle movement during exercise.
- Muscle tone or tonus is a state of partial contraction that maintains a person's posture.
- Isometric contraction does not cause muscle shortening or movement, such as in the motion of pushing against a fixed object like a wall.
- A twitch is a quick, jerky contraction of a whole muscle from one stimulus.
- Tetanic contraction is more sustained than a twitch and is caused by many stimuli in rapid succession. Tetany is continued contraction of a skeletal muscle.
- Fibrillation is uncoordinated contraction of muscle fibers.
- Convulsions are contractions of groups of muscles in an abnormal manner.
- Spasms are involuntary, sudden, and prolonged contractions.

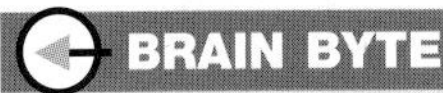

The strongest muscle is the masseter in the jaw.

Assessment Techniques

The muscular system can be assessed in numerous ways. With general inspection, the muscular system is assessed for asymmetry, deformity, swelling, or bruising. With systematic movement of body parts, muscle groups can be assessed for weakness. Reflex tests assess the neurologic functioning of the muscular system. The range of joint motion produced by skeletal muscles can be measured by using a protractor. Blood tests measuring enzymes may indicate muscular system damage. Electromyography (EMG) tests individual muscles through needles inserted into the muscle. A muscle biopsy may be used to assess for tissue disorders. The Gait Abnormality Rating Scale is used to determine the risk of falls in older adults.

DISORDERS OF THE Muscular System

Back pain, a common disorder, usually results from weakened muscles around the spine in the lower back. Recurrent back pain can be caused by a sedentary lifestyle, obesity, poor posture, or muscle tone. Back pain may also result from muscle strain or pressure on the sciatica nerve of the leg. The treatment includes bracing the back for support, heat applications, and exercises to strengthen the muscles. Medication may be used for pain or muscle spasm.

CASE STUDY 15-1 Your patient is lying on her back every time you come in the room. During her bath, you notice a red spot on her sacral area. What should you do?

Answers to Case Studies are available on the Evolve website: ***http://evolve.elsevier.com/Gerdin***

Contracture is a condition in which muscles remain contracted as a joint loses flexibility and ligaments and tendons shorten. Contractures result from gradual muscle wasting, called atrophy, because of a lack of movement of the muscles. Contractures can be prevented with range of motion (ROM) exercises. Treatment of severe contractures may involve surgical cutting of ligaments.

A *muscle cramp* is a sudden, involuntary contraction of a muscle producing pain. Cramps usually occur in the legs or feet. Cramps may result from exertion or unknown causes, as with the common cramps that occur at night. Treatment includes stretching and gentle pressure to relieve the pain.

CASE STUDY 15-2 Your friend suddenly has a cramp or "charley horse" in the calf of his leg while you are running. What should you do?

Answers to Case Studies are available on the Evolve website: ***http://evolve.elsevier.com/Gerdin***

Muscular *dystrophy* is a group of genetic diseases involving painless, gradual atrophy of muscle tissue. Duchenne muscular dystrophy, a severe X-linked form, occurs in 1 of every 3000 to 5000 boys. It can be detected with 95% accuracy during pregnancy. Becker muscular dystrophy is a milder form. Severe forms cause total disability, and others cause a mild disability. No cure has been found. Treatment may include medication to slow the progression of the disease, braces, or corrective surgery. Research in gene therapy is being conducted as a treatment for this disorder.

Fibromyalgia (fie-bro-my-AL-jee-uh) includes a group of muscle disorders affecting the tendons, ligaments, and other fibrous tissues. Common sites of pain include the neck, shoulders, thorax, lower back (lumbago), and thighs. Fibromyalgia does not cause inflammation. The person with fibromyalgia feels pain and tenderness after being exposed to cold, dampness, illness, or minor trauma. Generalized myalgia usually occurs in women. Treatment includes decrease in stress, rest, heat, massage, therapy to stretch the muscles, and exercise.

CASE STUDY 15-3 Your patient has been lying down in bed all day and complains of generalized muscle pain. What should you do?

Answers to Case Studies are available on the Evolve website: ***http://evolve.elsevier.com/Gerdin***

Gangrene (GANG-green) is caused by *Clostridium*, a bacterium that kills muscle tissue (Fig. 15-9). Gangrene begins when the bacteria enter an area of muscle tissue that has died. The bacteria destroy the surrounding living tissue. The condition may also result from a blocked blood vessel (thrombosis). The extremities are most often affected, but the gallbladder or intestines may become infected in some cases. Treatment includes removal of dead tissue, antibiotics, and medication against the toxins produced by the bacteria.

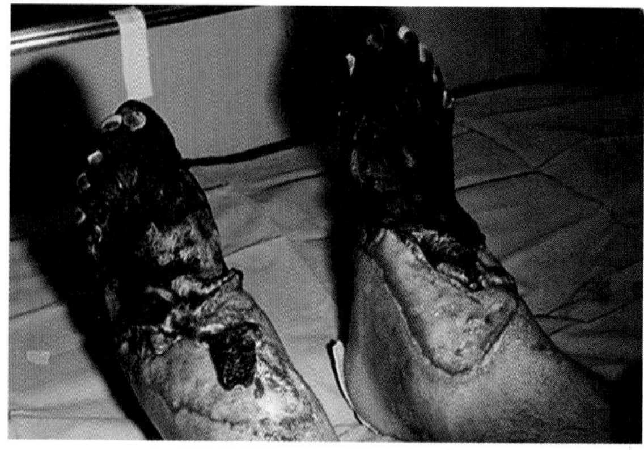

FIGURE 15-9 Gangrene is caused by an anaerobic bacterium, *Clostridium*. (Courtesy Cameron Bangs, MD. From Auerbach PS: *Wilderness medicine: management of wilderness and environmental emergencies*, ed 3, St. Louis, 1995, Mosby.)

A *hernia* (HER-nee-uh) is the abnormal protrusion of a body part into another body area. An example is the protrusion of the intestine through abdominal muscles in the groin area. Hernias may result from weakness in the muscles of the abdomen. Treatment may include bracing, a surgical procedure to restore proper positioning, and medication.

Myasthenia gravis (my-us-THEE-nee-uh GRAV-is) is a condition in which nerve impulses are not transmitted normally from the brain to the muscles. The cause of myasthenia gravis is not known, although it is considered to be an autoimmune disorder. Muscle weakness in different body areas eventually becomes severe, although remission may occur. No cure is available. Treatment may include medication, removal of the thymus, and maintaining life support if necessary.

Poliomyelitis (po-lee-O-my-eh-LI-tis) is a viral infection that results in paralysis of muscles. Polio can be prevented by a vaccine. No cure has been found. Treatment is directed toward relieving symptoms.

Muscle sprain (sprane) is traumatic injury to the tendons, muscles, or ligaments of a joint. It causes pain and swelling. Treatment includes alternating application of heat and cold, rest, and ultrasound.

Muscle strain (strane) is torn or stretched tendons and muscles, causing pain. It may occur if muscles are exerted too suddenly or for too long. In severe cases, muscles may break in two pieces, leaving a gap in the middle. Treatment includes stopping the activity, elevating the arm or leg, and applying ice to minimize swelling. Some treatments alternate cold and hot applications.

Pes planus (pez-PLANE-us) also called "flatfoot" or "fallen arches," may be congenital or result from weakened foot muscles. It causes extreme pain. Treatment includes corrective shoes, massage, and special exercises.

Tetanus (TET-uh-nus), commonly called "lockjaw," is caused by a bacterial infection. Muscle spasms may be severe and can result in death. Tetanus can be prevented by vaccination. No cure has been found. Treatment involves preventing complications of muscle spasm and life support.

Trichinosis (trik-i-NO-sis) is a parasitic infection caused by eating undercooked pork. The parasites form cysts in muscle tissues, especially the diaphragm and chest muscles. Infection causes pain, tenderness, and fatigue. The infection can be fatal if it affects the brain or heart. Treatment includes fluids, nutritional support, and medication to relieve pain, reduce fever, and kill the parasites.

Issues and Innovations

Sports Medicine

Many people think of sports medicine as a new health field, but actually it has long existed as a medical specialty. In 1928 the International Sports Medicine Federation was organized. In 1954 the American College of Sports Medicine was formed. It is the primary organization for this specialty in the United States. Sports medicine is involved in all sports and athletics. More than just treating sports injuries, trainers and doctors also direct the healthful development and training of athletes. Chapter 31 provides more information about career opportunities in athletic training.

Athletic injuries include strains, sprains, cuts, bruises, and similar conditions, many affecting the muscular system. Such injuries can be serious and take months to heal. Most sports injuries result from poor flexibility, overtraining, poor training methods, inadequate equipment, or muscle imbalance.

The field of biomechanics, the study of muscles in movement, applies the laws of mechanics and physics to human performance. Other methods of treatment for sports injury include ultrasound and electrical stimulation to increase circulation and promote healing.

Injecting a patient's own blood into an injured area has been shown to promote muscle repair and help regenerate tendon and ligament fibers. This procedure is called *platelet-rich plasma therapy*.

CASE STUDY 15-4 Your friend tells you that he does not need to stretch before running because he is young. What should you say?

Answers to Case Studies are available on the Evolve website: ***http://evolve.elsevier.com/Gerdin***

Fitness Fad

In 2008 the Centers for Disease Control and Prevention reported that more than 20% of the population of every state except Colorado was obese. Six states reported that more than 30% of their population were obese. They define obesity as a body mass index of 30 or more. They report that about half of young people age 12 to 21 do not regularly exercise actively. Regular exercise improves physical fitness and health and also promotes a feeling of well-being. People who exercise on a regular basis feel better about themselves and manage stress and tension more easily.

In the past 10 years, many new health clubs and spas have opened to provide facilities for exercise. When choosing an exercise club, some features to consider include the staff's credentials, how crowded or spacious the facilities are, the cleanliness of the club, and the contract terms.

Becoming too concerned with exercise is possible. For some people, exercise may come to take priority over family, work, and friends. Psychologists believe that this obsession results from the person becoming dependent on the "high" of exercise. This feeling results from a chemical called *endorphin* (en-DOOR-fin) that is released by the brain during exercise.

A person who has become obsessed with exercise feels he or she needs to work out daily to be even minimally functional. Such an "addicted" person feels withdrawal symptoms such as irritability and depression when not regularly exercising. A sign that a person has a problem is his or her continuing to exercise when ill or injured.

Summary

- Functions of the muscular system include movement, posture, protection of internal organs, transport of blood, and producing heat.

- Structures of the muscular system include the skeletal, visceral, and cardiac muscles. Skeletal muscles include the biceps, triceps, quadriceps, deltoid, masseter, and gracilis.
- Methods of assessment of the muscular system include inspection, electromyogram, and blood and reflex tests.
- Disorders of the muscular system include contractures, cramps, dystrophy, poliomyelitis, and gangrene.

Review Questions

1. Describe the six functions of the muscular system.
2. Identify the functional and structural units of the muscular system.
3. Describe three muscular system disorders that are caused by infectious agents.
4. Describe three methods used to assess the function of the muscular system.
5. List three benefits of maintaining a regular exercise program.
6. Use the following terms in one or more sentences that correctly relate their meaning: atrophy, contracture, posture, range of motion, and skeletal.

Critical Thinking

1. Investigate and compare the cost of at least three tests used in diagnosing disorders of the muscular system.
2. Investigate the function of at least five common medications used in the treatment of muscular system disorders.
3. List at least five occupations involved in the health care of muscular system disorders.
4. Classify the following muscle movements as voluntary or involuntary action:

Blinking	Laughing
Digestion	Pupil size
Eye movement	Respiration
Facial grimace	Snapping fingers
Heartbeat	Swallowing

5. Research rehabilitation training programs utilizing progressive-resistance and variable-resistance machines and other new treatments for sports injury.
6. Research and review an article regarding a recent development or treatment method relating to the muscular system.
7. Use the Internet to research and create a personalized fitness and activity calendar.
8. Use the Internet to compare the obesity rate of your state and the national trend.

Explore the Web

Fitness

CDC

http://www.cdc.gov/NCCDPHP/sgr/ataglan.htm

BAM

http://www.bam.gov/sub_physicalactivity/

Obesity

CDC

http://apps.nccd.cdc.gov/PASurveillance/StateSumV.asp

CHAPTER 16

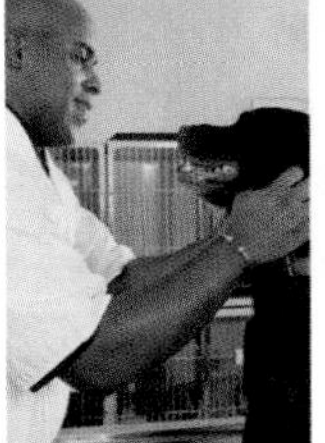
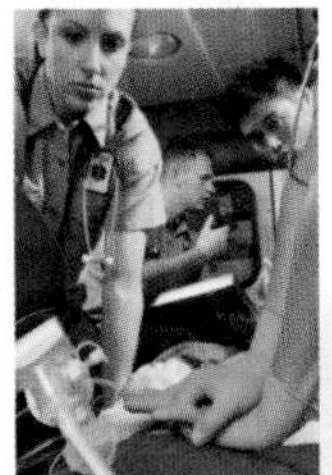
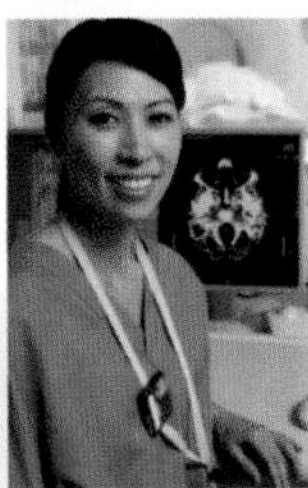

Digestive System

LEARNING OBJECTIVES

- Define at least 10 terms relating to the digestive system.
- Describe the four functions of the digestive system.
- Identify at least 10 digestive system structures and the function of each.
- Identify the location and function of three accessory organs of the digestive system.
- Identify at least three methods of assessment of the digestive system.
- Describe at least five disorders of the digestive system.

KEY TERMS

Alactasia *(a-lak-TAY-zee-uh)* Malabsorption or inability to absorb lactose caused by a deficiency of the enzyme lactase

Bile *(BY-uhl)* Fluid that helps digest fat in the small intestine; produced by the liver and stored in the gallbladder

Bolus *(BO-les)* Rounded mass of food

Bulimia *(buh-LEEM-ee-uh)* Excessive binge eating, which may be followed by self-induced vomiting or purging

Cholecystectomy *(ko-le-sis-TEK-to-me)* Surgical removal of the gallbladder

Chyme *(Kime)* Thick, semiliquid contents of stomach during digestion

Defecation *(def-ih-KAY-shen)* Evacuation of waste or fecal material from the rectum

Deglutition *(dee-gloo-TISH-en)* Act of swallowing

Emesis *(EM-eh-sis)* Act of vomiting, vomit

Endoscopy *(en-DOS-ko-pee)* Visual inspection of a body cavity using a scope

Enema *(EN-uh-muh)* Liquid instilled into rectum

Flatulence *(FLACH-uh-lents)* Excessive air or gas in stomach or intestines leading to distention of organs

Ingestion *(in-JES-chen)* Taking food or medicine into the body through the mouth

KEY TERMS cont'd

Jaundice *(JAWN-dis)* Yellow appearance resulting from bile pigment stored in the skin and sclera of the eyes

Mastication *(mas-tik-KAY-shen)* Process of chewing food

Peristalsis *(per-ih-STOL-sis)* Wavelike series of contractions of the digestive system that propels the contents

Sphincter *(SFINK-ter)* Ringlike band of muscle that closes a passage or opening

Villus *(VIL-es)* One of many tiny vascular projections on the surface of the small intestine

Digestive System Terminology*

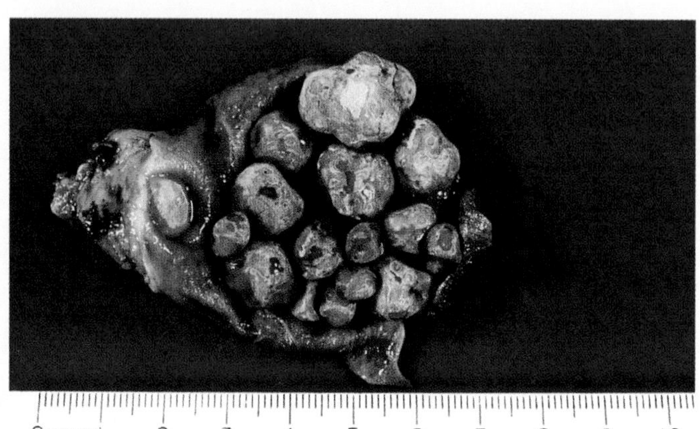

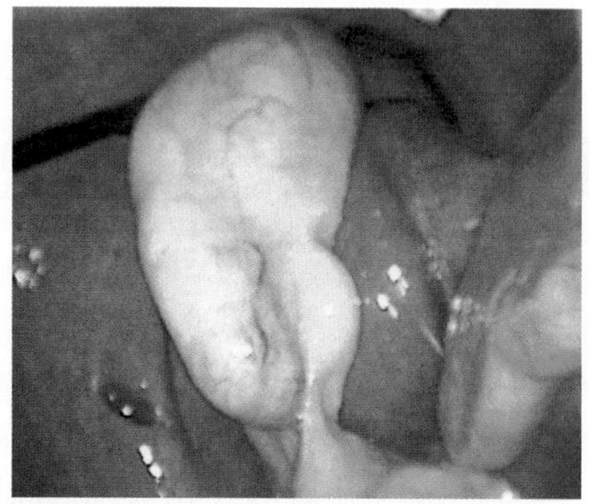

Gallbladder and gallstones. **A,** Surgery to remove gallstones is called a cholecystectomy. **B,** Laparoscopic view of gallbladder with yellow cholesterol gallstones. (From Patton KT, Thibodeau GA: *Anatomy & physiology,* ed 7, St. Louis, 2010, Mosby.)

Term	Definition	Prefix	Root	Suffix
Appendectomy	Removal of the appendix		append	ectomy
Cholecystectomy	Removal of the gallbladder	chole	cyst	ectomy
Colocentesis	Surgical puncture into the colon		colo	centesis
Enteritis	Inflammation of the intestines		enter	itis
Hematemesis	Vomiting of blood		hemat	emesis
Hepatitis	Inflammation of the liver		hepat	itis
Laparotomy	Incision into the abdomen		lapar	otomy
Peptic	Pertaining to digestion		pept	ic
Proctoscopy	Examination of the rectum		proct/o	scopy
Visceral	Pertaining to the organs		viscer	al

*A transition syllable or vowel may be added to or deleted from the word parts to make the combining form.

Structure and Function of the Digestive System

The digestive system consists of the organs that make up the alimentary canal, or digestive tract, from the mouth to the anus (Fig. 16-1). The digestive tract is about 30 feet long. It is not a sterile system like the other internal organs because it is open to the outside environment at both ends.

The main function of the digestive system, also called the *gastrointestinal system,* is to break down food to a form that can be used by body cells. The digestive process includes transportation of food and wastes, physical and chemical breakdown, absorption of digested food, and final elimination of wastes

Abbreviations of the Digestive System

Abbreviation	Meaning
ABD	Abdominal
BE	Barium enema
BM	Bowel movement
Cal	Calorie
cl liq	Clear liquid
FDA	Food and Drug Administration
GB	Gallbladder
GI	Gastrointestinal
NPO	Nothing by mouth
PO	By mouth (per os)

(Table 16-1). It also helps to maintain the proper amount of water, electrolytes, and other nutrients in the body.

Organs of the Digestive Process

Mouth

Food enters the alimentary canal at the mouth (**ingestion**). The teeth bite and chew the food to begin its physical breakdown. The tongue aids in tasting, chewing (**mastication**), and swallowing (**deglutition**) of food. The hard palate is the anterior roof of the

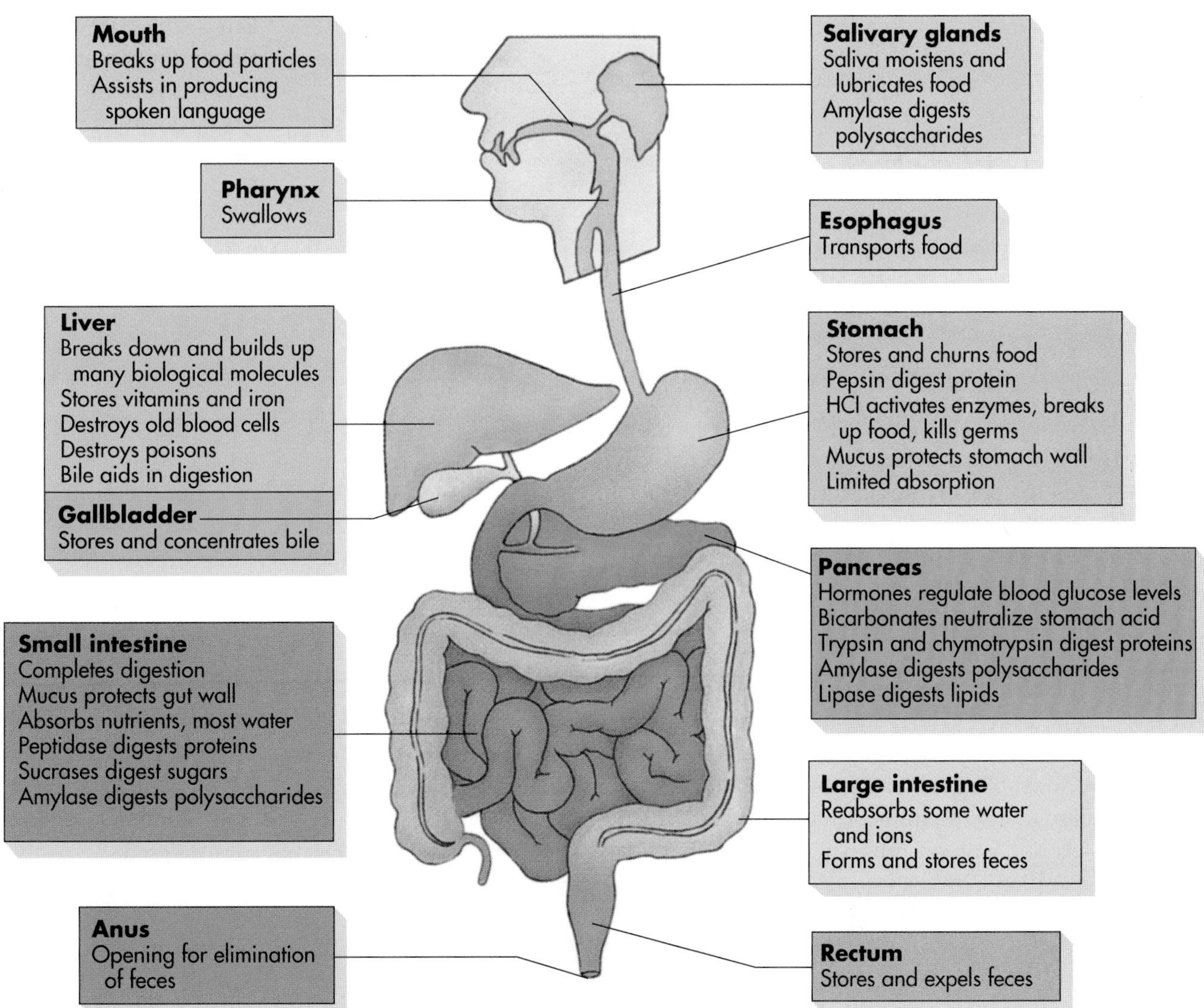

FIGURE 16-1 The digestive system is approximately 30 feet long. (From Patton KT, Thibodeau GA: *Anatomy & physiology*, ed 7, St. Louis, 2010, Mosby.)

TABLE 16-1
Digestive System

Organ	Size	Time for Food Passage	Enzymes Produced	Digestive Process
Mouth (salivary glands)		10-20 s (voluntary control)	Salivary amylase	Turn starch to glucose
			Mucus*	Lubricate
Pharynx			Mucus*	Lubricate
Esophagus	10-12 in (25-30 cm)	5-8 s	Mucus*	Lubricate
Stomach		1-4 h	Lipase	Digest fat
			Gastrin*	Stimulate hydrochloric acid
			Pepsinogen	Break down proteins
			Hydrochloric acid*	Dissolve minerals, kill bacteria
			Mucus*	Lubricate chyme, protect stomach lining
Pancreas			Pancreatin, trypsin	Break down protein
			Lipase	Break down fat
			Amylase, maltase	Break down starch
Liver	3 lb (1.4 kg)		Bile*	Break down fat
Small intestine		3-5 h	Sucrase, maltase	Break down sugar
Duodenum	10 in (25 cm)		Lactase	Break down lactose
Jejunum	8 ft (2.4 m)		Lipase	Break down fat
Ileum	12 ft (3.6 m)			
Large intestine	5 ft (1.5 m)	8-24 h	Mucus*	Lubricate
Appendix	3 in (7.5 cm)			Function unknown
Rectum	5 in (12.5 cm)	Voluntary control	Mucus*	Lubricate

*Not an enzyme.

mouth. Unlike the hard palate, the soft palate tissue is not attached to bone on the posterior portion of the mouth. The uvula is a small piece of tissue at the rear of the mouth that prevents food from entering the nasal cavity during swallowing.

As food is chewed it is mixed with saliva. Three salivary glands secrete an enzyme (amylase) that begins the chemical portion of the digestive process. An enzyme is a protein that increases the rate of a chemical activity in the body. The three salivary glands are the parotid, sublingual, and submandibular (Fig. 16-2). Amylase starts the transformation of starch to sugar. The portion of food mixed with saliva that is swallowed is called a **bolus**.

Pharynx

The pharynx, or throat, is divided into three portions called the *nasopharynx* (nose), *oropharynx* (mouth), and *laryngopharynx* (voice box). Food passes through the oropharynx from the mouth to the esophagus. The epiglottis is located at the junction of the esophagus and the oropharynx. The epiglottis is a small piece of tissue that closes off the trachea to prevent food and moisture from entering the respiratory tract.

Esophagus

The esophagus is a tubelike structure that carries food from the mouth to the stomach. The bolus of food moves down the esophagus to the stomach with a slow, wavelike motion. **Peristalsis** is a wave of contraction by which food is moved through the digestive system.

Stomach

In the stomach the food bolus mixes with hydrochloric acid and the enzymes pepsin and gastrin to become **chyme**. The stomach is a saclike muscular organ that

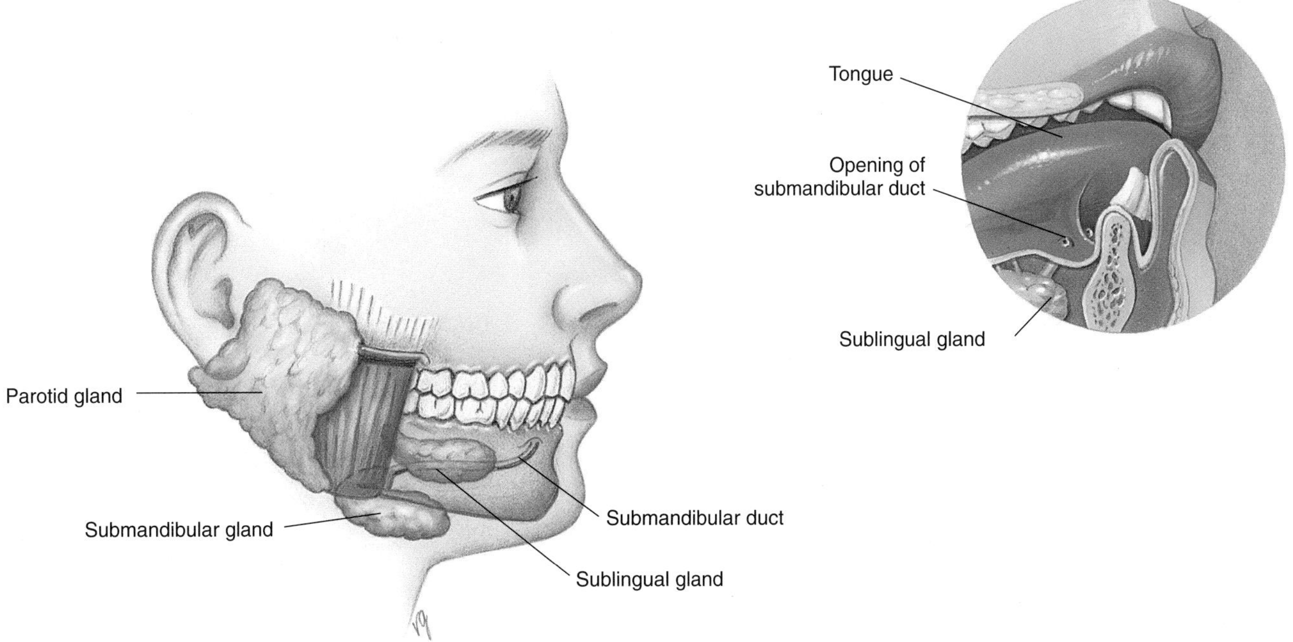

FIGURE 16-2 The salivary glands.

churns and squeezes food and continues its physical breakdown. Digestion of protein begins in the stomach. A few substances, such as glucose, some drugs, and alcohol, are absorbed directly into the blood through the stomach walls. The cardiac sphincter is a valve that prevents the chyme from flowing back into the esophagus. The pyloric sphincter controls the flow of the chyme into the intestines. It takes 1 to 4 hours for the stomach to empty the chyme into the intestines.

Small Intestine

From the stomach, the food enters the small intestine (Fig. 16-3). The small intestine is longer and narrower than the large intestine. It is lined with tiny threadlike projections of tissue called *villi* (singular, villus) that increase the area for absorption of nutrients. The three sections of the small intestine are the duodenum, jejunum, and ileum. The small intestine produces juices to aid the digestive process. Most absorption of digestive products occurs in the small intestine. When digestion is completed, carbohydrates have been reduced to sugar (monosaccharide and disaccharide). Protein has been changed to amino acid and dipeptide. Fats have been reduced to fatty acid and glyceride.

BRAIN BYTE

Large amounts and cool fluids empty from the stomach and are absorbed more quickly by the intestines than warm fluids. Fluids with high solutes empty slowly. After exercise, large amounts of cool, dilute fluids are best to replace what has been lost.

Large Intestine

The large intestine has three major portions, called the *ascending colon*, *transverse colon*, and *descending colon*. The appendix is a small tube of intestine descending from the side of the intestine with an unknown function in humans. Most of the water from ingested food is absorbed back into the blood through the walls of the large intestine, along with vitamins, electrolytes, and bile salts. The bacteria *Escherichia coli* (*E. coli*) normally reside in the large intestine and help to form feces and produce vitamin K.

The feces, or waste material, is collected in the rectum at the end of the large intestine and eliminated by defecation through the anus. Feces are composed of undigested food, bacteria, mucus, and water.

BRAIN BYTE

Within the colon, a typical person has more than 400 different species of bacteria.

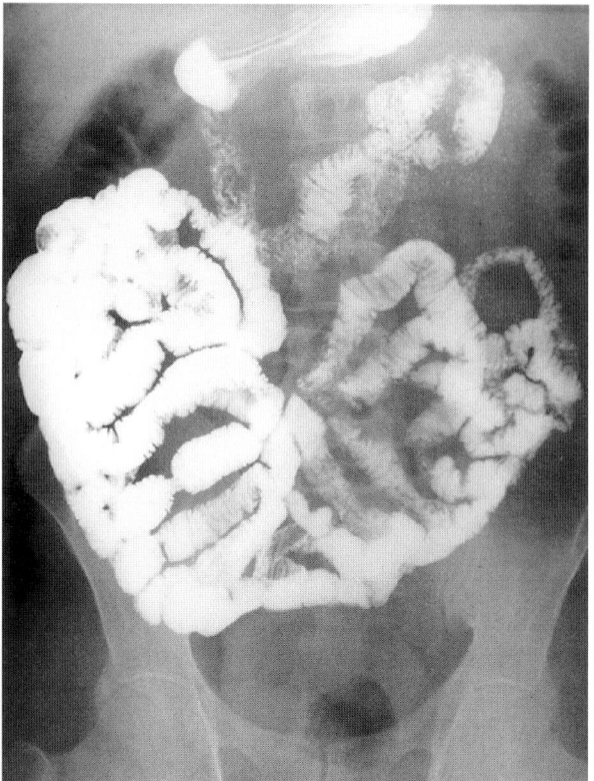

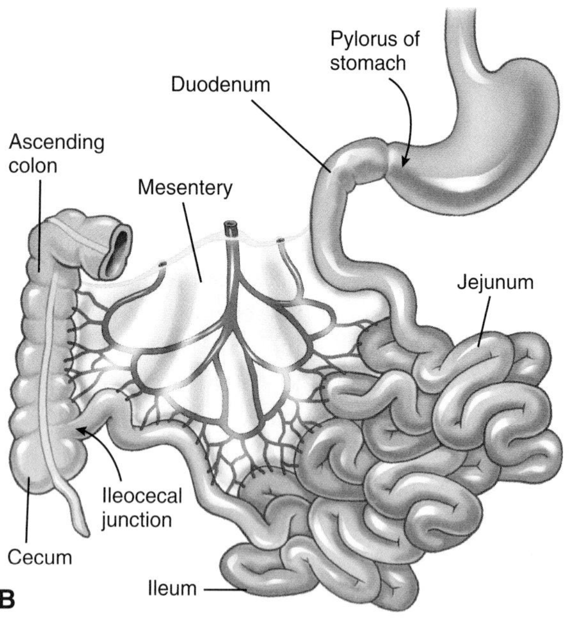

FIGURE 16-3 Small intestine. **A,** X-ray using barium. **B,** Stomach and intestines. (**A,** From Patton KT, Thibodeau GA: *Anatomy & physiology,* ed 7, St. Louis, 2010, Mosby. **B,** From *Mosby's dictionary of medicine, nursing & health professions,* ed 8, St. Louis, 2009, Mosby.)

Peritoneum

The peritoneum is a flat, serous (moist) membrane that surrounds the abdominal cavity. It lubricates and prevents friction between the organs. The mesentery is a fan-shaped projection of peritoneum that contains blood vessels and nerves. It provides support and helps to keep the abdominal organs in place by binding to them.

Accessory Organs of the Digestive System

The digestive system has three accessory organs; these organs aid the process of food breakdown. The exocrine, or ducted, organs carry digestive juices to the intestinal tract.

The pancreas is the only organ with both exocrine and endocrine functions. The exocrine function of the pancreas is to excrete digestive enzymes into the small intestine. The enzymes include pancreatin, trypsin, maltase, amylase, and lipase. Chapter 18 provides more information about the endocrine function of the pancreas.

The liver is the largest gland in the body. It has many important functions in addition to producing **bile** to assist in the digestion of fat. The liver converts glucose to a storage form called *glycogen*. It stores the fat-soluble vitamins (A, D, E, and K) and vitamin B12. It also breaks down many of the toxins taken into the body, including alcohol. It destroys old red blood cells, reprocesses the products, and synthesizes blood proteins. The liver also produces cholesterol, coagulation products, and antibodies.

The gallbladder, located adjacent to the liver, stores bile until the small intestine needs it for digestion of fatty food particles.

Assessment Techniques

Five types of assessment are commonly performed on the gastrointestinal system: radiography, **endoscopy**, gastric analysis, fecal analysis, and palpation and auscultation.

Radiography

Barium is an opaque substance that, when swallowed before radiographs (more commonly known as "x-rays") are taken, allows the structures of the esophagus, stomach, and small intestine to be seen. The rectum, colon, and lower portion of the small intestine can be evaluated on x-rays after a barium **enema**.

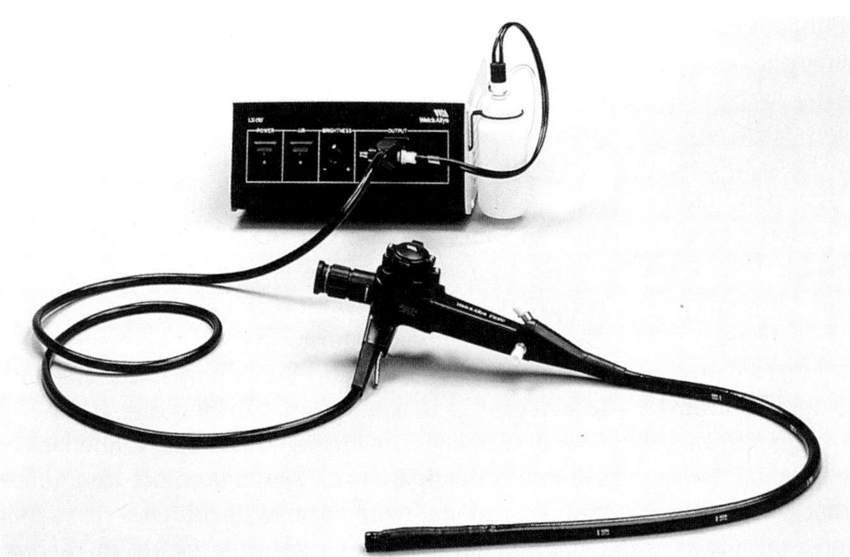

FIGURE 16-4 Endoscopy allows the health care worker to see inside the body. (Courtesy Welch Allyn, Skaneateles Falls, N.Y.)

The gallbladder can be assessed by using an ingested dye. The dye becomes part of the bile and aids visualization of the gallbladder on x-rays. Stones in the gallbladder may be seen as shadows.

Endoscopy

An endoscope is a small, flexible tube that can be inserted into body cavities, allowing the examiner to see body parts. Parts of the gastrointestinal system that can be assessed using an endoscope include the esophagus (esophagoscopy), stomach (gastroscopy), large intestine (colonoscopy), sigmoid colon (sigmoidoscopy), and rectum (proctoscopy) (Fig. 16-4).

Gastric Analysis

Gastric analysis is the study of the gastric juices in the stomach. A nasogastric tube is used to remove stomach contents. High levels of acid may indicate an ulcer, and low levels may be caused by anemia. Gastric analysis also may be performed using a special dye. The rate at which the dye appears in the urine is a measurement of the amount of stomach acid. Paracentesis or insertion of a needle into the abdominal cavity to remove fluids also may be performed to sample fluids outside the digestive tract.

Fecal Analysis

Stool specimens may be examined for the presence of microorganisms or blood (occult blood test). Watery or hard stools may indicate digestive disorders or an imbalance in diet and exercise. Black, tarry stools may indicate the presence of blood. Yellow, fatty stools may indicate a disorder of the liver.

Palpation and Auscultation

Feeling the abdomen (palpation) and listening to bowel sounds with a stethoscope (auscultation) are other methods of assessing the gastrointestinal system. A normal abdomen is flat and soft. Bowel sounds should be heard 5 to 35 times each minute.

DISORDERS OF THE Digestive System

Alactasia, also called *lactose intolerance*, is a common disorder. In individuals who do not produce enough of the enzyme lactase, unabsorbed lactose ferments in the intestines, leading to gas (**flatulence**), cramps, and diarrhea. Lactose, a form of sugar, is found in dairy products, such as milk. Treatment includes decreased lactose intake or dietary lactase supplements.

CASE STUDY 16-1 Your friend tells you that he does not want to go with you an afterschool event because he is embarrassed by the smell of his passing gas. What should you say?

Answers to Case Studies are available on the Evolve website: ***http://evolve.elsevier.com/Gerdin***

Appendicitis (ap-pen-dih-SI-tis) is inflammation of the appendix for unknown causes. It may be caused by a small piece of food that blocks the appendix passage or an infection. Appendicitis most often occurs between the ages of 10 and 30 and has a lifetime risk of 7%. The signs and symptoms of appendicitis vary greatly. The person with appendicitis may experience fever, pain in the right lower quadrant, and a high white blood cell count. The treatment is surgical removal of the appendix, called an *appendectomy*.

Cholecystitis (ko-le-sis-TIE-tis) is inflammation of the wall of the gallbladder. Stones formed from crystallized cholesterol, bile salts, and pigments also characterize it. The person with cholecystitis feels abdominal pain. Treatment includes diet changes to reduce fats. Stones may be dissolved nonsurgically by using bile acids or crushed with ultrasonic lithotripsy. In more severe cases, surgical removal of the gallbladder (**cholecystectomy**) is necessary. A laparoscopic cholecystectomy may be performed in some cases, preventing the need for major abdominal surgery.

Cirrhosis (ser-RO-sis) is a chronic degenerative condition of the liver accompanied by the formation of scar tissue. The person with cirrhosis may experience **jaundice**, skin lesions, demineralization of the bones, enlargement of the liver, anemia, and bleeding disorders. It may result from alcoholism and other infections (Fig. 16-5). The treatment is designed to relieve the symptoms, such as stopping any alcohol consumption and by diet modifications that allow the liver to rest. Cirrhosis can be fatal if the liver is severely damaged. It is the third most common cause of death of American adults 45 to 65 years of age and is usually related to alcoholism. Most deaths from cirrhosis in Asia and Africa are related to HBV.

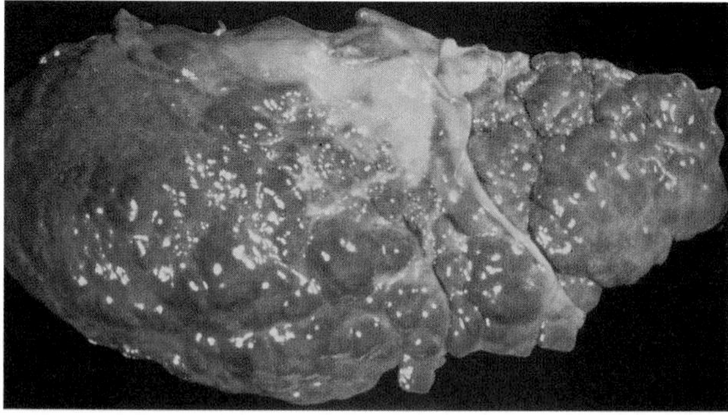

FIGURE 16-5 Chronic viral hepatitis is one of the causes of cirrhosis of the liver. (From Kumar V, Abbas AK, Fausto M: *Robbins and Cotran pathologic basis of disease*, ed 7, Philadelphia, 2005, Saunders.)

Colon (KO-lun) *cancer* is an abnormal growth in the large intestine. Warning signs of colon cancer include rectal bleeding, abdominal pain, and a change in bowel habits. An annual digital rectal examination and fecal occult blood test are recommended after the age of 50. Precancerous polyps can be removed to prevent cancer from occurring. Colon cancer can be treated by removal of the affected section and may require placement of an artificial anus or opening in the abdominal wall (colostomy).

Constipation (kon-stih-PAY-shun) is the inability to defecate. It is usually caused by a diet lacking in fiber or roughage, insufficient fluid intake, and lack of exercise. Constipation causes abdominal discomfort and distention. Treatment may include laxatives, but their frequent use may cause the bowel to become "lazy" and may be habit-forming.

CASE STUDY 16-2 Your patient tells you she does not drink water. She says she gets all the fluid she needs from food and other beverages. What should you say?

Answers to Case Studies are available on the Evolve website: ***http://evolve.elsevier.com/Gerdin***

Diarrhea (die-uh-REE-uh) is the passage of frequent and watery stools. It can be caused by infection, stress, or diet. Chronic diarrhea can lead to rectal tissue damage. Treatment includes a bland diet and medication (Table 16-2).

Diverticulitis (di-ver-tik-yoo-LIE-tis) is weakening of the colon wall leading to formation of a pouch (diverticula), causing infection or abscesses if fecal material is trapped. The cause is unknown. The person with diverticulitis experiences constipation, abdominal pain, loss of bowel sounds, and sometimes

TABLE 16-2
Bland Diet*

Eat	Avoid
Eggs	Raw fruits or vegetables
Meat	Carbonated beverages
Poultry	Spicy or seasoned foods
Fish	Rich desserts
Enriched fine cereals	
Milk	

*Mechanically, chemically, physiologically, and sometimes thermally nonirritating.

fever and rectal bleeding. Surgery may be required to remove the affected part.

Food poisoning is common and includes more than 250 illnesses transmitted by food. According to the CDC, *Campylobacter*, *Salmonella*, *E. coli*, and Norwalk viruses cause the most common food-borne illnesses. It also estimates 76 million cases and 5000 deaths each year. The person with food poisoning may experience headache, unrelenting diarrhea, vomiting (**emesis**), and fever. Treatment may include administration of antibiotics.

Gastritis (ga-strahy-Tis) is inflammation of the stomach lining, which may be caused by many factors, including the bacteria *Helicobacter pylori*. Symptoms of gastritis include stomach pain, heartburn, indigestion, and development of a peptic ulcer. Treatment for gastritis caused by *H. pylori* includes medications such as antacids to relieve symptoms, antibiotics to kill the bacteria, and proton pump inhibitors to heal the stomach lining.

Gastroesophageal reflux disease (**GERD**) (ga-stro-ih-sof-uh-GEE-uhl) occurs in approximately 60 million Americans each month. Over time this condition may lead to damage of the esophagus, difficulty swallowing, coughing, and an increased risk of throat cancer. Symptoms of GERD include frequent heartburn or chest pain, bitter taste in the mouth, difficulty swallowing, and frequent hoarseness or coughing. Treatment includes changes in the timing, type, and amount of food eaten and medications. If lifestyle changes and medication do not work, surgery may be used to improve the function of the esophageal sphincter that closes over the stomach.

CASE STUDY 16-3 Your patient asks for an antacid after eating lunch. When you ask if he is having heartburn, he says no, but he always takes antacids after eating to prevent it. What should you say?

Answers to Case Studies are available on the Evolve website: ***http://evolve.elsevier.com/Gerdin***

Halitosis, or bad breath, is caused by anaerobic bacteria that produce foul-smelling sulfur compounds on the surface of the tongue and in the throat. These bacteria assist in digestion by breaking down proteins found in specific foods, mucus or phlegm, blood, and in diseased or "broken-down" oral tissue. Factors that increase the production of these sulfur compounds include dry mouth, postnasal drip, a high-protein diet, and gum disease. Treatment of halitosis includes the use of compounds containing some combination of chlorine dioxide, oxychlorine, zinc compounds, and toothpaste that removes the odor. Treatment may also include scraping the tongue to remove the coating of white plaque.

Heartburn is a painful, burning sensation in the esophagus caused by the backflow of acidic chyme from the stomach. Losing excess weight, wearing loose clothing, and maintaining an upright position while eating can reduce this condition. Antacids may be used to neutralize the acid. Recurrent heartburn may indicate GERD.

A *hemorrhoid* (HEM-o-royd) is a painful, dilated vein in the lower rectum or anus. Hemorrhoids may be caused by straining to defecate, the pressure of an enlarged uterus during pregnancy, insufficient fluid intake, refined food, and abuse of laxatives. Treatment includes soaking the area with a sitz bath, fecal softeners, medication, and sometimes surgery.

Hepatitis (hep-uh-TIE-tis) is a viral infection of the liver. Hepatitis A, or contagious hepatitis, is transmitted in food or water by the feces of an infected person. Hepatitis B, or serum hepatitis, is transmitted in blood, saliva, and other body fluids. Hepatitis C, D, E (non-A, non-B), and G have also been described by researchers. Inflammation from the hepatitis B virus is generally more severe than hepatitis A. Inflammation of the liver may also result from infection by the Epstein-Barr virus, rubella, herpes simplex, and other viral diseases. With all types of hepatitis the person experiences abdominal pain, discolored feces, and yellowed skin, or jaundice (Fig. 16-6).

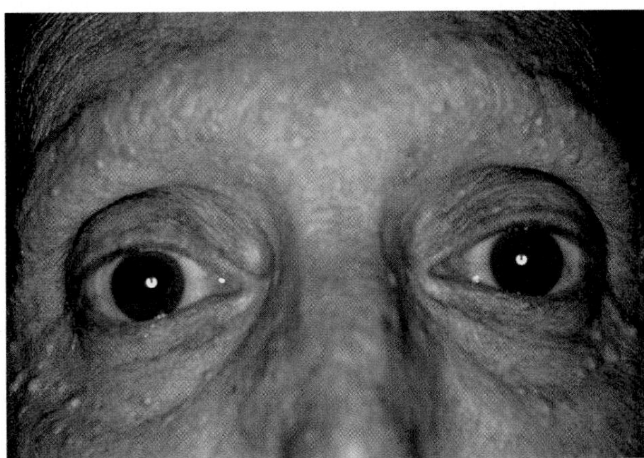

FIGURE 16-6 Jaundice, or yellow discoloration of the skin and other tissues, results from infection of the liver. (From Swartz MH: *Textbook of physical diagnosis*, ed 6, Philadelphia, 2010, Saunders.)

Treatment usually includes bed rest and a diet that is low in fat and high in vitamins. Vaccinations to prevent hepatitis are available for types A and B.

Inflammatory bowel disease (IBD), including Crohn's (krohnz) disease and ulcerative colitis (UL-ser-uh-tiv ko-LIE-tis), is a common condition of unknown cause. Crohn's disease is inflammation and ulceration, usually affecting the ileum or colon or both. It causes cramping, diarrhea, and bloody stools. According to the Crohn's and Colitis Foundation of America, as many as one million Americans have IBD. Recently a genetic abnormality that makes some families more likely to have it was identified. Ulcerative colitis involves the wall of the colon and rectum, leading to watery diarrhea containing blood, mucus, and pus. Emotion and stress can trigger the symptoms of IBD. Treatment may include diet changes, medication, and in severe cases, surgery to remove portions of diseased bowel.

Mumps is a highly contagious viral infection of the parotid glands, most common in 5- to 15-year-olds. The person with mumps experiences a painful swelling of the parotid glands and fever. In older persons, infection may damage the testes and ovaries, leading to sterility. Treatment is directed toward relieving symptoms.

Pancreatitis (pan-kree-uh-TIE-tis) may be a mild, acute, or chronic condition resulting from gallbladder stone blockage, disease, injury, or alcoholism. Gallbladder disease and alcoholism account for 80% of the cases of acute pancreatitis. The condition causes pain, vomiting, abdominal distention, and fever. Treatment includes a low-fat diet, monitoring of blood sugar, pain relief, and sometimes surgery.

Peritonitis (per-ih-toe-NIE-tis) is an inflammation of the abdominal cavity, caused by bacteria. The bacteria may enter this normally sterile area when the bowel is injured. The person with peritonitis experiences vomiting and abdominal pain. Treatment includes antibiotics.

Phenylketonuria (fen-il-kee-toh-NOO-ree-ah) is an inherited disease that can lead to mental retardation if untreated. About 1 in 8000 babies born in the United States each year has this condition, which is linked to a recessive gene. Phenylketonuria causes abnormal metabolism of some proteins. The infant first experiences irritability and restlessness. Damage to the brain from this condition can lead to convulsions. Treatment includes diet modification and monitoring of the blood levels of the proteins. Newborns are routinely screened for this disorder.

Pyloric stenosis (pie-LOR-ik steh-NO-sis) is a birth defect in which a constricted pyloric sphincter does not allow food to pass easily into the small intestine. According to the National Library of Medicine, two to three in 1000 infants are affected. The infant experiences projectile vomiting, diarrhea, dehydration, and weight loss. Pyloric stenosis can be corrected surgically.

Tay-Sachs (tay-SAKS) *disease* is a recessive genetic disorder in which fat cells accumulate in the body and cause damage to normal cells. The enzyme that metabolizes lipids is not produced in the child with Tay-Sachs disease. Symptoms appear between 3 and 6 months of age. The child experiences a progressive loss of muscle control, blindness, deafness, and paralysis as brain cells are destroyed by the accumulation of lipid compounds. No specific therapy for the condition exists, although supportive measures may be given. Tay-Sachs disease always leads to death, usually before age 3. The condition appears more often in people of Eastern European Jewish origin.

An *ulcer* (UL-ser) is an open sore on the lining of the digestive tract, affecting about one of every four adults in the United States (Fig. 16-7). Stomach (gastric) ulcers are called peptic ulcers. Ulcers can be caused

A

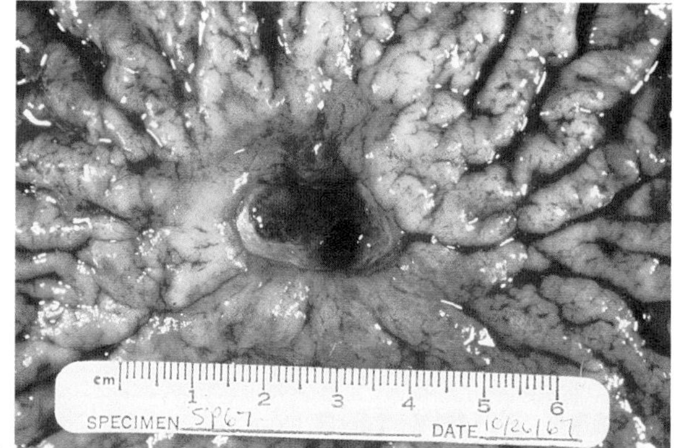

B

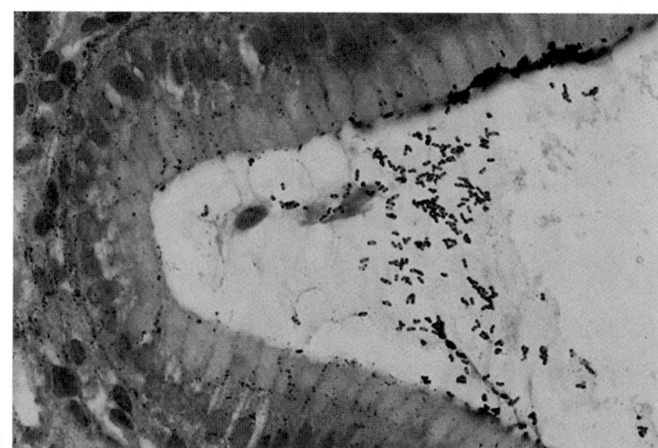

FIGURE 16-7 Ulcer. **A,** Gastric ulcer. **B,** Micrograph of *Helicobacter pylori* (black particles) infecting stomach mucosa (pink). (From Patton KT, Thibodeau GA: *Anatomy & physiology*, ed 7, St. Louis, 2010, Mosby.)

by emotional stress that increases the secretion of stomach acid. It is believed that most duodenal ulcers are caused by a bacterial infection. The bacterium, *H. pylori*, digests the stomach lining and increases the amount of acid production. The presence of the bacteria can be determined by blood tests for antibodies or a biopsy of stomach tissue. Tobacco, caffeine, aspirin, and alcohol can aggravate ulcers. The treatment includes a bland diet, reduced stress, and medication to decrease the amount of acid. If caused by bacteria, ulcers may be treated with antibiotics. Surgery to remove the affected tissue is sometimes necessary.

Issues and Innovations

Food-Borne Illness

The current trend of eating raw or rare fowl, fish, and beef is a serious health hazard. These foods are popularly sold as sushi, rare duck, steak tartare, and carpaccio. The U.S. Department of Agriculture (USDA) estimates that 37% of all fowl is infected with one or more of more than 2000 closely related *Salmonella* bacteria. The U.S. Food and Drug Administration (FDA) has found *Campylobacter* species in 20% of chickens and 83% of turkeys inspected. These bacteria cause diarrhea, vomiting, and fever. The condition may be mild or require medical attention. The USDA recommends that all meat be cooked to an internal temperature of 160° F to kill the bacteria. Another fad is to eat unpasteurized cheese. In 1985 in California, 80 people died from eating cheese that contained *Listeria monocytosis*. Although illegal, unpasteurized cheeses imported from Europe remain available in some stores. The CDC report more than 60 deaths each year from ingestion of the bacteria *E. coli* in undercooked meat. Contaminated by feces during the slaughtering process, ground beef is the most frequent food vector of *E. coli*. Other outbreaks have been linked to contaminated apple cider, lettuce, mayonnaise, salad dressing, and drinking water. *E. coli* can also cause infection through swimming in contaminated water and spread from infant to infant in daycare. The bacteria cause bloody diarrhea, and the infection can lead to kidney failure and formation of blood clots.

Some people are sensitive to a preservative ingredient called *sulfite*, which is added to some foods. The sulfite-sensitive person experiences headache, abdominal discomfort, and diarrhea about 10 minutes after eating it. Sulfites may cause constriction of the bronchial tubes, from which more than a dozen deaths have been reported. In 1986 the FDA prohibited the use of sulfites on fruits and vegetables. Since 1987 manufacturers have been required to list sulfite content on the labels of canned foods.

In 1995 the FDA approved irradiation of meat products to control disease-causing microorganisms. The approval applies to fresh and frozen red meats such as beef, lamb, and pork. The FDA concluded that irradiation does not compromise the nutritional quality of meat products. FDA had previously approved irradiation of poultry, pork, fruits, vegetables, grains, spices, seasonings, and dry enzymes used in food processing. Three methods of irradiation are used to sterilize food, including gamma rays, electron beams, and x-rays.

Eating Disorders

Experts estimate that almost two thirds of adults in the United States are overweight, and one third are obese. The body mass index (BMI) chart is an indicator of body fat (Fig. 16-8). It may overestimate fat in people with a muscular build, such as athletes. It may underestimate body fat in people who have lost muscle mass, such as older adults (Fig. 16-9). It is not intended for people from ages 2 to 20. Instead, "BMI-for-age" gender-specific charts are used (see Appendix II, Fig. II-4, *A* and *B*, see pp. 589–590). Other indicators of health risk resulting from weight include waist circumference and other factors. The risk of diseases associated with obesity increase when a man's waist circumference is more than 40 inches and a woman's waist circumference is more than 35 inches (Box 16-1). Other risk factors include high blood pressure, high low-density lipoprotein cholesterol, high triglycerides, high blood glucose, family history of heart disease, inactivity, and smoking.

The National Center for Health Statistics reports a continued increase in the percentage of children who are overweight. This increase may be caused by increased time watching television, fast foods, and lack of exercise. Literally hundreds of diets and programs for weight reduction are now available (Table 16-3). A trendy or "fad" diet may or may not be nutritionally sound. The healthiest and most successful programs include both calorie reduction and increased exercise.

Estimating the number of individuals affected by eating disorders is difficult because they are not reportable and are often kept secret by the individuals. Three well-documented disorders are bulimia, anorexia nervosa, and binge eating. **Bulimia** is an

Adult Body Mass Index Chart																	
BMI	19	20	21	22	23	24	25	26	27	28	29	30	31	32	33	34	35
Height	Weight in Pounds																
4'10"	91	96	100	105	110	115	119	124	129	134	138	143	148	153	158	162	167
4'11"	94	99	104	109	114	119	124	128	133	138	143	148	153	158	163	168	173
5'	97	102	107	112	118	123	128	133	138	143	148	153	158	163	158	174	179
5'1"	100	106	111	116	122	127	132	137	143	148	153	158	164	169	174	180	185
5'2"	104	109	115	120	126	131	136	142	147	153	158	164	169	175	180	186	191
5'3"	107	113	118	124	130	135	141	146	152	158	163	169	175	180	186	191	197
5'4"	110	116	122	128	134	140	145	151	157	163	169	174	180	186	192	197	204
5'5"	114	120	126	132	138	144	150	156	162	168	174	180	186	192	198	204	210
5'6"	118	124	130	136	142	148	155	161	167	173	179	186	192	198	204	210	216
5'7"	121	127	134	140	146	153	159	166	172	178	185	191	198	204	211	217	223
5'8"	125	131	138	144	151	158	164	171	177	184	190	197	203	210	216	223	230
5'9"	128	135	142	149	155	162	169	176	182	189	196	203	209	216	223	230	236
5'10"	132	139	146	153	160	167	174	181	188	195	202	209	216	222	229	236	243
5'11"	136	143	150	157	165	172	179	186	193	200	208	215	222	229	236	243	250
6'	140	147	154	162	169	177	184	191	199	206	213	221	228	235	242	250	258
6'1"	144	151	159	166	174	182	189	197	204	212	219	227	235	242	250	257	265
6'2"	148	155	163	171	179	186	194	202	210	218	225	233	241	249	256	264	272
6'3"	152	160	168	176	184	192	200	208	216	224	232	240	248	256	264	272	279
	Healthy Weight						Overweight					Obese					

FIGURE 16-8 Body mass index is one indicator of healthy weight for adults. (Courtesy Office of Disease Prevention and Health Promotion, U.S. Department of Health and Human Services, Washington, D.C.)

$$\frac{\text{Weight (lb)}}{\text{Height (in)} \times \text{height (in)}} \times 703 =$$

BMI
Below 18.5 = underweight
18.5 – 24.9 = normal
25.0 – 29.9 = overweight
30.0 and above = obesity

FIGURE 16-9 Body mass index formula. (From http://www.health.gov/dietaryguidelines/dga2005/healthieryou/html/personal_profile.html.)

eating disorder characterized by binge eating and purging. Binge eating, which is rapid and uncontrolled eating, may last a few minutes to several hours. Binge eaters have been known to consume more than 20,000 calories at one time. Binging is followed by self-induced vomiting (purging) or use of laxatives. Bulimia often affects teenagers but may occur in older women or men as well. It is often associated with anorexia nervosa. People with anorexia are often perfectionists who appear confident and in control. They actually lack confidence and perceive themselves as incompetent and overweight, even

BOX 16-1

Health Risks Associated with Excess Weight*

- Coronary heart disease
- Type 2 diabetes
- Cancers (endometrial, breast, and colon)
- Hypertension (high blood pressure)
- Dyslipidemia (for example, high total cholesterol or high levels of triglycerides)
- Stroke
- Liver and gallbladder disease
- Sleep apnea and respiratory problems
- Osteoarthritis (a degeneration of cartilage and its underlying bone within a joint)
- Gynecologic problems (abnormal menses, infertility)

*Overweight is defined as a body mass index (BMI) of 25 or higher; obesity is defined as a BMI of 30 or higher. (Courtesy Centers for Disease Control and Prevention, Atlanta, Ga.)

TABLE 16-3
Trendy Diets*

Name	Description
3-Day	Specific food plan for 3 days followed by normal eating for 4-5 days
Apple Cider	1-3 tsp of apple cider vinegar taken with each meal
Beverly Hills	Same types of foods eaten on alternate days
Biggest Loser	4-3-2-1 Pyramid (fruits/vegetables, protein, whole grains, fats or oils) making 45% carbohydrate, 30% protein, and 25% fat
Cabbage Soup	Diet restricted to cabbage soup and recommended foods, low calorie
Grapefruit	Small variety of food eaten with grapefruit at every meal
Hollywood Tapeworm	May have been marketed between 1900-1920 but considered an urban legend now
Jenny Craig	Three levels: food, mind, body program. Prepackaged meals with 50%-60% carbohydrate, 20%-25% protein, and 20%-25% fat
Low-carbohydrate (Atkins, South Beach)	Reduction of carbohydrates and eating more protein and fat
Low Fat	Reduction of fat from food intake
Master Cleanse	Drinking only a mixture of lemons, maple syrup, and cayenne pepper with no solid food
Mediterranean	High consumption of fruits, vegetables, bread, and cereals with olive oil. Low consumption of dairy products, eggs, poultry, and fish
Nutrisystem	Choice of more than 120 prepared foods for calorie-limited 5 meals a day. Diet approximately 55% carbohydrate, 25% protein and 20% fat.
South Beach	Low-carbohydrate diet
Weight Watchers	Point system used to track food with more movement, support, and better habits
Zone	30% protein, 30% fat, and 40% carbohydrates

*Trendy or fad diets may or may not be nutritionally sound. This is a brief description of a few.

when they are significantly underweight. They may be obsessive about food and exercise, strictly limiting their food intake. Anorexia nervosa has the highest death rate of any psychiatric illness (including major depression).

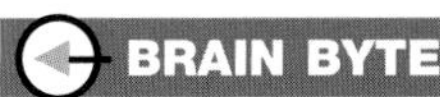

The mortality rate among people with anorexia nervosa has been estimated at 0.56% per year, which is about 12 times higher than the annual death rate due to all causes of death among girls and young women aged 15 to 24 in the general population.

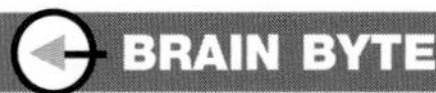

About 10% to 15% of people with anorexia nervosa or bulimia are males.

Purging may cause rashes, dry skin, and swollen salivary glands. Eventually bulimia can lead to destruction of the tooth enamel and tooth decay, irregular heart action, ulcers, colitis, muscle weakness and cramps, a perforated esophagus, and absence of a menstrual period. Resulting vitamin deficiencies and electrolyte imbalances lead to heart, liver, and kidney

CASE STUDY 16-4 You go into the restroom and notice that your friend is throwing up. You ask her if you can do anything to help, and she tells you nothing is wrong. She says she just ate too much breakfast and does not want to gain weight. What should you say?

Answers to Case Studies are available on the Evolve website: ***http://evolve.elsevier.com/Gerdin***

damage. Bulimia may result in death if untreated. Anorexia nervosa and bulimia are now considered addictions. They may be controlled with counseling and behavior modification programs.

Other conditions associated with eating disorders but not as well known include anorexia athletica (compulsive exercising), body dysmorphic disorder (excess concern about appearance), infection-triggered anorexia nervosa, orthorexia nervosa (concern with eating only "pure" foods), sleep-eating disorder, and rumination syndrome (food is ingested and regurgitated to be swallowed again). Prader-Willi syndrome is a genetic condition that causes a compulsion to eat constantly. Pica is the desire to eat nonfood items like dirt, clay, plaster, or paint chips. To reduce caloric intake, some individuals may chew food and spit it out before swallowing. Many of these conditions are part of the behavior of people with the better known eating disorders.

Designer Foods

When it was approved in 1989, the FDA called the new biotechnologically engineered "Flavr Savr" tomato as safe as tomatoes bred by conventional means. It was the first whole food to be genetically altered. The developing company, Calgene, began sales of the Flavr Savr in 1994. Genetic alteration of the tomato decreases production of the enzyme that causes ripening, causing the tomato to soften more slowly. The Flavr Savr can be left on the vine longer than conventionally grown tomatoes, producing a more "homegrown" taste.

Since that time, corn, potato, cotton, squash, cucumber, watermelon, papaya and other products have been genetically altered. Most alterations have been made so that the crops are more resistant to pests and herbicides. "Golden rice" is one product that has been bioengineered to contain beta-carotene. This product may be used to combat vitamin A deficiency and blindness. Another type of rice has been bioengineered to contain iron.

Biotechnology may soon enter the market of aquaculture. A genetically engineered salmon developed by Aqua Bounty Farms can grow from egg to market size in 12 to 18 months. In conventional breeding, this normally requires 2 to 3 years.

The industry disputes concerns that have been raised by the introduction of biotechnologically engineered foods. These concerns include the death of monarch butterflies caused by the pollen from genetically engineered corn. Although the monarch caterpillars do not feed on corn, genetically engineered corn pollen has been found on milkweed and other plants that are the food source for the monarch. It is carried by the wind. There has also been concern that crops in Mexico have crossbred with bioengineered crops in the United States. This has not been proven. The USDA has produced "terminator," or sterile, seeds as part of its research. When the plant grows, it does not produce seeds for a new generation. The concern about this technology is that one company or country could become the only source for seeds to grow a plant.

Summary

- The main function of the digestive system is to break down food to a form that can be used by the body cells.
- Structures of the digestive system include the mouth, esophagus, stomach, intestines, rectum, and anus.
- Accessory organs of the digestive system include the pancreas, liver, and gallbladder.
- Methods of assessment of the digestive system include endoscopy, fecal analysis, gastric analysis, palpation, and auscultation.
- Disorders of the digestive system include alactasia, appendicitis, cholecystitis, cirrhosis, and colon cancer.

Review Questions

1. Describe the four functions of the digestive system.
2. Identify the location and function of each of the following parts of the digestive system:
   Cardiac valve — Esophagus
   Colon — Small intestine
3. List the function and organ of production for five enzymes used by the digestive system.
4. Describe the location and function of the three accessory organs of the digestive system.
5. Describe the usage of barium enemas, gastric analysis, and endoscopic procedures in assessing the function of the digestive system.
6. Describe three digestive system disorders.
7. Describe the effects of anorexia and bulimia on the body.
8. Use the following terms in one or more sentences that correctly relate their meaning: bile, cholecystectomy, emesis, and jaundice.

Critical Thinking

1. Investigate and compare the cost of at least three tests used in diagnosing disorders of the digestive system.
2. Investigate the function of at least five common medications used in treatment of the digestive system.
3. List at least five occupations involved in the health care of digestive system disorders.
4. Use a telephone directory to investigate the prevalence of treatment programs for eating disorders in the community.
5. Research and review an article regarding a recent development of treatment method relating to the digestive system.
6. Use the Internet to compare the long-term effectiveness of three trendy or fad diet plans.
7. Use the Internet to research the risks and benefits of genetically modified foods.
8. Use the Internet to research and describe the economic consequences of obesity.

Explore the Web

Trendy or Fad Diets

WebMD

http://www.webmd.com/diet/guide/the-truth-about-fad-diets

MedlinePlus

http://www.nlm.nih.gov/medlineplus/diets.html

Genetically Modified Food

World Health Organization

http://www.who.int/foodsafety/publications/biotech/20questions/en/

Human Genome Project

http://www.ornl.gov/sci/techresources/Human_Genome/elsi/gmfood.shtml

Obesity

CDC

http://www.cdc.gov/obesity/causes/health.html
http://www.cdc.gov/obesity/causes/economics.html

CHAPTER 17

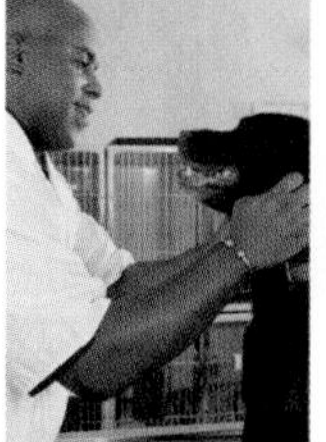
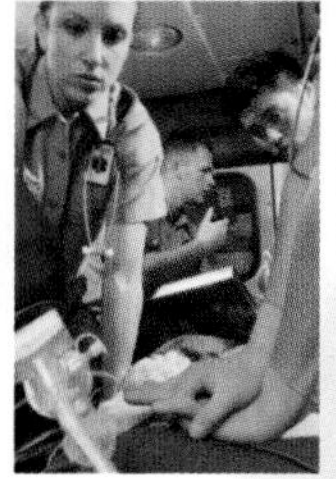
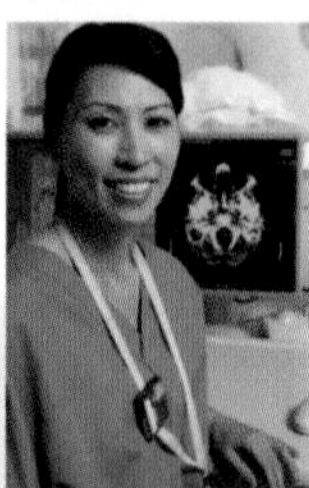

Urinary System

LEARNING OBJECTIVES

- Define at least 10 terms relating to the urinary system.
- Describe the two functions of the urinary system.
- Identify four structures of the urinary system.
- Identify the function of at least three structures of the kidney.
- Identify at least five components normally found in urine.
- Describe the possible cause of at least five abnormal components of urine.
- Describe at least three methods used to assess disorders of the urinary system.

KEY TERMS

Albuminuria *(al-buh-min-OO-ree-uh)* Excess protein in the urine

Anuria *(uh-NOO-ree-uh)* Complete suppression of excretion by kidneys; absence of urine

Dialysis *(die-AL-ih-sis)* Separating particles from a fluid by filtration through a semipermeable membrane

Diuresis *(die-uh-REE-sis)* Increased excretion of urine

Dysuria *(dis-YOO-ree-uh)* Painful or difficult urination

Glycosuria *(glie-ko-SOO-ree-uh)* Presence of sugar in urine

Hematuria *(hem-uh-TOO-ree-uh)* Presence of blood in urine

Micturition *(mik-tuh-RISH-en)* Passage of urine; urination

Oliguria *(ol-ig-OO-ree-uh)* Excretion of diminished amount of urine in relation to fluid intake

Polyuria *(pol-ee-YOO-ree-uh)* Passage of large amount of urine in given time

Pyuria *(pie-YOO-ree-uh)* Pus in the urine

Urinalysis *(yoo-rin-AL-ih-sis)* Physical, chemical, or microscopic examination of urine

Urination *(yoo-rin-AY-shen)* Discharge or passage of urine

Void *(voyd)* To empty, urinate, or defecate

Urinary System Terminology*

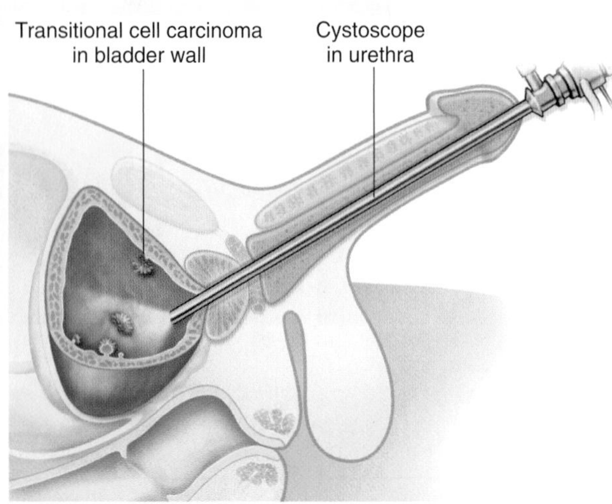

By inserting a scope through the urethra, a cystoscopy shows abnormalities of the bladder. (From Patton KT, Thibodeau GA: *Anatomy & physiology*, ed 7, St. Louis, 2010, Mosby.)

Term	Definition	Prefix	Root	Suffix
Cystocele	Tumor or swelling of the bladder		cyst/o	cele
Cystoscopy	Examination of the bladder		cyst/o	scopy
Lithotomy	Incision into a stone		lith	otomy
Nephrology	Study of the kidney		nephr	ology
Nephropexy	Fixation of the kidney		nephr/o	pexy
Nocturia	Urination at night	noct	uria	
Pyelonephrectomy	Removal of the kidney pelvis	pyel/o	nephr	ectomy
Pyuria	Pus in the urine	py	uria	
Renal	Pertaining to the kidney		ren	al
Renal calculus	Kidney stone		calculus	

*A transition syllable or vowel may be added to or deleted from the word parts to make the combining form.

Abbreviations of the Urinary System

Abbreviation	Meaning
amt	Amount
BRP	Bathroom privileges
cath	Catheter
cysto	Cystoscopy
FF	Force fluids
I&O	Intake and output
IVP	Intravenous pyelogram
KUB	Kidneys, ureter, bladder
qns	Quantity not sufficient
sp gr	Specific gravity

Structure and Function of the Urinary System

The urinary system has two primary functions:

- To regulate the chemical composition of body fluids
- To remove body wastes by filtering blood (excretion)

The urinary system filters about 180 L of blood plasma daily. On average 1.0 to 1.5 L of urine is formed and excreted daily to remove waste products. The amount of urine formed is controlled largely by hormones. An increase in the antidiuretic hormone, from the pituitary gland, decreases the amount of water excreted by the kidneys. An increase in the amount of aldosterone, from the adrenal gland, conserves sodium in the plasma, causing water to be retained. The urinary system consists of two kidneys, ureters, the bladder, and the urethra (Fig. 17-1).

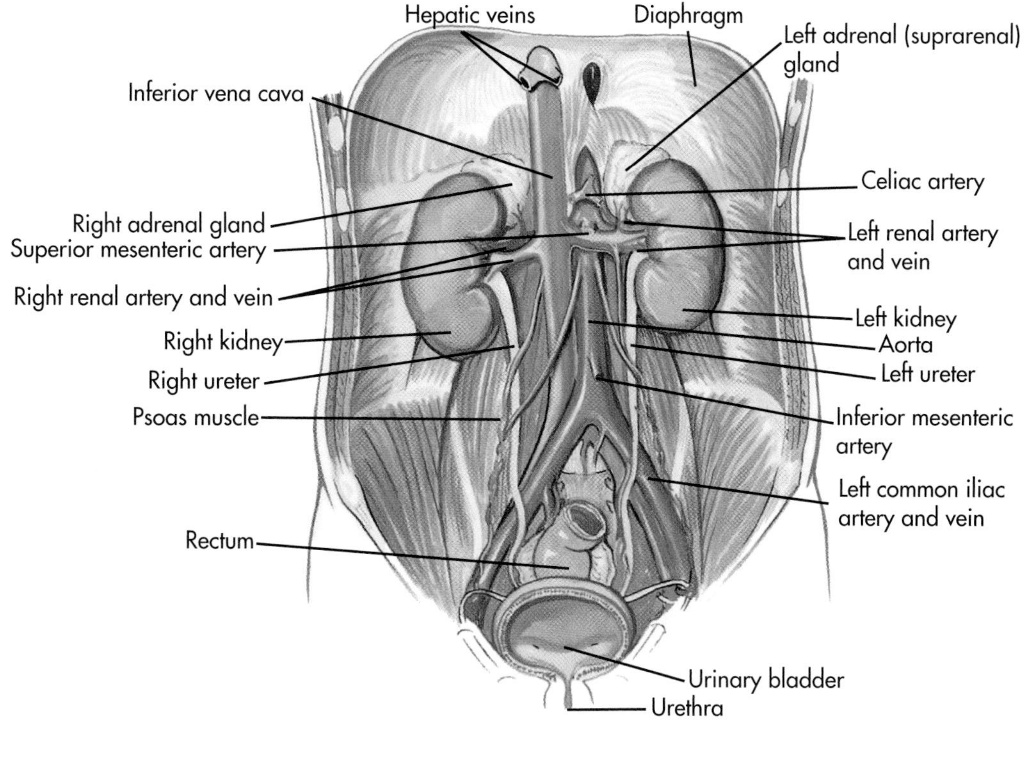

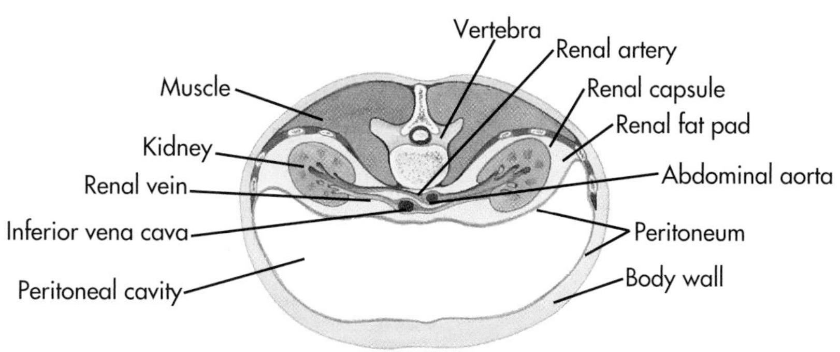

FIGURE 17-1 The urinary system. (From Patton KT, Thibodeau GA: *Anatomy & physiology*, ed 7, St. Louis, 2010, Mosby.)

Kidneys

The basic structural unit of the urinary system is the kidney. Each kidney is about 4 inches (10 cm) long and 2 inches (5 cm) wide and weighs about 150 g. Each kidney contains about one to two million nephrons, the tiny structures that filter the blood (Fig. 17-2). The nephron is the location of formation of urine and is the functional unit of the urinary system. The process by which the urine is filtered in the nephron is complex (Table 17-1). The kidney has three layers (Fig. 17-3):

- The cortex, the outer layer, is composed of soft, granular, reddish brown tissue.
- The medulla is deep red.
- The renal pelvis is the funnel-shaped innermost structure that collects and temporarily stores urine as it is formed.

Inside the renal pelvis is the hilum, which serves as a passageway for lymph vessels, nerves, the renal artery, and renal vein.

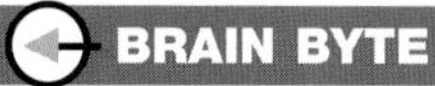

The kidneys filter about 440 gallons of blood every day.

Ureters

The ureters, small tubes composed of smooth muscle tissue, move the urine from the kidney to the bladder

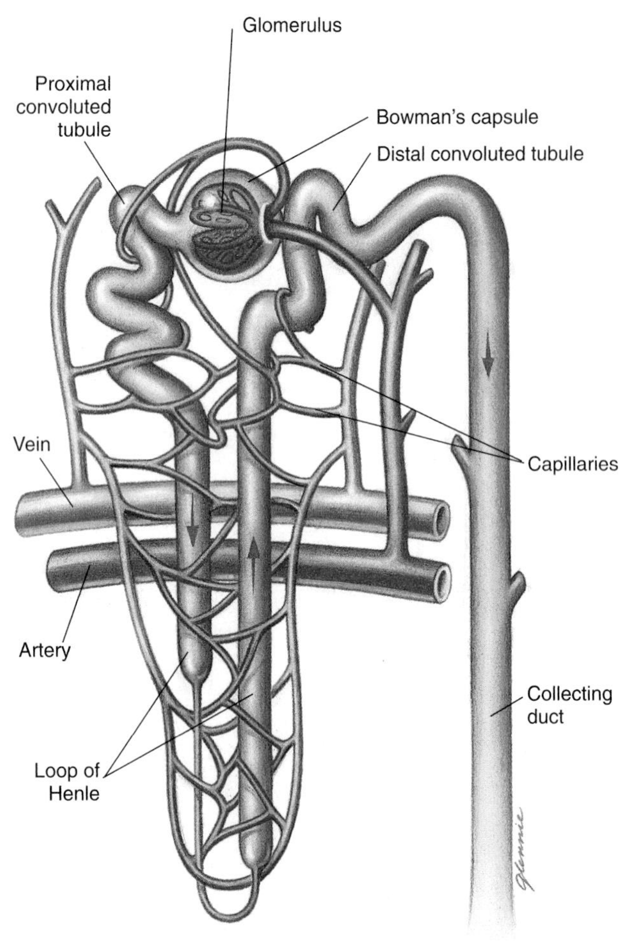

FIGURE 17-2 The nephron.

TABLE 17-1
Nephron Function

Section of Nephron	Function
Renal arterioles	Carry blood to nephron
Bowman's capsule	Filters out water, glucose, and electrolytes (Na^+, Cl^-)
Proximal tubule	Reabsorbs glucose, some electrolytes (Na^+, Cl^-), and water
Loop of Henle	Secretes urea, reabsorbs electrolytes (Na^+, Cl^-), and water
Distal tubule	Secretes ammonia, some electrolytes (K^+, H^+), and some drugs
Collecting duct	Reabsorbs electrolytes (Na^+) and urea; secretes ammonia and electrolytes (K^+, H^+)
Renal venules	Return blood to the body

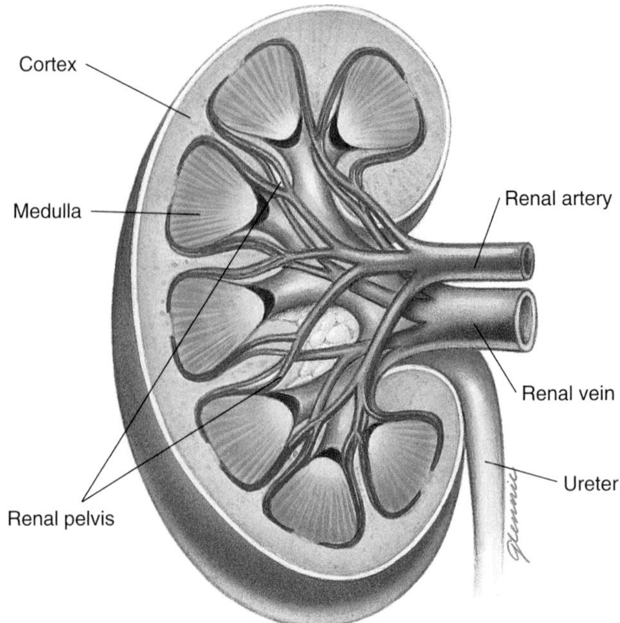

FIGURE 17-3 The kidney.

with peristaltic motion. Each ureter is about 10 to 12 inches (25 to 30 cm) long. At the junction with the bladder, a valvelike narrow region of the ureter prevents urine from flowing back to the kidneys.

Bladder

The bladder, a smooth muscular sac that expands as it fills with urine, can hold up to 1 L. When the bladder fills, nerves in the muscular wall are stimulated and cause the urge to urinate. **Urination** is also called **voiding** or **micturition**.

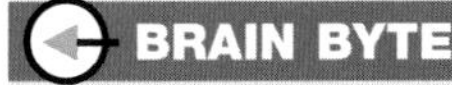

There is no scientific evidence to support the common scuba-diving myth that applying urine relieves the sting of a jellyfish.

Urethra

The urethra moves urine from the bladder to be excreted from the body. It is about 1.0 to 1.5 inches (5 cm) long in the female and runs through the vulva. In the male it is 8 inches (20 cm) long and runs through the penis. At the end of the urethra is an opening called the *urinary meatus*, through which urine passes to the outside of the body.

Urine Formation

Each minute about 600 mL of blood plasma enters the nephrons of each kidney through the renal arteries. In the glomerulus of the nephron, particles are filtered from the blood to be eliminated from the body. Water, glucose, vitamins, amino acids, and chloride salts are reabsorbed into the blood in the renal tubules. Ammonia, potassium, hydrogen ions, and some drugs are secreted into the urine by tubular cells using the process of active transport. The blood leaves the kidneys through the renal veins.

Urine normally consists of 95% water. The remaining 5% includes waste products from the breakdown of protein, hormones, electrolytes, pigments, toxins, and any abnormal components (Table 17-2). Urine is normally sterile in the kidneys and bladder.

Assessment Techniques

The primary methods of assessing the urinary system are urinalysis and examinations such as radiography and cystoscopy. Urodynamic testing, another method, measures the force of the urine flow through the system, evaluating the bladder's efficiency.

Urinalysis

Urinalysis is a series of tests that determine urine composition. These tests can detect many body disorders. Urinalysis assesses the urine color, clarity, pH, specific gravity, odor, and volume. It can also determine the components that are not normally found in urine.

Urine color normally varies from yellow to amber or straw. Dark or red urine may indicate the presence of bile or blood. Some drugs may color urine, turning it blue, orange, or other colors.

CASE STUDY 17-1 You are helping a patient use the bedpan and notice that her urine is green. What should you do?

Answers to Case Studies are available on the Evolve website: *http://evolve.elsevier.com/Gerdin*

TABLE 17-2
Characteristics of Urine

Characteristic	Normal	Abnormal
Volume	1-1.5 L/day	Polyuria (>2.0 L/day) Oliguria (<0.5 L/day)
Odor	None	Sweet (sugar) Ammonia (old) Offensive (bacteria)
Color	Yellow, straw, amber	Red (blood, infection, some drugs) Brown (bile) Orange, blue (drugs)
Turbidity	Clear	Cloudy (pus, bacteria, cells, fat, phosphates)
pH	4.8-7.4 (average 6)	Alkaline (phosphates, vegetarian diet)
Specific gravity	1.002-1.040	High (dehydration) Low (diuresis)

Abnormal Component	Possible Cause
Sugar (glycosuria)	Diabetes mellitus
Protein (albuminuria)	Renal disease
Ketones (ketonuria)	Incomplete fat metabolism, diabetes mellitus
Blood (hematuria)	Infection, injury
Pus (pyuria)	Infection
Bacteria (bacteriuria)	Infection
Casts	Dead cells, injury

The clarity of urine is normally clear. Cloudy composition may indicate mucus or bacteria in the urine. Alkaline urine contains calcium and may appear cloudy.

The pH of urine should be in the range of 4.8 to 7.4 (average 6.0) or slightly acidic. The acidity helps to prevent bacterial growth. Vegetarian diets may lead to a slightly more alkaline composition.

Specific gravity is a measurement of the density of a liquid. The normal specific gravity of urine is 1.002 to 1.040. Dehydration might lead to a higher measurement, and a condition such as diabetes insipidus would lead to a lower specific gravity.

Urine that is fresh should have no odor. An ammonia smell indicates that the specimen is old. A fruity odor may indicate the presence of sugar caused by uncontrolled diabetes mellitus. A foul or putrid smell indicates the presence of bacteria. The normal urine output in 24 hours is 1 to 1.5 L. **Anuria**, or no urine output, may indicate kidney malfunction or low blood pressure. **Oliguria**, or less than 0.5 L urine output daily, may be caused by retention of urine or dehydration. Output of more than 2 L is called **polyuria**. **Diuresis**, a temporary increase in the amount of urine output, can be caused by ingestion of certain beverages, drugs, or increased fluid intake.

CASE STUDY 17-2 Your friend tells you that she cannot come to your slumber party because she has enuresis. What should you say?

Answers to Case Studies are available on the Evolve website: ***http://evolve.elsevier.com/Gerdin***

Abnormal components of urine include sugar (**glycosuria**), proteins such as albumin or globulin (**albuminuria**), blood (**hematuria**), pus (**pyuria**), casts, and ketones. The presence of sugar and waste products of fat metabolism (ketones) may indicate uncontrolled diabetes mellitus. Proteins may appear during pregnancy. Urine may contain blood or pus as a result of infection or injury of the urinary system. Casts are dead cells and waste materials that indicate injury to the urinary tract.

Other Examinations

Radiological examination of the kidneys, ureters, and bladder (KUB) may be used to detect the presence of stones in the system. In a procedure called *intravenous pyelogram* (IVP), blockage in the urinary system can be seen. In this procedure, an opaque liquid called a *contrast medium* is injected into a blood vessel. A series of x-rays is then taken as the liquid passes through the system.

Another procedure used to examine the bladder is called *cystoscopy*. To view the inside of the bladder and urethra, a cystoscope is inserted in the urethra and the bladder is inflated with water or air. Minor surgical procedures such as taking tissue samples for biopsy are performed with the cystoscope.

Urodynamic tests determine the force of the flow of urine through the system. The rate may be measured with uroflowmetry. Bladder and sphincter muscle control can be assessed with the use of electromyography.

BRAIN BYTE

Urine therapy, urotherapy, or urinotherapy includes drinking urine and applying it to skin is an alternative medical practice.

DISORDERS OF THE Urinary System

Cystitis (sis-TIE-tis) is inflammation of the bladder caused by many different types of bacteria. Cystitis more commonly occurs in women than in men because of the shorter length of the urethra. The leading causative organism is *Escherichia coli*, or *E. coli*, which, through poor hygiene, may be carried from the rectum to the urinary tract. The person with cystitis may experience painful urination or **dysuria**, the urge to urinate frequently, or blood in the urine, known as *hematuria*. Treatment usually includes an increase in fluid intake and antibiotics. Although cystitis may also be caused by tumors or calculi, many cases can be prevented by using good hygiene practices.

Edema (eh-DEE-ma) is an abnormal accumulation of fluid in the tissue intercellular space (Fig. 17-4). This area may be swollen locally in one part of the body or throughout all tissues of the body (systemic). Edema caused by kidney (renal) failure is systemic. It may be treated by use of **dialysis** and diuretic medication.

Nephritis (neh-FRY-tis), which is inflammation of the kidneys, may occur as a result of illness or chronic cystitis. *Pyelonephritis* (pie-eh-lo-neh-FRY-tis) is an inflammation of the kidney pelvis and the nephron. Symptoms are similar to those of cystitis but more

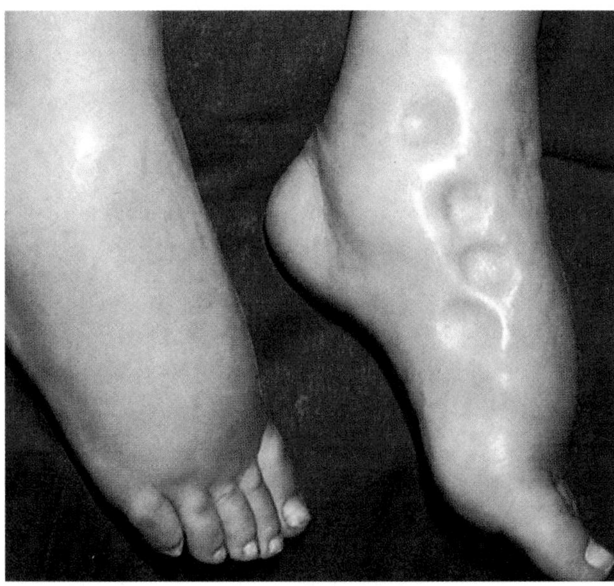

FIGURE 17-4 Finger-shaped depressions that do not rapidly refill indicate pitting edema. (From Patton KT, Thibodeau GA: *Anatomy & physiology*, ed 7, St. Louis, 2010, Mosby.)

commonly involve back pain. Untreated nephritis can cause permanent damage to the kidney tissues. Treatment includes antibiotics and increased fluid intake.

Renal calculus (REE-nul KAL-kyoo-lus) is a kidney stone. Kidney stones occur in about 1 of 1000 people. Calculi are composed of uric acid and calcium salts. Although the specific cause is not known, a lack of adequate fluid intake and large doses of vitamins, especially vitamin C, may lead to kidney stone formation. The person with a kidney stone feels extreme pain when an area of the kidney or ureter is blocked by the stone. Treatment depends on the location and size of the stone and might include surgical removal. Lithotripsy (LITH-o-trip-see) has become an alternative treatment.

CASE STUDY 17-3 Your friend tells you that he cannot drink milk because he once had a kidney stone and does not want to develop another. What should you say?

Answers to Case Studies are available on the Evolve website: ***http://evolve.elsevier.com/Gerdin***

Renal (REE-nul) *failure,* the absence of urine formation, can be acute or chronic. When the kidneys fail, nitrogen wastes and fluids build up in the tissues, leading to many complications, such as congestive heart failure, and may be fatal. Acute renal failure may result from trauma, toxins, or hemorrhage. It is often treated with restriction of fluids, antibiotics, and diuretic medications. Acute renal failure is often reversible. Chronic renal failure may result from other conditions, such as high blood pressure, diabetes mellitus, and autoimmune disorders. Chronic renal failure develops slowly and may have initial symptoms of sluggishness, fatigue, and mental slowness. The condition is eventually called *end-stage renal disease* when the kidneys have lost all function. Renal failure results in 80,000 deaths in the United States each year. Treatment includes special diet considerations, diuretic medications, dialysis, and transplantation. In children, chronic renal insufficiency is treated with growth hormone.

Uremia (yoo-REE-mee-uh) is a condition in which the kidneys do not filter the blood. Waste products and urea stay in the blood and tissues, preventing nutrients and oxygen from entering the cells. Uremia may result from trauma, hypotension, nephritis, renal failure, and other conditions. The person suffering from uremia may experience nausea, vomiting, headache, and coma. White crystals, called *uremic frost,* may form on the skin as the body attempts to excrete the uremic waste. Treatment may include a restricted diet and dialysis to remove the waste products.

Urethritis (yoo-rih-THRIE-tis) is acute or chronic inflammation of the urethra. It may be caused by bacteria or chemical irritation from agents such as bubble bath. The person experiences frequent, painful urination and a red and painful urinary meatus (mee-AY-tus) and surrounding tissues. Urethritis can lead to a narrowing or stricture of the urethra resulting from the formation of scar tissue. Treatment may include antibiotics, sitz baths, and an increase in fluid intake.

Urinary incontinence (in-KON-tih-nens) is the inability to control urination. A number of factors, including lack of muscle control, immobility, or spinal cord or neurologic damage may cause urinary incontinence. Treatment may include retraining the bladder, drugs, or surgery.

Urinary retention is the inability to urinate when the urge is felt or the bladder is full. Retention may result from an obstruction, drugs, trauma, or neurologic disorders. The affected person may experience abdominal pain, distention, and excretion of small amounts of urine. Treatment focuses on the underlying cause and may include inserting a tube (catheterization) to empty the bladder.

Urinary tract infections, usually caused by bacteria, may affect the bladder, kidneys, or prostate. The person with a urinary tract infection may experience fever; lower back pain; and frequent, painful, and bloody urination. Antibiotics and sitz baths may be used to relieve the infection and discomfort.

BRAIN BYTE

Women are at greater risk of developing a urinary tract infection because their urethra is shorter.

CASE STUDY 17-4 Your friend needs to use the restroom to urinate in every class. She tells you that she also feels burning when she urinates. What should you say?

Answers to Case Studies are available on the Evolve website: ***http://evolve.elsevier.com/Gerdin***

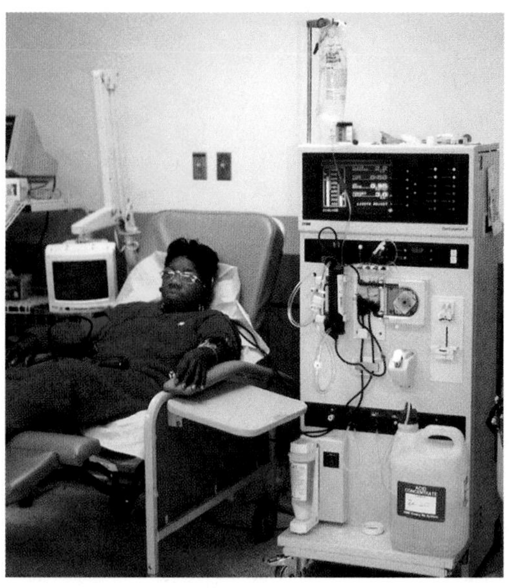

FIGURE 17-5 Dialysis typically takes several hours several times a week. (From Lewis SM, Heitkemper MM, Dirksen SR: *Medical-surgical nursing: assessment and management of clinical problems,* ed 6, St. Louis, 2004, Mosby.)

Issues and Innovations

Dialysis

Dialysis is the filtration of body fluids through a semipermeable membrane or machine instead of the kidneys to remove excess water and waste. Hemodialysis is the filtration of the blood by using an artificial membrane. Blood is removed from a vein, filtered slowly through the machine, and returned to the body. It may take several hours to complete the process. Hemodialysis may be required two or three times weekly to replace failed kidney function (Fig. 17-5). The procedure is expensive and carries the risk of infection and damage to blood cells. Patients who must use dialysis to treat kidney disease experience many lifestyle changes (Table 17-3).

Another form of dialysis uses the peritoneal membrane of the abdomen as the filter to remove the wastes from body fluid. Continuous abdominal peritoneal dialysis requires insertion of a cannula into the abdominal cavity. A solute of glucose and salts is poured into the abdominal cavity to combine with the waste products. The fluid is then drained out of the cavity by gravity. Peritoneal dialysis can be performed in the home, although a risk of infection exists because of the opening into the body cavity. Other complications include the development of scar tissue called *adhesions* in the abdomen.

In some cases dialysis may be completed at home. One of five types of home dialysis is continuous ambulatory peritoneal dialysis, which uses the peritoneum to filter wastes and does not use any machinery. A surgically implanted tube is filled with a dialysate solution that cleans the waste in the peritoneum. The solution is manually put in and removed from the abdomen with this type of home dialysis. Continuous cycling peritoneal dialysis uses the same type of implanted tube and a filtering machine that can be attached at night to remove and instill the dialysate fluid.

Conventional home hemodialysis may be performed at home if the hemodialysis machine and training are available. This is usually performed two or three times a week. Daily home hemodialysis uses the same technique and equipment as conventional home hemodialysis but is performed daily. Nocturnal home hemodialysis uses the same techniques as conventional hemodialysis but is performed at night during sleep.

Kidney Transplant

Kidney transplant is another method of restoring kidney function. Drawbacks include the difficulty of matching tissues, expense, and shortage of donor kidneys. Although the cost of kidney transplant is high, this cost is still less than the cost of treating a patient with kidney failure by using dialysis over a period of 3 years (Table 17-4). Kidney dialysis costs about $66,000 annually. The donor program pays the cost of donation of organs for transplant.

TABLE 17-3
Lifestyle Changes of Dialysis*

Area	Change	Possible Solution
Blood count	Anemia, trouble sleeping	Plan activities for peak energy, limit fluids, rest periods, light exercise regularly, avoid heavy lifting
Emotion	Feeling "blah" before dialysis and "wrung out" after	Adjust activities to days when feeling good
Fluid retention	Weight gain, high blood pressure, headache, leg cramps	Adjust diet and restrict fluid intake to gain less than 2 lb daily
Mouth	Dry mouth, bad breath	Rinse mouth, chew gum, suck sugar-free candy
Skin	Dry skin, brittle hair, itching, bruising, sunburn more easily	Mild soap, shampoo, lotion, diet change, medication for itching, protective clothing

*Changes may or may not occur because people do not all react the same way to treatment.

TABLE 17-4
Estimated U.S. Average 2008 Cost of Transplants*

Organ	Cost
Heart	$ 787,700
Single lung	$ 450,400
Double lung	$ 657,800
Heart-lung	$ 1,123,800
Liver	$ 523,400
Kidney	$ 259,000
Pancreas	$ 275,200
Intestine	$ 1,121,800

*This estimated cost of transplant includes medical and non-medical items. These are divided into categories including pre-transplant, procurement, hospital, physician, posttransplant and immunosuppressants. From United Network for Organ Sharing (UNOS), http://transplantliving.org.

Many factors are used to determine who receives a kidney when it becomes available. The length of time the recipient has been on the waiting list, blood type, tissue type, and medical condition are considered. Geographic location is also a determining factor in the selection of the candidate. Local waiting lists at hospitals and a national list exist. The United Network for Organ Sharing (UNOS) maintains the national list.

Kidney transplantation is now routine and has a success rate of 94% from cadaver donors and 98% from living donors. According to the National Kidney Foundation (NKF), 4573 kidney patients, 1506 liver patients, 371 heart patients, and 234 lung patients died in 2008 while waiting for organ transplants. The shortage of donors, both living and cadaver, is a concern for health professionals. As of 2010, the NKF reported that 104,748 patients were waiting for transplant organs.

Kidneys are one of 22 organs that are being regrown by the Wake Forest Institute for Regenerative Medicine in North Carolina. In this regenerative medicine process, cells are taken from the patient's body, cultivated in Petri dishes, and layered into three-dimensional models of the organ. This procedure has been used successfully to create bladders.

Lithotripsy

Extracorporeal shock wave lithotripsy uses high-energy pressure or sound waves sent through the kidney to break apart or disintegrate kidney stones. The "shock wave" may be sent through water or air. Two types of shock wave therapy are available. The original method sent the shock waves through water. The patient was placed in a tub of water for this technique. A newer procedure passes the shock waves through padded cushions on a table. In this method the patient is not placed in water. With both techniques, two fluoroscopic or ultrasound monitors are used to position the lithotripsy machine in order to target the stone precisely. Up to 2000 "shocks" may be necessary to dissolve a stone. Although the procedure may occasionally cause bleeding or heart irregularities, it may prevent the need for surgery to remove the stone (Fig. 17-6). Another procedure, called *tunnel surgery*, may be used when lithotripsy is not recommended. In this method a small incision is made into the kidney from the back. A tube is then inserted in the kidney to remove the stones.

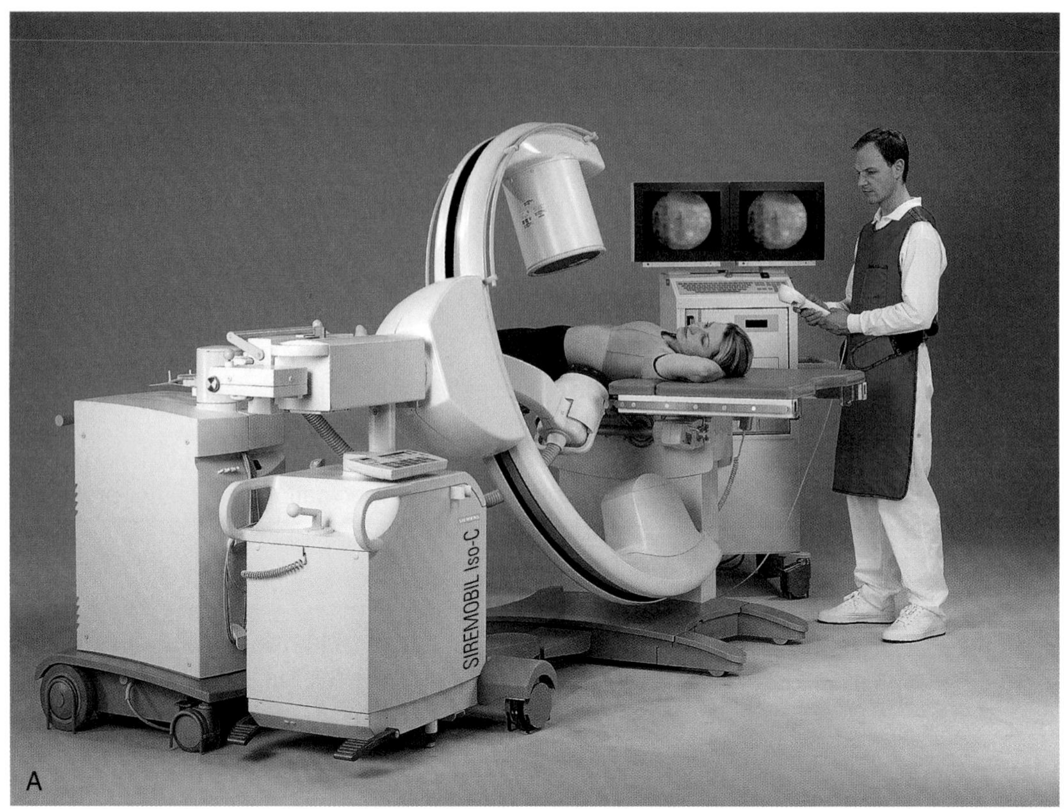

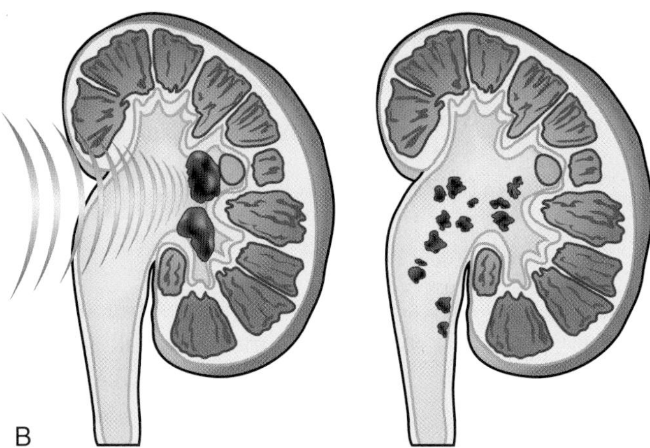

FIGURE 17-6 **A,** Lithotripsy allows removal of kidney stones without surgery. (**A,** Courtesy Siemens Medical Systems, Inc.) **B,** Kidney stones are broken into small pieces using shock waves.

Summary

- The functions of the urinary system include regulating the composition of body fluids and removing wastes by filtering the blood.
- Structures of the urinary system include the kidneys, ureters, bladder, and urethra.
- Structures of the kidney include glomerulus, Bowman's capsule, loop of Henle, and collecting duct.
- Components normally found in urine include water, yellow coloring, and a pH of about 6.
- Abnormal components of urine and their possible causes include sugar (diabetes), protein (renal disease), blood (injury), ketones (diabetes), and bacteria (infection).
- Methods used to assess the urinary system include urinalysis, radiography, and cystoscopy.

Review Questions

1. Describe the two functions of the urinary system.

2. Describe the function of the four structures of the urinary system.
3. Describe the function of the structures of the kidney.
4. Describe the location and function of each of the following parts of the urinary system:

bladder	renal pelvis
cortex	ureter

5. List five components normally found in urine.
6. List five abnormal components of urine and one possible cause of each.
7. Differentiate between peritoneal dialysis and hemodialysis.
8. Describe three methods of assessment of the urinary system.
9. Use the following terms in one or more sentences that correctly relate their meaning: diuresis, glycosuria, polyuria, and urination.

Critical Thinking

1. Investigate and compare the cost of at least three tests used in diagnosing disorders of the urinary system.
2. Investigate the function of at least five common medications used in treatment of the urinary system.
3. List at least five occupations involved in the health care of urinary system.
4. Investigate the recommended dietary needs after renal failure.
5. Investigate and compare the cost of dialysis and kidney transplant. What other factors might be considered in choosing the method of treatment for renal failure?
6. List five beverages that act as diuretics.
7. Investigate the function of each part of the nephron.
8. Use the Internet to research recent developments or treatment methods relating to the urinary system.
9. Use the Internet to research and compare the possible types of dialysis.
10. Use the Internet to research sports drinks and water intoxication.

Explore the Web

Dialysis

Medline
http://www.nlm.nih.gov/medlineplus/dialysis.html

National Kidney and Urologic Diseases Information Clearinghouse (NKUDIC)
http://kidney.niddk.nih.gov/kudiseases/pubs/kidneyfailure/index.htm

Sports Drinks

About.com
http://sportsmedicine.about.com/od/hydrationandfluid/a/Hyponatremia.htm

HowStuffWorks.com
http://health.howstuffworks.com/water-intoxication.htm

CHAPTER 18

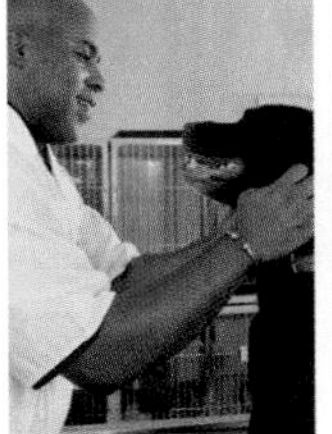
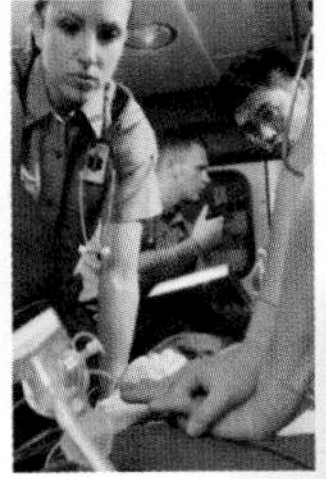
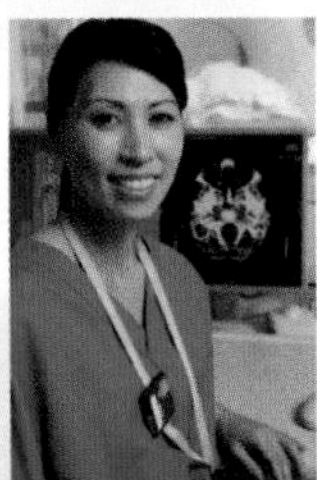

Endocrine System

LEARNING OBJECTIVES

- Define 10 terms relating to the endocrine system.
- Describe the function of the endocrine system.
- Identify at least nine endocrine system structures.
- Identify at least one hormone produced by each of the 10 endocrine glands.
- Describe at least three methods used to assess the function of the endocrine system.
- Describe at least five disorders of the endocrine system.

KEY TERMS

Basal metabolic rate *(BAY-sal met-uh-BOL-ik rayt)* Minimal energy expended for respiration, circulation, peristalsis, muscle tone, body temperature, and glandular activity of the body at rest

Endocrine *(EN-do-krin)* Glands that secrete internally into blood or lymph

Exophthalmos *(ek-sof-THAL-mus)* Abnormal protrusion of eyeball

Gonadotropin *(go-NAD-o-trope-in)* Any hormone that stimulates the reproductive organs

Hormone *(HORE-mone)* Chemical substance produced in the body that has specific regulatory effect on the activity of a specific organ

Hyperglycemia *(hi-per-glie-SEE-mee-uh)* Abnormally high sugar content in the blood

Hypoglycemia *(hi-po-glie-SEE-mee-uh)* Abnormally low sugar content in the blood

Immunoassay *(im-yoo-no-AS-say)* Quantitative determination of antigenic substances by examination of blood

Polydipsia *(pol-ee-DIP-see-uh)* Excessive thirst persisting for long periods

Polyphagia *(pol-ee-FAY-jee-ah)* Excessive hunger

Polyuria *(pol-ee-YOO-ree-uh)* Passage of a large volume of urine in a given time

Prostaglandin *(pros-tah-GLAN-din)* Lipid molecule that has hormone-like effect; tissue hormone

Puberty *(PYOO-ber-tee)* Period during which the secondary sexual characteristics begin to develop and the capability of sexual reproduction is attained

Endocrine System Terminology*

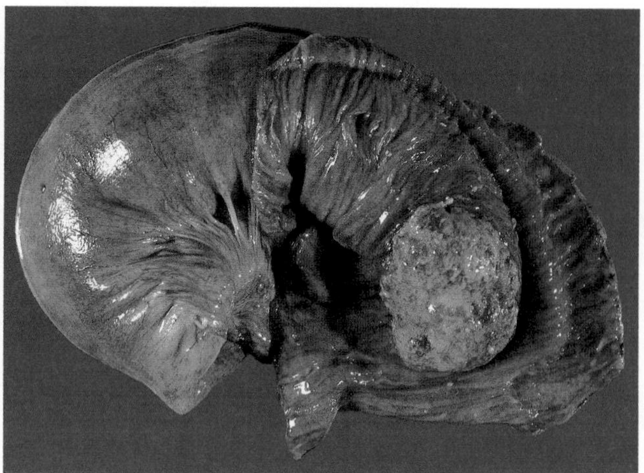

An adenoma may be benign or cancerous, like this adenocarcinoma of the intestines. (From Cooke RA, Stewart B: *Colour atlas of anatomical pathology,* ed 3, Sydney, 2004, Churchill Livingstone.)

Term	Definition	Prefix	Root	Suffix
Acromegaly	Enlargement of the extremities		acro	megaly
Adenoma	Tumor of a gland		aden	oma
Adenomalacia	Softening of a gland		aden/o	malacia
Adrenalectomy	Removal of the adrenal gland		adrenal	ectomy
Endocrine	To secrete inside	endo	crine	
Hyperglycemia	Too much sugar in the blood	hyper	glyc	emia
Pancreatitis	Inflammation of the pancreas		pancreat	itis
Polyphagia	Excessive hunger	poly	phagia	
Polyuria	Excessive excretion of urine	poly	uria	
Thyroidectomy	Removal of the thyroid		thyroid	ectomy

*A transition syllable or vowel may be added to or deleted from the word parts to make the combining form.

Abbreviations of the Endocrine System

Abbreviation	Meaning
ADH	Antidiuretic hormone
ANS	Autonomic nervous system
BMR	Basal metabolic rate
DM	Diabetes mellitus
FSH	Follicle stimulating hormone
GH	Growth hormone
SIADH	Syndrome of inappropriate antidiuretic hormone
STH	Somatotropic hormone
TH	Thyroid hormone
TSH	Thyroid-stimulating hormone

Structure and Function of the Endocrine System

The primary function of the **endocrine** system is to produce hormones that monitor and coordinate body activities (Fig. 18-1). **Hormones** are chemical messengers secreted by the endocrine glands. Each type of hormone moves through the blood to its own target cells, which react specifically to it. The endocrine glands secrete hormones directly into the bloodstream. Hormones may be proteins, glycoproteins, polypeptides, amino-acid derivatives, or lipids.

Hormones may be divided into two classes on the basis of their composition and the way they influence their target organs:

- Nonsteroid hormones are proteins that work as "first-messengers." They act on cells of the target organ to cause them to produce or release a second messenger molecule.
- Steroid hormones influence the target organ independently.

Hormones may also be divided into categories on the basis of their function:

- Tropic hormones target other endocrine structures to increase their growth and secretions.
- Sex hormones influence reproductive changes.
- Anabolic hormones stimulate the process of building tissues.

TABLE 18-1
Endocrine Glands and Hormones*

Gland	Hormone	Function
Pituitary	Somatotropin (or growth hormone [GH])	Promotes tissue growth and development
Pineal	Melatonin	Supports the biological clock
Thyroid	Thyroxine (TH)	Regulates the metabolic rate
Parathyroid	Parathyroid hormone (PTH)	Regulates calcium and phosphates in the bloodstream and bones
Thymus	Thymosin	Stimulates development of T cells
Adrenal	Epinephrine	Regulates autonomic nervous system response
Pancreatic islets	Insulin	Regulates blood sugar
Ovaries	Estrogen	Regulates female sexual characteristics
Testes	Testosterone	Regulates male sexual characteristics

*Most of the endocrine glands secrete more than one hormone with functions not listed here.

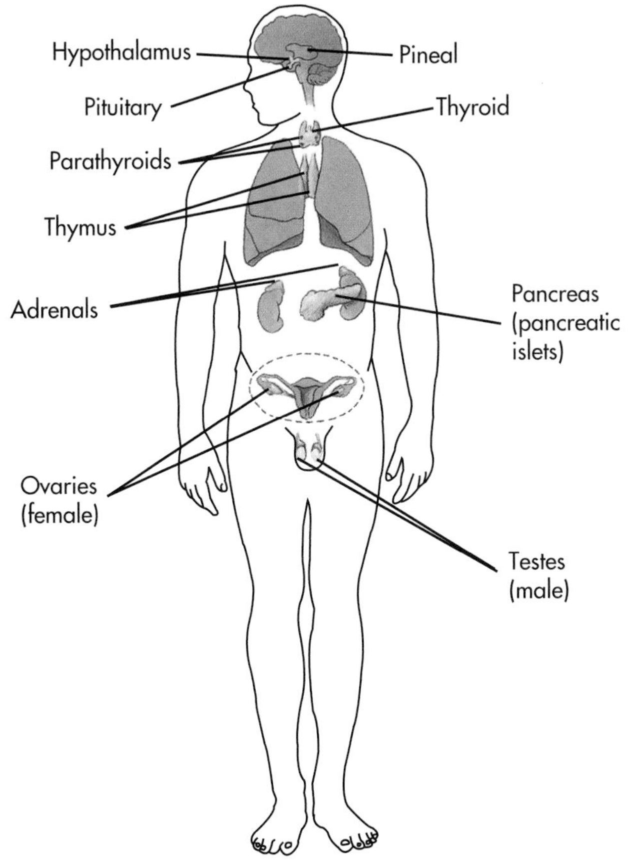

FIGURE 18-1 The endocrine system. (From Patton KT, Thibodeau GA: *Anatomy & physiology*, ed 7, St. Louis, 2010, Mosby.)

Hormones direct many body processes, including growth, metabolism, and reproductive functions (Table 18-1). Hormones regulate the body's reaction to stress and maintain the internal environment (homeostasis). The importance of hormones in the body can be demonstrated by the numerous and diverse disorders that occur when the amount of hormone produced is either too great (hypersecretion) or too little (hyposecretion). The quantity of hormones in the blood is monitored through a negative feedback mechanism, which stimulates more secretion when needed (Fig. 18-2). Additionally, the autonomic nervous system controls and stimulates the secretion of the hormones of the adrenal gland.

Glands and their Hormones

Hypothalamus

The hypothalamus is a structure located above the pituitary gland that translates nervous system impulses into endocrine system messages. It regulates the secretions of the pituitary adenohypophysis by secreting neurohormones that stimulate or inhibit pituitary hormones. For example, the hypothalamus produces a growth hormone–releasing hormone that stimulates the pituitary to release growth hormone.

Pituitary

The pituitary gland (hypophysis) is sometimes called the "master" gland because the hormones that it produces regulate the secretion of other glands (Fig. 18-3). It is located at the base of the brain and is divided into two parts: the anterior and posterior.

The anterior pituitary (adenohypophysis) gland produces seven hormones:

- Thyroid-stimulating hormone (TSH) stimulates the growth and secretion of the thyroid gland.

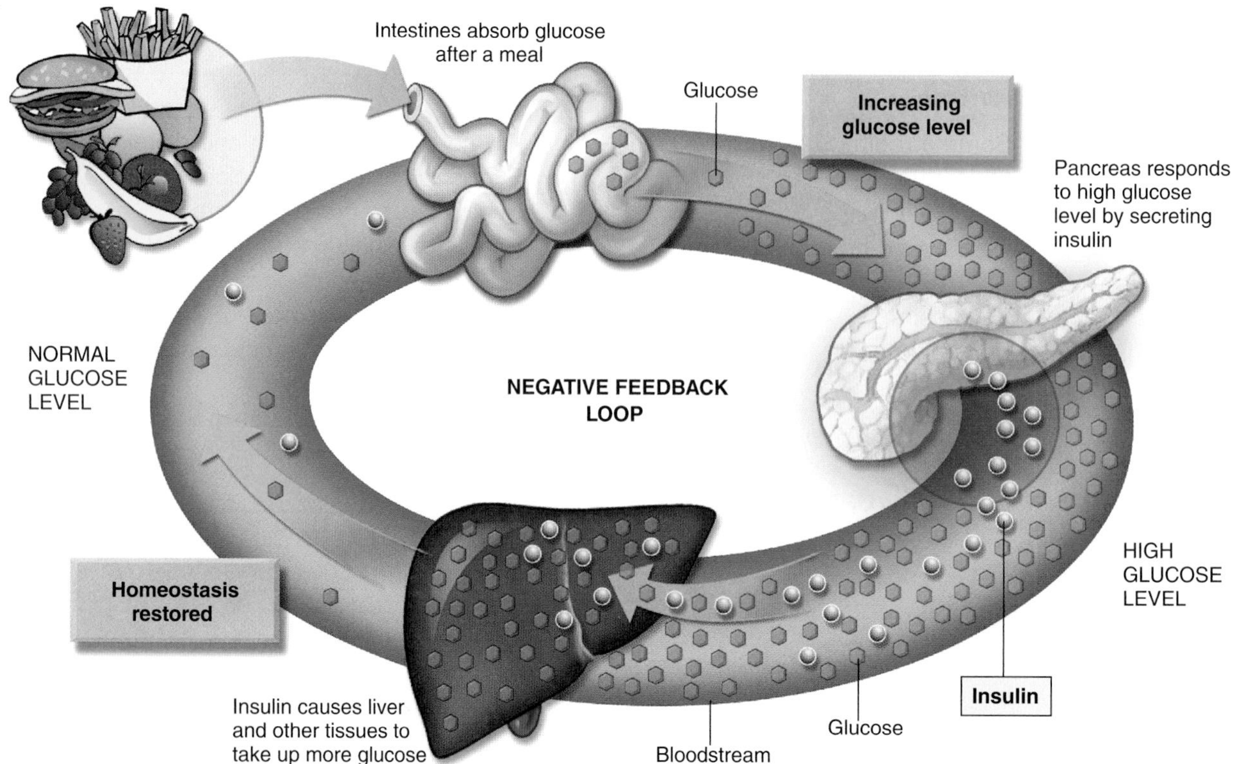

FIGURE 18-2 The triggered factor for the negative feedback mechanism of hormone control may be the concentration of a hormone or other substance such as calcium in the blood.

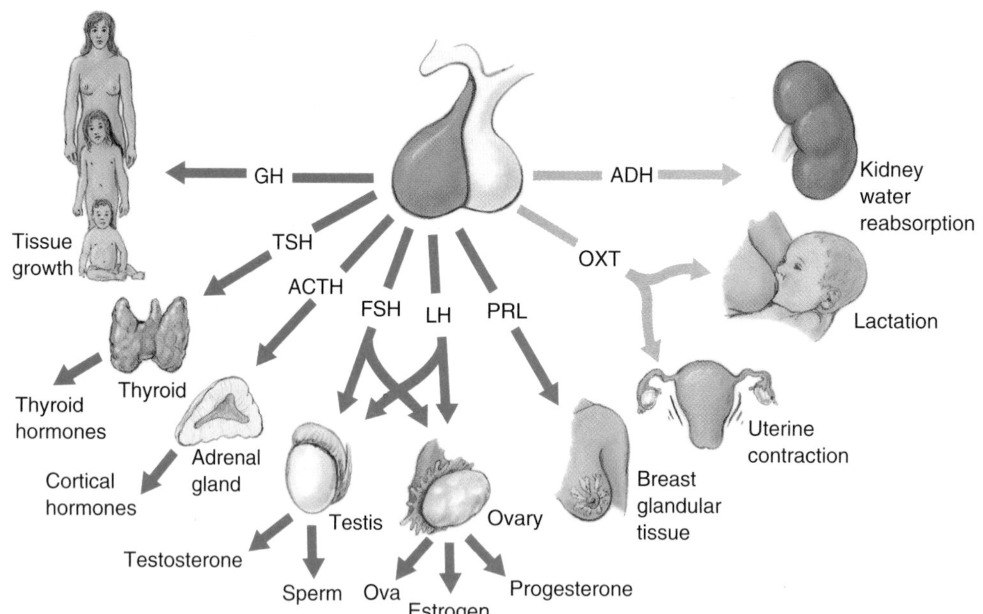

FIGURE 18-3 Effects of hormones from the pituitary gland. (From Applegate E: *The anatomy and physiology learning system,* ed 3, St. Louis, 2006, Saunders.)

BRAIN BYTE

Although the pituitary gland is called the "master" gland because its hormones control other glands, the hypothalamus releases chemicals that stimulate the release of pituitary hormones.

- Adrenocorticotrophic hormone (ACTH) stimulates the growth and secretion of the adrenal cortex.
- Follicle-stimulating hormone (FSH) stimulates the growth of the ovarian follicle, production of estrogen in females, and production of sperm in males.

- Luteinizing hormone (LH) stimulates ovulation and the formation of the corpus luteum in the menstrual cycle.
- In males the LH, called *interstitial cell-stimulating hormone*, stimulates the secretion of testosterone.
- Lactogenic hormone (prolactin) stimulates the secretion of milk and influences maternal behavior.
- Somatotropic hormone, also called the *growth hormone*, accelerates the growth of the body.

The posterior pituitary (neurohypophysis) produces two hormones:

- Antidiuretic hormone (ADH), or vasopressin, maintains water balance by increasing the reabsorption of water by the kidneys.
- Oxytocin (Pitocin) promotes the ejection of milk and stimulates uterine contractions during pregnancy.

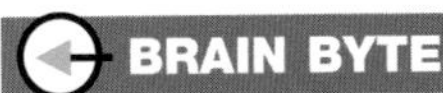

Endocrine disruptors are chemicals that mimic a natural hormone and trigger overproduction or underproduction of hormones.

Pineal Body

The pea-sized pineal body is a gland located deep within the brain. It produces the hormone melatonin. Melatonin regulates the release of substances in the hypothalamus of the brain that influence secretion of the pituitary **gonadotropins**, or sex hormones. It is believed that melatonin inhibits the activity of the ovaries and LH secretion. Thus it influences the menstrual cycle and onset of **puberty**. Melatonin is also believed to be involved in the regulation of the "biological clock," or the body's physiologic reaction to changes in light and dark.

Thyroid

The thyroid, a butterfly-shaped gland with two lobes, is located in the neck. The thyroid produces hormones that regulate body metabolism. They are called *thyroxine* and *tri-iodothyronine*. Iodine is required for production of both of these hormones. Calcitonin, another hormone produced by the thyroid, decreases the amount of calcium in the blood.

Parathyroid

The parathyroids are actually four tiny glands attached to the back of the thyroid gland. They secrete parathyroid hormone, which also affects the amount of calcium in the blood. This hormone increases the blood's calcium level by breaking the bonds of calcium and phosphorus compounds in the bones. It also increases the rate of phosphorus excretion by the kidneys.

Thymus

The thymus is a butterfly-shaped gland located above the heart. It produces the hormone thymosin, which stimulates the lymphoid organs to produce T lymphocytes or antibodies in newborns and young children. The thymus gland provides additional immunity until it disintegrates and is replaced with fatty tissue at the time of puberty.

Pancreas

The pancreas, located behind the stomach, produces the hormones insulin and glucagon. Insulin regulates the transportation of sugar, fatty acids, and amino acids into the cells. It also participates in protein synthesis. The action of glucagon opposes that of insulin by increasing the blood sugar level. The pancreas is the only gland that has both endocrine and exocrine functions. Chapter 16 provides more information about the exocrine function of the pancreas.

Adrenal Glands

The adrenal glands are located above the kidneys. Each gland can actually be divided into two layers, called the *adrenal cortex* and *adrenal medulla*. The adrenal cortex produces about 30 hormones, including glucocorticoids, mineralocorticoids, and androgens. Three of the most important hormones of the cortex are cortisol, aldosterone, and androgen. Glucocorticoids produce an anti-inflammatory response, metabolize food, and make new cells. Mineralocorticoids control the body's fluid level and electrolyte balance by influencing the rate of excretion of mineral salts (sodium and potassium) by the kidneys. Androgenic hormones stimulate the development of male sexual characteristics, including increased body size, and affect the buildup of protein tissues (anabolism).

The adrenal medulla produces epinephrine (adrenalin) and norepinephrine. Epinephrine initiates the "fight or flight" reaction to stress. Epinephrine increases heart rate, blood pressure, and blood sugar, and it decreases the blood flow to the internal organs.

Gonads

The gonads are the primary sexual glands. In the female the ovaries produce estrogen and progesterone. The ovaries are located in the lower abdomen beside the uterus. Estrogen and progesterone stimulate breast development, hair placement, and menstruation. Estrogen also initiates ovulation. Progesterone assists in the normal development of pregnancy.

In the male the primary sexual organs are the testes, located in the external scrotal sac. The testes produce the hormone testosterone. Testosterone stimulates secondary characteristics of the male, including a lowered voice, body hair growth, and muscular development.

Prostaglandins

Prostaglandins are fatty hormones that are produced by tissues throughout the body that influence the tissues surrounding the area. At least 16 types have been identified. Prostaglandins are known to decrease blood pressure, cause fever, increase hydrochloric acid secretion in the stomach, increase uterine contraction during pregnancy, and influence intestinal peristalsis. These "tissue hormones" are broken down quickly in the body.

Hormonal Changes of Puberty

Puberty is the time during which the body matures sexually. Hormones of the pituitary gland direct the changes that occur during puberty. These stimulate the gonads to secrete the hormones that cause the testes and ovaries to mature. In males the testes enlarge. In females the menstrual cycle (menarche) begins. Both acquire the ability to reproduce. Chapter 21 provides more information about the reproductive system.

The adrenal gland secretes the hormones that begin the development of secondary sexual characteristics, those body features that are different in males and females but do not directly affect reproduction. In the male the voice deepens and facial hair begins to grow. In the female the breasts enlarge and fatty tissue is deposited around the hips. In both males and females, height and weight increase. Emotional changes, which have been attributed to hormonal changes, may also occur during this growing time.

Hormonal Changes of Pregnancy

With the onset of pregnancy, many hormonal changes occur that influence the appearance and function of the woman's body. The placenta, or interfacing organ between the fetal and maternal circulation, produces a hormone called *human chorionic gonadotropin* (HCG), which stimulates the development and secretions of the ovaries to maintain the uterine lining. HCG can be detected in the urine and is used for pregnancy testing.

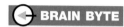

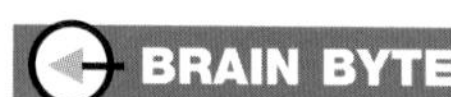

Injections of HCG are used as part of a rapid weight loss program called Simeons therapy.

The increased estrogen and progesterone from the ovaries are maintained until the placenta begins to produce these hormones for the duration of the pregnancy. Progesterone increases the mobility of the pelvic and lower bones of the back to allow the birthing process and may result in backache. Dilation of the ureters and renal pelvis may lead to urinary frequency. Progesterone also decreases the mobility and tone of the gastrointestinal tract and causes relaxation of the pyloric sphincter. It may cause heartburn and constipation.

During pregnancy the pituitary and thyroid glands increase in size, resulting in a higher metabolic rate. The adrenal gland secretions increase, especially aldosterone. An increase in the plasma level of insulin may be due to an increase in lipids or fats in the blood. Additionally, the destruction of insulin is faster during pregnancy, which may lead to a condition called "gestational" diabetes in which the woman's pancreas cannot produce enough insulin. The changes in the hormonal levels during early pregnancy may also be responsible for the nausea and vomiting called "morning sickness."

Hormonal Changes of Menopause

Menopause, or climacteric, is the term used to describe the time during which the female stops menses. Menopause occurs after a decrease in secretion of the gonadotropins FSH and LH. This change leads to a decrease in the secretion of the hormone estrogen by the ovaries. Hot flashes, periods of feeling extreme heat, are the only universal symptoms of menopause. Estrogen replacement therapy may be given after menopause in some instances.

Assessment Techniques

Hormonal disorders except diabetes mellitus (types 1 and 2) and thyroid disease are rare. Thyroid function may be assessed by using the **basal metabolic rate** and protein-bound iodine studies. However, results of both of these tests can be affected by many other factors. Several newer methods now used for assessment of the endocrine disorders include **immunoassay**, radioiodine uptake studies, and glucose tolerance testing.

- Basal metabolic rate is the amount of energy necessary to maintain the functions of a resting body, including circulation, respiration, digestion, and cell metabolism. The basal metabolic rate is measured by a test called *indirect calorimetry*, which measures the amount of oxygen consumed.
- Protein-bound iodine is a blood test to measure the amount of proteins attached to thyroxine. Test results may be influenced by cough syrups, iodine used in tests, diuretics, steroids, and pregnancy.
- Immunoassay is a chemical test in which a blood specimen is mixed with a specific agent. The number of antigens formed indicates the presence of certain hormones.
- Radioiodine uptake involves drinking radioactive iodine and measuring the iodine absorbed by the thyroid with a Geiger counter. The rate that the thyroid removes the iodine from the blood indicates how well it is functioning.
- The glucose tolerance test assesses the function of the pancreas, using urine and blood specimens. Glucose is given and specimens are compared over time. This measures the efficiency of the insulin production of the pancreas.

DISORDERS OF THE Endocrine System

Acromegaly (ak-ro-MEG-uh-lee) is an enlargement of the bones of the hands, feet, and jaws (Fig. 18-4). It results from an increased secretion of somatotropic (so-mah-to-TROP-ik) hormone, usually caused by a pituitary tumor. Heavy perspiration, oily skin, excess body hair, high blood pressure, and other symptoms may also result. Treatment includes surgical removal of the tumor or radiation to destroy gland tissue.

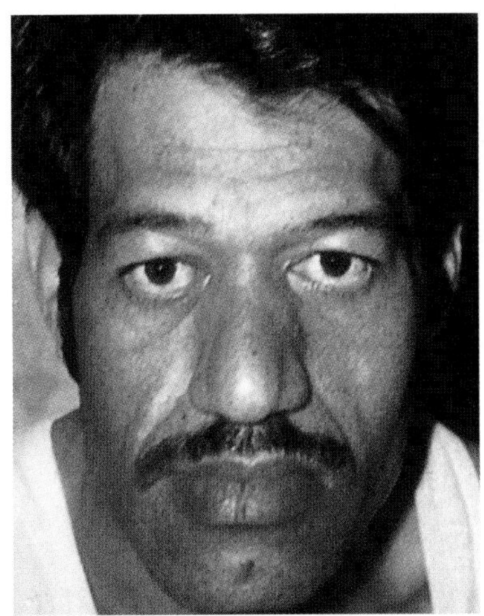

FIGURE 18-4 Acromegaly is characterized by enlargement of the bones of the hands, feet, and jaws with an increase in the soft tissue covering them. (Courtesy Henry M. Seidel, MD.)

Addison (AD-ih-sun) *disease* is caused by hyposecretion of the hormones produced by the cortex of the adrenal gland. The person with Addison disease experiences excessive skin pigmentation, decreased blood sugar, and decreased blood pressure, which result in muscle weakness, fatigue, gastrointestinal disturbances, and dehydration. Treatment includes administration of cortisone, a decrease in sodium intake, and monitoring the level of potassium and sodium in the blood.

Cretinism (KREE-tin-izm) is a condition resulting from a congenital deficiency of thyroid secretion, or hypothyroidism (hi-poe-THI-royd-izm). The basal metabolic rate and mental and physical growth are decreased. Early indications of hypothyroidism include jaundice, excessive drowsiness, and a hoarse cry. Hypothyroidism can be treated by oral administration of thyroxine, and early treatment can minimize mental and physical damage.

Cushing (KOOSH-ing) *syndrome* is a disorder that causes hyperactivity of the adrenal glands, which has been triggered by oversecretion of the pituitary hormone ACTH. The person with Cushing syndrome has a redistribution of fat, giving a distinctive "moon face" and "buffalo hump" appearance (Fig. 18-5). Sexual dystrophy, increased blood pressure, unusual hair growth (hirsutism), and easy bruising also result. Treatment depends on the cause of the hormone imbalance. If the cause is a tumor, it is surgically removed.

Diabetes insipidus (die-uh-BEE-tez in-SIP-i-dus) results from an acquired or inherited decrease in the

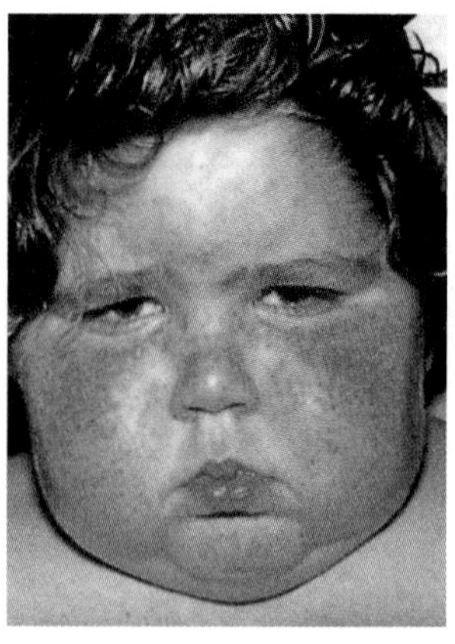
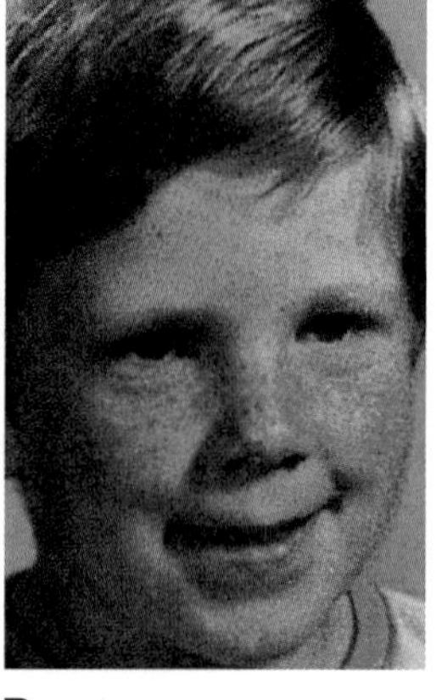

A B

FIGURE 18-5 **A,** This boy shows the fatty "moon face" of Cushing syndrome. **B,** The same boy 4 months after treatment. (From Patton KT, Thibodeau GA: *Anatomy & physiology*, ed 7, St. Louis, 2010, Mosby.)

pituitary hormone ADH. The main sign is an increase in urine production (polyuria) that leads to an intense thirst (polydipsia), weakness, constipation, and dry skin. Treatment includes giving ADH by injection or nasal spray.

CASE STUDY 18-1 You are helping admit a patient to the hospital for fatigue and weight loss. He has lost 64 lb in 2 years even though he is eating more. He also complains of being thirsty and irritable all the time. What should you do?

Answers to Case Studies are available on the Evolve website: ***http://evolve.elsevier.com/Gerdin***

Diabetes mellitus (die-uh-BEE-tez mel-LIE-tus) is a complex disorder of carbohydrate, fat, and protein metabolism resulting from insufficient insulin production by the pancreas. Its cause is unknown. The person with diabetes mellitus experiences unusual thirst (polydipsia), increased urine output (polyuria), and unusual hunger (polyphagia) (Table 18-2). Hyperglycemia may result, which is a greater-than-normal amount of glucose in the blood, causing nausea, headache, coma, and, if untreated, eventual death.

Two main types of diabetes mellitus exist. Type 1 can occur at any age and results when the pancreas does not produce insulin. Treatment includes injection of insulin to meet this need. Type 2 diabetes is linked with obesity. The pancreas does not produce enough insulin to meet the need of the body. Treatment may include oral hypoglycemic medication and weight

TABLE 18-2
Signs and Symptoms of Diabetes Mellitus

Hyperglycemia	Hypoglycemia
Increased thirst	Weakness
Increased urination	Trembling
Weight loss	Drowsiness
Increased appetite	Headache
Nausea	Confusion
Vomiting	Dizziness
Fatigue	Double vision
Ketoacidosis	Insulin shock

loss. Having a blood glucose level that is higher than normal but not high enough to be classified as diabetes is called prediabetes. The Centers for Disease Control and Prevention (CDC) estimates that 57 million Americans were prediabetic in 2007.

BRAIN BYTE

According to the CDC, people with prediabetes can reduce the onset of type 2 diabetes by 58% with lifestyle changes, including at least 7% weight loss and at least 150 minutes of physical activity per week.

CASE STUDY 18-2 Your friend who has diabetes tells you she is feeling faint and needs something to eat quickly. What should you do?

Answers to Case Studies are available on the Evolve website: ***http://evolve.elsevier.com/Gerdin***

Dwarfism (DWARF-izm) is usually characterized by a normal trunk and head with shortened extremities. It results from hyposecretion of the growth hormone of the pituitary gland, which has been caused by a tumor, infection, genetic factors, or trauma (Fig. 18-6). If discovered in the development years, dwarfism can be treated with injections of a somatotropic hormone (growth hormone) for 5 years or longer. Dwarfism does not affect intelligence.

Gigantism (ji-GAN-tizm), or giantism (see Fig. 18-6), is an excessive growth of the long bones caused by hypersecretion of the somatotropic hormone. Treatment may include hormones to control growth and perhaps removal or destruction of the pituitary if diagnosed early.

Graves (grayvz) *disease* is caused by hyperthyroidism (hi-per-THIE-royd-izm) or thyrotoxicosis (thie-ro-

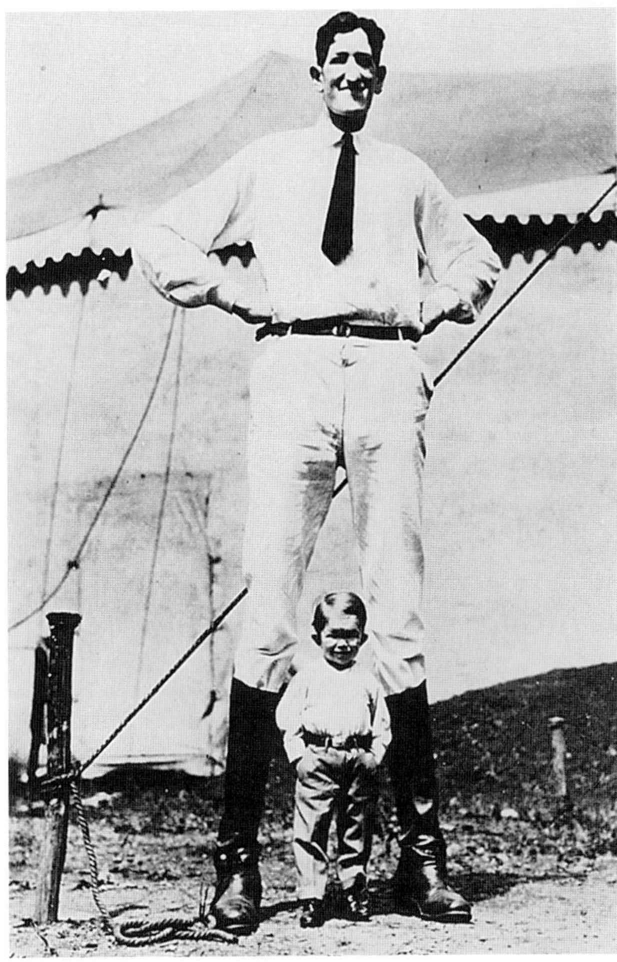

FIGURE 18-6 Dwarfism results from low levels of pituitary growth hormone during the early years and is the opposite of the condition of gigantism. (Courtesy Ewing Galloway.)

tok-sih-KO-sis). The person with Graves disease experiences nervousness; rapid pulse; weight loss; irritability; sensitivity to heat; increased basal metabolic rate and blood sugar; and sometimes **exophthalmos**, or protruding eyeballs. Treatment includes removal of part or all of the thyroid and administration of drugs to decrease the thyroxine level. Adults older than 40 years can be given radioactive iodine to destroy thyroid tissue.

Hyperparathyroidism (hi-per-pare-ah-THIE-roid-izm) causes hypercalcemia (hi-per-kal-SEE-mee-uh), an increased calcium blood level. It can cause kidney stone formation. The calcium is taken from the bones, which can lead to fractures and deformities. This condition is often caused by an adenoma (ad-uh-NO-mah), a glandular tumor, and treatment requires its removal.

Hypoglycemia (hi-po-glie-SEE-mee-uh) results from increased insulin production by the pancreas. The low blood sugar causes fatigue, tremors, cold sweats, headache, and weight disturbances. Treatment includes a diet that is low in carbohydrates and high in protein.

Hypoparathyroidism (hi-po-par-uh-THIE-roid-izm) is a decreased secretion of parathyroid hormone that causes tetany. Blood calcium levels are decreased, interrupting function of the nerves. The sufferer experiences a convulsive twitching. Death may result if the respiratory muscles are affected. Treatment is giving oral supplements of vitamin D, calcium, and parathormone.

Hypothyroidism (hi-po-THIE-royd-izm) results from an insufficient production of thyroxine. It may be caused by an autoimmune disorder, iodine deficiency, or malfunction of the pituitary gland or hypothalamus. Hypothyroidism is most often caused by *Hashimoto disease* (thyroiditis). Hashimoto disease is an autoimmune disorder in which the body attacks the thyroid gland. The thyroid enlarges to compensate for the deficiency, resulting in goiter (GOY-ter) (Fig. 18-7). This leads to increase in fat tissue and sluggishness. Myxedema (mik-seh-DEE-muh) is the most severe form of hypothyroidism. The person with myxedema experiences edema, obesity, lethargy, decreased heart rate, decreased intelligence, sensitivity to cold, and coarse skin. Treatment includes administration of oral thyroid extract.

CASE STUDY 18-3 You are helping to admit a patient to the hospital for chronic tiredness and difficulty concentrating. She also complains of weight gain and constipation. She tells you she is chilly and needs another blanket. What should you do?

Answers to Case Studies are available on the Evolve website: ***http://evolve.elsevier.com/Gerdin***

Syndrome of inappropriate antidiuretic hormone **(SIADH)** involves water intoxication and the dilution of intracellular and extracellular body tissues, usually resulting from lung cancer. Antidiuretic hormone production is increased in the pituitary gland. SIADH can lead to convulsions and death. Treatment is removal of the cancer, restriction of fluids, and drug therapy.

Virilism (VIR-i-lizm) results from increased secretion in the adrenal glands. Adrenal virilism may be present at birth due to congenital adrenal hyperplasia. It may also develop later in life due to a tumor. The female may develop male sexual characteristics, including facial hair, broad shoulders, and small

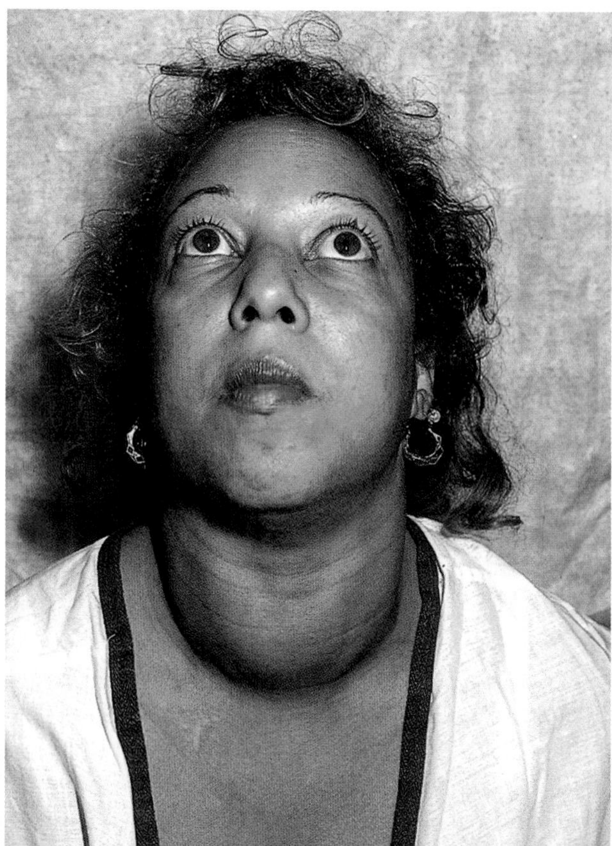

FIGURE 18-7 Simple goiter is a painless enlargement of the thyroid gland that may result from inadequate iodine intake in the diet. (From Swartz MH: *Textbook of physical diagnosis,* ed 6, Philadelphia, 2010, Saunders.)

breasts. Treatment focuses on the cause of hypersecretion by the gland.

Issues and Innovations

Diabetes

According to the CDC, 23.6 million people, or about 8% of the U.S. population, have diabetes. Of the 8%, it is estimated that 5.7 million people have not been diagnosed. In 2007 there were 1.6 million new cases diagnosed in people 20 years or older. In the same population, diabetes was the leading cause of new cases of blindness, kidney failure, and lower-extremity amputations not caused by trauma (Fig. 18-8). In 2006 it was the seventh leading cause of death. The International Diabetes Federation is an umbrella organization of more than 200 national diabetes associations in more than 160 countries. Their statistics indicate that diabetes rates are highest in India, China, and the United States and can be considered an epidemic.

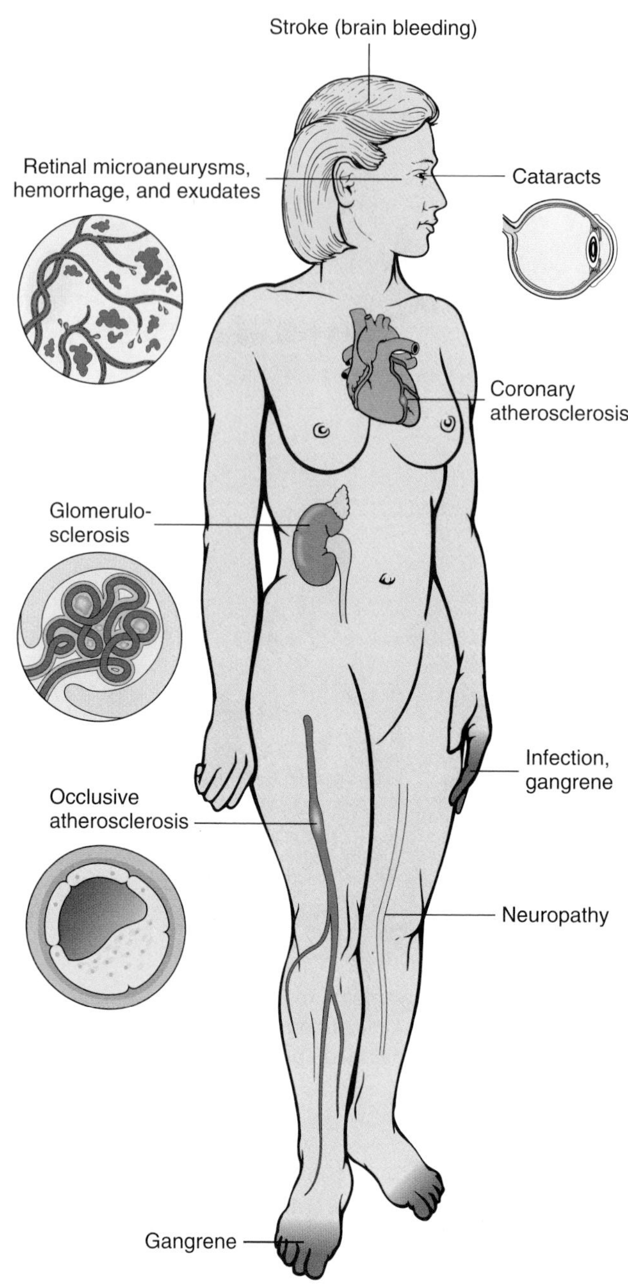

FIGURE 18-8 Complications of diabetes mellitus. (From Damjanov I: *Pathology for the health professions,* ed 3, St. Louis, 2006, Saunders.)

Exubera, a new form of insulin that can be taken with an inhaler, was approved by the U.S. Food and Drug Administration and became available in 2006. Exubera can be used by patients who have either type 1 or type 2 diabetes. A Canadian company, Generex Biotechnology Corporation, has developed an insulin medication that can be sprayed into the buccal mucosa or mouth. The Generex Oral-lyn is in clinical trials. Transplantation of a donor pancreas has been used with varied success.

In 2002 Florida became the first state to offer screening for diabetes mellitus to all newborns. The newborns will be monitored throughout their lifetime. The purpose of this program is to identify newborns with genetic risk for developing type 1 diabetes and refer them to clinical trials and research designed to end the disease.

Another clinical trial in Florida is using infusion of cord stem cells into children with type 1 diabetes. Using the children's own cells, the researchers are comparing this treatment with standard insulin injection. Preliminary results indicate that infusion of cord blood stem cells is safe and may slow the progression of type 1 diabetes in children.

Steroid Abuse

Abuse of hormones continues to be a problem, especially by athletes hoping for better performance. In 2008 a National Institute of Drug Abuse survey indicated that 1.4% of eighth and tenth grade students and 2.2% of high school students had tried steroids. Performance-enhancing or "ergogenic" steroids are commonly abused. These include somatotropin, or growth hormone, and androgenic anabolic steroids such as testosterone. The benefit, if any, from use of these hormones in sports training is far less than the health risk imposed. The effects of even a short use of these steroids can be long lasting or permanent.

Synthetic growth hormone was developed to treat children with a deficiency of this pituitary hormone. Some athletes believe that supplementing exercise with growth hormone will improve performance, but such improvement has not been shown scientifically. It is known that an oversupply of the hormone in adults leads to physical changes of acromegaly.

Androgenic anabolic steroids, including synthetic drugs similar to the hormone testosterone, have been banned by most major sports organizations. Muscle growth can be increased with use of anabolic steroids, but the risks and complications far exceed the benefits. Effects on men include early baldness, stunted growth, changes in liver structure, liver tumors, decreased sperm production, testicular atrophy, enlarged breasts, and increased risk of cardiovascular disease. Effects on women include menstrual irregularities, complete loss of menstrual cycle (amenorrhea), abnormal hair placement (hirsutism), baldness, and irreversible deepening of the voice. Bad breath, severe acne, headache, dizziness, hypertension, mood swings, and aggressiveness ("roid rages") are commonplace in both sexes.

CASE STUDY 18-4 You notice that one of your friends has more facial hair and is adding muscle weight and seems aggressive most of the time. What should you do?

Answers to Case Studies are available on the Evolve website: ***http://evolve.elsevier.com/Gerdin***

In 1988 anabolic steroids were classified as a controlled substance by federal law. Conviction for the selling of steroids results in a minimum sentence of 5 years in prison. The use of steroids may result in 1 to 6 years in prison.

Summary

- The function of the endocrine system is to produce hormones that monitor and coordinate body activities.
- Endocrine system structures include the pineal, hypothalamus, thyroid, pituitary, and thymus glands, as well as others.
- The hormone produced by the thyroid gland (thyroxine) regulates body metabolism.
- Methods used to assess the endocrine system include basal metabolic rate, protein-bound iodine blood tests, and radioactive uptake.
- Disorders of the endocrine system include acromegaly, cretinism, Cushing syndrome, diabetes insipidus, and diabetes mellitus.

Review Questions

1. Describe the functions of the endocrine system.
2. Describe the location and function of each of the following parts of the endocrine system:
   adrenal medulla — pituitary
   pineal body — prostaglandin
3. Describe three tests used to assess the function of the endocrine system.
4. Describe three changes that occur during puberty as a result of hormonal changes.
5. Describe three changes that occur during pregnancy as a result of hormonal changes.
6. List five side effects and risks of using androgenic anabolic hormones.
7. Use the following terms in one or more sentences that correctly relate their meaning: endocrine,

hormone, hyperglycemia, polyphagia, and polyuria.

Critical Thinking

1. Investigate and compare the cost of at least three tests used to diagnose disorders of the endocrine system.
2. Investigate the function of at least five common medications used in treatment of the endocrine system.
3. List at least five occupations involved in the health care of endocrine system disorders.
4. Compare the difference between the conditions of being a dwarf or midget.
5. Investigate and describe the function of the following exocrine glands: lacrimal, mammary, salivary, and sudoriferous.
6. Use the Internet to research the incidence of steroid abuse in sports and the methods used to combat this problem. Create a pamphlet that describes the issue.
7. Use the Internet to research and review an article regarding a recent development or treatment method relating to the endocrine system.
8. Use the Internet to research and write a report on CDC success stories for diabetes prevention in Alaska, North Dakota, or Texas.

Explore the Web

Diabetes Success Stories

CDC
http://www.cdc.gov/chronicdisease/resources/publications/AAG/ddt.htm

CDC
http://www.cdc.gov/diabetes/

IDF Diabetes Atlas
http://www.diabetesatlas.org/

Steroid Abuse

National Institute on Drug Abuse
http://www.drugabuse.gov/students.html

U.S. Department of Justice
http://www.deadiversion.usdoj.gov/pubs/brochures/steroids/professionals/index.html

CHAPTER 19

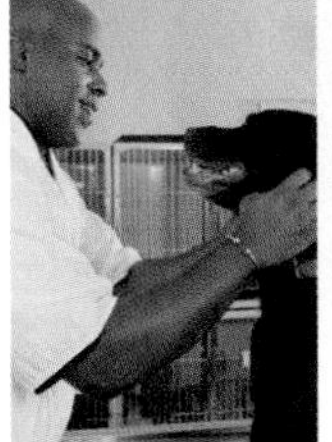
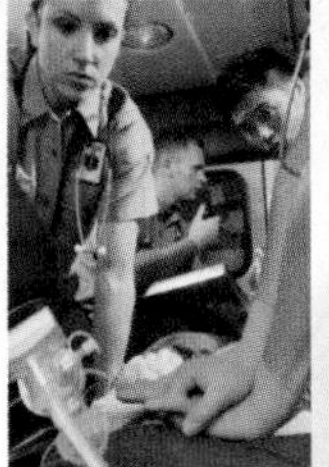
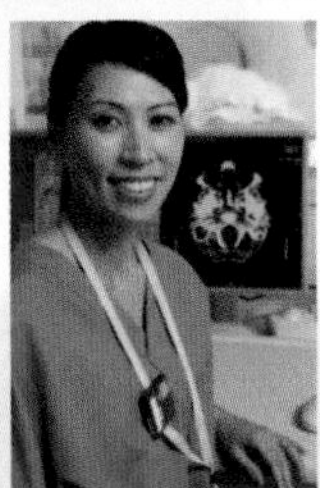

Nervous System

LEARNING OBJECTIVES

- Define at least 10 terms relating to the nervous system.
- Describe the function of the nervous system.
- Identify at least 10 structures of the nervous system.
- Identify at least three methods used to assess the function of the nervous system.
- Describe at least five disorders of the nervous system.

KEY TERMS

Cerebrospinal fluid *(se-ree-bro-SPY-nal FLOO-id)* Fluid contained in the brain's ventricles, intracranial spaces, and central canal of the spinal cord

Dementia *(de-MEN-shee-uh)* Organic loss of intellectual function

Epilepsy *(EP-ih-lep-see)* Transient disturbances of brain function

Impulse *(IM-puls)* Sudden pushing force; activity along nerve fibers

Intracranial *(in-tra-KRAY-nee-uhl)* Situated within the cranium

Ischemia *(is-KEE-mee-uh)* Insufficient blood to a body part caused by a functional constriction or actual obstruction of a blood vessel

Meninges *(me-NIN-jeez)* Three membranes that surround and protect the brain and spinal cord

Myelography *(my-eh-LOG-rah-fee)* X-rays of the spinal cord after injection of a contrast medium

Neurotransmitter *(noo-ro-TRANS-mit-er)* Chemical messenger, released from the axon of one neuron, that travels to another nearby neuron

Polyneuritis *(pol-ee-noo-RIE-tis)* Inflammation of many nerves at once

Reflex *(REE-fleks)* An involuntary action in response to a stimulus

Regenerate *(re-JEN-uh-rate)* Natural renewal of a structure, as of lost tissue or part

Senile *(SEE-nile)* Pertaining to or characteristic of old age, especially physical or mental deterioration accompanying aging

Nervous System Terminology*

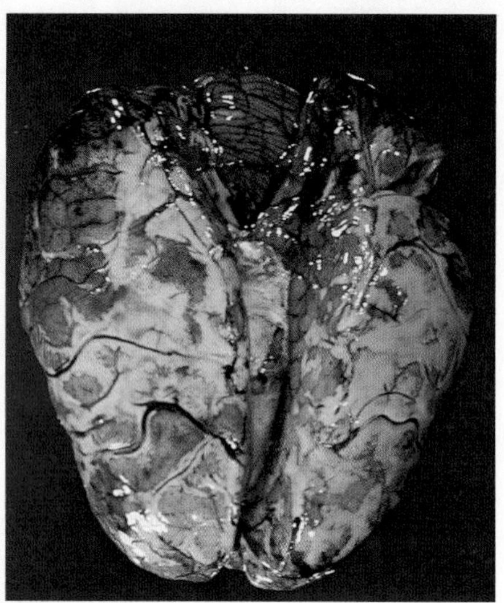

The surface of this brain shows pus from bacterial meningitis. (Courtesy of Dr. John J. Kepes, Kansas City, Kansas. In Damjanov I: *Pathology for the health professions*, ed 3, St. Louis, 2006, Saunders.)

Term	Definition	Prefix	Root	Suffix
Anesthesia	Without sensation	an	esthes	ia
Cerebrospinal	Pertaining to the brain and spine	cerebro	spin	al
Craniotomy	Incision into the skull		crani	otomy
Encephalotomy	Incision into the brain		encephal	otomy
Hypnotic	Pertaining to sleep		hypnot	ic
Insomnia	Lack of sleep	in	somn	ia
Meningitis	Inflammation of the meninges		mening	itis
Microencephaly	Small brain	micro	encephal	y
Neuralgia	Nerve pain		neur	algia
Neurology	Study of the nerve		neur	ology

*A transition syllable or vowel may be added to or deleted from the word parts to make the combining form.

Abbreviations of the Nervous System

Abbreviation	Meaning
CAT	Computerized axial tomography
CNS	Central nervous system
CSF	Cerebrospinal fluid
CVA	Cardiovascular accident
H/A	Headache
MRI	Magnetic resonance imagery
NICU	Neurointensive care unit
PERLA	Pupils equally reactive to light
REM	Rapid eye movement
TIA	Transient ischemic attack

Structure and Function of the Nervous System

The nervous system is one of the most complex and interesting body systems. It is also one of the least understood. New discoveries are made almost daily about the capabilities of the nervous system.

The function of the nervous system is to sense, interpret, and respond to internal and external environmental changes to maintain a steady state in the body (homeostasis). The nervous system is divided into two major structures: the central nervous system (CNS) and the peripheral nervous system (PNS) (Fig. 19-1).

The CNS is made up of the brain and spinal cord (Fig. 19-2). It functions as the coordinator of the body's full nervous system and contains the nerves that control connections between **impulses** coming to and

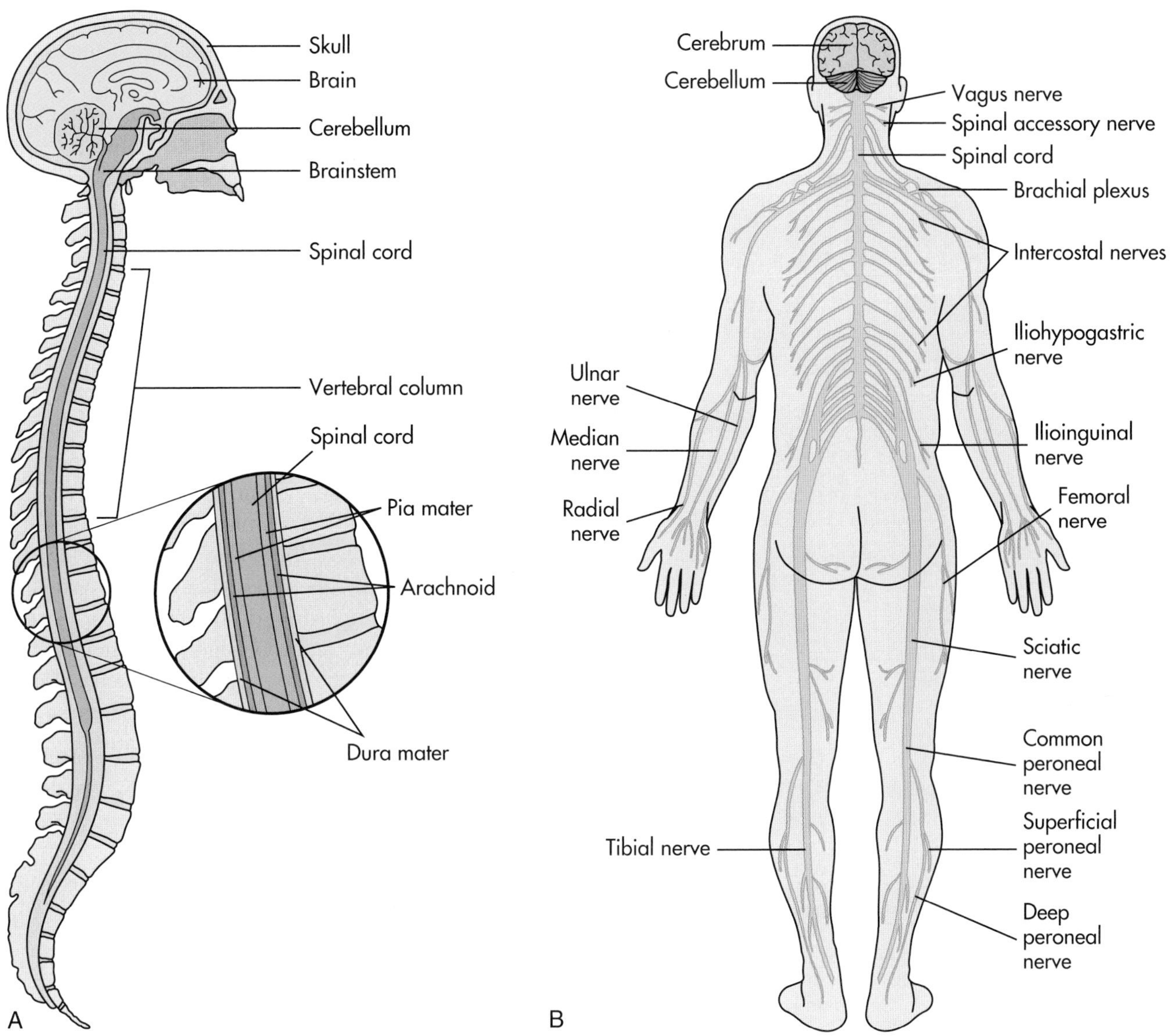

FIGURE 19-1 Divisions of the nervous system. **A,** The central nervous system. **B,** The peripheral nervous system. (From Sorrentino SA: *Mosby's textbook for nursing assistants*, ed 7, St. Louis, 2008, Mosby.)

from the brain and the rest of the body. The CNS plays a crucial role in maintaining a healthy, normally functioning body. Because nervous tissues are delicate and easily damaged, tough membranes called **meninges** surround the tissues. The nervous tissue and meninges are further protected by bones (vertebrae and cranium).

The PNS consists of 12 pairs of cranial nerves and 31 pairs of spinal nerves (Table 19-1) that reach all parts of the body. The cranial nerves originate in the brain, and the spinal nerves emerge from the spinal cord. The spinal cord nerves can act independently from the brain in some **reflex** reactions (Fig. 19-3). Other reflex reactions of the nervous system may lead to the release of glandular secretions.

The organs of the PNS contain sensory (afferent) and motor (efferent) neurons (Fig. 19-4). Afferent neurons, or nerves, carry messages from the sensory cells of the body to the brain. Efferent, or motor, nerves carry messages from the brain to the body organs or parts. The connecting nerves (interneurons) of the CNS carry messages from afferent nerves to efferent nerves. Efferent nerves are classified as voluntary (somatic) or involuntary (autonomic).

The autonomic (involuntary) nervous system (ANS) is a part of the PNS (Fig. 19-5). It has two parts: the sympathetic system and the parasympathetic system. The sympathetic nerves are stimulated in situations that require action, such as the "fight or flight" reaction. The parasympathetic functions in response

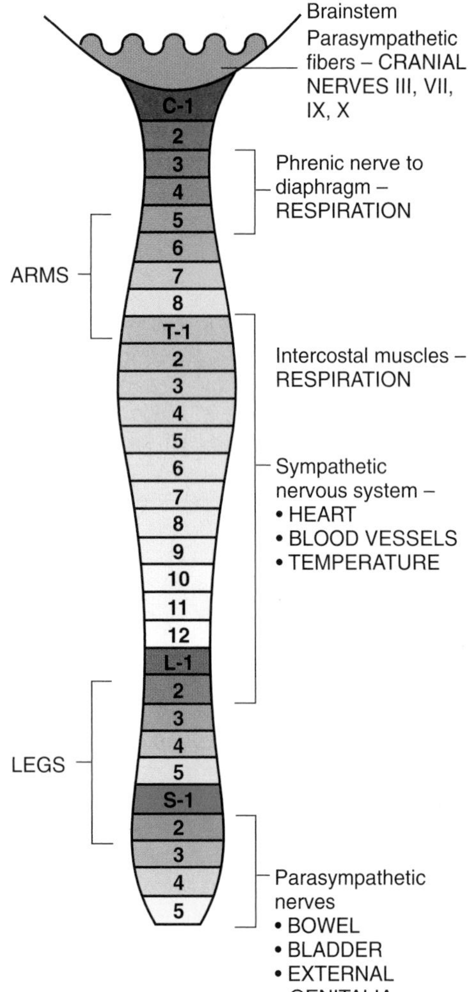

FIGURE 19-2 Functional areas of the spinal cord. (From Gould BE, Dyer R: *Pathophysiology for the health professions*, ed 4, St. Louis, 2011, Saunders.)

to normal, everyday situations. For example, the parasympathetic system would stimulate the digestion of food and slow the heart rate, whereas the sympathetic system would inhibit digestion and increase the heart rate.

Neuron

The basic structural unit of the nervous system is the nerve, which is a bundle of fibers that carries impulses. Nerve fibers consist of neuron cells, which are the functional unit of the nervous system. The three main

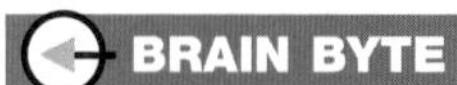

The human brain has about a 100 billion neurons that, if lined up, would be 600 miles long.

types of neurons are afferent, efferent, and interneuron. Each carries messages, or impulses, to and from the body's organs.

The neuron has several important parts (Fig. 19-6). The dendrites receive impulses and transmit them to the cell body. The cell body, which contains the nucleus of the neuron, transmits the impulse to the axon. The axon transmits the impulse away from the cell body to the dendrite of the next neuron. These impulse transmissions can travel more than 130 meters per second or 300 miles per hour.

Some neurons outside the CNS have a white, fatty substance covering the axon called *myelin*. Myelin, also called *white matter*, is arranged in bundles called *Schwann cells*. Layers of Schwann cells wrap around the axon forming the myelin sheath. The myelin sheath is covered with a membrane called the neurilemma. It is believed that *neurilemma* enables the axons to repair and **regenerate** themselves. Axons in the CNS, called *gray matter*, do not have neurilemma and therefore cannot repair or regenerate themselves. Another benefit of the myelin sheath is the microscopic spaces between the Schwann cells. These are called the *nodes of Ranvier*, and they greatly increase the speed of impulse transmission.

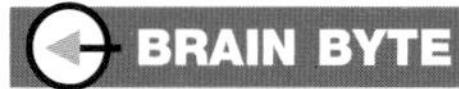

Neurons are the largest cells in the body and do not perform mitosis.

Neuroglia

Neuroglia, often called *glia*, are special nervous tissue cells that act as "glue" to support, bind, repair, and protect neurons. An estimated 900 billion neuroglia are in the body. They can be divided into four major types:

- The astrocytes, star-shaped cells, are believed to help transfer substances from the blood to the brain. They make up what is known as the blood-brain barrier.
- The oligodendroglia in the CNS and Schwann cells in the PNS help to develop the myelin sheath.
- The microglia destroy and engulf bacteria and fight infection.
- The ependymal cells line the cavities of the nervous system, producing and circulating fluid in the system.

Neuroglia may become cancerous when they divide to make new cells.

TABLE 19-1
Functions of the Peripheral Nervous System

Nerve		Function
Cranial Nerves		
I	Olfactory	Smell (S)
II	Optic	Vision (S)
III	Oculomotor	Raise eyelids, move eyes, focus lens, control pupil size (M)
IV	Trochlear	Rotate eyes (M)
V	Trigeminal	Facial and head sensation, control muscles in floor of mouth for chewing (B)
VI	Abducens	Move eyes laterally (M)
VII	Facial	Taste in anterior of mouth, control facial expression (B)
VIII	Acoustic (auditory)	Hearing and balance (S)
IX	Glossopharyngeal	Taste and swallowing (B)
X	Vagus	Control muscles of speech, swallowing, and of thorax and abdomen; feeling from pharynx, larynx, and trachea (B)
XI	Spinal accessory	Move neck and back muscles (M)
XII	Hypoglossal	Move tongue (M)
Spinal Nerves		
C1-8 Cervical (8 pair)		Neck and head movement; elevation of shoulders; movement of arms, hands, and diaphragmatic breathing
T1-12 Thoracic (12 pair)		Intercostal muscles of respiration and abdominal contractions
L1-5 Lumbar (5 pair)		Leg movement
S1-5 Sacral (5 pair)		Sphincter muscles of anus and urinary meatus; foot movement

S, Sensory; *M,* motor; *B,* both sensory and motor functions.

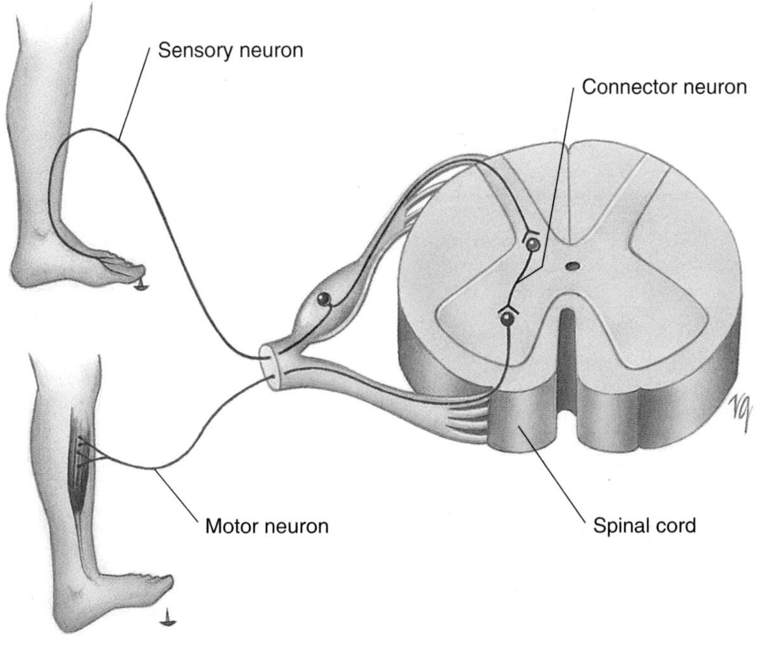

FIGURE 19-3 The spinal reflex arc. The motor response to injury is a reflex action controlled by the spinal nerves.

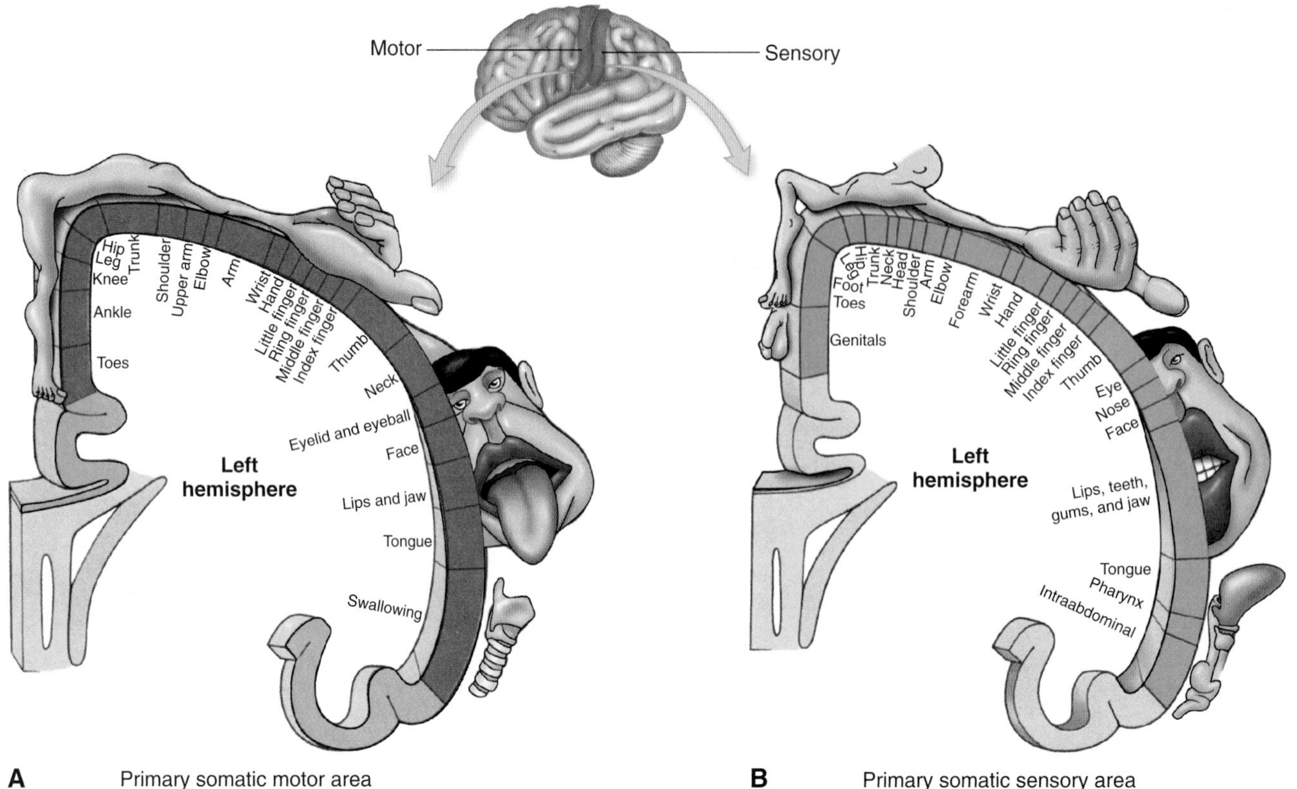

FIGURE 19-4 Somatic **(A)** and motor **(B)** sensory areas of the brain. The exaggerated images show the amount of cortical areas involved in processing the information. (From Patton KT, Thibodeau GA: *Anatomy & physiology*, ed 7, St. Louis, 2010, Mosby.)

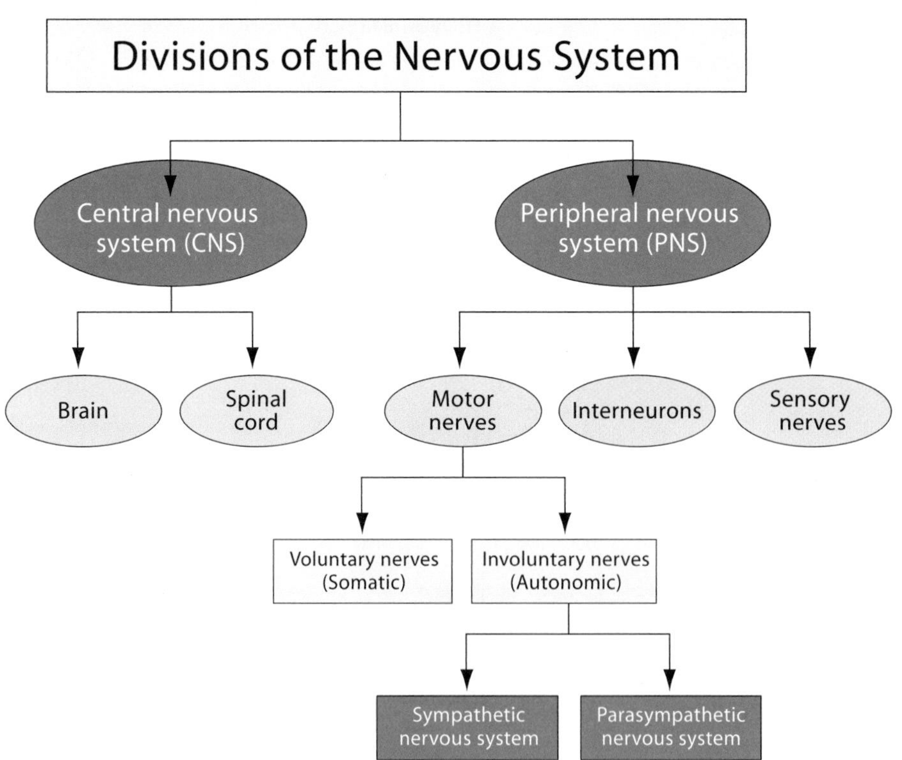

FIGURE 19-5 The nervous system may be divided into parts on the basis of their functions.

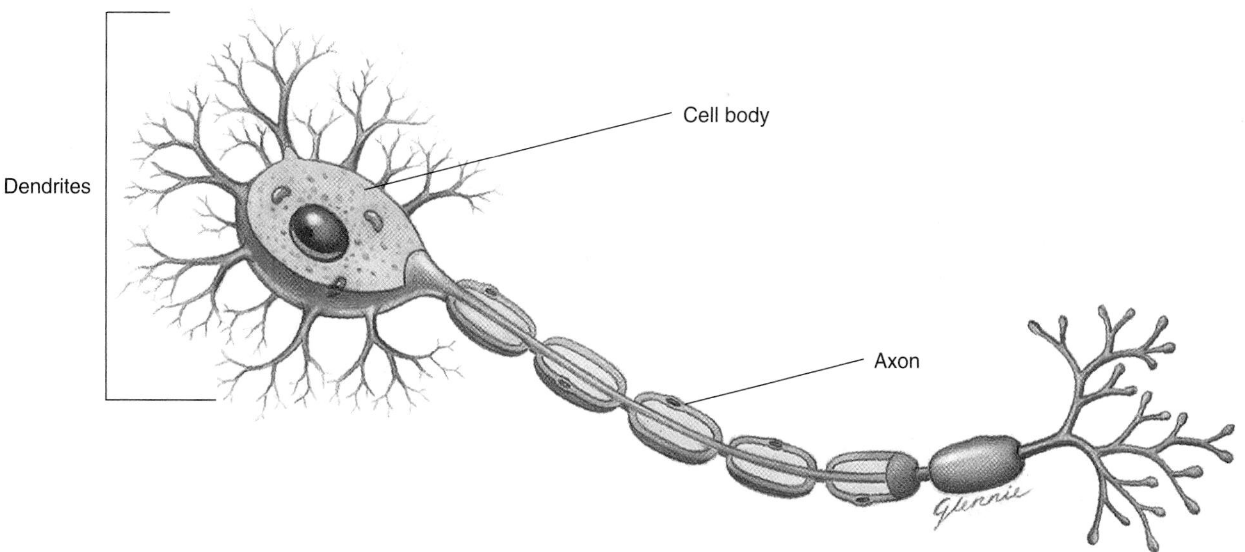

FIGURE 19-6 Neuron.

Synapse

A synapse is the space between two neurons. Neurons may be as close as one millionth of an inch to each other but still not touch. One neuron may send messages to up to 10,000 other neurons through the synapse. Impulses from one neuron are transmitted across the synapse to another neuron by a chemical called a **neurotransmitter**. The two most common neurotransmitters are acetylcholine and norepinephrine. One neurotransmitter may have different effects in varied synapses. More than 100 chemical messengers used by the nervous system have been identified.

Ganglia

Ganglia are groups of nerve tissue, principally nerve cell bodies, located outside the CNS. These cell bodies have some increased ability to transmit impulses compared with nerve cells because they are clustered together in the ganglion.

Plexus and Dermatome

Four major networks of interwoven spinal nerves, called *plexuses*, provide impulses to specific regions of the body. They are called the *cervical*, *brachial*, *lumbar*, and *sacral* plexuses on the basis of the location of the spinal nerves that are involved in each group.

Sensations on the skin surface are controlled by specific spinal nerves. For example, the second cervical spinal nerve senses afferent messages on the top of the cranium. These areas are called *dermatomes*.

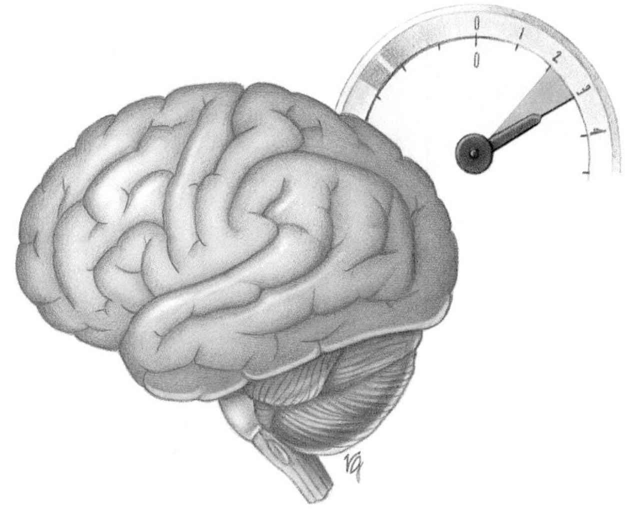

FIGURE 19-7 The brain weighs 2 to 3 lb.

Brain

The brain is the largest structure of the nervous system and one of the largest organs of the body (Fig. 19-7). It weighs about 2 to 3 lb (0.9-1.4 kg). It uses about 20% of the blood flow from the heart. The brain's cells can survive only 4 to 6 minutes without oxygen and glucose from the blood.

The brain is covered by three layers of membranes called *meninges*: the dura mater, arachnoid, and pia

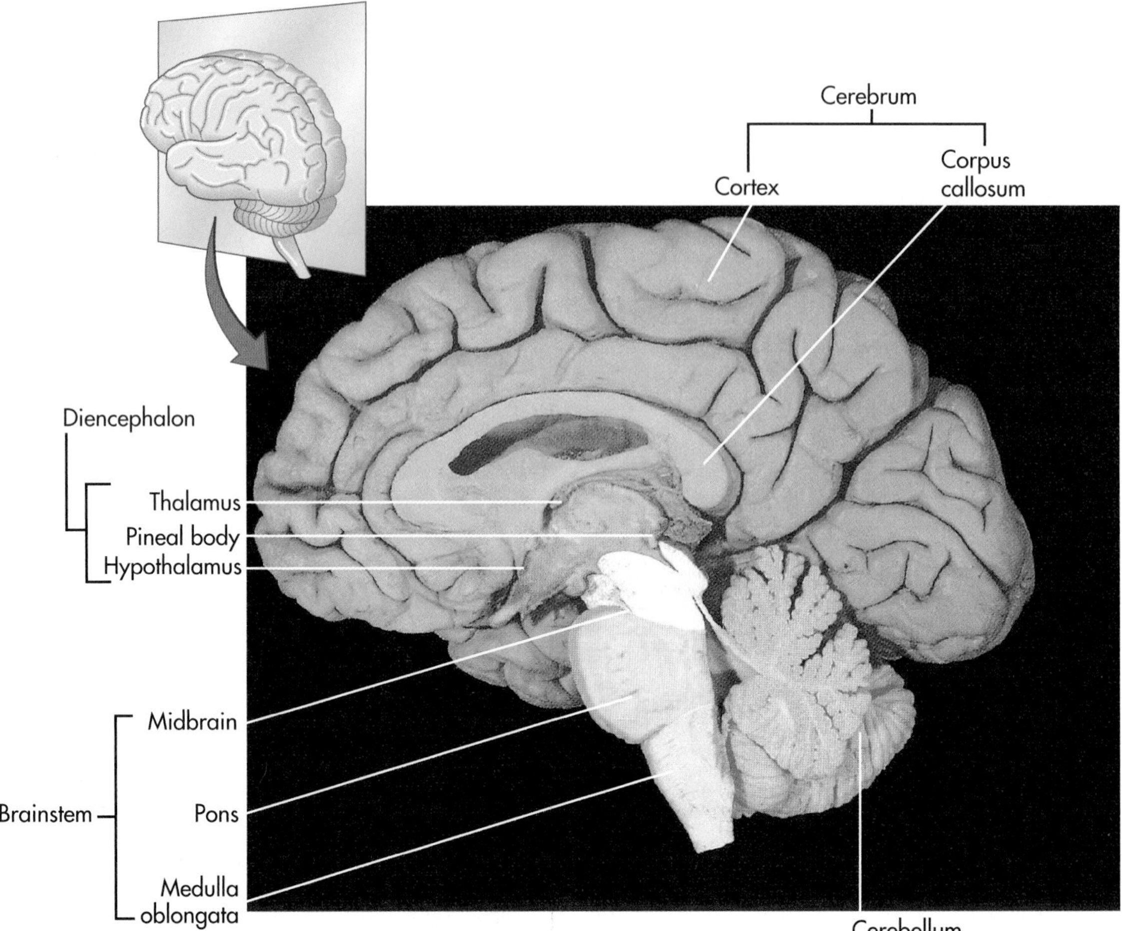

FIGURE 19-8 The parts of the brain. (From Patton KT, Thibodeau GA: *Anatomy & physiology*, ed 7, St. Louis, 2010, Mosby.)

mater. The pia mater is the innermost layer attached to the brain and spinal cord. The arachnoid is the middle layer and acts as a channel for **cerebrospinal fluid** (CSF). The dura mater is a leathery outer layer.

The brain has four lined cavities, called *ventricles*. The inner layers of the brain, spinal cord, and ventricles are filled with a clear fluid called CSF. This fluid acts as a cushion to protect the brain from injury and carries nutrients to, and wastes from, the CNS cells.

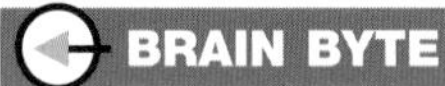

BRAIN BYTE

At any time, only 4% of brain cells are active.

The four major areas of the brain are the cerebrum, the diencephalon, the cerebellum, and the brainstem. The cerebrum is the largest area and is divided into two hemispheres. It is concerned with reasoning and the senses. Each of the hemispheres is further divided into lobes and sections on the basis of function (Fig. 19-8). The right hemisphere controls many of the functions of the left side of the body; the left hemisphere controls the right side. One side usually has more influence over the overall body functions.

The diencephalon contains the hypothalamus and the thalamus. The hypothalamus regulates and coordinates the activity of the autonomic nervous system. It also controls hormone secretion and appetite. The thalamus transfers sensory impulses to the sensory areas of the cerebral cortex.

BRAIN BYTE

After the age of 20, humans tend to lose 1 g of brain weight each year.

The cerebellum directs coordination, muscle tone, and equilibrium. The brainstem includes the pons, medulla, and midbrain. It maintains the heartbeat, respiration, and blood pressure. Some areas of the

TABLE 19-2
Functions of the Brain

Brain Part	Function
Cerebrum	
Frontal lobe	Personality, behavior, memory, reasoning, emotion
Broca's area	Speech
Sensory cortex	Sensations of heat and pain
Motor cortex	Controls movement
Angular gyrus	Written language
Wernicke's area	Understanding written or spoken language
Parietal lobe	Understanding speech or choosing words
Temporal lobe	Hearing and understanding speech and printed words, memory of music and visual scenes
Occipital lobe	Vision and its interpretation
Cerebellum	Coordination of voluntary movement, balance
Brainstem	
Pons	Breathing, relaying impulses between cerebellum and medulla
Medulla	Control of involuntary movements, heartbeat, blood pressure, respiration, and swallowing
Midbrain	Visual and auditory reflex

brain have been identified with specific functions (Table 19-2).

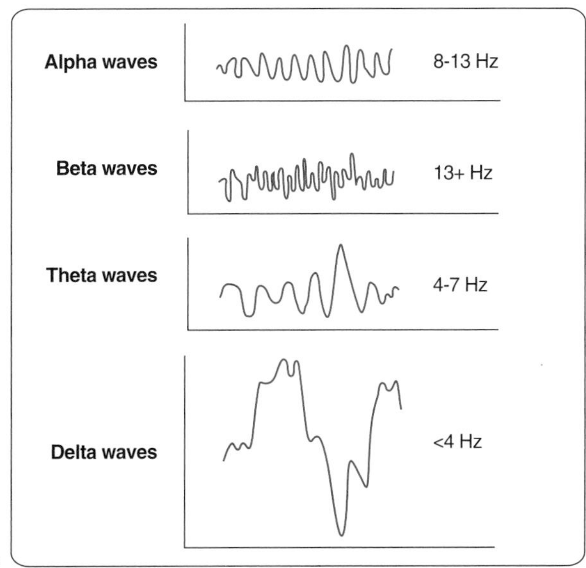

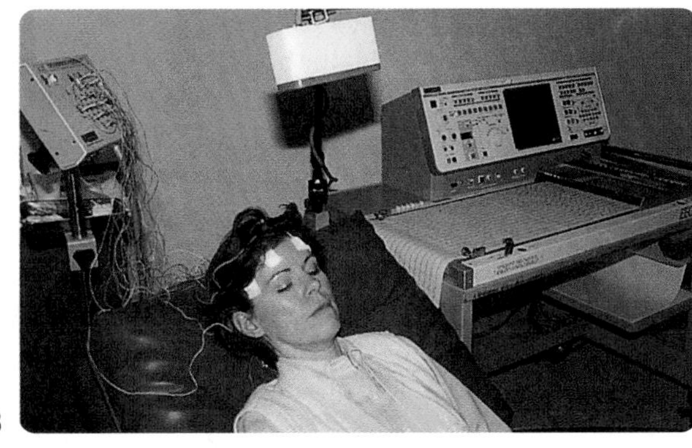

FIGURE 19-9 **A,** Electroencephalogram showing wave types. **B**, Scalp electrodes detect electrical voltage changes in the cranium. (From Thibodeau GA, Patton KT: *Human body in health and disease*, ed 5, St Louis, 2010, Mosby.)

Assessment Techniques

Evaluation of the nervous system includes assessment of the following:
- Mental status
- Cranial nerve function
- Motor and sensory nerve function
- Reflexes
- Coordination
- Gait (walking)
- Balance
- Internal body processes
- Blood flow to the brain

Primary methods of testing to assess the nervous system include the following:
- Electroencephalography is a simple, painless test that measures the electrical activity of the brain and aids in the location and treatment of disorders (Fig. 19-9). Encephalography may be used in surgery by applying the electrodes directly to the brain tissue.
- Lumbar puncture assesses CSF for blood, foreign cells, infection, and chemical imbalances. Lumbar puncture is performed by a physician using strict sterile technique to avoid introduction of microorganisms into the spinal column.
- **Myelography** is a type of x-ray of the interior of the spinal cord used to detect growths or displacement of the vertebral column.
- Nerve conduction velocity tests the speed of impulses through nerves. This test stimulates nerves on a surface electrode placed on the skin and

records the time necessary to conduct the information to another electrode. This test may be used to diagnose nerve damage.

- Computed tomography (CT) is a special radiographic technique that uses scanning equipment to reconstruct sectional slices of the body at any angle to detect abnormalities.
- Positron emission tomography is a type of CT using radioactive isotopes introduced into brain cells to detect disorders related to chemical functions.
- Magnetic resonance imagery (MRI) determines the movement of ions in tissue cells by measuring energy changes cause by radio waves (Fig. 19-10). MRI is so sensitive that white matter and fluid in the brain can be seen.
- Network spinal analysis is a technique used by chiropractors. It is based on the Epstein Model of Somatic Awareness. Palpation, observation, and thermography studies are used along with traditional medical testing to locate and correct functional or structural disorders (subluxation) of the spinal column.
- Blood flow to the brain may be tested using magnetic resonance angiography, computed tomography angiography, or cerebral angiography. These tests are used to determine the risk of a stroke occurring.

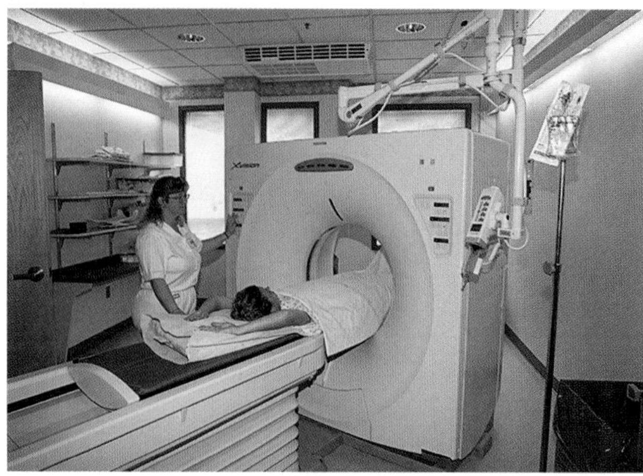

FIGURE 19-10 Magnetic resonance imagery allows the visualization of the body without use of radiation. (From Elkin MK, et al: *Nursing intervention and clinical skills*, ed 4, St. Louis, 2008, Mosby.)

BOX 19-1

Warning Signs of Alzheimer Disease*

- Memory loss that disrupts daily life
- Challenges in planning or solving problems
- Difficulty completing familiar tasks at home, at work, or at leisure
- Confusion with time or place
- Trouble understanding visual images and spatial relationships
- New problems with words in speaking or writing
- Misplacing things and losing the ability to retrace steps
- Decreased or poor judgment
- Withdrawal from work or social activities
- Changes in mood and personality

*Alzheimer's Association (http://www.alz.org/alzheimers_disease_10_signs_of_alzheimers.asp).

DISORDERS OF THE Nervous System

Alzheimer (AHLZ-hi-mer) *disease* is the most common form of **senile dementia**, but it also occurs in middle-aged adults. It is reported by the Alzheimer's Association that as many as 5.3 million Americans have Alzheimer disease, which is more than twice the number in 1980. Although the specific cause is unknown, several forms have been identified, at least one of which is genetically linked. The person with this condition experiences a progressive loss of memory and intellectual impairment (Box 19-1). No single diagnostic test for Alzheimer disease exists. The Mini-Mental State Examination may be used to help with identification of the condition. Lesions caused by deposit of plaque on brain cells can be seen on autopsy. Also, a positron emission tomography scan may be used to identify it. Treatment helps the person control the symptoms, but no cure is known. One area of research for treatment is the use of granulocyte-colony stimulating factor to stimulate growth of blood stem and white blood cells.

Cerebrovascular (se-ree-bro-VAS-kyoo-lar) *accidents*, commonly called *strokes* or *CVAs*, are cardiovascular disorders that directly affect the neurological system. According to the American Heart Association statistics for 2006, about 795,000 Americans have a stroke each year. A CVA is caused by loss of oxygen, or **ischemia**, to an area of the brain when a clot blocks a vessel or when a vessel breaks. The extent of damage depends on the area of the brain that is affected, and the stroke victim may experience mental or physical dysfunction. Prevention of a stroke includes controlling risk factors, such as hypertension, diabetes, and heart disease. Treatment may include anticoagulants, angioplasty, or clot-dissolving drug tissue plasminogen activator. Treatment is also designed to help the person recover from or cope with functional losses caused by tissue death, such as the ability to walk or talk.

Creutzfeldt-Jakob (KROITS-felt ya-kob) *disease* (CJD) is a rare degenerative brain disorder. It can be hereditary but may also be caused by an infectious protein, or prion. It is then commonly called "mad cow disease." Humans may become infected by eating the meat of diseased cows. The incubation period for the disorder can be years. Symptoms may include depression, difficulty walking, and dementia. In 1986 the first case of bovine spongiform encephalopathy, or mad cow disease, was found. The suspected cause of mad cow disease is feeding the cattle meat and bone meal products. As of 2009 a new type of mad cow disease had killed 166 people in the United Kingdom and 44 in other countries. All prion diseases are fatal, and there is no effective treatment available.

Down syndrome is one of the most common causes of mental retardation and the most common disorder of human chromosomes. The genetic disorder is caused by the presence of an extra chromosome. The resulting characteristics include short stature, short neck, broad hands and feet with stubby fingers and toes, a large protruding tongue, and mental retardation. The degree of mental retardation varies greatly, but the average mental age that is reached is 8 years. Individuals with Down syndrome are also more likely to have respiratory infections, heart defects, and leukemia. No cure exists.

Encephalitis (en-sef-uh-LIE-tis) is inflammation of the brain caused by a virus, bacteria, or chemical agent. Encephalitis is usually an acute condition characterized by fever, headache, extreme irritability of the nervous system, and disorientation. Encephalitis may lead to convulsions and death. Treatment depends on the exact cause and may include antibiotics and precautions to reduce stimulation.

Guillain-Barré (ge-YAN bar-RAY) *syndrome* is also called infectious **polyneuritis**. The cause is unknown, but it may appear shortly after a viral immunization or infection. The person with this condition experiences muscle weakness that rapidly moves from the legs to the face. Total paralysis of respiratory function may result. Treatment is supportive to maintain vital life functions. About 95% of the Guillain-Barré cases have complete recovery in a few weeks to several months.

Headache is a common condition resulting from several different causes. However, headache can be the symptom of another, more serious disorder and should be investigated when occurring frequently. Tension headaches are directly related to stress. The muscles around the occipital area of the brain may constrict the blood flow to the area. Tension headaches are usually dull and steady in nature. They can be relieved with nonprescription analgesics. Treatment includes relaxation techniques, massage of the neck and back muscles, and application of heat such as a hot shower.

Migraine headaches are vascular headaches of unknown cause. The pain results from the narrowing of blood vessels in the brain. Migraine headaches are generally throbbing, located in one area on one side of the brain, and involve gastrointestinal disturbances such as vomiting. They may last several days. Treatment includes avoiding triggering factors such as certain foods. Relief from migraine headaches may require prescription medicine.

Sinus headaches result from the swelling of the membranes that line the sinus cavities. The pain is usually dull and shifts with head movement. Decongestants and nonprescription analgesics relieve this headache pain.

Head injury may occur when the brain impacts the skull as a result of a blow or rapid movement. Depending on the location of the injury, the person who experiences such an injury may experience nausea, confusion, increased blood pressure, and drowsiness. Treatment includes surgical relief of pressure on the brain if necessary. The person is assessed for neurologic damage after a head injury for at least 24 hours.

Huntington disease is a degenerative neural disorder that affects brain tissues. The condition usually appears between the ages of 35 and 50. The person with Huntington disease first experiences loss of balance and coordination and then progressively involuntary movements and dementia. Death occurs 10 to 20 years after the disease appears. An autosomal dominant gene causes the disease. If one parent has the gene for the disease, each child has a 50% chance of receiving it. The appearance of this gene can now be identified with gene mapping, allowing for counseling of families with a history of the disorder. No treatment is available.

CASE STUDY 19-1 Your friend tells you that Huntington disease runs in her family, and she may get genetic testing for it. What should you say?

Answers to Case Studies are available on the Evolve website: ***http://evolve.elsevier.com/Gerdin***

Hydrocephalus (hi-dro-SEF-uh-lus) occurs when more CSF is produced than is absorbed into the circulatory system. The excess fluid increases intracranial pressure and may enlarge the head. It may be caused by developmental defects, infection, trauma, or a tumor in the cranial space. Treatment includes removal of the excess fluid by a tube inserted into the intracranial space.

Intracranial (in-tra-KRAY-nee-uhl) *tumors* may be benign or malignant. Tumors of the nervous system usually involve neuroglia, blood vessels, or membranes rather than neurons. A neuroma (noo-RO-ma) generally refers to a benign or noncancerous growth. A glioma would be more likely to be malignant or cancerous. It is also possible for a growth to be metastatic, originating from cells that have then been transported to the brain by the lymph vessels from another part of the body. Any type of growth can disrupt nervous system function, with symptoms depending on the portion of the brain or nerves that is compressed by the growth. Treatment may include surgical removal, radiation, or chemotherapy and varies with the location and type of growth.

Meningitis (men-in-JIE-tis) is a serious inflammation of the meninges caused by a bacterium, virus, or fungus. The person can experience a high fever, stiff neck, vomiting, severe headache, and convulsions. Damage to the nervous system may result in blindness, loss of hearing, paralysis, or retardation. Some cases of meningitis are self-limiting and require treatment only to relieve symptoms. In severe cases, treatment varies with the cause and usually includes antibiotics.

CASE STUDY 19-2 You hear there is a case of meningitis in one of the local schools. What should you do?

Answers to Case Studies are available on the Evolve website: ***http://evolve.elsevier.com/Gerdin***

Meningocele (me-NING-go-seel) is a birth defect that occurs when the membranes covering the brain or spinal cord protrude through a congenital defect in the skull or spinal column (Fig. 19-11). If treated rapidly with surgery to correct the defect, the damage done to the spinal cord and nerves can be minimized. The cause of meningocele is unknown. However, folic acid deficiency may play a part in neural tube defects. Environmental factors and a viral cause have also been theorized as a cause.

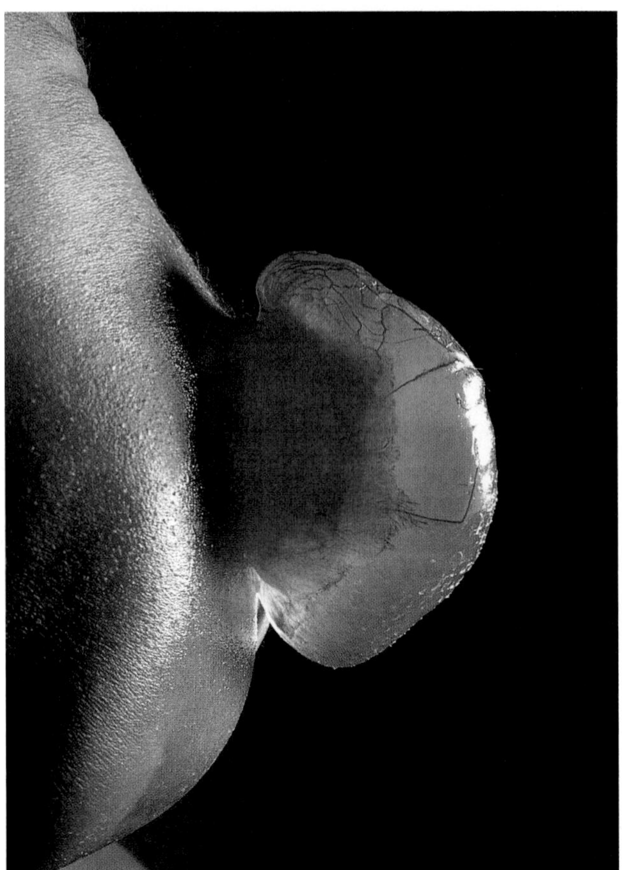

FIGURE 19-11 Protrusion of meninges, cerebrospinal fluid, and nerve tissue in a meningocele. (From Cooke RA, Stewart B: *Colour atlas of anatomical pathology*, ed 3, Sydney, 2004, Churchill Livingstone.)

Multiple sclerosis (skle-RO-sis) results from a defect in electrical transmission of the neurons caused by degeneration of the myelin sheath. Multiple sclerosis usually appears in adults 20 to 40 years of age. The cause is unknown. Most scientists believe that the loss of myelin is caused by a virus or an autoimmune process. The person with multiple sclerosis may first experience double vision or diplopia (di-PLO-pee-uh), loss of sensation, stiff extremities, or progressive loss of muscle control. Multiple sclerosis is treated with medication such as steroids and other medications to help control the symptoms and disabilities. No cure is available.

Narcolepsy (NAHR-kuh-lep-see) is a chronic sleep disorder that causes excessive sleepiness and may

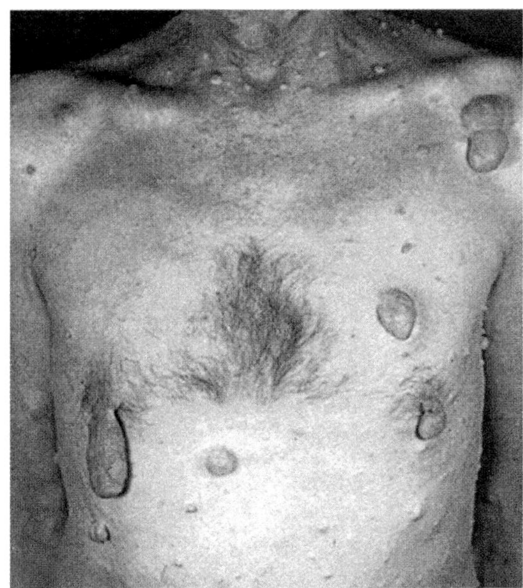

FIGURE 19-12 Tumors of nervous system tissue develop with neurofibromatosis. (From Patton KT, Thibodeau GA: *Anatomy & physiology*, ed 7, St. Louis, 2010, Mosby.)

result in frequent daytime sleep attacks. Symptoms of narcolepsy may include extreme drowsiness every 3 to 4 hours, dreamlike hallucinations, sleep paralysis, and sudden loss of muscle control leading to an inability to move. The cause of narcolepsy is believed to be related to brain proteins, including orexin and hypocretin. Narcolepsy runs in families, and researchers have identified genes associated with it. There is no known cure for narcolepsy. Treatment is designed to control the symptoms.

Neural (NOO-ral) *tube defect* is a defect in the formation of the skull and spinal column caused primarily when the neural tube fails to close during the development of the embryo. Severe mental and physical disorders usually are present as well. Prenatal testing during the fourteenth to sixteenth week can determine whether a neural tube defect is present. Infection of the CSF is the main concern after birth. In some cases, surgery may be performed to correct the deformity.

Neurofibromatosis (noo-ro-fi-bro-mah-TOE-sis), also called *von Recklinghausen* (REK-ling-how-zen) *disease*, is caused by a defect in an autosomal dominant gene. It affects more than 100,000 people in the United States. The condition may be caused by genetic mutation in about half of the cases. The condition first causes large tan spots on the skin. Small benign tumors of nervous tissue develop with increased age (Fig. 19-12). The tumors may cause loss of hearing or blindness if located in the ears and eyes. In many cases the symptoms are mild and life expectancy is normal. Although no treatment exists, unsightly tumors can be removed surgically.

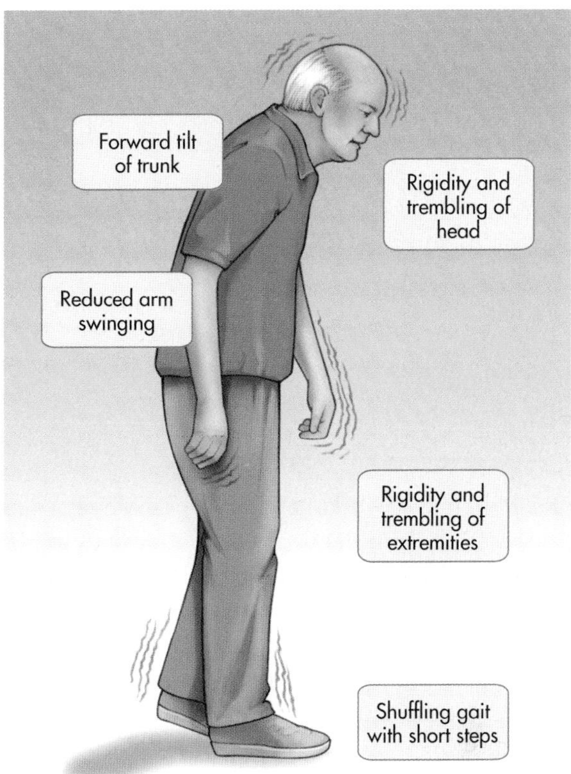

FIGURE 19-13 The signs of Parkinsonism include rigidity and trembling of the head and extremities. (From Thibodeau GA, Patton KT: *Human body in health and disease*, ed 4, St Louis, 2005, Mosby.)

Parkinson (PAR-kin-sun) *disease* commonly affects people older than 50 years of age (Fig. 19-13). It results from degeneration of certain brain cells and is sometimes called "shaking palsy." A decrease in secretion of the neurotransmitter dopamine, which has no known cause, is responsible for this degeneration. A person with Parkinson disease gradually feels stiffness and tremors, leading to uncontrolled muscular movement and rigidity. Treatment includes medication to decrease the symptoms. Drug therapy is usually successful but has many side effects. Surgery may be performed in some cases.

Poliomyelitis (po-lee-o-mi-uh-LIE-tis) is caused by a virus that spreads from the nose and throat to neural tissue. The virus destroys neural cell bodies and leads to temporary paralysis. Vaccination prevents the infection and has minimized the incidence of polio. Treatment of the disease includes measures to prevent deformity caused by loss of muscle function.

BOX 19-2

Types of Seizures

Generalized
- Absence
- Atonic
- Tonic-clonic
- Myoclonic

Partial
- Simple
- Complex

Sciatica (sie-AT-ih-ka) is characterized by constant pain radiating from the back and buttocks to the leg. Movement may also be limited in the affected leg. The cause is usually a rupture of an intervertebral disk and osteoarthritis (os-tee-o-ar-THRI-tis), producing pressure on the nerve or other nerve injury. Treatment of sciatica requires finding the cause of the pain and controlling it.

A *seizure* (SEE-zher) may result from injury, infection, or epilepsy. More than 40 types of seizure are classified into two groups (Box 19-2): (1) partial seizures involving part of the brain and (2) generalized seizures involving the whole brain. Absence seizures, also called petit mal (PET-ee mahl) seizures, cause a lapse of consciousness for several seconds. Febrile and chemical seizures may result from drugs. Grand mal (grand mahl) seizures are a series of distinctive tonic and clonic spasms that last several minutes. In the tonic portion of the seizure, the muscles are contracted rigidly. The clonic phase involves involuntary muscle movements. Seizures may cause injury from uncontrolled movement. Seizures can often be controlled successfully with medication.

CASE STUDY 19-3 You enter a patient's room and observe that he is having a seizure. What should you do?

Answers to Case Studies are available on the Evolve website: ***http://evolve.elsevier.com/Gerdin***

Sleep disorders include more than 100 identified conditions, such as insomnia, apnea, hypersomnia, sleep terrors, restless leg syndrome, and sleep walking. The cause and treatment of the disorders are varied. Some suggestions for improving sleep patterns are to reduce caffeine and exercise before sleep. Other suggestions include developing consistent sleep habits, such as a set bedtime and activities. Medication may be used in some cases.

CASE STUDY 19-4 You fall asleep every day after eating lunch. Your habit is causing you to be reprimanded and you even worry about driving until you have had a short nap. What should you do?

Answers to Case Studies are available on the Evolve website: ***http://evolve.elsevier.com/Gerdin***

Spina bifida (SPI-nuh BIF-i-da) is a birth defect involving a malformed spinal column resulting from neural tube defects. Seventy-five percent of spina bifida cases result from myelomeningocele or a neural tube defect. In the United States, 7 of every 10,000 babies are born with this defect each year. Spina bifida is partly hereditary but is also affected by the pregnant woman's diet and environment. Folic acid supplements before and during pregnancy reduce the risk of spina bifida occurring. At birth the infant's spinal column is not closed completely over the spinal cord. The condition may cause problems with bowel and bladder control or paralysis. The opening can be closed surgically to minimize damage.

Spinal cord injuries affect 12,000 people in the United States each year. According to the Spinal Cord Injury Statistical Center, the average age at injury is 40.2 years. About 80.9% of the injuries occur in males. About 42.1% of spinal cord injuries result from automobile accidents, 26.7% from falls, and 15.1% from violence. Most spinal injuries resulting from trauma occur in the cervical and lumbar area of the spinal column, which have the greatest mobility. Injuries to the cervical spine may cause quadriplegia (tetraplegia). In the lumbar region, paraplegia may result. The severity of the injury is diagnosed by using x-ray, CT scan, and/or MRI. Treatment may include steroids to reduce the swelling in the cord and management to prevent complications resulting from lost sensory and motor function.

Transient ischemic attacks (TIAs) are often called "little strokes" and are caused by a decrease in blood to an area of the brain resulting from a small clot that temporarily lodges in a vessel. The person may experience slurred speech, numbness, or vision disturbances that usually disappear within a few days. Because the symptoms disappear, the condition may

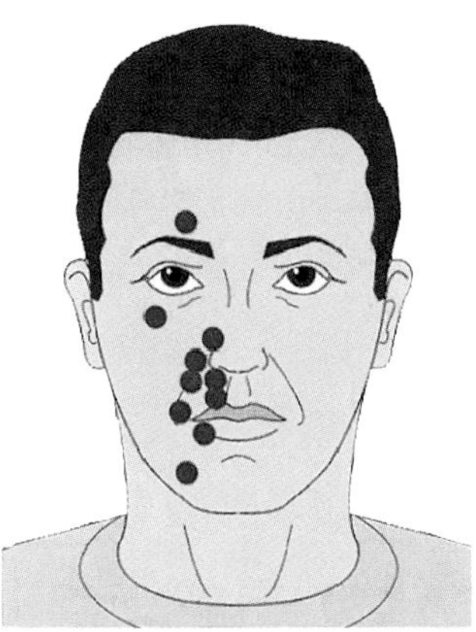
Pain zones in
trigeminal neuralgia.

FIGURE 19-14 One method used to relieve the pain of trigeminal neuralgia is surgically to remove the ganglion on the end of the nerve. (From Patton KT, Thibodeau GA: *Anatomy & physiology*, ed 7, St. Louis, 2010, Mosby.)

go unrecognized. TIAs may indicate an impending irreversible CVA, which can be prevented with anticoagulants or vascular surgery to clear blocked blood vessels.

Trigeminal neuralgia (tri-JEM-in-al noo-RAL-jee-ah), also called *tic douloureux* (tik doo-loo-ROO), is characterized by sudden, intense, unpredictable pain on one side of the face (Fig. 19-14). The pain is caused by pressure on or deterioration of the trigeminal facial nerve. Treatment may include medication or surgery.

Issues and Innovations

Memory Research

The storage and recall of information constitutes one of the most specialized functions of the nervous system. Three components of memory include sensory memory, short-term memory, and long-term memory. Sensory memory holds information for 20 to 30 seconds. Short-term memory is information retained for several minutes to several hours. The same information can be converted by repetition to long-term memory that may be retained for years. It is believed that information is stored in different areas of the brain according to whether the method of input is visual, auditory, or touch related (kinesthetic). These areas are interconnected by chemical messengers for more efficient retrieval of information.

Researchers have also determined that memories are retained differently and in separate areas of the brain. For example, discursive or declarative information such as a multiplication table is stored in a different area than procedural information such as how to ride a bike or dance. An aphasic (without speech) injury might allow a person to remember the name of living things but not nonliving things. The temporal lobe is believed to store long-term memory. The hippocampus is the site for facts, events, novelties, and spatial relations.

The method that the brain uses to store and recall information is not clearly understood, but ribonucleic acid may play a role. Most research on memory uses a marine slug named Aplysia or people who have sustained neurologic changes resulting from injury or illness as subjects. The slugs are used for memory research because their ganglia are large and their behavior patterns are limited. The slugs do have the capacity to retain short-term memories of environmental changes. Researchers believe that the slug's memories result from a biochemical change in the synapse receptors. To create a new memory, the synapse reacts differently to the neurotransmitters it receives. In 2005 the National Human Genome Research Institute announced that it will sequence the genome of this slug.

Neuroscientists believe that the 100 billion neurons of the brain communicate in a complicated network. Any single neuron may be connected to as many as 10,000 other neurons. Computer networks have been designed to try to simulate the action of the brain. Researchers hope to discover how the brain rearranges the connections to store new information and restore operations after damage to some neurons.

Parkinson Correction

Parkinson disease is a progressive neurologic disorder characterized by three distinct functional changes. These three changes include slowness of movement (bradykinesia), tremor, and rigidity. According to the National Parkinson Foundation, 60,000 new cases are diagnosed each year. The usual treatment involves a series of drugs that alleviate symptoms and assist the body to make the neurotransmitter dopamine, which is missing in Parkinson patients.

The first transplant of adrenal gland cells to the brain in the United States was performed in 1987. Adrenal cells and fetal brain cells may be used to replace or stimulate the function of an area of the brain called the *substantia nigra* (sub-stan-shah NYE-grah) that normally produces dopamine. Researchers in Mexico who first performed the procedure reported a striking improvement in the condition. In the United States, implantation of fetal tissue has been limited because of a ban on fetal tissue research that was imposed in 1988. In 1993 the federal government lifted the ban on fetal tissue research, opening the way for more research in this area.

Effectiveness of fetal tissue transplant to cure Parkinson disease cannot be fully demonstrated. Only a few transplants have been completed, and varied techniques were used in the procedure. Additionally, the supply of fetal tissue for transplant is limited. Another cell transplant technique that has been used is retinal pigment epithelial cells. These cells produce and release dopamine.

Deep brain stimulation has been approved by the U.S. Food and Drug Administration for cases that do not respond to medication. Electrodes are implanted in the brain and attached to a pulse generator. The pulse generator is inserted into the chest, and the electrodes are placed under the skin to the brain. The generator is programmed externally and can reduce the tremors, slowness, and gait problems.

In 2009 results from a clinical trial using autologous neural stem cells to treat Parkinson disease were published. The technique uses the patient's own neural stem cells to produce neurons and then puts them pack into the brain. Because the cells were mature and not rejected by the body, the patients did not need immunosuppressant drugs. The study indicated that the patient's motor skills improved by more than 80% for at least 3 years following treatment.

Summary

- The function of the nervous system is to sense, interpret, and respond to internal and external environmental changes to maintain homeostasis.
- Structures of the nervous system include the CNS and PNS and their parts.
- Methods of assessment of the nervous system include electroencephalography, lumbar puncture, myelography, CT, and positron emission tomography.
- Disorders of the nervous system include CVAs, encephalitis, spina bifida, headache, and Huntington disease.

Review Questions

1. Describe the function of the nervous system.
2. Identify the parts of the neuron.
3. Describe the location and function of each of the following parts of the nervous system:
   Autonomic nervous system
   Parasympathetic nervous system
   Sympathetic nervous system
4. Describe the function of each of the 12 cranial nerves.
5. List the function of the following parts of the brain: frontal lobe, medulla, occipital lobe, parietal lobe, pons, and temporal lobe.
6. Describe three nervous system disorders that are caused by a pathogenic organism.
7. Describe three methods used to assess the function of the nervous system.
8. Use the following terms in one or more sentences that correctly relate their meaning: epilepsy, impulse, myelography, and reflex.

Critical Thinking

1. Investigate and compare the cost of at least three tests used in diagnosing disorders of the nervous system.
2. Compare and contrast Creutzfeldt-Jakob and Parkinson disease. Draw a Venn diagram to show their similarities and differences.
3. Investigate the function of at least five common medications used in treatment of the nervous system.
4. List at least five occupations involved in the health care of nervous system disorders.
5. Use the Internet to research and investigate the methods used to regain use of the brain following injury.
6. Use the Internet to research and review an article regarding a recent development or treatment method relating to the nervous system.
7. Use the Internet to research and create a pamphlet or poster describing methods to improve the lifestyle of an Alzheimer patient.
8. Use the Internet to research and describe the current use of stem cells in treatment of a neurological disorder.
9. Use the Internet to investigate the amount of sleep needed by teenagers. Prepare a poster, pamphlet or essay about sleep disorders including methods for maintaining good sleep hygiene.

Explore the Web

Alzheimer Disease

Alzheimer's Association

http://www.alz.org/living_with_alzheimers_caring_for_alzheimers.asp

WebMD

http://www.webmd.com/alzheimers/guide/alzheimers-disease-living-managing

Stem Cell Research

National Institutes of Health

http://www.ninds.nih.gov/research/stem_cell/index.htm

Sleep

WebMD

http://www.webmd.com/sleep-disorders/guide/understanding-sleep-problems-symptoms

National Institutes of Health (NIH)

http://science.education.nih.gov/supplements/nih3/sleep/guide/info-sleep.htm

CHAPTER 20

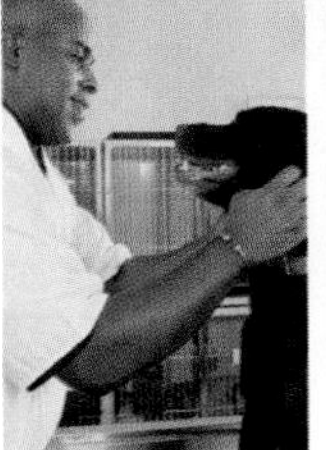
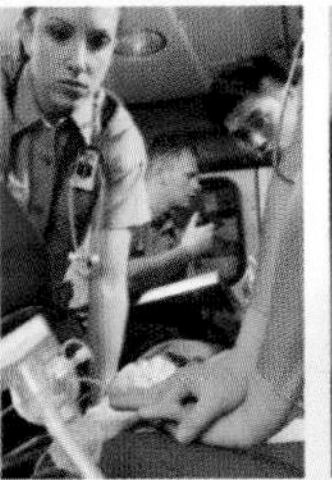
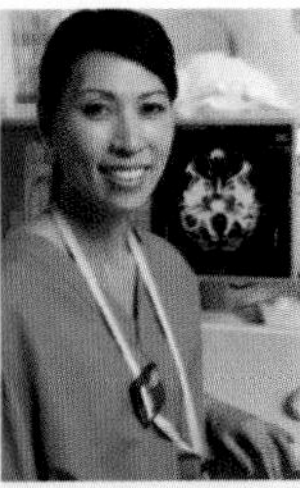

Sensory System

LEARNING OBJECTIVES

- Define at least 10 terms relating to the sensory system.
- Describe the function of the sensory system.
- Identify at least 10 sensory system structures and the function of each.
- Identify at least three methods of assessment of the sensory system.
- Describe at least five disorders of the sensory system.

KEY TERMS

Accommodation *(uh-kom-uh-DAY-shun)* Focusing of the eye for varied distances

Auditory *(AW-dih-tore-ee)* Pertaining to the sense of hearing

Converge *(kon-VERJ)* When two eyes move in a coordinated fashion toward fixation on the same near point

Cutaneous *(kyoo-TAY-nee-us)* Pertaining to the skin

Equilibrium *(ee-kwih-LIB-ree-um)* State of balance

Gustatory *(GUS-tuh-tore-ee)* Pertaining to the sense of taste

Intraocular *(in-truh-OK-yoo-lar)* Within the eye

Labyrinth *(LAB-ih-rinth)* System of communicating canals in the inner ear

Olfactory *(OLE-fak-tore-ee)* Pertaining to the sense of smell

Receptor *(ree-SEP-tor)* Specific type of cell that responds to a specific stimulus

Refraction *(ree-FRAK-shun)* Deviation of light when passing through a medium to another medium of a different density

Stimulus *(STIM-yoo-lus)* Any agent that produces a reaction in a receptor

Vision *(VIZH-un)* Act or faculty of seeing; sight

Sensory System Terminology*

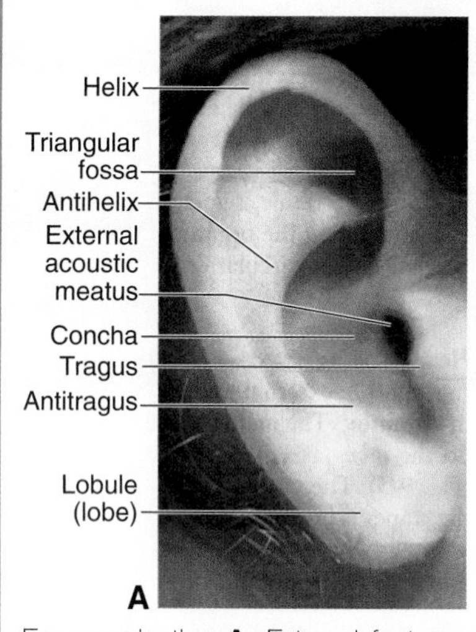

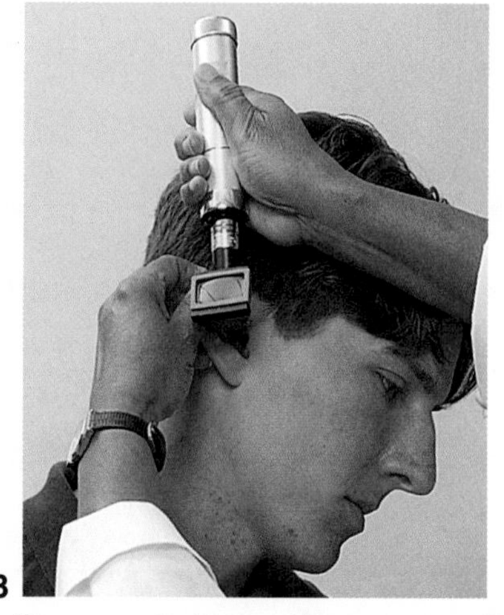

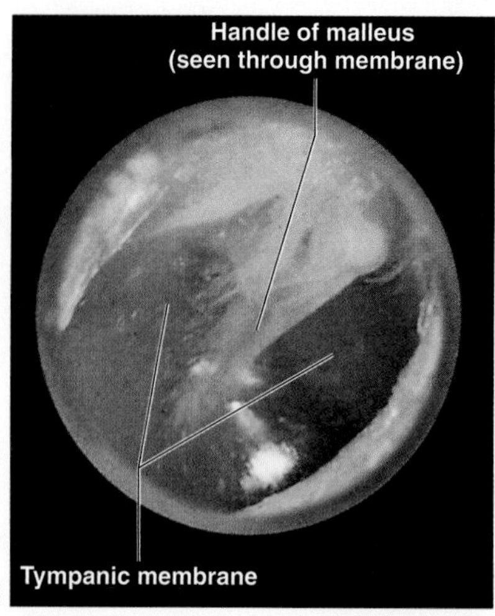

Ear examination **A,** External features. **B,** Otoscope. **C,** Tympanic membrane. (From Patton KT, Thibodeau GA: *Anatomy & physiology*, ed 7, St. Louis, 2010, Mosby.)

Term	Definition	Prefix	Root	Suffix
Gustatory	Pertaining to taste		gusta	tory
Intraocular	Within the eye	intra	ocul	ar
Kinesthetic	Pertaining to the sense of movement		kinesthest	ic
Nasal	Pertaining to the nose		nas	al
Ocular	Pertaining to the eye		ocul	ar
Olfactory	Pertaining to the sense of smell		olfac	tory
Ophthalmologist	Specialist in the eye and its disorders		opthalmal	ogist
Otoscope	Instrument used to view the ear	oto	scope	
Retinopathy	Disease of the retina		retin	opathy
Tympanitis	Inflammation of the eardrum		tympan	itis

*A transition syllable or vowel may be added to or deleted from the word parts to make the combining form.

Abbreviations of the Sensory System

Abbreviation	Meaning
aq	Aqueous
EENT	Ears, eyes, nose, throat
o.d.	Right eye
oint	Ointment
Ophth	Ophthalmology
o.s.	Left eye
o.u.	Both eyes
PERLA	Pupils equally reactive to light
REM	Rapid eye movement
RK	Radial keratotomy

Structure and Function of the Sensory System

The sensory system consists of **receptors** in specialized cells and organs that perceive changes (stimuli) in the internal and external environment. The stimuli cause nerve impulses that are sent to the brain for interpretation. Environmental stimuli are perceived with the senses of **vision**, hearing, touch, taste, position, and balance. Specialized organs of the senses include the eye, ear, tongue, nose, and skin.

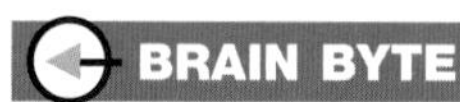

Some scientists believe there are nine senses instead of five. They include four internal senses: pain, balance, thirst, and hunger.

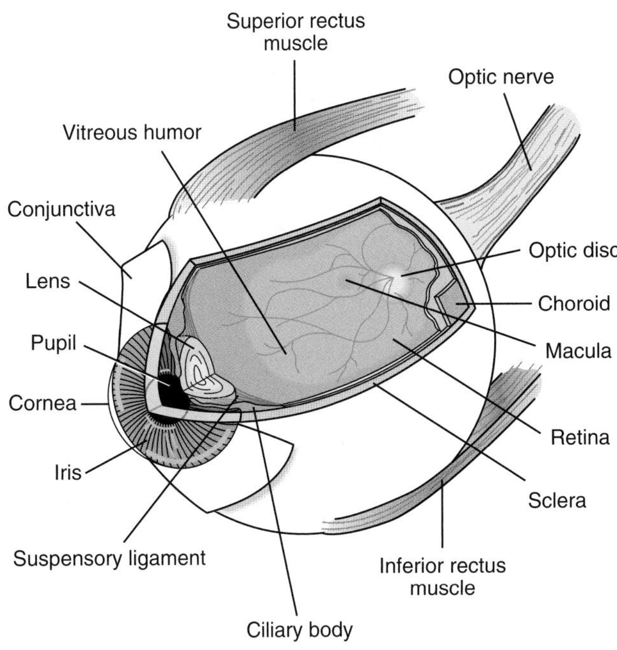

FIGURE 20-1 Structures of the eye. (From Sorrentino SA: *Mosby's textbook for nursing assistants*, ed 7, St. Louis, 2008, Mosby.)

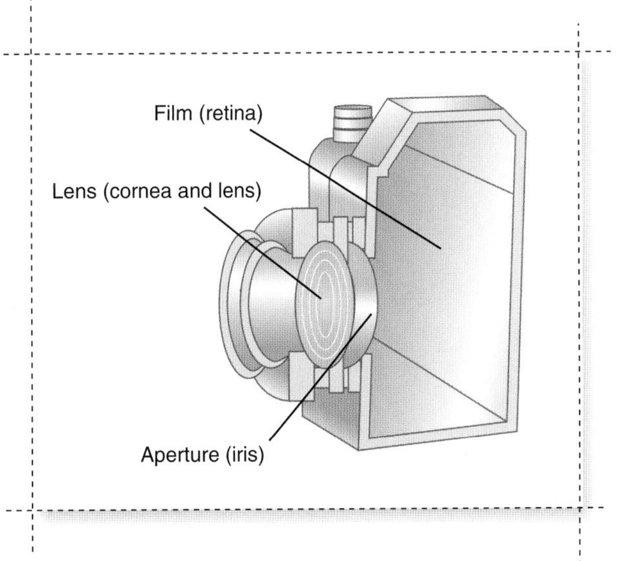

FIGURE 20-2 The eye functions like a camera.

Eye

The eyes are considered the most important sensory organ because 90% of the information about the environment reaches the brain from the eyes. The external structures of the eye are shown in Fig. 20-1. The orbital cavity is composed of bones that protect and adipose tissue that cushions the eye. When the eyelids and eyelashes close or "blink," they protect the eye from injury. The conjunctiva is a mucous membrane that protects and lubricates the eyelids and part of the eye. The lacrimal apparatus forms tears that keep the eye moist and lubricated. Movement of the eye is controlled by the extrinsic muscles. Only one fifth of the eye is actually exposed to the environment.

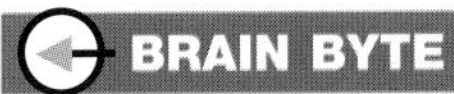

BRAIN BYTE

Most people blink every 2 to 10 seconds.

The internal structures of the eye are also shown in Fig. 20-1. The sclera is a tough, white tissue that supports and gives structure to the eye. The sclera is continuous with the transparent cornea that covers the iris and pupil. The cornea focuses light rays on the retina at the back of the eye. The blood supply for the eye originates in the choroid, iris, and ciliary muscles. The iris and ciliary muscles are the intrinsic muscles of the eye.

The eyeball is not solid but is divided into sections, the anterior and posterior cavities. The anterior cavity is filled with a clear watery fluid called aqueous humor. The posterior cavity is filled with a semisoft gelatin-like substance called vitreous humor. Both the aqueous and vitreous humor help maintain the shape of the eye.

The opening called the pupil is in the choroid layer. The iris is a round, colored muscle that surrounds the pupil. The iris contracts and relaxes to adjust the amount of light entering the eye through the pupil. The lens is a convex, transparent tissue located directly behind the pupil that focuses and directs incoming light on the retina of the eye. The amount of light admitted into the eye is regulated by the movement of the iris.

Vision is similar to the action of a camera, beginning with **refraction**, the process of the lens bending light rays as they enter the eye to focus on the retina (Fig. 20-2). The eye changes the shape of the lens to focus near and far through the process of **accommodation**. The pupil constricts to focus the object on the retina and protect it from receiving too much light. The eyes **converge** on the object so that single binocular vision occurs and only one object is seen.

Specialized cells called *rods* and *cones* in the retina absorb the light. The retina of each eye contains 100 million rods and 7 million cones. Rods are sensitive to dim light. Cones react to bright light and allow color distinction through three types of pigments that are

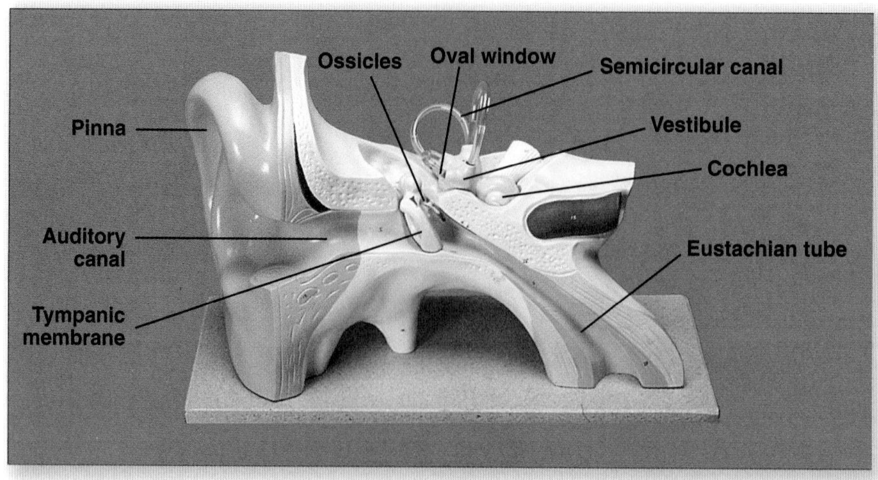

FIGURE 20-3 Structures of the ear.

sensitive to different wavelengths of light. The three photopigments recognize the colors: green, red, and blue. The impulses released by the pigments in the rods and cones are transmitted to the brain by the optic nerve.

Ear

The auditory or acoustic sense (hearing) is the primary function of the ear. A second function of the ear is to help maintain equilibrium. The ear has three parts, called the *external*, *middle*, and *inner ear* (Fig. 20-3).

The external ear channels the incoming sound waves or vibrations. The auricle or pinna is the flap of tissue on the side of the head that collects and transmits sound waves through the ear or auditory canal to the eardrum (tympanic membrane). Specialized glands in the ear canal produce earwax (cerumen) that protects the middle ear from entry of foreign particles.

The middle ear is an air-filled chamber that begins with the tympanic membrane, which changes sound waves into mechanical movements. Auditory bones (ossicles) transmit the sound vibrations. These three bones are called the *hammer (malleus)*, *anvil (incus)*, and *stirrup (stapes)*. The ossicles amplify and transmit the sound to the inner ear. Two openings into the inner ear are the membrane-covered round window and the oval window, which touches the stapes. Another opening between the middle ear and pharynx is called the *eustachian tube*. The eustachian tube has two main functions. It allows the pressure of air in the middle ear to be equalized with the air pressure of the environment. Additionally, fluids and mucus from the middle ear are drained to the nasopharynx. Swallowing and yawning open the eustachian tube for these purposes.

The inner ear contains a series of canals called *bony labyrinth*, which includes the cochlea, semicircular canals, and vestibule with the membranous labyrinth inside it. The movement of fluid and hair cells lining the cochlea converts the mechanical vibrations from the ossicles to neural impulses. Each ear contains 16,000 hair cells. Each hair cell has 100 stereocilia or bristles that transmit impulses to the auditory cranial nerves. The semicircular canals contain a clear fluid called *endolymph* that gives a sense of balance when the body is in motion. Two chambers called the *saccule* and *utricle of the vestibule* maintain static or resting equilibrium.

Hearing is a result of interpretation of sound waves. Sound waves are described by their amplitude (volume) and pitch (frequency). A sound is perceived when the tympanic membrane is vibrated or the hairs in the cochlea are stimulated. Sound waves may be transmitted through the air, bone, or fluid.

Tongue

Taste, or the gustatory sense, is perceived by specialized cells located in projections (papillae) on the tongue called *taste buds*. Taste buds are chemoreceptors. The five tastes perceived by the tongue are sweet, sour, bitter, salty, and umami (Fig. 20-4). Umami, described as "meatiness," is a response to glutamic acid found in processed meats, cheese, and many Asian foods. Each taste bud has 50 to 100 taste cells. These cells respond to all five types of taste. All areas

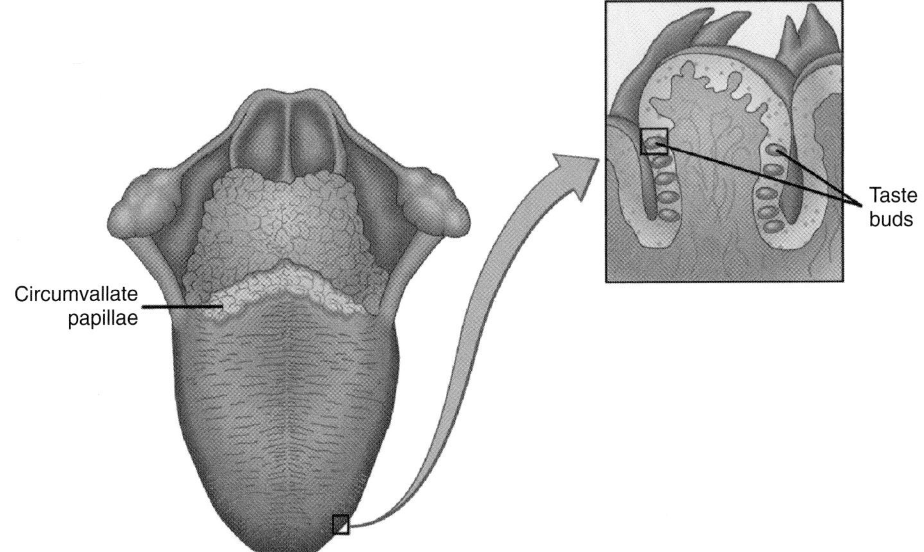

FIGURE 20-4 Taste buds are located on the tongue. (From Patton KT, Thibodeau GA: *Anatomy & physiology*, ed 7, St. Louis, 2010, Mosby.)

of the tongue sense all five of the tastes. As more research is completed, new "tastes" may be identified. It is possible that "metallic" is also a primary taste. Before a taste can be sensed, the substance must be dissolved in fluid or saliva. The particular flavor of an item is identified by smell as well as taste.

Nose

The olfactory sense, or smell, originates in olfactory receptor cells in the nose that immediately transmit impulses to the brain through the olfactory cranial nerves (Fig. 20-5). The nasal cavity is divided into two sections by the septum. Each side of the nose is further divided into three passageways by bony projections called turbinates. Specialized epithelial tissue near the roof of the nasal cavity contains the olfactory cells. Olfactory receptor neurons are stimulated by chemicals (gases) in the air. When the receptors reach a threshold, the olfactory bulb reacts and an impulse is transmitted to the brain. Air that is inhaled also circulates into the paranasal sinuses surrounding the nasal cavity.

The sense of smell is 10,000 times more sensitive than taste. More than 5000 distinct smells can be perceived. However, these smells result from a mixture of only 30 primary or "pure" odors. Some examples of primary odors include floral, putrid, and peppermint. Smells can reduce stress, affect blood pressure, recall memories, and aid in the sense of taste.

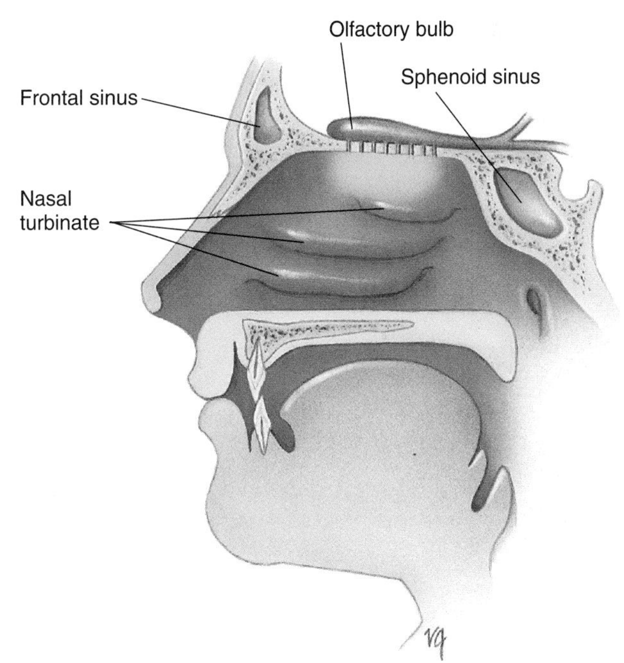

FIGURE 20-5 The nose and surrounding structures.

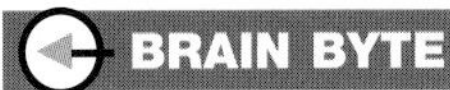

BRAIN BYTE

Smell is sometimes called the "emotional brain" because it can be linked to memories, feelings, and work performance.

Skin

The cutaneous senses of the skin perceive touch, pressure, temperature, and pain through five specialized

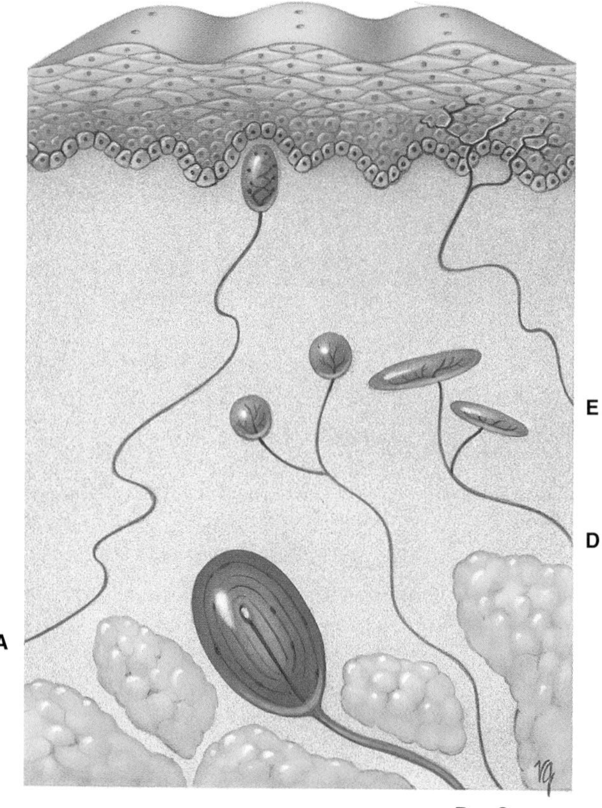

FIGURE 20-6 Nerve receptors of the skin. **A,** Meissner's corpuscle (touch). **B,** Pacinian corpuscle (pressure). **C,** Krause's end-bulb. **D,** Ruffini nerve endings (warmth). **E,** Free nerve endings (pain).

cells located in the skin (Fig. 20-6). Touch, or the tactile sense, is the perception of textures such as smooth, rough, sharp, dull, soft, and hard. Light touch and motion near the skin are perceived by Meissner's corpuscles. Pacinian corpuscles, commonly found in deeper tissues of the tendons and ligaments, sense deep pressure. End-bulbs of Krause sense cold, low-frequency vibration, and two-point discrimination. Corpuscles of Ruffini sense heat, deep pressure, and continuous touch. Pain receptors, also called *nociceptors*, are distributed throughout the skin, mucous membranes, skeletal muscles, and internal organs. Pain receptors are free nerve endings that respond to more than one type of stimulus. The brain has no pain receptors. Pain is the only type of nerve receptor found in visceral organs.

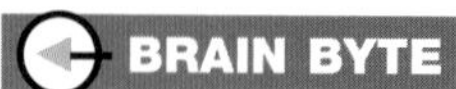
BRAIN BYTE

Pain perception is influenced by both physical and psychological factors.

CASE STUDY 20-1 You are caring for a patient who complains of pain even though she has been given all of the ordered medication. You notice that she is sweating and slightly hot when you touch her. What should you do?

Answers to Case Studies are available on the Evolve website: ***http://evolve.elsevier.com/Gerdin***

The sensation of stretching or knowing the position of muscles is determined by muscle spindles and Golgi tendon receptors. Muscle spindles in skeletal muscles sense the length of the muscles. Golgi tendon receptors, located in areas where muscles join to tendons, sense the tension of the muscle. These two proprioceptors help to maintain muscle tone and posture.

CASE STUDY 20-2 You are starting a new exercise program that consists of swimming laps every day. You notice that you are getting pains in your arm and leg muscles when you swim. What should you do?

Answers to Case Studies are available on the Evolve website: ***http://evolve.elsevier.com/Gerdin***

Assessment Techniques

Sight

Inner structures of the eye are examined by using an ophthalmoscope (Fig. 20-7). The pupils are usually dilated to allow better visualization.

Visual acuity is assessed with a Snellen chart that shows letters or shapes identified from a distance. Normal vision (emmetropia) is 20/20 vision. This measurement indicates that a character of the designated size can be identified from a distance of 20 feet. A measurement of 20/100 would indicate that a person with normal vision would be able to identify the character at 100 feet, but the person being tested can identify it at 20 feet. A measurement of 20/200 is considered legal blindness. Near vision may be tested with a Jaeger chart. Defective visual acuity can be corrected with eyeglasses or contact lenses.

Pressure of the inner eye, or intraocular pressure, is measured by using a tonometer, which can detect glaucoma. It measures the force necessary to indent

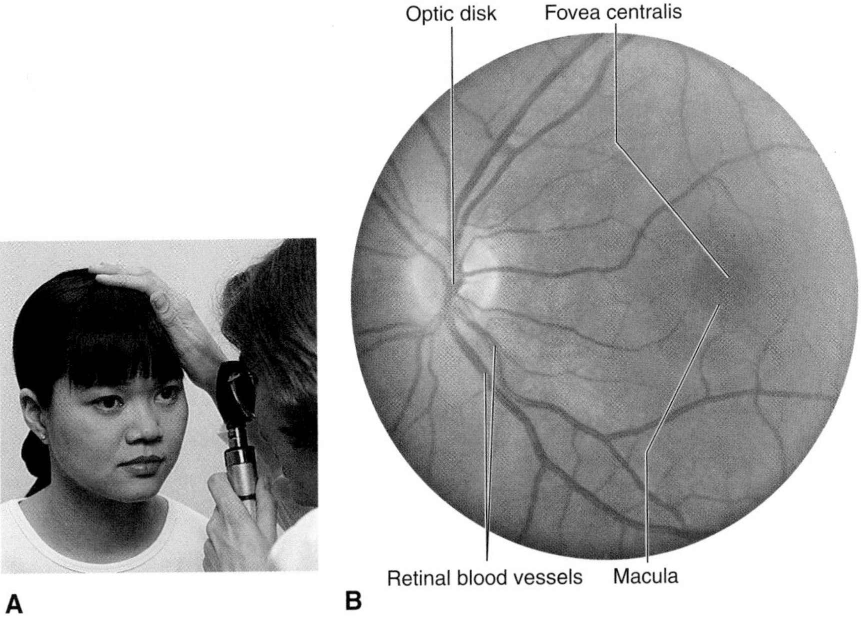

FIGURE 20-7 Eye examination. **A,** Ophthalmoscope. **B,** Retina.

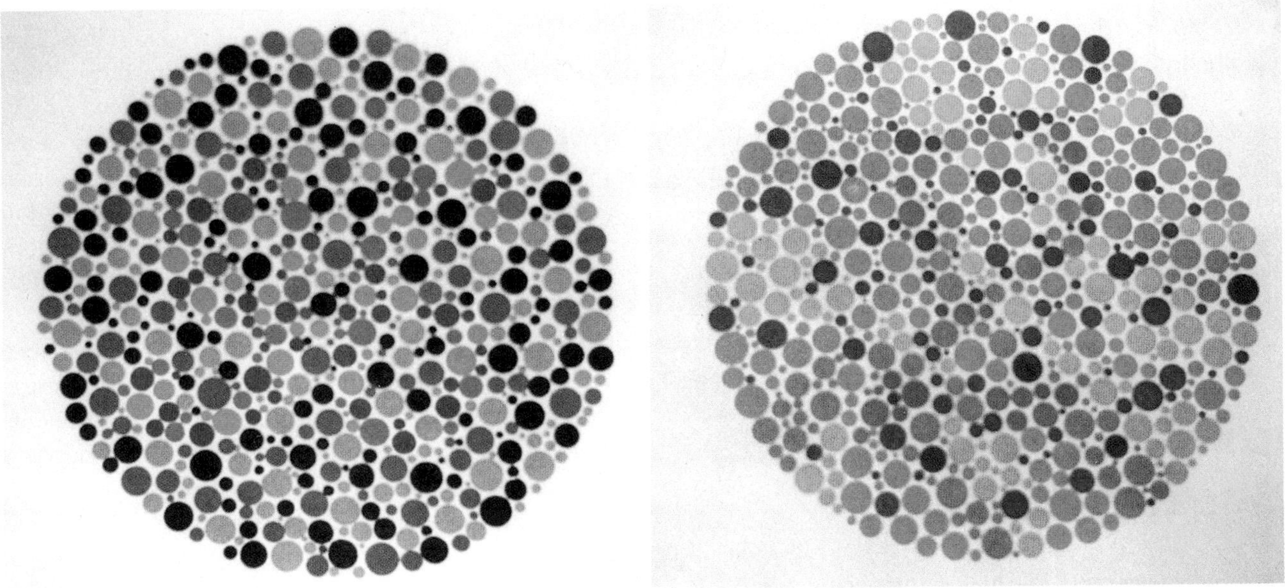

FIGURE 20-8 The most common type of color blindness is characterized by the inability to distinguish reds from greens. (From Kinn ME, Woods M: *The medical assistant*, ed 8, Philadelphia, 1999, Saunders; modified from Ishihara S: *Tests for colour-blindness*, Tokyo, Japan.)

the cornea with a plunger. The pressure is usually 13 to 19 mm Hg.

A "slit-lamp" is used to view the anterior eye for scratches or deformities. The eye is viewed through a binocular microscope, on which the patient rests the chin to prevent movement of the eyes.

The visual field, or space in which a person can see peripherally, is measured as the patient indicates that flashing pinpoints of light in the peripheral field are viewed while concentrating on a central point.

Defects in color determination may be tested with a color blindness chart (Fig. 20-8).

Hearing

The instrument used to view the structures of the ear is called an *otoscope*. Hearing ability can be measured by using an audiometer that emits specific sounds of varied intensity and frequency through the air. Hearing ability may also be assessed by using

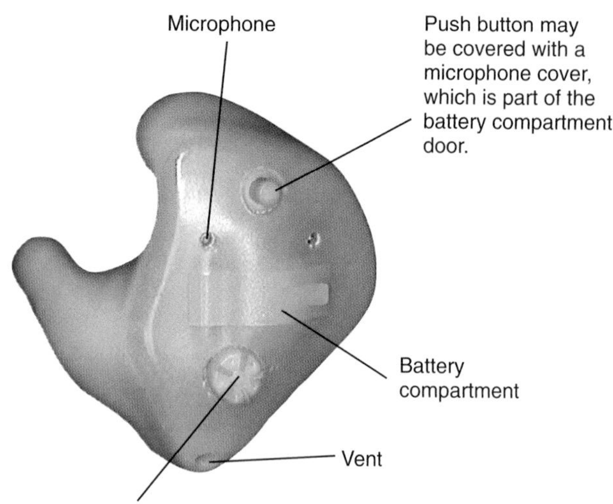

FIGURE 20-9 Hearing Aid. (Courtesy Siemens Hearing Instruments, Inc., Piscataway, NJ. In Sorrentino SA: *Mosby's textbook for nursing assistants*, ed 7, St. Louis, 2008, Mosby.)

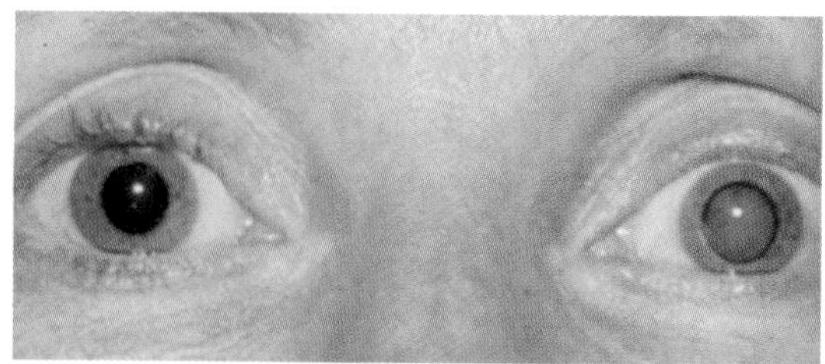

FIGURE 20-10 Cataracts cause blurred or partial vision. (From Patton KT, Thibodeau GA: *Anatomy & physiology*, ed 7, St. Louis, 2010, Mosby.)

CASE STUDY 20-3 Your friend says that her aunt is color blind but that she has been told that is not possible because only males can be color blind. What should you say?

Answers to Case Studies are available on the Evolve website: ***http://evolve.elsevier.com/Gerdin***

a vibrator on the mastoid process to measure bone conduction of sound waves. Normal hearing is in the range of 10 to 100 dB. Defective hearing can be corrected in some cases with a hearing aid that amplifies the sound (Fig. 20-9). Impedance testing emits sound directly into the ear canal to measure the flexibility of the tympanic membrane. The Rinne test uses a tuning fork to assess transmission of sound through the ear structures. Weber's test uses a tuning fork to test for unilateral or one-sided hearing loss.

DISORDERS OF THE Sensory System

Achromatism (ah-KRO-mah-tizm), also called *color blindness*, is a common inherited defect. Monochromatism is complete color blindness in which only grays are seen. Color blindness results from a recessive gene located on the X chromosome. It results when one or more of the three photopigments that assess color is defective. A person affected by monochromatism sees the color but cannot interpret it correctly. Green color blindness is most common; red is the second most common. Red-green color blindness is also possible. Blue color blindness is uncommon. There is no treatment for color blindness, although the person must learn to make adjustments for it. For example, the type of traffic signal at an intersection may be determined by placement of the lights rather than the color.

Amblyopia (am-blee-OH-pee-uh), also called *"lazy eye,"* is poor vision in one eye often resulting from better vision in the other eye during infancy or early childhood. Exercises, corrective lenses, patching of the eye that has better vision, and surgery to shorten muscles around the eye may be used for treatment in young children. After 6 to 9 years of age, the development of the visual system is complete and the condition cannot be corrected.

Anacusis (an-ah-KYOO-sis), or *hearing loss*, can be either perceptive or conductive. Sensorineural (sen-so-ree-NOO-ral) hearing (perceptive) loss results from damage to neural tissues. Central nervous system tissue does not repair, so this type of hearing loss cannot be corrected. Transmission hearing loss (conductive) may result from otosclerosis (o-to-skle-RO-sis). Hearing loss may also result from infection or trauma to ear structures. Treatment of conductive hearing loss may include surgery or use of hearing aids.

Astigmatism (uh-STIG-muh-tizm) is a congenital defect of the eyeball that may increase with age. Imperfect curvature of the cornea results in blurred vision. Treatment is use of corrective lenses.

Cataract (KAT-uh-rakt) is a clouding of the lens that causes blurred or partial vision (Fig. 20-10). The cause is unknown. Cataracts are not contagious and, if treated, do not cause permanent blindness. If untreated, cataracts may cause blindness. Some research indicates that antioxidants taken in food or supplements help to prevent cataracts from occurring.

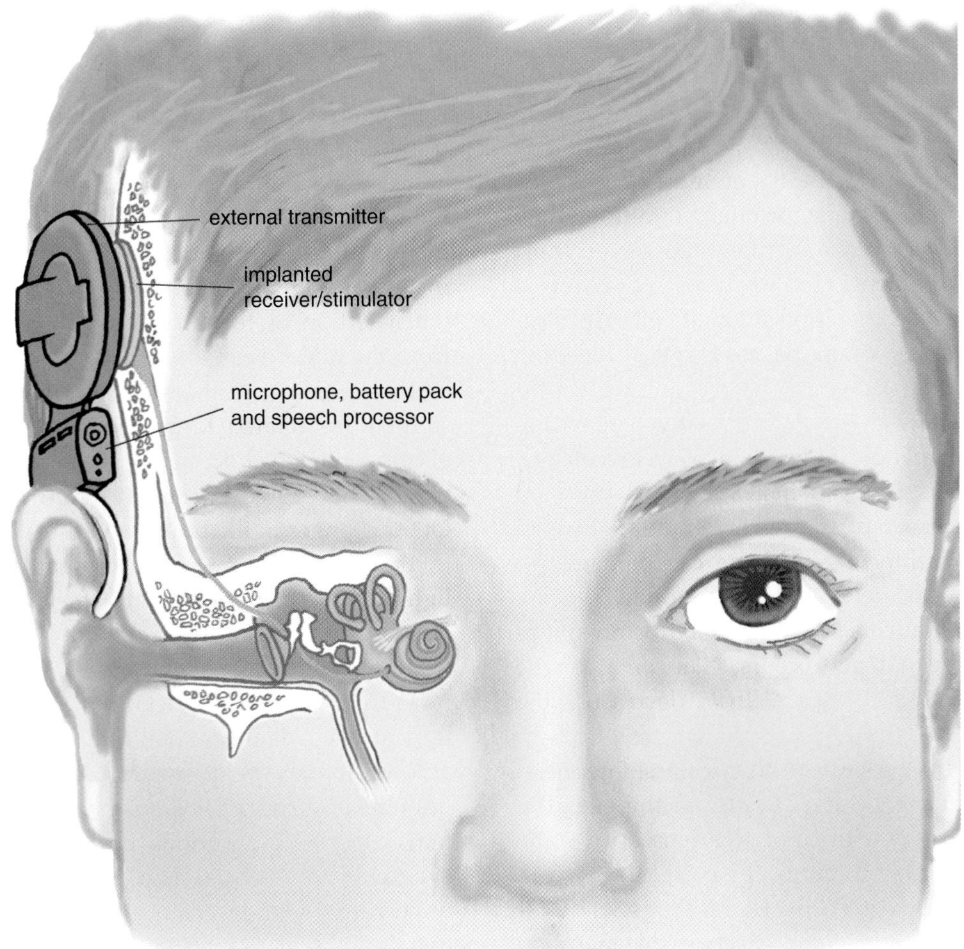

FIGURE 20-11 Cochlear implant. (Courtesy of Stephanie Freese, artist, and American Scientist, *The Magazine of Sigma Xi*, The Scientific Research Society. In Gould BE, Dyer R: *Pathophysiology for the health professions*, ed 4, St. Louis, 2011, Saunders.)

Cataracts can be corrected by surgical replacement of the cloudy lens.

Conjunctivitis (kon-junk-tih-VIE-tis), also called *pink eye*, is bacterial or viral inflammation of the eyelid. Conjunctivitis is extremely contagious. It causes reddening of the eyelids and sclera with pus formation. The pus may lead to closure of the eye, especially in the morning. Conjunctivitis is treated with antibiotics.

Deafness is the complete loss of hearing in one or both ears. It can be inherited or caused by complications at birth, disease, excessive noise or ototoxic drugs. In 2005 the World Health Organization (WHO) estimated that 278 million people in the world were deaf. A cochlear implant (CI) is an electronic device used to treat profound deafness and severe hearing loss (Fig. 20-11). The device has an external part with a microphone, speech processor, and transmitter and an internal part with a receiver, stimulator, and electrodes. Unlike a hearing aid, a cochlear implant does not amplify sound. Instead, it gives the deaf person a representation of sound by stimulating the auditory nerve. Cochlear implants have caused some controversy because some people feel that they threaten deaf culture and communities.

Diabetic retinopathy (die-ah-BET-ik ret-in-OP-ah-thee) is a common condition of damaged blood vessels in the retina caused by uncontrolled diabetes mellitus. Visual loss results. According to the American Diabetes Association, diabetes is the leading cause of blindness in people 20 to 74 years of age. The person may not notice the symptoms until the damage is so severe that it causes perceptible loss of vision. Treatment may not be necessary or may include laser surgery. The most important treatment is to control the diabetic condition to prevent damage.

Diplopia (dih-PLO-pee-uh), or double vision, results from muscle imbalance or paralysis of an extraocular muscle. It may also result from a problem with the sixth cranial nerve. Treatment of diplopia is to correct the cause.

Epistaxis (ep-ih-STAK-sis), or nosebleed, may result from disease, trauma, or other conditions such as hypertension, leukemia, or rheumatic fever. Most nosebleeds can be controlled easily with pressure at the base of the nose and application of cold. Application of heat (cautery) may be used to seal bleeding vessels.

Glaucoma (glaw-KO-muh) is a relatively common eye disorder in people older than 35 years of age. Glaucoma results from an increase in the pressure inside the eye, caused by trauma or hereditary factors. The increased intraocular pressure can damage the optic disc and optic nerve and cause "tunnel" vision. A person with glaucoma may feel pain or no symptoms at all until damage occurs. Glaucoma can be controlled with medication that decreases the pressure.

Hyperopia (hi-per-O-pee-uh), or farsightedness, results from a congenital deformity in the eye. The condition is treated with corrective lenses. In some cases, hyperopia may be surgically corrected.

Macular degeneration is the leading cause of blindness in people 65 and older. Macular degeneration results in a slow or sudden painless loss of central vision. The first symptom may be visual distortion from one eye. Recent research indicates that high doses of antioxidant vitamins and zinc may slow vision loss. Treatment may include laser surgery.

Ménière (men-ee-EER) *disease* is a collection of fluid in the labyrinth of the ear leading to dizziness (vertigo), ringing in the ear or tinnitus (TIN-ih-tus), pressure, and eventual deafness. The cause is unknown. Treatment includes medication, drainage of the fluid, or surgery.

Myopia (my-O-pee-uh), or nearsightedness, results from a congenital deformity in the eye. Treatment is corrective lenses. Procedures that may be used to correct vision by changing the shape of the eye include radial keratotomy (kare-uh-TOT-o-mee), photorefractive keratotomy, and laser (LASIK) treatment. It is also possible to implant corrective lenses in the eyes in some cases.

Night blindness, or poor vision in dim light, results from a deficiency in the rods of the retina. This may be caused by insufficient vitamin A, cataracts, a birth defect, or inflammation of the retina. Treatment may include supplementation of the diet with vitamin A.

Otitis media (o-TIE-tis MEE-dee-uh) is a middle ear bacterial or viral infection common in young children (Fig. 20-12). It often appears in conjunction with a throat infection. The person feels pressure or pain in the ear. Otitis media may lead to hearing loss. Treatment includes antibiotics to cure the illness and may include myringotomy (meer-ing-GOT-o-me), which is the insertion of tubes to relieve pressure and fluid from the middle ear.

Presbyopia (pres-bee-O-pee-uh) is a type of farsightedness related to aging. The eye becomes less elastic, and the fluid in the eye decreases. This can usually be treated effectively with corrective lenses. Other changes in the fluid may result in small clumps in the vitreous humor called floaters or flashes of light in the field of vision. These are not usually serious but should be monitored by periodic eye examination.

Retinal detachment (RD) may be due to injury or uncontrolled diabetes mellitus. It may occur gradually, or it may be a medical emergency requiring immediate surgery. The person with a detached retina may experience a sudden appearance of light with eventual loss of visual field. Retinal detachment may be corrected with laser surgery or cryopexy (freezing) that forms scar tissue that holds the retina in place. The most common treatment is scleral buckle. With this treatment, a sponge or band is attached to the sclera to hold the retina in place.

Rhinitis (rie-NIE-tis) is inflammation of the lining of the nose caused by allergic reaction, viral infection, sinusitis, or chemical irritants. Symptoms include drainage of nasal fluids, tears, and sneezing. Treatment depends on the cause and includes medication. Seasonal rhinitis (hay fever) may be caused by pollen in the air.

Ruptured eardrum may result from infection, an explosion, a blow to the head, or a sharp object inserted into the ear. The person experiences a slight pain and discharge from the ear. Healing usually occurs quickly. Scar tissue can form and result in hearing loss if the condition is chronic.

Sinusitis (sie-nus-I-tis) is a chronic or acute inflammation of the cavities of the cranium. Sinusitis is usually caused by the spread of infection from the nasal passages to the sinuses or by nasal obstructions, which block the normal sinus drainage. The infected person experiences nasal discharge, sneezing, swelling below the eyes, and headache. Treatment may

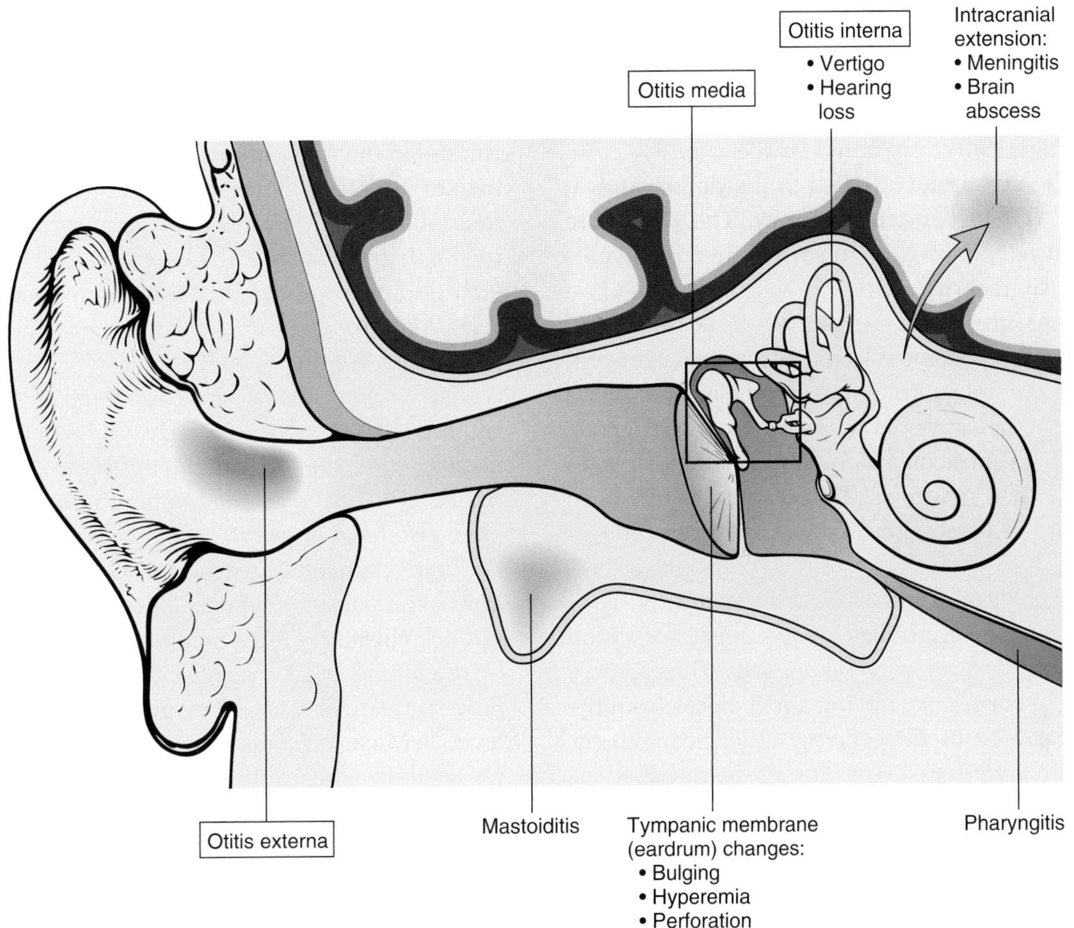

FIGURE 20-12 Otitis media is a common among young children. (From Damjanov I: *Pathology for the health professions*, ed 3, St. Louis, 2006, Saunders.)

include medications or, in severe chronic cases, may require surgical correction of deformities.

Strabismus (strah-BIZ-mus) is a condition in which both eyes do not focus on the same point or direction. Strabismus may be caused by brain injury, a tumor, or infection, but it is often the result of amblyopia. It may also be an inherited condition in which both eyes cannot be fixed on an object at the same time. Esotropia (es-o-TRO-pee-uh), or "crossed eyes," is the condition in which the muscles pull the eyes inward. Exotropia (ek-so-TRO-pee-uh) is the condition in which the muscles pull the eyes outward. Strabismus can be treated with eye exercises, patching, and corrective lenses. Surgery may be performed to correct the extraocular eye muscles.

A *sty* (stie) is caused by bacterial infection of the sebaceous glands of the eyelid. The sty contains pus and usually drains in 3 or 4 days. The person experiences pain, redness, and swelling. Treatment includes hot compresses, sometimes incision to drain the sty, and antibiotics.

Issues and Innovations

Visual Correction by Surgery

Radial keratotomy has been a popular microscopic surgery that makes eight incisions into the cornea of the eye. These incisions cause a flattening of the cornea that corrects the refraction error causing myopia, or nearsightedness. The angle and depth of the cuts are calculated by computer and performed by an ophthalmologist. A 10-year study concluded in 1994 by the U.S. National Eye Institute reported that the procedure was successful in two thirds of cases. However, it also reported that 43% of those who had surgery later developed farsightedness.

Another surgical procedure is called *epikeratophakia*. This procedure involves freezing a donor cornea and then cutting it like a contact lens. A prescription correction can be provided with the cornea. The cornea is surgically implanted in the eye. In 4 to 6 months, the eye tissue attaches to the donor cornea, and improved visual acuity results. The procedure has been used successfully to correct myopia, hyperopia, and cataract disorders.

Intacs are intracorneal rings that can be implanted to the cornea to reshape it to repair myopia. This procedure is reversible with removal of the inserts. Intacs are made of the same plastic used in contact lenses. PRELEX is an intraocular lens implant that replaces the lens with a new one. This technique has been used to correct presbyopia, as well as hyperopia and myopia.

In 1995 the Food and Drug Administration approved a computer-controlled laser surgery for vision repair called *photorefractive keratectomy*. This surgery reshapes the cornea by shaving small pieces from the surface. It can be used to correct either nearsightedness or farsightedness. The cornea is reshaped as pieces of the cornea are removed by the laser. The main benefit of this procedure is that it does not weaken the cornea as might occur in radial keratotomy. Other laser surgeries include laser in situ keratomileusis (LASIK) and laser thermal keratoplasty.

Noise Pollution

Noise in the environment can damage the nerve endings and cells in the inner ear. The ossicles of the ear amplify incoming sound 25 times before it reaches the inner ear. Hearing loss in industrial settings with strong noise pollution has been documented and has led to legislation to lower noise levels.

Loud music can also damage the cells in the inner ear. Once damaged, these cells cannot be repaired and the hearing loss is permanent. Environmental studies indicate that protection of the ears is necessary with sound greater than 85 dB. Exposure to 2 hours of noise at 100 dB is known to cause some degree of permanent hearing loss. Even portable stereos with earphones can produce sound as loud as 115 dB.

Most people do not notice hearing loss until they cannot understand normal speech or they develop ringing in the ear (tinnitus). A sensation of fullness or buzzing in the ear after a concert or similar exposure to a loud noise indicates that damage has been done to the hair cells in the inner ear. This is called a "temporary threshold shift." In some cases, the hair cells may repair, but repeated exposure leads to permanent hearing loss.

The volume of music is too high if it causes a ringing sensation or headache. It is too loud if a normal conversation cannot be heard. Because the ringer is in the earpiece, some cordless telephones have also been found to cause permanent damage to hearing when placed near the ear as it is ringing. Electronic noise-canceling devices are used in headphones worn by airline pilots and can be purchased by the public. In 2006 Apple Computers developed an iPod software program to limit the maximum volume level because of concern about the damage of the noise while using ear buds. Chapter 34 provides more information regarding the environmental hazards of noise pollution.

Studies have confirmed that even casual use of cellular phones can damage the DNA in sensitive areas of the brain. Dr. Henry Lai of the University of Washington conducted a study that indicates that even low-level exposure to radiofrequency electromagnetic fields and radio frequencies can cause DNA damage to brain cells of rats, resulting in loss of short and long-term memory and slower learning. He also concluded that the damage is cumulative. Research has provided extensive information on biological responses to power-frequency electric and magnetic fields. A strong link to development of cancer or other health problems due to electromagnetic frequency exposure has not been established. In 2009 the National Cancer Institute reported that research has not consistently linked cell phone use and cancer but suggested further study before drawing conclusions about the effect.

CASE STUDY 20-4 Your friend tells you that she can hear music from your player even though you are wearing ear buds. She says you will go deaf. What should you say?

Answers to Case Studies are available on the Evolve website: ***http://evolve.elsevier.com/Gerdin***

Summary

- The function of the sensory system is to perceive changes in the internal and external environment with specialized receptors.
- Sensory system structures include the eye, ear, tongue, nose, and skin.

- Methods of assessment of the sensory system include use of the Snellen chart, otoscope, and Rinne test.
- Disorders of the sensory system include conjunctivitis, epistaxis, glaucoma, macular degeneration, and rhinitis.

Review Questions

1. Describe the function of each of the five sensory organs.
2. Describe the location and function of each of the following parts of the sensory system:

   corpuscles of Ruffini — optic nerve
   iris — ossicle
   Meissner's corpuscles — pupil
   olfactory receptors
3. Describe three methods of assessment of the sensory system function.
4. Describe the method by which radial keratotomy changes the vision of the eye.
5. Describe how hearing is damaged by noise.
6. Use the following terms in one or more sentences that correctly relate their meaning: accommodation, intraocular, receptor, stimulus, and vision.

Critical Thinking

1. Investigate and compare the cost of at least three tests used in diagnosing disorders of the sensory system.
2. Investigate the function of at least five common medications used in treatment of sensory system disorders.
3. List at least five occupations involved in the health care of sensory system disorders.
4. Investigate the current surgical techniques for correction of eye disorders with the use of laser technology.
5. Use the Internet to research and describe the styles and cost of hearing aids.
6. Use the Internet to research and describe a recent development or treatment method relating to the sensory system.
7. Use the Internet to research and describe deaf culture and communities.
8. Use the Internet to research and describe the effect of noise pollution or electromagnetic fields on sensory functions.

Explore the Web

Deaf Culture

National Association of the Deaf
http://www.nad.org/

PBS—Sound and Fury
http://www.pbs.org/wnet/soundandfury/culture/index.html

Alexander Graham Bell Association for the Deaf and Hard of Hearing
http://nc.agbell.org/NetCommunity/Page.aspx?pid=550

Noise Pollution

Noise Pollution Clearinghouse (NPC)
http://www.nonoise.org/

Environmental Protection Agency (EPA)
http://www.epa.gov/air/noise.html

Electromagnetic Fields

Centers for Disease Control and Prevention
http://www.cdc.gov/niosh/topics/EMF/

National Institute of Health—INTERPHONE Study
http://www.ncbi.nlm.nih.gov/pubmed/17636416

National Institutes of Health—National Cancer Institute
http://www.cancer.gov/cancertopics/factsheet/Risk/cellphones

CHAPTER 21

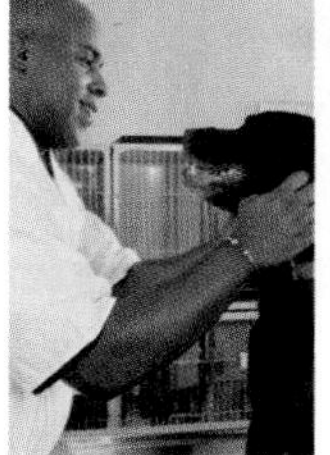
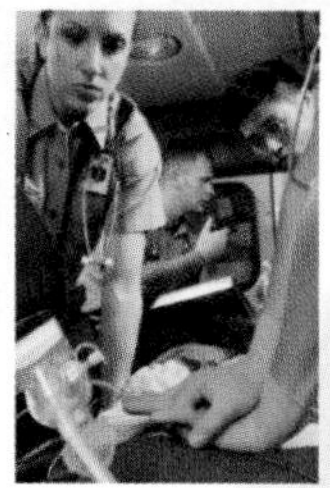
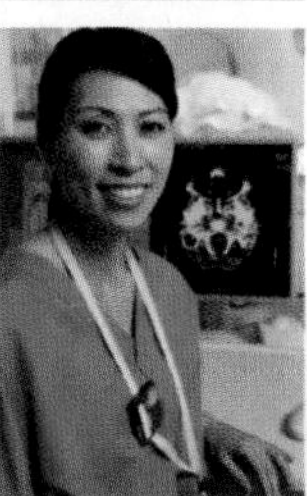

Reproductive System

LEARNING OBJECTIVES

- Define at least 10 terms relating to the reproductive system.
- Describe the function of the reproductive system.
- Identify at least 10 reproductive system structures and the function of each.
- Identify at least three methods of assessment of the reproductive system.
- Describe common patterns of growth and development of the neonate.
- Describe at least five disorders of the reproductive system.

KEY TERMS

Conception *(kon-SEP-shun)* Onset of pregnancy; union of sperm and egg (ovum)

Ectopic *(ek-TOP-ik)* Located away from normal position

Erectile *(e-REK-til)* Capable of becoming rigid and elevated when filled with blood

Fertile *(fer-TIL)* Capacity to conceive or induce conception

Fibroid *(FIE-broyd)* Tissue composed of threadlike, fibrous structure

Genital *(JEN-ih-tal)* Reproductive organ

Gestation *(jes-TAY-shun)* Development of young from conception to birth; pregnancy

Intercourse *(IN-ter-kors)* Sexual union

Lactation *(lak-TAY-shun)* Production and secretion of milk by the mammary glands (breasts)

Mammography *(ma-MOG-ruh-fee)* Radiologic view of breasts

Menses *(MEN-seez)* Normal flow of blood and uterine lining that occurs in cycles in women

Menstrual cycle *(MEN-stroo-al)* The recurring cycle of change of the reproductive organs induced by hormones in women

Ovulation *(o-vyoo-LAY-shun)* Release of the egg (ovum) from the ovary

Sterile *(ster-IL)* Being unable to produce offspring

Reproductive System Terminology*

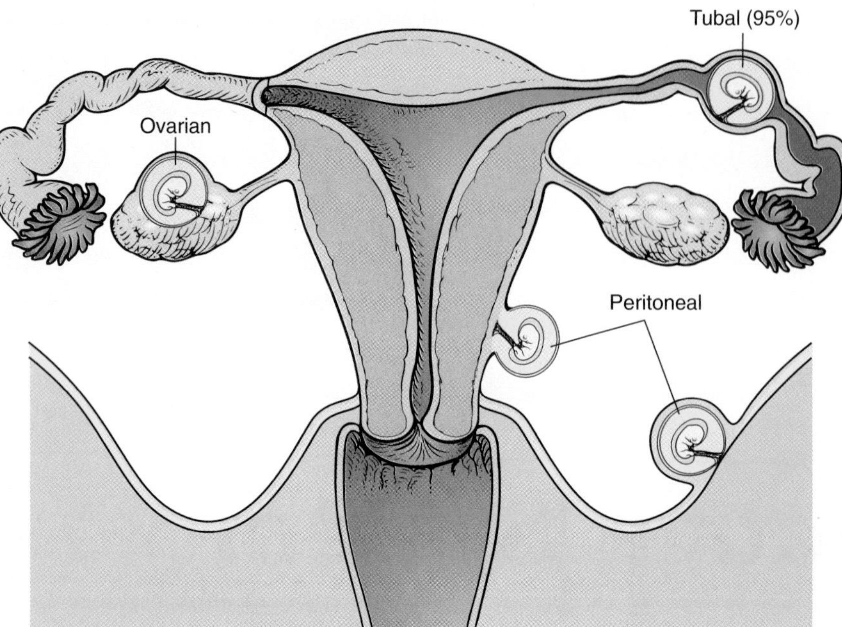

Ectopic pregnancy. (From Damjanov I: *Pathology for the health professions*, ed 3, St. Louis, 2006, Saunders.)

Term	Definition	Prefix	Root	Suffix
Antenatal	Before birth	ante	nat	al
Colporrhaphy	Repair of the vagina		colpo	rrhaphy
Ectopic	Outside of the normal location		ectop	ic
Gynecology	Study of women		gyn/ec	ology
Hysterectomy	Removal of the uterus		hyster	ectomy
Mammography	Picture of the breast		mammo	graphy
Orchiectomy	Removal of the testes		orchi	ectomy
Prostatectomy	Removal of the prostate		prostat	ectomy
Uteropexy	Fixation of the uterus		uter/o	pexy
Vasectomy	Removal of a vessel		vas	ectomy

*A transition syllable or vowel may be added to or deleted from the word parts to make the combining form.

Abbreviations of the Reproductive System

Abbreviation	Meaning
circ	Circumcision
cx	Cervix
D&C	Dilation and curettage
del	Delivery
Gyn	Gynecology
Lap	Laparotomy
OB	Obstetrics
PEDS	Pediatrics
PMS	Premenstrual syndrome
TAH	Total abdominal hysterectomy

Structure and Function of the Reproductive System

The function of the reproductive system is to produce offspring. The male and female reproductive organs (gonads) are different in structure to accomplish this function. Puberty is the age at which the reproductive organs mature sufficiently to allow reproduction.

The reproductive organs of both the male and female produce sex cells called *gametes*. The combination of genes of the female gamete (ova) and male gamete (sperm) is called *fertilization* (Fig. 21-1). From the time of **conception** to 2 weeks, the fertilized ovum is called a *zygote*. From 2 to 8 weeks' **gestation**, the growing cells are called an *embryo*. From 8 weeks to birth, the unborn baby is called a *fetus*. During the first 30 days of life, the infant is considered to be a neonate.

Male Organs of Reproduction

The organs of reproduction of the male are shown in Fig. 21-2. The testes, about 4 to 5 cm long, produce the sperm. The testes also secrete an androgenic hormone (testosterone), causing the appearance of secondary sexual characteristics such as facial and body hair, deepened voice, increased muscle mass, and thickening of the bones.

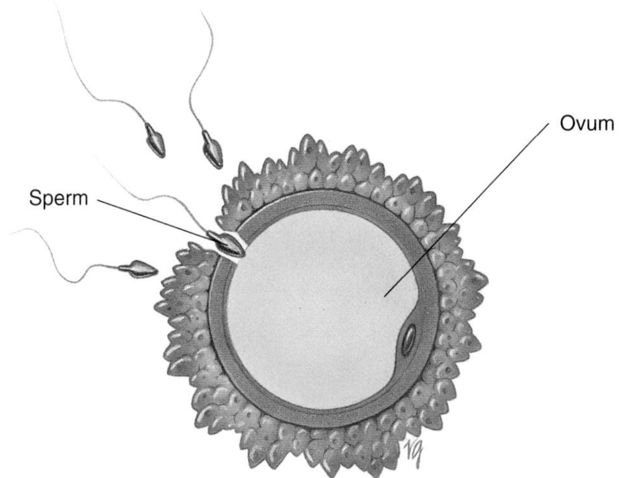

FIGURE 21-1 Fertilization.

The epididymis is a tube on the surface of each testis that stores the sperm while they mature. Sperm are transported by the vas deferens into the ejaculatory duct below the bladder. The seminal vesicle adds fluid that increases the volume and nourishes the sperm. The prostate gland, located below the bladder, secretes a fluid that protects the sperm.

The penis becomes rigid and elevated when filled with blood (**erectile**). The penis encloses the urethra. The glans penis is covered with a loose-fitting, retractable casing called the *foreskin* (prepuce), which may be removed (circumcision). Both semen and urine are excreted through the urethra, but the systems operate separately. Semen is a thick, white secretion that contains the sperm and fluid. Expulsion of semen is called *ejaculation*. Approximately 200 million sperm are in each ejaculation.

The National Cancer Institute (NCI) recommends a monthly self-examination of the testes to detect testicular cancer (Fig. 21-3). For 2009, the NCI estimated that 8400 new cases and 380 deaths occurred as a result of testicular cancer in the United States. Testicular cancer represents about 1% of all cancers in men. However, it is the most common form of cancer in men between 15 and 40 years of age.

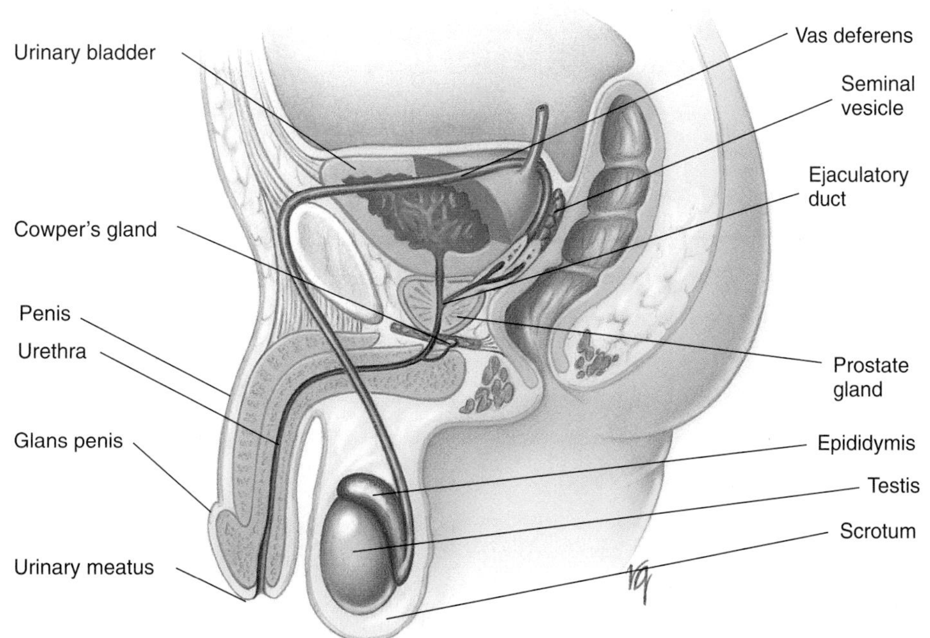

FIGURE 21-2 Male reproductive system.

Female Organs of Reproduction

The organs of reproduction in the female are shown in Fig. 21-4. The ovaries are glands that produce eggs (ova) and the hormones estrogen and progesterone.

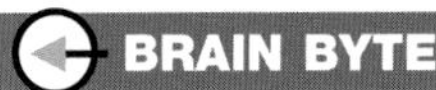

The ovaries of a newborn girl contain about 600,000 immature eggs.

The hormones prepare an egg (ovum) for fertilization, regulate the **menstrual cycle**, and help maintain pregnancy by promoting the growth of the placenta.

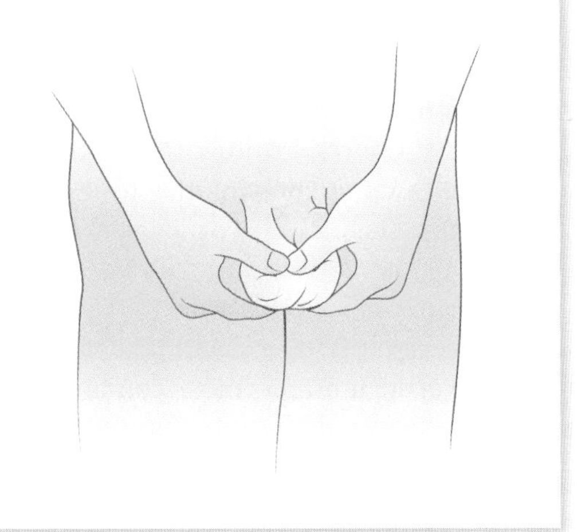

FIGURE 21-3 Testicular self-examination.

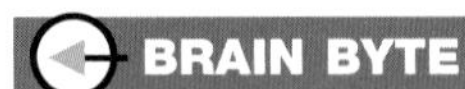

The largest cell in the female body is the egg.

The fallopian tubes (oviducts) transport the mature ovum from the ovary to the uterus. Fertilization usually occurs in the fallopian tubes during the 5 days required for the ovum to move to the uterus. If the ovum is not fertilized, it degenerates and is excreted as part of the menstrual cycle.

The uterus is a muscular structure about the size of a small finger. The zygote is implanted in the uterus after conception. The cervix, or neck of the uterus, thins and opens for delivery of a fetus. The inner layer of the uterus, called the *endometrium*, is shed during each menstrual cycle.

The vagina is a muscular tube that extends from the cervix to the exterior of the body. It is the site of sexual **intercourse** and the passageway (birth canal) for delivery of the fetus.

The external structures of the female reproductive system are collectively called the *vulva* (Fig. 21-5). The labia majora are folds of adipose tissue that protect the vaginal opening. The mons pubis is a pad of fat that joins the labia majora. The labia minora are pinkish folds of skin between the labia majora.

The clitoris is a small projection of erectile tissue located between the labia minora. The Bartholin glands secrete mucus and a lubricating fluid into the vaginal opening. The mammary glands (breasts) enlarge during puberty. The mammary glands have a

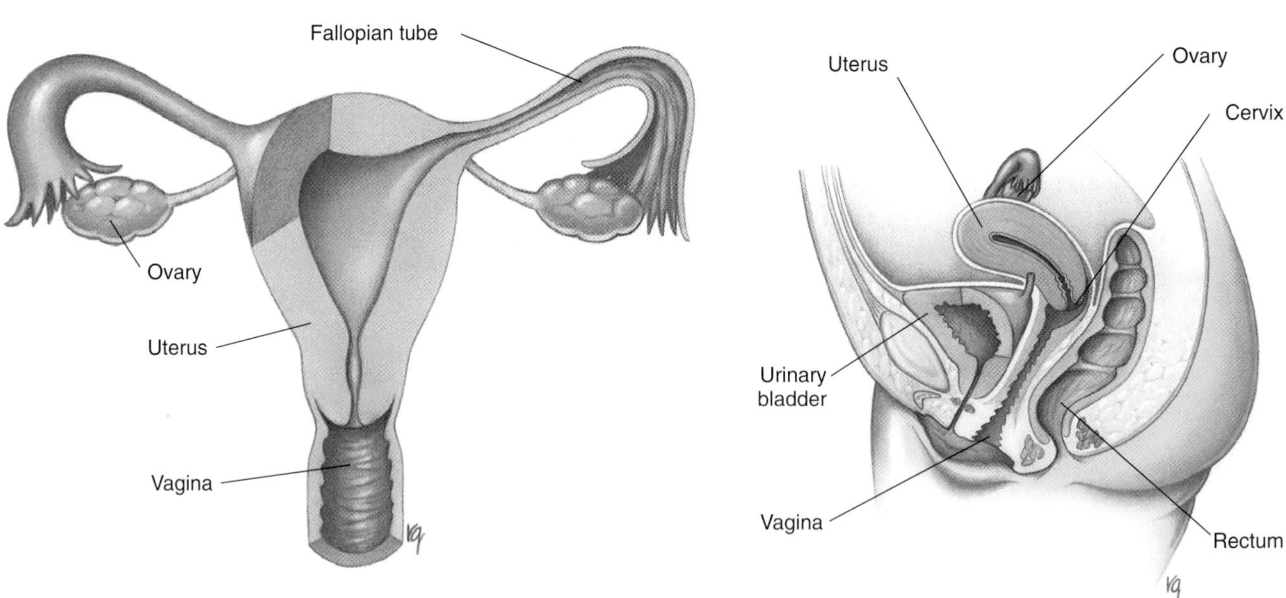

FIGURE 21-4 The internal structures of the female reproductive system.

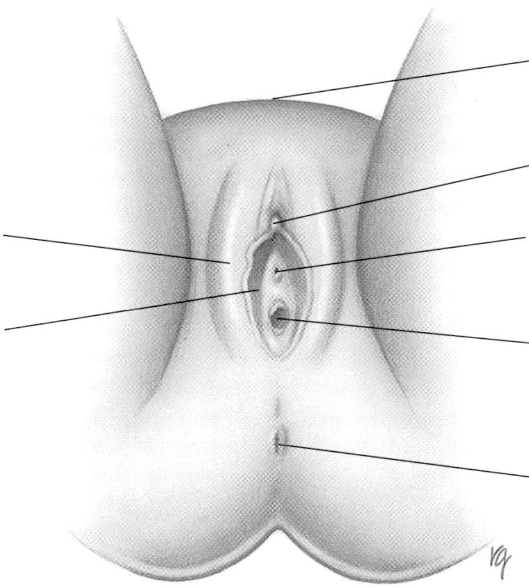

Mons pubis
Clitoris
Labia majora
Urethral meatus
Labia minora
Vaginal opening
Anus

FIGURE 21-5 The external structures of the female reproductive system.

system of ducts that secrete milk (**lactation**) after pregnancy.

Menstrual Cycle

The shedding of blood tissues of the uterus (menstruation) in the female signals the onset of puberty at about 10 to 16 years of age. The menstrual cycle, which lasts about 28 days, is a complex process of hormone secretion and tissue changes in the uterus (Table 21-1). A mature ovum is released from an ovary on about the 14th day of each cycle (Fig. 21-6). Some women experience pain a few hours after **ovulation** called *mittelschmerz*. This "middle pain" is believed to be caused by irritation of the peritoneum. If the released ovum is not fertilized, the lining of the uterus (endometrium) is released from the body along with the ovum. The sloughing of this bloody tissue, or **menses**, lasts from 3 to 7 days. The menstrual cycle continues until 45 to 50 years of age. The cessation of the cycle is called *menopause* (climacteric). Reduction in hormone production that occurs with menopause may cause a variety of symptoms, including "hot flashes," or transient periods of feeling warm. Reduced levels of both estrogen and pituitary gonadotropins occur with menopause. Without these hormones, the woman's ability to conceive or reproduce ceases.

Endometrial ablation is the removal or destruction of the lining of the uterus. Methods used to destroy the tissue include laser beam, heat, electricity, freezing, and microwave. It is an alternative to hysterectomy used to control heavy, prolonged menstrual bleeding. The procedure reduces or stops the menstrual cycle.

Pregnancy

Growth of an offspring in the uterus lasts about 280 days (9 months), or through the period of pregnancy. Pregnancy results from the union of the ovum and sperm, usually in the fallopian tube. The fertilized egg is known as a zygote for about 3 days. It is then considered to be the morula and enters the uterus. As a blastocyst, it implants in the uterine wall and is considered an embryo through the eighth week. From the eighth week until birth, it is considered a fetus.

Changes in the female reproductive system during pregnancy include an increase in muscle mass of the uterus and an elongation of the vagina. The uterus increases to 16 times its normal size during pregnancy. The secretions, vascularity, and elasticity of the cervix and vagina also increase in preparation for the delivery of the fetus.

The amniotic sac is a membrane that surrounds the fetus in the uterus. The sac is filled with fluid to cushion and protect the fetus against infection and temperature changes. A portion of the uterus forms the placenta, which filters the blood of the mother to provide oxygen and nutrients for the fetus.

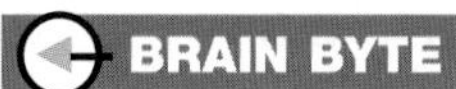

In the uterus, prior to birth, the infant's body is covered by a thin layer of hair called lanugo.

TABLE 21-1
Menstrual Cycle

Day(s)	Hormone Activity	Change in System
1	Pituitary secretes FSH Pituitary secretes LH	Follicle cells mature and produce estrogen Promotes estrogen production
2	Estrogen increases	Uterine lining begins to thicken; secondary sexual characteristics are maintained
3-13	No hormone activity	No change in system
14	Pituitary secretes FSH and LH	Mature follicle ruptures causing release of ovum (ovulation)*; follicle of ovary becomes corpus luteum
15	Corpus luteum secretes	Lining of uterus becomes more vascular; secretions of pituitary inhibited progesterone and estrogen
16-23	No hormone activity	No changes in system
24	No hormone activity	Corpus luteum degenerates if ovum is not fertilized
25	Progesterone and estrogen	Blood vessels to uterine lining constrict; tissues disintegrate and slough secretion decreases
26-27	No hormone activity	No changes in system
28	No hormone activity	Menses begin and last approximately 5 days

*If the ovum is fertilized after leaving the ovary, it is implanted in the rich uterine wall. The corpus luteum continues to secrete progesterone throughout the pregnancy to maintain the uterine wall and inhibit the secretion of pituitary hormones.
FSH, Follicle-stimulating hormone; *LH*, luteinizing hormone.

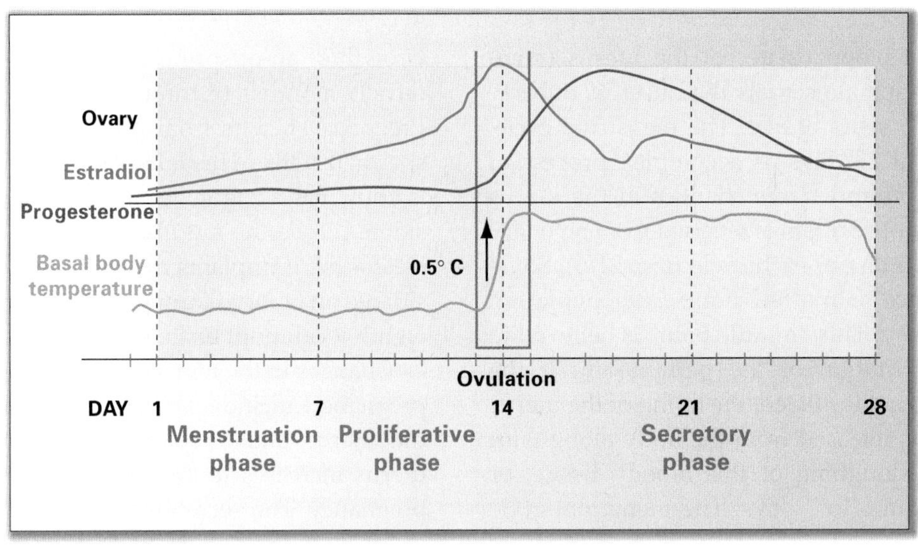

FIGURE 21-6 The menstrual cycle.

An infant born before the 37th week of pregnancy or weighing less than 2500 g (5 ½ lb) or (5 lb, 8 oz.) is considered premature. About 10% of babies in the United States fall in this category. Although there is no single cause for premature birth, some influencing factors have been identified. These include social, environmental, economic, and nutritional deficits. The cost of care for a premature neonate ranges from $12,000 to $150,000.

Labor and Delivery

Labor is muscle contractions that signal the onset of delivery of the fetus. Labor consists of three stages. In the first stage, muscle contractions of the uterus cause the amniotic sac to rupture and the cervix to open (dilate) to about 10 cm in diameter, allowing passage of the fetus. The second stage of labor is delivery of the baby, called *parturition*. Delivery of the afterbirth, or placenta, takes place about 15 minutes later and is the third stage of labor.

In the first 6 to 8 weeks after delivery of the baby, the mother is considered to be postpartum. During this time, the uterus shrinks back to normal size and the hormonal balance of the body is reestablished.

Growth and Development

The physical and psychological stage of the newborn (neonate) changes rapidly from the moment of birth. *Growth* refers to the changes that can be measured by changes in height and weight, as well as changes in body proportions. *Development* describes the stages of change in psychological and social functioning. These changes occur in spurts throughout the lifespan. At birth the baby, or neonate, is about 19 to 21 inches long and weighs 7 to 8 lb. The head is one fourth the length of the body compared with the adult ratio of one eighth. For the first 4 weeks, the baby is referred to as a *neonate*.

Assessment Techniques

Many disorders of the reproductive system can be assessed by palpation. Others are determined by blood tests, tissue culture, or by visual examination of the organs.

The most common methods of assessment of the male reproductive system are palpation and inspection of the organs (Box 21-1). Most disorders of the male reproductive system are treated by a physician specializing in urinary conditions (urologist). Cystoscopy can be used to view some of the reproductive structures. A blood test that measures a prostate-specific antigen may be used to detect prostate cancer.

Disorders of the female reproductive system are treated by a specialist called a *gynecologist*. The vagina can be opened with an instrument called a *speculum* to allow inspection of the cervix. With a Papanicolaou (Pap) smear, a few cells of the cervix are removed and studied microscopically to detect any potentially cancerous cells. Women older than 35 years of age should have a Pap smear every 1 to 3 years.

Many abnormalities of the breast may be first discovered by self-examination (Box 21-2). **Mammography** is an x-ray technique used to visualize breast tissue to detect any possible cancerous changes early. Digital imaging software used in computerized mammograms can eliminate some errors in the reading. Although there is some disagreement regarding how frequently a mammogram should be performed, the American Cancer Society (ACS) recommends that women have a yearly mammogram starting at age 40. Mammography may be followed by a biopsy to determine whether breast tissue is cancerous (Fig. 21-7). In 2009 the United States Preventative Services Task Force (USPSTF) changed its guidelines for mammography to no longer recommend routine screening for women between 40 and 49 years of age. The ACS responded by renewing their annual screening recommendation for women beginning at age 40. The ACS states that the data show that lives are saved with this screening, but the USPSTF states that not enough lives are saved to warrant the cost of routine testing.

Several tests can be used to detect abnormalities of the fetus during gestation. These include amniocentesis, ultrasonography, and chorionic villus sampling.

BOX 21-1

Testicular Self-Examination*

1. While standing in front of a mirror, check for swelling on the scrotum.
2. Examine each testicle with both hands. Roll the testicle between the thumb and fingers. This should not be painful.
3. The epididymis may be confused with a lump but is located behind the testicle.
4. If you feel a lump, see a physician.

*Perform once a month after a warm bath or shower.

BOX 21-2

Breast Self-Examination*

1. In a supine position, flatten the right breast by placing a pillow under the right shoulder. Place the right arm behind the head.
2. Use the middle three fingers of the left hand to palpate for lumps using a circular rubbing motion from the center of the breast out.
3. Press firmly to feel through layers of the breast tissue.
4. Palpate the chest and axilla for lumps.
5. Repeat the procedure for the left breast.

*Complete once a month, 2–3 days after the menstrual cycle.

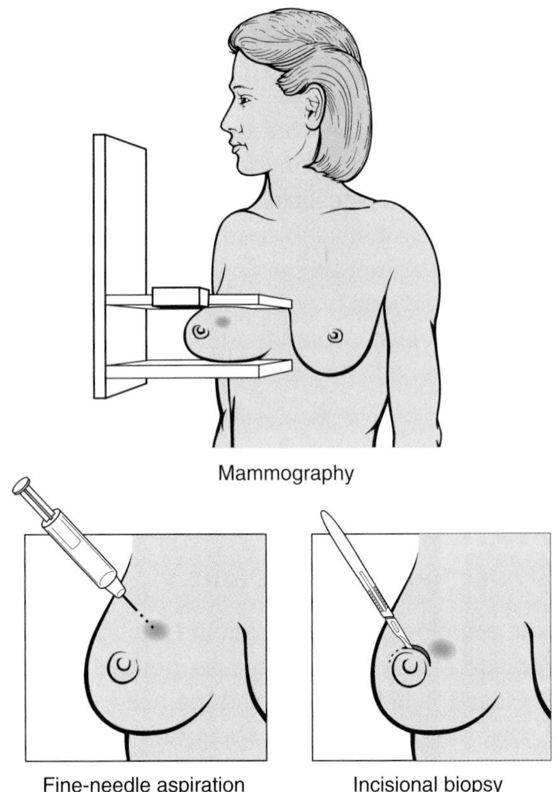

FIGURE 21-7 Examination for breast cancer. (From Damjanov I: *Pathology for the health professions*, ed 3, St. Louis, 2006, Saunders.)

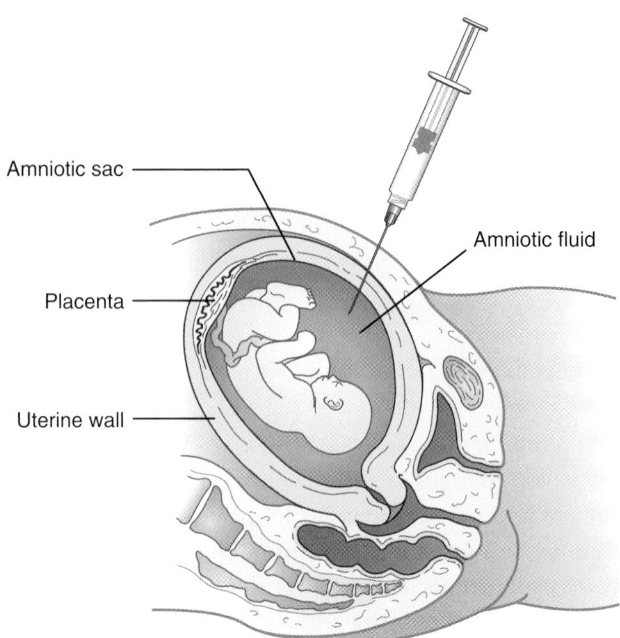

FIGURE 21-8 Amniocentesis. (From Bonewit-West K: *Clinical procedures for medical assistants*, ed 7, St. Louis, 2008, Saunders.)

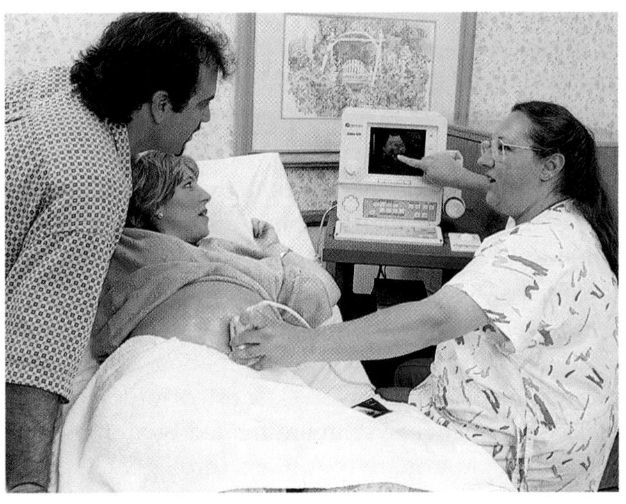

FIGURE 21-9 The ultrasound shows an image of the fetus during pregnancy. (From Gorrie TM, McKinney ES, Murray SS: *Foundations of maternal newborn nursing*, ed 2, Philadelphia, 1998, Saunders.)

Amniocentesis is a procedure that removes a small amount of amniotic fluid between the 16th and 20th week (Fig. 21-8). This fluid can be used to detect fetal abnormalities. Ultrasonography uses high-frequency sound waves to visualize structures deep in body cavities (Fig. 21-9). Some evidence indicates that frequent sonograms (five or more) during pregnancy may lead to low birth weight. Chorionic villi are tiny vascular fibrils that help to form the placenta. Sampling of these fibrils by using laparoscopy allows prenatal evaluation of the fetus. This procedure is often done in earlier stages of pregnancy than amniocentesis. Chorionic villus sampling may cause birth defects such as missing fingers and toes in the unborn infant when performed early in the pregnancy.

DISORDERS OF THE Reproductive System

Benign prostatic hypertrophy (be-NINE pros-TAT-ik hi-PER-tro-fee) is an age-associated condition in men in which the prostate grows and may stiffen, causing blockage of the urethra (yoo-REE-thrah). Men with this condition may experience difficult and frequent urination and bloody urine, known as hematuria (hem-uh-TOO-ree-uh). Treatment may include surgical removal of part or the entire gland to remove the blockage.

Cancer of the female reproductive system occurs in several ways. With the exception of skin cancer, breast

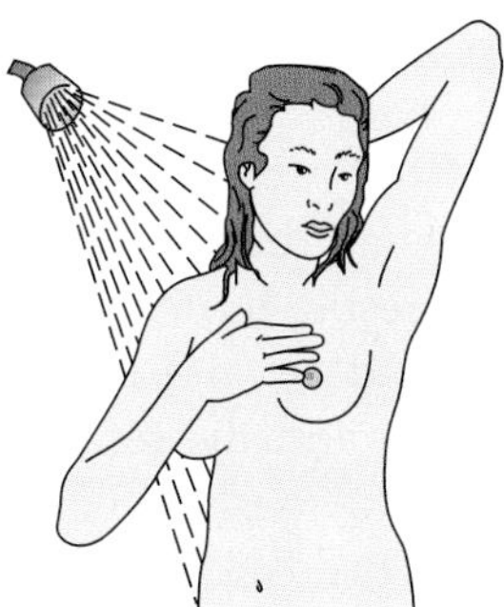

FIGURE 21-10 Breast self-examination. (From Kinn ME, Woods M: *The medical assistant*, ed 8, Philadelphia, 1999, Saunders.)

cancer is the most common cancer in women. Second to lung cancer, it is the second most common cause of death in women. According to the ACS, about one in eight women in the United States will be diagnosed with breast cancer in their lifetime. The chance of dying of breast cancer is 1 in 35.

Breast cancer can be painless and will spread, or metastasize (meh-TAS-tah-size), to other areas of the body if not detected early. Breast cancer can be detected by regular palpation for growths and with mammography (Fig. 21-10; and see Box 21-2). Less than 1% of breast cancers occur in men; however, the outcome for treatment is usually not as successful in men as it is in women.

CASE STUDY 21-1 Your friend tells you she is destined to have breast cancer because she has all of the risk factors except the gene that causes it. What should you say?

Answers to Case Studies are available on the Evolve website: ***http://evolve.elsevier.com/Gerdin***

Endometrial cancer is the most common cancer in the reproductive organs of women, with a lifetime chance of 1 in 40. Cervical cancer is associated with a history of sexually transmitted infection (STI), smoking, and multiple sexual partners. Cervical cancer can be detected early with a Pap smear. Treatment for invasive cervical cancer may include surgery, radiation, and biologic therapy or chemotherapy.

Cancer of the prostate is the second leading cause of death in men older than 50 years of age. According to the ACS, there were 192,280 new cases and 27,360 deaths resulting from cancer of the prostate in 2009. It is a slow-growing cancer that may show no symptoms for years. The affected person may experience a urinary disorder. Treatment may include removal of cancerous tissue and radiation.

Cancer of the testis, usually occurring in men 15 to 40 years of age, appears as a painless swelling of the scrotum. Rapid spread, or metastasis, is possible. Testicular cancer can be treated with surgery, radiation therapy, and chemotherapy. A survival rate greater than 95% has been reported for testicular cancer that is detected early.

CASE STUDY 21-2 Your friend says while he was showering he noticed that his testicles are not the same size. He says he also has some pain the groin area. What should you say?

Answers to Case Studies are available on the Evolve website: ***http://evolve.elsevier.com/Gerdin***

Chancroid (SHANG-kroid) is a contagious bacterial infection characterized by painful sores (ulcers) on the **genital** area. The person may also have enlarged, painful lymph nodes, fever, and headaches. Chancroid is associated with poor hygiene and is transmitted by sexual contact. Treatment includes antibiotic medication and cleansing of the lesions.

Chlamydia (klah-MID-ee-uh), caused by the bacteria *Chlamydia trachomatis*, is the most commonly reported STI or disease according to the National Institute of Allergy and Infectious Diseases (NIAID). An estimated three million new cases occur each year. *Chlamydia* infection causes symptoms similar to those of gonorrhea, including painful urination and a discharge in both sexes. One of every two women infected has no symptoms. Pelvic inflammatory disease (PID) is a serious complication of chlamydial infection and may result in infertility in women. A pregnant woman may pass the infection to the newborn during delivery, leading to neonatal problems such as eye infections or pneumonia. *Chlamydia* can be treated successfully with antibiotics in 95% of cases.

Cryptorchidism (kript-OR-kid-izm) is the failure of the testes to descend into the scrotal sac before birth (Fig. 21-11). The undescended testes often descend later without intervention. If not descended by age 5, treatment may include hormone supplementation. Surgical correction, known as *orchiopexy* (OR-kee-o-pek-see), is possible but may result in reduced **fertility**.

An *ectopic pregnancy* is one that occurs in an abnormal location in the body. In **ectopic** pregnancies,

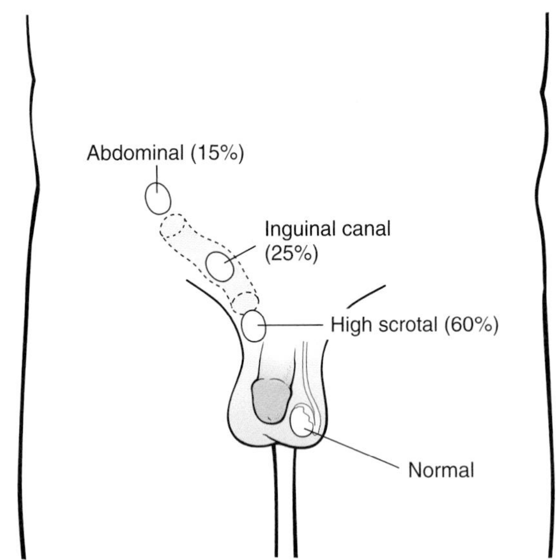

FIGURE 21-11 Cryptorchidism. (From Damjanov I: *Pathology for the health professions*, ed 3, St. Louis, 2006, Saunders.)

the embryo or fetus does not usually survive and the condition can be life-threatening to the woman if rupture results in internal bleeding. Ectopic pregnancies are now more common because of the greater incidence of STIs, which damage the fallopian tubes. Ectopic pregnancies are associated with PID and the use of an intrauterine device and some birth control pills. The person may experience lower abdominal pain, mild vaginal bleeding, and abdominal tenderness on palpation. Treatment is surgical removal of the embryo and, possibly, affected reproductive organs.

Endometriosis (en-do-mee-tree-O-sis) is growth of endometrial tissue in an area other than the uterus. The tissue continually grows and sheds, leading to abnormal bleeding and pain and sometimes to infertility. Treatment includes medication with pain relievers and steroids and possibly surgical removal of the affected organs.

Erythroblastosis fetalis (e-rith-ro-blas-TO-sis fet-AL-is) is a condition that may develop in an Rh+ fetus of an Rh– mother who has developed antibodies against the Rh blood protein in a prior pregnancy. Antibodies from the mother cross the placenta and attack the blood of the fetus. The condition leads to red cell destruction, jaundice, respiratory distress, and plaque formation in the brain of the fetus. Development of the Rh antibodies can be detected with a Coomb's test and blocked with an injection of RhoGAM. Treatment of the affected fetus can be done while the fetus is still in the uterus and at birth with transfusion.

Fetal alcohol syndrome (FAS) and *fetal alcohol effect* (FAE) include a group of physical and mental birth defects that result from damage to the fetus by alcohol consumed by the mother. The alcohol crosses the placenta, and the fetus's liver is unable to remove it quickly. An estimated 0.5 to 2 of every 1000 live births in the United States involves FAS each year with FAE three times as prevalent. The affected infant is often premature with a smaller head and brain, low birth weight, and typical facial features of the disorder. In addition to learning and behavior problems, the infant may also suffer seizures and heart defects. No safe level of alcohol consumption by the expectant mother is recommended to prevent this disorder. No cure is available for the affected child. Children affected with FAE and FAS are often placed in programs for children with special needs because of learning and behavioral problems and may need anticonvulsive medication or even brain surgery.

Fibroid tumors or *fibromyomas* are benign uterine growths found in 50% of women older than 50 years of age. The person may experience bleeding or no symptoms. Treatment may include surgical removal if the tumors cause symptoms.

Genital warts are caused by one type of human papilloma virus called *Condylomata acuminata*. According to Planned Parenthood, about 1% of the American population contracts genital warts each year. About two thirds of the people having sexual contact with people who have genital warts develop them. Warts on the external genitalia can be treated by surgical removal, freezing (cryotherapy), chemical or electrical burning, or injection of the warts with interferon. Although treatment removes the warts, it does not kill the virus, so they often reappear.

Gonorrhea (gon-or-REE-uh) is a bacterial infection and is one of the most prevalent STIs. According to the NIH, 355,991 new cases were reported in 2007. Because not all cases are reported, it is estimated that the real number may be closer to one million. The most common symptom is painful urination and a white to yellowish green discharge from the urethra. The female often experiences no symptoms but may have dysuria or pain in the abdomen. Gonorrhea can lead to sterility and arthritis if untreated. Gonorrhea may result in blindness in infants born to infected mothers. Treatment includes penicillin, but penicillin-resistant strains of gonorrhea are increasing.

Herpes simplex (HER-peez SIM-pleks) *virus* (HSV-2), or *genital herpes*, is the most common STI, affecting an estimated 30 million Americans. According to the CDC, 16.2% of people aged 14 to 49 years of age have herpes simplex virus 2. Herpes is caused by a virus that results in blisters, which open into painful sores. Herpes lesions appear in episodes, triggered by factors such as sunlight, friction, emotional stress, and fever. Herpes is spread by sexual contact or secretions from open lesions. Women who have herpes lesions can transfer the virus to their infants during birth, causing mental retardation or death. No cure exists, but new treatment includes an antiviral medication that controls symptoms. In 2009, the National Institute of Allergy and Infectious Diseases (NIAID) and GlaxoSmithKline partnered in a clinical study of the vaccine Herpevac.

Human papilloma virus (HPV) newly infects an estimated six million Americans each year according to the CDC. More than 40 types of HPV have been identified. HPV infection often does not cause visible symptoms. It may appear as genital warts. HPV is the most important risk factor for development of cervical cancer. HPV may be treated by cryotherapy, burning (electrocautery), injection of interferon, or application of chemicals. Treatment removes the warts but does not eliminate the virus. In 2006 a vaccine to prevent HPV was approved for use in the United States by the FDA. The vaccine prevents infection by four strains of HPV, including the two types that are responsible for 70% of cervical cancer cases. It also blocks other strains of HPV that are responsible for about 90% of genital wart cases.

Klinefelter (KLINE-fel-ter) syndrome is a defect appearing in males who carry an extra chromosome resulting in a karyotype of XXY. Males with this syndrome may develop breast tissue, tall stature, small testicles, below-normal intelligence, and sterility. No treatment is available.

Leukorrhea (loo-ko-REE-uh) is a whitish vaginal discharge. A slight discharge is normal in the menstrual cycle when the ovum is released (ovulation) and just before menstruation (Fig. 21-12). Any change in the color, odor, or character of the discharge may indicate a disorder. An excessive discharge may occur as a result of infection. Leukorrhea may be accompanied by redness, painful urination, or discomfort. Treatment of leukorrhea depends on the cause.

Menstrual (MEN-stroo-ul) *disorders* may result from endocrine, metabolic, and nutritional imbalances. Painful menstrual cramping, called *dysmenorrhea* (dis-men-o-REE-a), is often due to hormonal imbalance and faulty uterine structure. Excessive bleeding, or menorrhagia (men-o-RAY-jee-ah), or no bleeding, known as *amenorrhea* (a-men-o-REE-uh), may also occur. Menorrhagia may occur as a result of benign fibromas of the uterus. Amenorrhea may result from hormone imbalances, structural deformities, weight loss, and excessive exercise. Treatment depends on the severity and cause but may include surgical removal of the uterus in severe cases of menorrhagia.

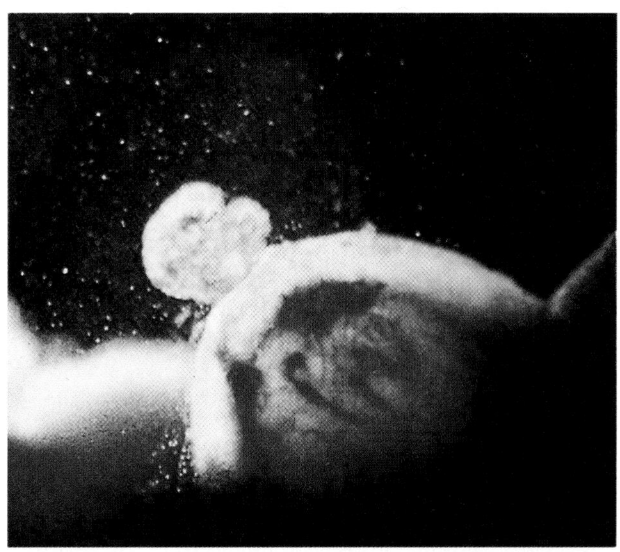

FIGURE 21-12 Ovulation. (From Patton KT, Thibodeau GA: *Anatomy & physiology*, ed 7, St. Louis, 2010, Mosby.)

CASE STUDY 21-3 Your friend is a distance runner. She tells you that besides being healthy and thin, a great benefit for her is that she no longer has periods. What should you say?

Answers to Case Studies are available on the Evolve website: ***http://evolve.elsevier.com/Gerdin***

Orchitis (or-KI-tis) is an inflammation of the testes usually resulting from STI or mumps. The person may experience swelling, redness, and pain in the scrotum. Treatment may include elevation of the scrotum, ice packs, and pain-relieving medication.

Pelvic inflammatory (PEL-vik in-FLAM-ah-tore-ee) *disease* (PID) is relatively common, particularly in teenage women. Approximately one million women develop PID each year. Development of PID is usually associated with infection by gonorrhea or chlamydia and can become chronic. It affects all the reproductive organs of the pelvis and causes scarring of the fallopian tubes. The woman experiences lower abdominal pain, fever, vaginal discharge, and menstrual disorders. According to the NIAID, an estimated 100,000 women become infertile each year as a result of PID. Ectopic pregnancy may result from damage to the fallopian tubes. Diagnosis can be done rapidly with a biotechnology technique called *polymerase chain reaction*. Treatment includes antibiotics and sometimes surgery.

Phimosis (fih-MO-sis) is a narrowing (stenosis) of the foreskin of the glans penis. Usually caused by infections, phimosis may interfere with urination and cause redness, swelling, pain, and pus formation. Treatment includes antibiotics, soaking, and surgical removal of the foreskin (circumcision).

Premenstrual (pre-MEN-stroo-al) *syndrome* (PMS) is a common collection of up to 150 symptoms occurring 3 to 14 days before the beginning of the bleeding part (menses) of the menstrual cycle. The woman may experience irritability, depression, impaired concentration, headache, and edema (eh-DEE-ma). The symptoms vary greatly and disappear with the menses. Several hypotheses have been offered to explain the symptoms of PMS, including hormonal or biochemical imbalance and poor nutrition. Treatment includes diet modification to eliminate sugar, caffeine, alcohol, nicotine, and processed foods. Vitamin B, calcium, magnesium, and chromium are prescribed in some cases. Exercise and stress-reduction training may also be helpful. Evidence indicates that a brain chemical (serotonin) may affect a severe and disabling form of PMS called *premenstrual dysphoric disorder (PMDD)*. The FDA has approved three medications for treatment of PMDD.

Pubic (PYOO-bik) *lice* are yellow-gray parasites found in the pubic hair. They become dark when engorged with blood. They are usually transmitted sexually, but they can also be spread through clothes and bed linen. They cause itching. Treatment includes medicated shampoo, cream, or lotion to kill the parasites.

Sexually transmitted diseases (STD) or *infections* (STI) affect men and women of all social and economic backgrounds. More than 30 STDs have been identified. The CDC estimates there are more than 19 million new cases each year, with half in people age 15 to 24. Some common STIs are chlamydia, herpes simplex, HPV, gonorrhea, and syphilis. Other STDs include trichomoniasis, hepatitis B, scabies, AIDS, and pubic lice.

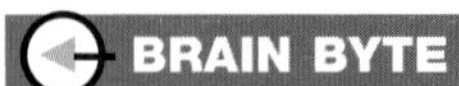

BRAIN BYTE

The cost of STDs to the U.S. health care system is estimated to be as much as $15.9 billion annually.

CASE STUDY 21-4 Your friend tells you that she is taking birth control pills so she will not have to worry about getting human immunodeficiency virus (HIV) and other STIs. What should you say?

Answers to Case Studies are available on the Evolve website: ***http://evolve.elsevier.com/Gerdin***

Syphilis (SIF-ih-lis) is caused by a spirochete (SPY-ro-keet) bacteria, *Treponema pallidum* (trep-o-NEE-mah PAL-ih-dum), and it occurs in three stages. Painless sores, or chancres, first appear 10 to 90 days after infection and disappear in a few weeks in the second stage. The infection spreads into the bloodstream and causes fever, swollen glands, and rash that disappear in 10 to 14 days. Third-stage syphilis may appear years later as the nervous system tissue is damaged, leading to death in one third of untreated cases. Unfortunately, the rate of syphilis infection increased by 11.8% between 2005 and 2006. Syphilis may cause birth defects in the infants of mothers with syphilis. Syphilis can be successfully treated with antibiotics.

Trichomonas vaginalis (trik-o-MO-nas VAJ-ih-nal-es) is a parasitic protozoa. The infected person may have no symptoms or may experience a foul-smelling, yellowish green discharge and redness of the vulva, urinary frequency, or painful urination (dysuria). Treatment includes oral medication.

Vaginitis (vaj-ih-NIE-tis) is a nonspecific infection that may cause a scant, gray, foul-smelling discharge. Treatment includes antibiotics such as ampicillin.

Yeast infection is an overgrowth of yeast in the vagina that appears as a curdy, cheeselike discharge. This infection commonly occurs in women who are diabetic or are taking medication such as antibiotics, steroids, or commercial douches that alter the pH of the vagina. Treatment includes antifungal, or mycostatic (MY-ko-stat-ik), medication or potassium hydroxide.

Issues and Innovations

Alternatives in Conception

Technological advances have given people many choices regarding reproduction. Effective birth control

TABLE 21-2
Contraceptive Methods

Method	Effectiveness	Description
Abstinence	100%	Refraining from sexual activities that could result in pregnancy
Barrier methods	88%	Condoms cover the erect penis to collect sperm entry into uterus
	84%	Diaphragms cover the entrance to the cervix with a soft cap that prevents the sperm from entering; best used with spermicidal jelly; must be individually fitted and checked yearly
	79%	Spermicidal agents are chemicals in creams, jellies, suppositories, or foams inserted into the vagina before intercourse to kill sperm cells
	73%-92%	Cervical cap inserted 1 hour before intercourse, blocking entry of sperm
Birth control pills	94%-97%	Contain estrogen and progesterone hormones to prevent ovulation or progesterone only to prevent implantation of the ovum; not recommended in some women because of health risk; Depo-Provera developed in 1992 as a synthetic form of progesterone
Implanon	99%	Flexible, plastic implant inserted under the skin of the upper arm; effective for 3 years
IUD	94%	Inserted into uterus by doctor; IUD scrapes lining of uterus to prevent implantation of ovum
"Natural" methods	60%-75%	Rhythm method, or fertility awareness, requires abstention during ovulation by counting days or checking body temperature
	81%-96%	Withdrawal is the removal of the penis before ejaculation
Norplant	99%	Capsules implanted under the skin of the upper arm containing a synthetic progesterone that stops ovulation; effective for 5 years. Still used in developing countries although use discontinued in United States
Ortho Evra	99%	Thin, plastic patch stuck to skin once a week for 3 weeks followed by patch-free week
RU486	100%	Abortifacient drug (mifepristone) taken orally up to 9 weeks of pregnancy along with prostaglandin, resulting in abortion of fetus 1 to 1.5 weeks later; ban against use lifted in United States in 1993; also used for treatment of breast cancer, endometriosis, glaucoma, and brain tumors
Tubal ligation	99.6%	Surgical cutting of the fallopian tubes of the woman so that the ovum does not reach the uterus; may be reversed in 25% of cases
Vasectomy	99.8%	Surgical cutting of the vas deferens of the man so that sperm does not leave the testes; may be reversed in about 50% of cases

IUD, Intrauterine device.

methods have been developed to prevent pregnancy (Table 21-2). The United States continues to have a higher rate of teenage pregnancy and abortion than other industrialized countries. The CDC reported a 4.19% rate of pregnancy for mothers aged 15 to 19 in 2006. The effectiveness of contraceptive methods varies a great deal (Fig. 21-13). Abortion remains a controversial moral and legal issue.

Assisted reproductive technology (ART) refers to the treatment of sperm and eggs to increase the chance of reproduction. The most common types of ART include in vitro fertilization, in which the egg and sperm are mixed outside of the body and then transferred to the uterus. The first "test tube" infant was born in England in 1978, with hundreds more now living throughout the world. The procedure involves removal of eggs from the ovary with a surgical needle. The egg is incubated and then joined with sperm cells. Some of the fertilized eggs are then implanted by laparoscopy into the uterus of the female who will

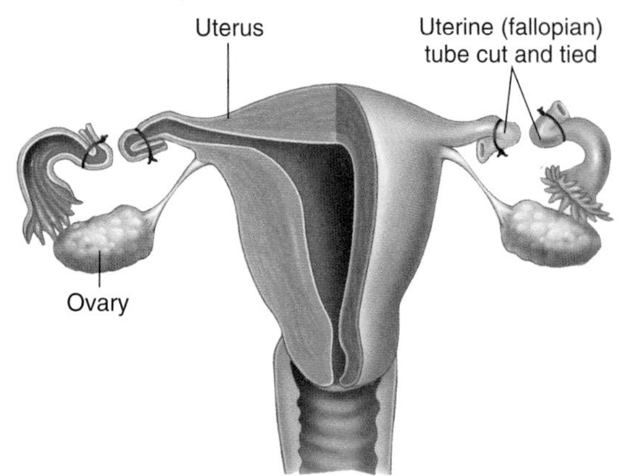

FIGURE 21-13 Tubal ligation. (From Patton KT, Thibodeau GA: *Anatomy & physiology*, ed 7, St. Louis, 2010, Mosby.)

carry the pregnancy. An ethical concern of this method relates to the status of the unused embryos, which can be frozen and implanted later or discarded. Intracytoplasmic sperm injection is the injection of a single sperm into an egg. The egg is then implanted in the uterus or fallopian tube. Gamete intrafallopian transfer occurs when eggs are placed in a thin tube with the sperm. The mixture is then injected into the woman's fallopian tube. Zygote intrafallopian transfer mixes the sperm and eggs outside of the body and then places them in the fallopian tubes. In 2006 about 1% of children born in the United States were conceived by using ART.

The issue of surrogacy has become an ethical and legal concern. In surrogacy the sperm and ovum are artificially fertilized and implanted in a woman who agrees to give the infant to the couple after birth. A fee is usually given to the woman for bearing the child. Surrogate mothering is an alternative for women for whom pregnancy is a health risk or impossibility. In some cases, the woman bearing the child has been reluctant to give the infant to the couple as agreed. Some states have passed laws to make surrogacy illegal.

In 2009 the March of Dimes reported that one of eight infants born in the United States are premature or less than 37 weeks of gestation. With innovations such as the drugs used to replace pulmonary surfactant in the care of premature infants, a fetus can now survive outside the uterus (called *viability*) at a much younger age, even at less than 20 weeks' gestation.

Surgery has also been successful to correct a defect in a fetus as early as the 21st week of gestation. The fetus is partially removed from the uterus in a procedure similar to a cesarean section and replaced after the surgical correction is completed. "Closed" fetal procedures are more common and use ultrasound to place a needle in the uterus or umbilical cord to treat the fetus. Some closed fetal procedures include transfusion in cases of Rh blood incompatibility, removal of excess lung fluid, administration of heart medication, and clearing urinary system obstructions.

Infertility

Infertility is defined as the inability to conceive after 1 year of trying. About one of every 10 women is infertile because of abnormalities in the reproductive system or problems with production of gametes. About one third of cases of infertility are caused by problems in the woman, and another third is caused by the man. The remaining third are unknown or a result of problems in both the man and woman. Factors that increase the risk of infertility include age, smoking, stress, alcohol use, athletic training, weight, and STIs. The tendency of couples to delay childbearing until their late 20s or early 30s may also be a factor.

Redefining the Sexes

Changes in family structure and sexual orientation have become more common lifestyle alternatives. These gender roles remain a controversial issue, such as relations between members of the same gender (homosexual) or both genders (bisexual). Transvestites dress in the clothes of the opposite gender. Transgender refers to an individual whose "gender identity" or self-identification is not the same as the "assigned sex" or physical structures.

Some people have surgeries to change their sexual appearance (transsexual). The person who seeks transsexual treatment is given hormones to produce secondary sexual characteristics, such as voice and hair changes and breast tissue growth. Plastic surgery cosmetically changes genital structure. Internal reproductive organs and the genetic makeup of the cells are not changed. Sexual intercourse is possible for the transsexual, but conception is not possible.

Summary

- The function of the reproductive system is to produce offspring.
- Reproductive structures of the man include the testes, prostate gland, penis, ejaculatory duct, and seminal vesicle.

- Reproductive structures of the woman include the ovaries, fallopian tubes, vagina, uterus, and cervix.
- Methods to assess the reproductive system include self-examination, mammography, cystoscopy, and chorionic villus sampling.
- Growth and development of the neonate change rapidly after birth and occur in spurts throughout the lifespan.
- Disorders of the reproductive system include STDs, cancers, ectopic pregnancies, erythroblastosis fetalis, and fetal alcohol syndrome.

Review Questions

1. Describe the function of the reproductive system.
2. Describe the location and function of each of the following parts of the reproductive system:

cervix	penis
fallopian tube	uterus
ovary	vagina

3. Describe three reproductive system disorders that are caused by a pathogen.
4. Describe three methods used to assess the reproductive system.
5. Differentiate between the effectiveness of three methods of contraception.
6. Describe three methods of assisted reproductive technology and the circumstances that might lead to the choice of each method.
7. Describe the development of the newborn from conception to neonate.
8. Use the following terms in one or more sentences that correctly relate their meaning: conception, fertility, gestation, and intercourse.

Critical Thinking

1. Investigate and compare the cost of at least three tests used in diagnosing disorders of the reproductive system.
2. Investigate the function of at least five common medications used in treatment of the reproductive system.
3. List at least five occupations involved in the health care of reproductive system disorders.
4. Investigate the cost of in vitro fertilization.
5. Investigate the current legal issues regarding contracts for surrogate mothers.
6. Investigate the postpartum disorder sometimes called the "blues."
7. Use the Internet to research the frequency of occurrence and cause of sudden infant death syndrome, commonly known as SIDS.
8. Use the Internet to research and review an article regarding a recent development or treatment method relating to the reproductive system.
9. Use the Internet to research the vaccine used to prevent infection of HPV. Write a paragraph to support or oppose the recommendation to administer the drug to girls between the ages of 11 and 12.
10. Use the Internet to research STIs. Create a poster, pamphlet, or essay to describe the cause and effect of a common STI.

Explore the Web

HPV Vaccine

CDC

http://www.cdc.gov/std/hpv/STDFact-HPV-vaccine-hcp.htm#vaccrec

Sexually Transmitted Infections

NIH

http://www3.niaid.nih.gov/topics/sti/

CDC

http://www.cdc.gov/std/

UNIT THREE

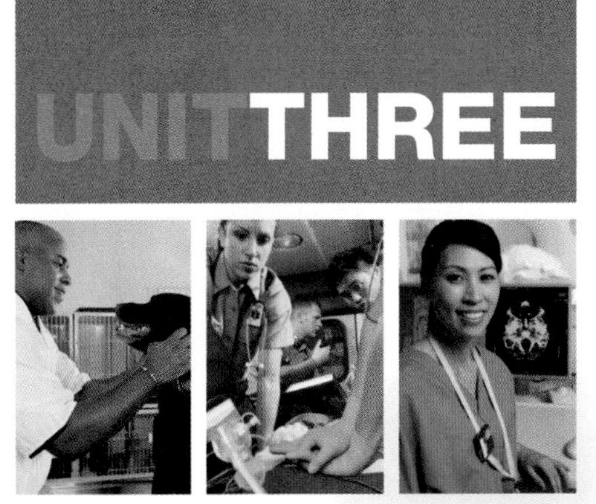

Career Clusters

CHAPTER 22

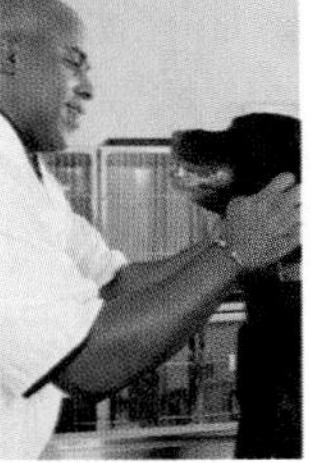

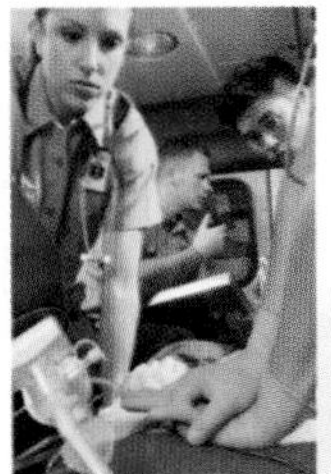

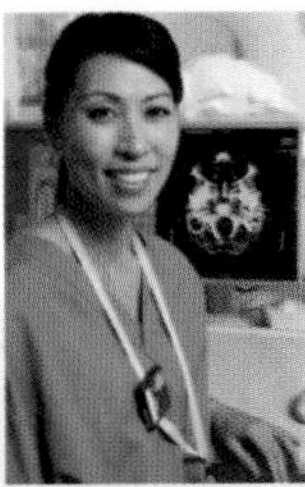

Laboratory Careers

LEARNING OBJECTIVES

- Define at least 10 terms relating to laboratory careers.
- Specify the role of selected laboratory health care workers including personal characteristics, levels of education, and credentialing requirements.
- Differentiate between pathogenic and nonpathogenic microorganisms.
- Identify six groups of organisms that may be pathogenic in humans.
- Describe the conditions that are favorable for growth of microorganisms.
- Identify three ways in which the skin serves as a defense against infection.

KEY TERMS

Donor *(DOE-ner)* Person who supplies living tissue or who furnishes blood or blood products for transfusion to another person

Fomite *(FOE-mite)* Inanimate object capable of carrying germs

Immunity *(im-YOO-nih-tee)* High level of resistance to certain microorganisms or diseases

Infection *(in-FEK-shun)* Invasion and multiplication of pathogenic microorganisms in the body tissues

Microorganism *(mie-cro-ORG-un-izm)* Microscopic living organism, microbe

Nonpathogenic *(non-path-o-JEN-ik)* Microorganism that does not produce disease

Pathogen *(PATH-o-jen)* Microorganism that produces disease

Phagocyte *(FAY-go-site)* Cell that surrounds and destroys microorganisms and foreign particles

Phlebotomy *(fle-BOT-uh-mee)* Incision into a vein to withdraw blood

Recipient *(re-SIP-ee-int)* One who receives tissue from another, such as in a blood transfusion

Sterile *(STARE-ul)* Free from all living microorganisms

Laboratory Careers Terminology*

Term	Definition	Prefix	Root	Suffix
Aerobic	Pertaining to air		aerob	ic
Antitoxin	Against poisoning	anti	toxin	
Microbiology	Study of life on the microscopic level	micro	bio	ology
Microorganism	Small living thing	micro	organism	
Nonpathogen	Does not originate (cause) disease	non	path/o	gen
Pathogen	Originates (causes) disease		path/o	gen
Pathologist	One who studies disease		path	ologist
Phagocyte	Cell that eats	phag/o	cyte	
Urinalysis	Test to study urine		urin	alysis
Zoologist	One who studies animals		zoo	o/logist

*A transition syllable or vowel may be added to or deleted from the word parts to make the combining form.

Abbreviations for Laboratory Careers

Abbreviation	Meaning
ABC	Aspiration, biopsy, cytology
AFB	Acid-fast bacillus
bl wk	Blood work
BUN	Blood, urea, nitrogen
CPK	Creatine phosphokinase
ESR	Erythrocyte sedimentation rate
H&H	Hemoglobin and hematocrit
SMAC	Sequential multiple analysis computer
spG	Specific gravity
UA	Urinalysis

BOX 22-1

Laboratory Careers

Blood donor unit assistant
Chemistry technologist
Cleaner, laboratory equipment
Cytologist
Cytotechnologist
Dairy technologist
Feed research aide
Histologic technician
Histopathologist
Immunohematologist
Laboratory assistant, culture media
Laboratory sample carrier
Medical laboratory assistant
Medical laboratory technician
Medical technologist
Medical technologist, chief
Microbiology technologist
Pathologist
Phlebotomist
Poultry scientist
Zoologist

Careers

Laboratory careers include workers with a broad range of interests and abilities (Box 22-1). Life scientists use advanced biomedical technology to assist with diagnosis and treatment of patients, as well as monitoring public health. Opportunities in this area include clinical laboratory, blood banking, research, and related fields in life science (Table 22-1).

Clinical Laboratory Science

Laboratory personnel do not usually have contact with the patient. The laboratory provides a clean, well-lighted, and controlled working environment with regular hours. Most of the laboratory work is done while sitting. Excellent vision and manual dexterity are necessary to perform laboratory work. In 1988 the Clinical Laboratory Improvement Amendments standards were established by Congress to ensure quality laboratory testing. Facilities that perform testing on human specimens must comply with these standards and obtain a certificate from the Department of Health and Human Services. Among other requirements, the personnel of certified laboratories must meet specific educational qualifications.

Health Careers in Practice

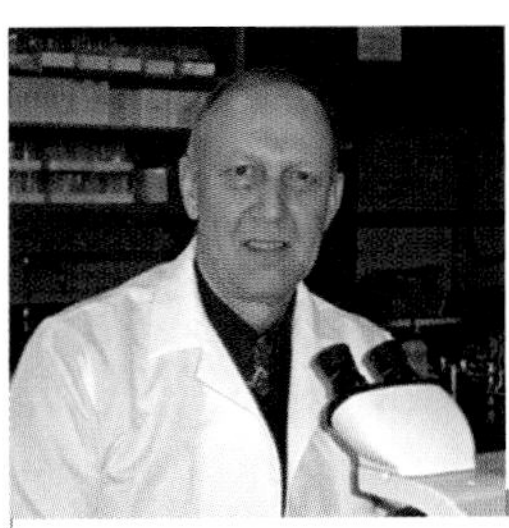

ROB HUBERT

LABORATORY COORDINATOR
DEPARTMENT OF ANIMAL SCIENCE, MICROBIOLOGY PROGRAM
IOWA STATE UNIVERSITY, AMES, IOWA

Educational background: Bachelor of Science in Biology from Iowa State.

A typical day at work/job duties include: During the academic year most of my days are filled with teaching six sections of general microbiology lab and two sections of microbiology lab for life science and health science majors. In addition to teaching, I am also responsible for laboratory preparations, including maintaining and developing the various bacterial cultures. I use the summer months for developing, testing, and refining new laboratory exercises as well as improving the existing laboratory procedures. Occasionally I have the pleasure of supervising a student taking on an independent project for credit in the microbiology program. Throughout the year I also provide laboratory support and hands-on assistance for the undergraduate microbiology club, which conducts special events such as open houses and workshops as part of departmental outreach.

The most gratifying part of my job: Without a doubt the best, most gratifying part of my job is the close interaction with the students. I love seeing them get excited about microbiology, especially those who admit to me after the course that they expected it to be "just another lab class they needed to graduate." After taking the course I have seen a number of students add microbiology as a second major and sometimes change their major to microbiology—it doesn't get much better than that!

The biggest challenge(s) I face in doing my job: The greatest challenge with regard to my teaching role is to change the attitude that the field of microbiology is boring and obscure (i.e., interesting and useful only to "science nerds"). Once my students realize the scope of the field and the way microbes affect virtually every aspect of our lives, their passive attitudes change and real education begins.

What drew me to my career? I simply love biology—every aspect of it.

Something I learned in my early education that I currently use in my career or that caused me to be interested in my career is: I fell in love with biology as a result of my high school biology teacher whose enthusiasm motivated me never to narrow my interest and become a master of only one area of biology but to always keep a wider perspective. I am always fascinated by the fact that all the different fields and areas of biology are interconnected, but at the same time they are diverse and unique.

The pathologist is a medical doctor who examines specimens of body tissue, fluids, and secretions to diagnose disease (Fig. 22-1). Other medical practitioners rely on the pathologist as a consultant who determines the effectiveness of treatments and the cause of death. The pathologist must first complete medical school and then obtain specialized education and training in this area. Hospitals, medical schools, all levels of government, and private industry employ pathologists. In many hospitals the pathologist supervises the laboratory.

The laboratory technologist, also called the *clinical laboratory scientist*, performs clinical laboratory testing and analyzes the results, using independent judgment. For example, the technologist cross-matches blood to be used for transfusion. The technologist calibrates the equipment and assists in determining the accuracy and utility of new tests and procedures under the supervision of the pathologist or laboratory supervisor. Technologists usually complete a bachelor's degree followed by a training program of up to 1 year long (Table 22-2). The Board of Registry for Laboratory

Technologists requires a baccalaureate degree and an examination to become a certified technologist. Licensure of technologists is required in some states.

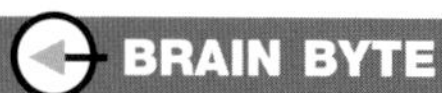

BRAIN BYTE

Employment for clinical laboratory workers is expected to grow by 14% between 2008 and 2018.

Several areas of specialization are possible for the laboratory technologist. The microbiology technologist may collect the specimen directly from the patient or receive materials from an autopsy. The technologist then grows and isolates the **microorganisms** to assist with their identification (Fig. 22-2). Cytotechnologists specialize in the preparation and screening of cells for diagnosis after collection by scraping, brushing, or aspirating body cells from an organ or site (Fig. 22-3). These microscopic cells may be used to diagnose cancer, infectious agents, or inflammation.

TABLE 22-1
Laboratory Career Opportunities

Career	Education Required
Laboratory assistant	1-2 yr hospital training, college, or vocational school
Laboratory technician	Associate degree or specialized training
Clinical laboratory scientist or medical technologist	Bachelor's degree and specialized training
Pathologist	Medical doctor degree and specialized training

Chemistry technologists analyze body fluids and wastes. Other areas of specialization are the study of blood (hematology) and the study of resistance to **pathogens** (immunology).

Medical laboratory technicians (MLTs), also called *clinical laboratory technicians,* perform daily tasks under the supervision of the laboratory technologist or pathologist. The responsibilities include preparation of tissue slides and performance of simple blood tests. The MLT obtains blood samples, prepares tissue slides, analyzes body specimens, and performs cell counts and urinalysis. Technicians complete at least 2 years of training. To qualify for the MLT certification examination through the American Society for Certified Pathologists, an associate degree from an accredited college or university program or 5 years of full-time acceptable clinical laboratory experience is necessary. Some states require certification or licensure for technicians.

BRAIN BYTE

As technology advances, the work of laboratory workers is less hands-on and more analytical.

MLTs may specialize in one area, such as histology. This involves the preparation of tissues for diagnosis, research, and teaching purposes. Histology technicians may work in many different settings, including the hospital, forensics laboratories, immunopathology research, veterinary practice, or marine biology. Histology technicians may be certified and must be licensed in some states. The certified histologic technician must complete an associate degree and 1 year of acceptable experience in histopathology or 3 years of experience under the supervision of a certified pathologist.

TABLE 22-2
Laboratory Career Educational Cost and Earnings

Career	Educational Cost*	Earnings†
Medical laboratory technologist	Bachelor of science in clinical laboratory science, University of Arizona; Tuition (in state) $8237 Room and board $9024 Books and supplies $1000 Travel $1682 Other $2438	Median annual salary: Tucson, Ariz.—$52,670

*(2010-2011) https://financialaid.arizona.edu/money/estimated-cost.aspx.
†http://data.bls.gov:8080/oes/datatype.do.

COLLEGE HOSPITAL
4567 BROAD AVENUE
WOODLAND HILLS, MD 21532

PATHOLOGY REPORT

Date:	June 20, 2008	**Pathology No.:**	430211
Patient:	Molly Ramsdale	**Room No.:**	1308
Physician:	Harold B. Cooper, M.D.		
Specimen Submitted:	Tumor, right axilla		

FINDINGS

GROSS DESCRIPTION: Specimen A consists of an oval mass of yellow fibroadipose tissue measuring 4 x 3 x 2 cm. On cut section, there are some small, soft, pliable areas of gray apparent lymph node alternating with adipose tissue. A frozen section consultation at time of surgery was delivered as NO EVIDENCE OF MALIGNANCY on frozen section, to await permanent section for final diagnosis. Majority of the specimen will be submitted for microscopic examination.

Specimen B consists of an oval mass of yellow soft tissue measuring 2.5 x 2.5 x 1.5 cm. On cut section, there is a thin rim of pink to tan-brown lymphatic tissue and the mid portion appears to be adipose tissue. A pathological consultation at time of surgery was delivered as no suspicious areas noted and to await permanent sections for final diagnosis. The entire specimen will be submitted for microscopic examination.

MICROSCOPIC DESCRIPTION: Specimen A sections show fibroadipose tissue and nine fragments of lymph nodes. The lymph nodes show areas with prominent germinal centers and moderate sinus histiocytosis. There appears to be some increased vascularity and reactive endothelial cells seen. There is no evidence of malignancy.

Specimen B sections show adipose tissue and 5 lymph node fragments. These 5 portions of lymph nodes show reactive changes including sinus histiocytosis. There is no evidence of malignancy.

DIAGNOSIS: A & B: TUMOR, RIGHT AXILLA: SHOWING 14 LYMPH NODE FRAGMENTS WITH REACTIVE CHANGES AND NO EVIDENCE OF MALIGNANCY.

Stanley T. Nason, MD

Stanley T. Nason, MD

FIGURE 22-1 The pathologist examines specimens to diagnose disease. (Modified from Diehl MO, Fordney MT: *Medical transcription: techniques and procedures*, ed 5, Philadelphia, 2003, Saunders. In Bonewit-West K, Hunt S, Applegate E: *Today's medical assistant: clinical & administrative procedures*, St. Louis, 2009, Saunders.)

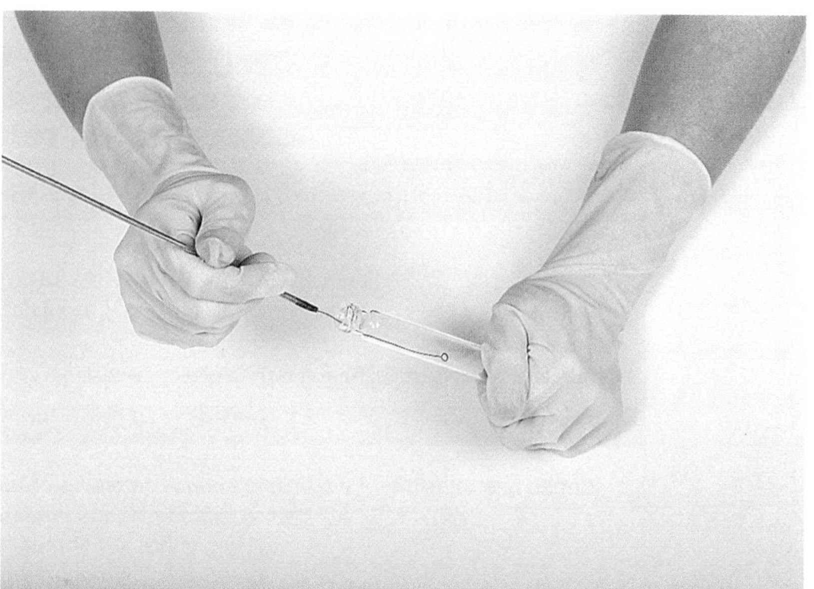

FIGURE 22-2 Care must be taken not to touch the loop to the sides of the test tube during transfer of microorganisms.

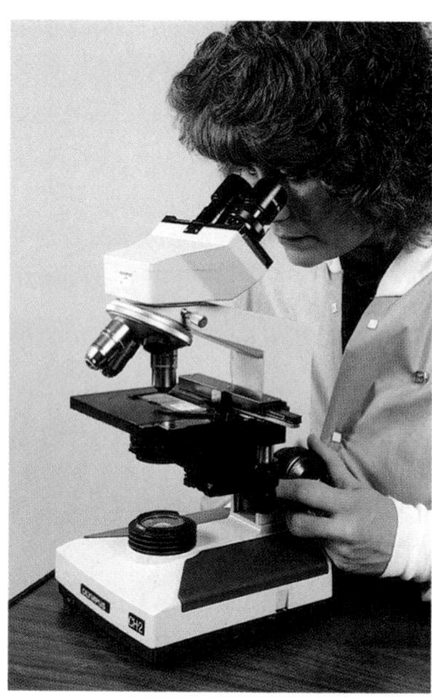

FIGURE 22-3 The microscope allows the health care worker to study many microorganisms. (From Klieger D: *Saunders textbook of medical assisting*, St. Louis, 2005, Elsevier.)

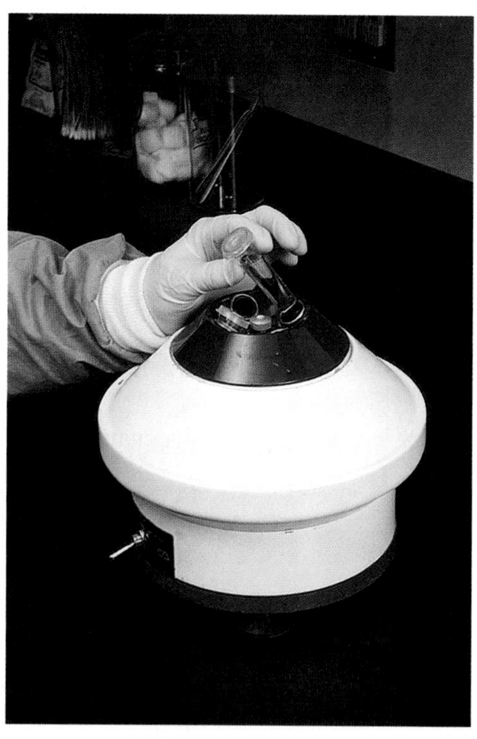

FIGURE 22-4 The phlebotomist uses a centrifuge to process blood. (From Klieger D: *Saunders textbook of medical assisting*, St. Louis, 2005, Elsevier.)

Medical laboratory assistants (MLAs) perform routine tests under the supervision of the technologist or other qualified personnel. Areas of testing that are performed by the assistant may include urinalysis, hematology, serology, and bacteriology. MLAs complete 1 year of training in a hospital or 2 years in college or vocational programs. Certification is possible after successful completion of an accredited program and a registry examination. Phlebotomists obtain and process blood specimens to aid in the diagnosis and treatment of disease (Fig. 22-4). Phlebotomists may be trained on the job or in community college or vocational programs.

Blood Banking

Careers in blood banking include **donor** recruitment, collection, and processing of donor blood, testing and typing of blood, laboratory supervision, and teaching. Specialists in blood bank technology select donors, draw blood, classify (type) blood, and run pretransfusion tests to ensure the safety of the **recipient**. Blood bank specialists act as a resource in solving blood-related problems. Applicants as blood bank specialists must have a baccalaureate degree and certification as a medical technologist. The blood bank specialist program of study is 12 months long. After successful completion of the program and examination, the blood bank specialist may be qualified for certification.

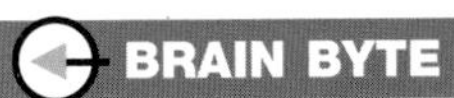

The American Red Cross supplies about 45% of the blood supply in the United States.

CASE STUDY 22-1 You are going to draw some blood for lab tests. You ask your patient whether he has been fasting. He says he has had nothing except coffee with cream and no sugar. What should you say?

Answers to Case Studies are available on the Evolve website: ***http://evolve.elsevier.com/Gerdin***

Life Science

Life scientists are researchers who study living organisms and life processes including growth and reproduction. Many areas of specialization are possible in research and development in the health care industry. The educational requirements for research are a master's degree or doctoral-level preparation. Medical research is conducted in the areas of biology, anatomy, biochemistry, genetics, physics, physiology, and microbiology. Life scientists are responsible for the development of new drugs, plant varieties, methods of treatment, and methods of environmental protection. Biotechnologists or genetic engineers explore the genetic design of plants and animals. Chapter 35 provides more information regarding career opportunities in biotechnology. About one fourth of life scientists work for the federal government, and one third work in private industry. Universities and similar agencies employ others.

Microbiologists study bacteria, algae, viruses, and other microorganisms that cause disease or that may be used to prevent it. Some accomplishments of microbiological research include the development of vaccines for polio and other diseases. Microbiologists also help to determine the method of transmission of diseases. Clinical microbiologists work in a medical, veterinary, or laboratory setting to identify microorganisms in specimens. This may include the development of new drugs. Microbiologists usually work in a laboratory of a hospital or private industry such as pharmaceuticals. Microbiologists may begin work with a 4-year university degree. Higher salary offers are given to employees with a master's or doctoral degree. Most researchers and supervisors in microbiology hold a doctoral degree. Licensure is not required of microbiologists. Specialty areas of microbiology include virology, mycology, and immunology.

Virologists specialize in researching the method by which viruses infect cells and cause disease. More recently, virologists have helped develop viruses that are used to transport and manipulate genetic material. Mycologists study fungal organisms such as molds and yeast.

CASE STUDY 22-2 Your friend tells you that she had laboratory work done a week ago, but no one has called, so she assumes everything is fine. What should you say?

Answers to Case Studies are available on the Evolve website: ***http://evolve.elsevier.com/Gerdin***

Immunologists use the body's defense mechanisms (antibodies) to fight disease. Biotechnology techniques used by the immunologist include cell typing and tissue culturing to produce transplant skin or tumor grafts. Recombined or genetically manipulated cells can be implanted directly into the body in a process called *cell fusion*. Commercially produced tissue cultures can be used for grafts. Cell cultures that are being developed include liver, connective tissue, bone marrow, and blood vessels. An artificial pancreas tissue has been developed and is currently being tested.

Biochemists study the chemical nature of living things. In cells the work involves the methods of reproduction, growth, and metabolism. Biochemists analyze and research the effect of hormones, enzymes, serums, and foods on the tissues and organs of animals. Some areas of study for biochemists include processes such as aging, tooth decay, and viral infection. Clinical biochemists may work in medical laboratories or private industry such as pharmaceuticals. A master's or doctoral degree is preferred for positions in biochemistry. Licensure for biochemists is not required. Certification may be required for jobs in hospitals.

Biochemistry technologists use specimens such as urine, spinal fluid, blood, and gastric juices to study the hormonal and chemical composition that might cause disease. Technologists work under the supervision of a biochemist. Education and training may include a 2-year associate degree or vocational program. A position as a research or laboratory assistant may be available for individuals with a bachelor's degree.

Content Instruction

Laboratory health care workers provide a picture of the patient's health status at one point in time. This may be done with a variety of laboratory tests. Many of the complex processes of the body are possible because a constant balance is maintained in chemical and electrical components of the cells. When an imbalance occurs, laboratory tests may indicate the cause. Because the normal values of many laboratory tests vary from one person to another, they are given in ranges. The result of a test may be affected by age, gender, pregnancy, medication, diet, exercise, and other differences in lifestyle. Chapter 12 provides more information about the normal values of laboratory tests dealing with blood. Information about urinalysis testing is found in Chapter 17.

Microbiology

Microbiology is the study of life forms that can be seen only with powerful magnification. Microorganisms (microbes) are present in the air and on the surfaces of all objects. Many microorganisms live on the surface of or inside the body without causing harm (**nonpathogenic**). When an animal harbors or hosts a microorganism without self-injury, it is called a *carrier*.

Microorganisms that usually live in a certain location of the body are considered normal flora (Table 22-3). Microorganisms may be nonpathogenic in

TABLE 22-3
Microorganisms Normally Found in the Body*

Location	Microorganism	Action
Skin	*Corynebacterium* spp. *Propionibacterium* spp. *Staphylococcus epidermis* *Streptococcus aureus*	Underarm odor
Mouth and throat	*Actinomyces* spp. *Bacillus* spp. *Candida albicans* *Fusobacterium* spp. *Lactobacillus* spp. *Staphylococcus viridans* *Streptococcus* spp.	Tooth decay and plaque formation
Upper respiratory tract	*Corynebacterium* spp. *Hemophilus* spp. *Neisseria* spp. *Staphylococcus* spp. *Streptococcus* spp.	
Intestines	*Bacteroides* spp. *Bifidobacterium* spp. *Clostridium* spp. *Escherichia coli*	
Genital tract	*Corynebacterium* spp. *Lactobacillus* spp. *Staphylococcus* spp. *Streptococcus* spp.	Maintains acidic environment

spp., Multiple species.
*Blood, urine, and the internal body systems are normally sterile, or free from all microorganisms.

certain circumstances but cause disease (pathogenic) in others. For example, *Escherichia coli* (*E. coli*) is normally found in the intestines but is pathogenic if it enters the urinary tract.

Some microorganisms are always present (resident), and some are found temporarily (transient). Microorganisms that damage the host organism on or in which they live are called *parasites*. Microorganisms can be further separated into groups that can live in the presence of oxygen (aerobic) and those that cannot (anaerobic). Most microorganisms survive well in conditions for growth such as warmth, darkness, moisture, and a source of food. The size of microorganisms is an important factor in determining a method of prevention of illness (Table 22-4).

Infection is a state of disease caused by the presence of pathogenic microorganisms in the body. For a microorganism to cause disease, several factors must be present (Fig. 22-5). A portal of entry for the organism must exist, and the microorganism must have a mode of transmission or method of transfer. Infectious microorganisms may be transferred by direct contact or in droplets of water in the air. They may be transferred by other animals, plants (vectors), and fomites. **Fomites** include countertops, eating utensils, linens, and other inanimate objects. There is a period before the infection shows its effects (incubation) and a period during which the microorganism is able to cause an infection in another (communicability).

TABLE 22-4
Relative Size of Organisms and Structures

Organism or Structure	Size in Microns*
Virus	0.01-0.05
Rickettsia	0.2-0.5
Bacteria	0.5-1.5
Red blood cell	5
Lymphocyte	5-8
Human sperm (without tail)	60
Human egg	100
Human hair (width)	100
Paramecium (protozoan)	200

*1 Micron = 1 micrometer = 0.001 mm = 10^{-6} m.

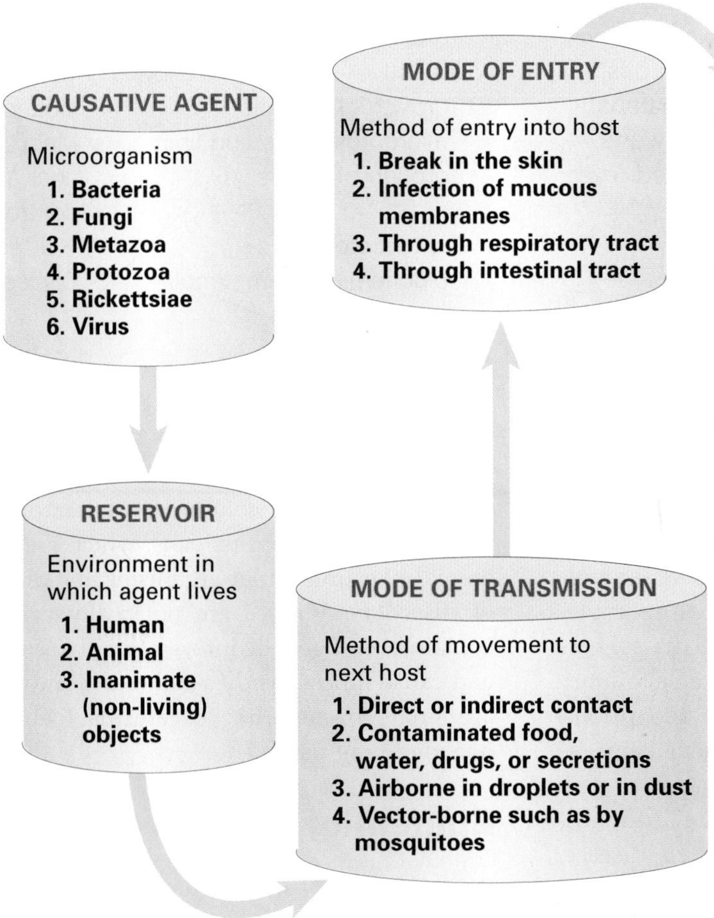

CAUSATIVE AGENT
Microorganism
1. Bacteria
2. Fungi
3. Metazoa
4. Protozoa
5. Rickettsiae
6. Virus

RESERVOIR
Environment in which agent lives
1. Human
2. Animal
3. Inanimate (non-living) objects

MODE OF TRANSMISSION
Method of movement to next host
1. Direct or indirect contact
2. Contaminated food, water, drugs, or secretions
3. Airborne in droplets or in dust
4. Vector-borne such as by mosquitoes

MODE OF ENTRY
Method of entry into host
1. Break in the skin
2. Infection of mucous membranes
3. Through respiratory tract
4. Through intestinal tract

INCUBATION PERIOD
Time for infection to develop once microorganism has entered the host

PERIOD OF COMMUNICABILITY
Time during which the infection may be transferred to another

HOST
Organism that is susceptible to infection

FIGURE 22-5 Infectious process.

TABLE 22-5
Pathogenic Microorganisms and Their Associated Diseases

Type of Microorganism	Examples of Diseases
Bacteria	Anthrax, boils, botulism, bronchitis, carbuncles, cholera, diphtheria, dysentery, gangrene, gonorrhea, leprosy, meningitis, osteomyelitis, pertussis, pink eye, pneumonia, scarlet fever, sinus infection, sore throat, syphilis, tetanus, tonsillitis, trench mouth, tuberculosis, typhoid fever, urinary tract infection
Fungi, mold, yeast	Athlete's foot, histoplasmosis, ringworm, thrush, vaginitis
Protozoans	African sleeping sickness, amebic dysentery, malaria
Metazoans	Hookworm, intestinal diarrhea, pinworm, tapeworm, trichinosis
Viruses	Acquired immunodeficiency syndrome (AIDS), chickenpox, cold sores, genital herpes, hepatitis, measles, mumps, poliomyelitis, rabies, warts
Rickettsiae	Rocky Mountain spotted fever

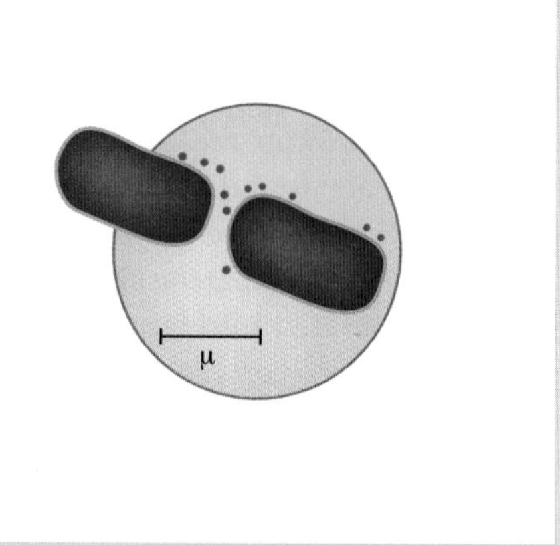

FIGURE 22-6 Bacterium surrounded by viruses.

TABLE 22-6
Types of Media

Purpose	Example
Growth—provides nutrients for microorganism growth	Nutrient agar, blood agar, tryptic soy agar
Differential—change in agar indicates microorganism growth	Triple sugar iron agar, citrate agar, urea agar
Selective—ingredients allow growth of specific microorganisms and limit growth of others	Phenylethyl alcohol agar, MacConkey agar, potato dextrose agar
Test—determines biochemical or metabolic trait of bacteria	PKU test agar, DNase test agar

DNase, deoxyribonuclease; *PKU*, phenylketonuria.

Six major groups of organisms cause disease in humans: bacteria, fungi, protozoans, metazoans, viruses, and rickettsiae (Table 22-5). Bacteria are the most common cause of human disease and infection. Bacteria are single-celled organisms that are neither animals nor plants (Fig. 22-6). Bacteria are placed into smaller groups according to their shape. Bacilli are rod-shaped microorganisms. Cocci are round, and spirilla are spiral shaped. Bacteria may grow as single cells or clump together in colonies. Cultures or samples of bacteria are grown on a variety of media such as nutrient agar or broth (Table 22-6). Clinical laboratory personnel may also identify metazoans and prions. Metazoans are microscopic animals that may be parasites in humans. Prions are misshapen protein molecules that may appear in brain tissue. Prion diseases in humans include Creutzfeld-Jacob disease, Gerstmann-Sträussler-Scheinker syndrome, and fatal familial insomnia.

The fungi group contains yeast and molds. Fungi grow in groups or colonies on other organisms, so they are parasitic. Protozoans, which are protists, are animal-like, unicellular organisms that cause a variety of disorders. Viruses are not really cells, but they contain bits of genetic information that can reproduce and cause illness inside a cell of the body. Rickettsiae are small, bacteria-like organisms that cannot live outside living tissue.

Epidemiology

Epidemiology is the study of diseases occurring in human populations. The field of epidemiology has expanded from this original goal to the study of contagious (communicable) diseases. Epidemiology now includes study of the distribution, causative factors, and prevalence of infectious, chronic, and degenerative diseases. This includes cardiovascular disorders, cancer, arthritis, mental illness, congenital defects, nutritional disorders, and accidents. Some diseases known to result from contaminated environmental resources include cholera, typhoid, malaria, and typhus. With modern advancements in the control of the environment, these diseases are unusual in developed countries such as the United States.

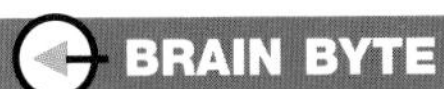

Employment for epidemiologists is expected to grow by 15% between 2008 and 2018.

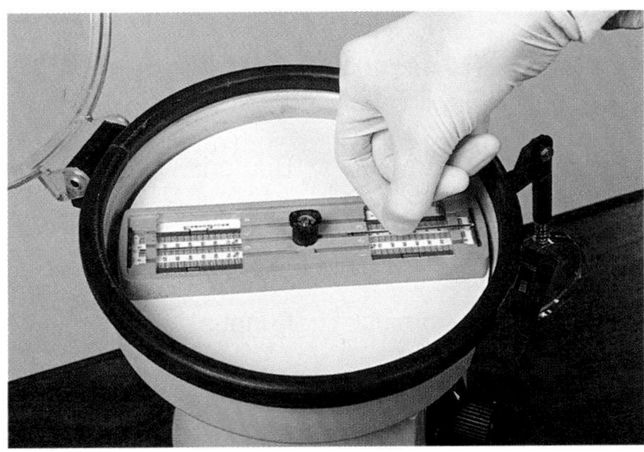

FIGURE 22-7 Blood and other body fluids are separated using a centrifuge. (From Bonewit-West K: *Clinical procedures for medical assistants*, ed 7, St. Louis, 2008, Saunders. In Bonewit-West K, Hunt S, Applegate E: *Today's medical assistant: clinical & administrative procedures*, St. Louis, 2009, Saunders.)

When enough individuals in a community are immunized against a disease, those who are not vaccinated may be protected by herd or community immunity. The size of the reservoir or source for the pathogen is reduced. When a disease reemerges after it has been eliminated, it may be due to an increase in the number of people who are not vaccinated. An example of this occurred in the United States in 1989-1991 when measles increased after a second dose of the vaccine was not given to school-age children. During that time 55,000 people became infected with measles and 123 died.

Epidemiologic studies use demographic data, such as the number of times a condition occurs (prevalence), in relation to the total number of people in the community. Information from epidemiologic studies is provided to health care workers to help control and prevent the spread of disease. The ratio of sick (morbidity) to well individuals and death rate (mortality) are considered. These figures are based on census information gathered by departments of vital statistics. More than 40 diseases must be reported to the CDC so that measures may be taken to control their spread. Methods of control may include sanitation measures to destroy the host or passive carrier of the pathogen (reservoir), immunization, or limiting exposure by quarantine. Immunization against some childhood diseases is a legal requirement for admission to school.

Communicable diseases are those caused by specific organisms that are capable of producing a contagious disease. Infectious disease is the concern of the entire community. An epidemic is an outbreak of disease that affects a large number of people in one area. Infectious diseases can be caught by direct contact with another person, by indirect contact, or through the air. Other infectious diseases are transmitted by vectors, or carriers, such as animals or insects (Table 22-7).

Organisms causing infectious disease adapt and evolve at a rapid rate. New diseases are discovered or rediscovered each year. The emergence of the human immunodeficiency virus identified in 1959 is one example. The Lyme disease disorder was first documented in 1975 and the Hanta virus in 1976. In 1993 the parasite *Cryptosporidium* was found in the water supply in Milwaukee, Wisconsin. About 400,000 people became ill from it. Another 300 people in the Northwest became ill with a strain of *E. coli* in undercooked meat. Two microorganisms that have evolved to form more harmful strains are the tuberculosis and streptococcus bacteria. In 1995 the Ebola virus reappeared in Africa for the first time since 1976. The host and cure for this deadly virus that causes massive hemorrhaging in its victims remain unknown.

Secretions Analysis

One of the most common methods of studying secretions is through separation of the liquid and solid portions of a specimen by using centrifugal force (Fig. 22-7). The specimen is spun at a high speed to cause the formed, or solid, part to settle as sediment on the bottom of the tube. Either portion can then be visualized with a microscope or used for testing to identify cells and microorganisms.

TABLE 22-7
Causes, Reservoirs, and Modes of Transportation of Communicable Diseases

Disease	Causative Agent	Reservoir	Mode of Transmission
Botulism	Bacteria	Soil, water, intestinal tract of animals, fish	Ingestion of contaminated canned foods
Cholera	Bacteria	People	Ingestion of contaminated water, feces, vomitus, food
Coccidioides immitis (valley fever)	Fungus	Soil	Inhalation of spores
Conjunctivitis	Bacteria	People	Contact with discharge from infected area or from airborne droplets (respiration)
Epstein-Barr (mononucleosis)	Virus	People	Person-to-person contact with saliva, nasal secretions
Herpes zoster (chickenpox)	Virus	People	Direct contact, airborne droplets
Malaria	Protozoa	People	Mosquito bite
Rocky Mountain spotted fever	Rickettsia	Ticks	Tick bite
Trichomoniasis	Protozoa	People	Direct contact
Typhus	Rickettsia	People	Body lice

Clinical chemistry deals with the analysis of the serum portion of blood, urine, spinal fluid, and other body fluids. Many tests can be done on these types of specimens, including tests for the presence of drugs, microorganisms, electrolytes, and enzymes.

Hematology is the study of the components of formed, or solid, elements of blood and blood-forming tissues. Whole blood (formed elements) includes the red and white blood cells and platelets. Chapter 12 provides more information regarding the structure and function of blood. Blood can be collected in small amounts by using a finger puncture (Fig. 22-8). Larger specimens are obtained with venipuncture, or **phlebotomy**. Serology is the study of antibody reactions in serum, whole blood, or urine.

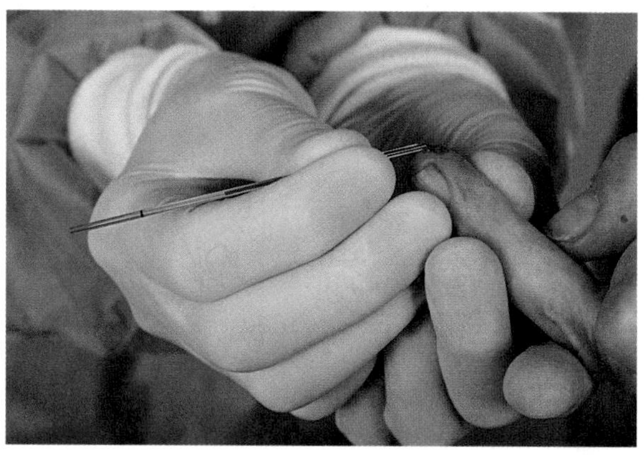

FIGURE 22-8 Small samples of blood are collected using a capillary tube. (From Bonewit-West K: *Clinical procedures for medical assistants*, ed 7, St. Louis, 2008, Saunders. In Bonewit-West K, Hunt S, Applegate E: *Today's medical assistant: clinical & administrative procedures*, St. Louis, 2009, Saunders.)

CASE STUDY 22-3 You are going to draw blood for lab tests. Your patient tells you that she is extremely afraid of needles. What should you do?

Answers to Case Studies are available on the Evolve website: ***http://evolve.elsevier.com/Gerdin***

Immunology is the study of how the blood cells prevent disease caused by microorganisms. The work of the blood bank portion of the laboratory is also known as *immunohematology*. This is a specialized branch of immunology that studies and identifies blood groups. More than 300 blood factors are used to cross-match blood before it is used for transfusion. Blood component therapy separates blood into parts that can be used for specific conditions. For example, plasma, platelets, and the proteins serum albumin and gamma globulin can be separated from red blood cells. New technology includes intrauterine transfusion of blood to unborn infants to treat blood disorders. Stored or refrigerated blood is good for only 35 days, but frozen blood can be kept up to 3 years. Blood

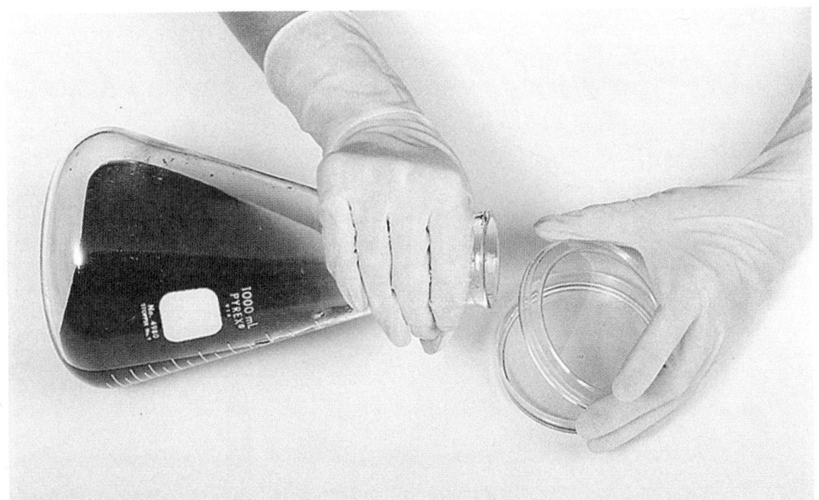

FIGURE 22-9 The agar media may be sterilized separately from the sterile Petri dish if sterile technique is used during transfer.

banks store and provide blood for replacement in surgery or illness. Chapter 12 provides further information regarding tests performed by the blood bank.

Defense Systems of the Body

Humans have several methods of defense against pathogenic microorganisms. The first line of defense is the skin. The skin surface is acidic and dry and acts as a barrier to prevent microorganisms from entering the body. A second defense mechanism is the action of phagocytic cells of the immune system. **Phagocytes** react to a microorganism as a foreign body. They surround and digest it, if possible. The immune system also prevents infection by producing antibodies and antitoxins to combat the action of pathogens that enter the body. **Immunity** is the ability to resist or overcome infection caused by microbes. Immunity can be either inborn or acquired. An individual is born with an innate (inborn) immunity to some organisms. Acquired immunity results when the body produces cells or antibodies to combat a specific organism once exposure occurs. Laboratory tests can determine the type of microorganism causing an infection, whether antibodies have been formed, and the most effective treatment when the body's defenses fail. Immunity to some microorganisms results from administering a vaccine. A vaccine contains a form of the organism that has been treated so that it will increase immunity but not cause the illness.

Performance Instruction

One of the skills used by the laboratory personnel is the preparation of bacterial cultures. This includes using **sterile** technique to prepare growth media and transfer microorganisms. Agar is a growth medium on which bacteria can grow and may be made of nutrients from seaweed, potato, or blood. Agar plates are prepared by using sterile technique to prevent contamination by undesired microorganisms (Fig. 22-9). The microorganism to be cultured or grown may be transferred to the agar plate by using a sterilized loop or culture swab (Fig. 22-10). After the transfer of bacteria or inoculation of the plate is completed, it is labeled with the name of the patient, date, and time of collection and placed in an incubator. After the microorganism has grown on the plate, the colonies may be counted or sampled for identification (Fig. 22-11). (See Skill List 22-1, Transferring Bacteria; Skill List 22-2, Preparing an Agar Plate; and Skill List 22-3, Making a Streak Plate, pp. 362-364)

CASE STUDY 22-4 Your friend tells you she does not donate blood because she does not want to get any infection from the needles. What should you say?

Answers to Case Studies are available on the Evolve website: ***http://evolve.elsevier.com/Gerdin***

Clinical laboratory workers may also use a microscope to identify bacteria. Microscopes are delicate instruments that require special handling and care (Fig. 22-12). Care must be taken to prepare slides so that no air bubbles are formed and they are not contaminated by debris (Fig. 22-13). They also use microscopes to identify urine particles. The specimen is placed in a centrifuge before viewing to separate solid particles from the liquid portion. The laboratory

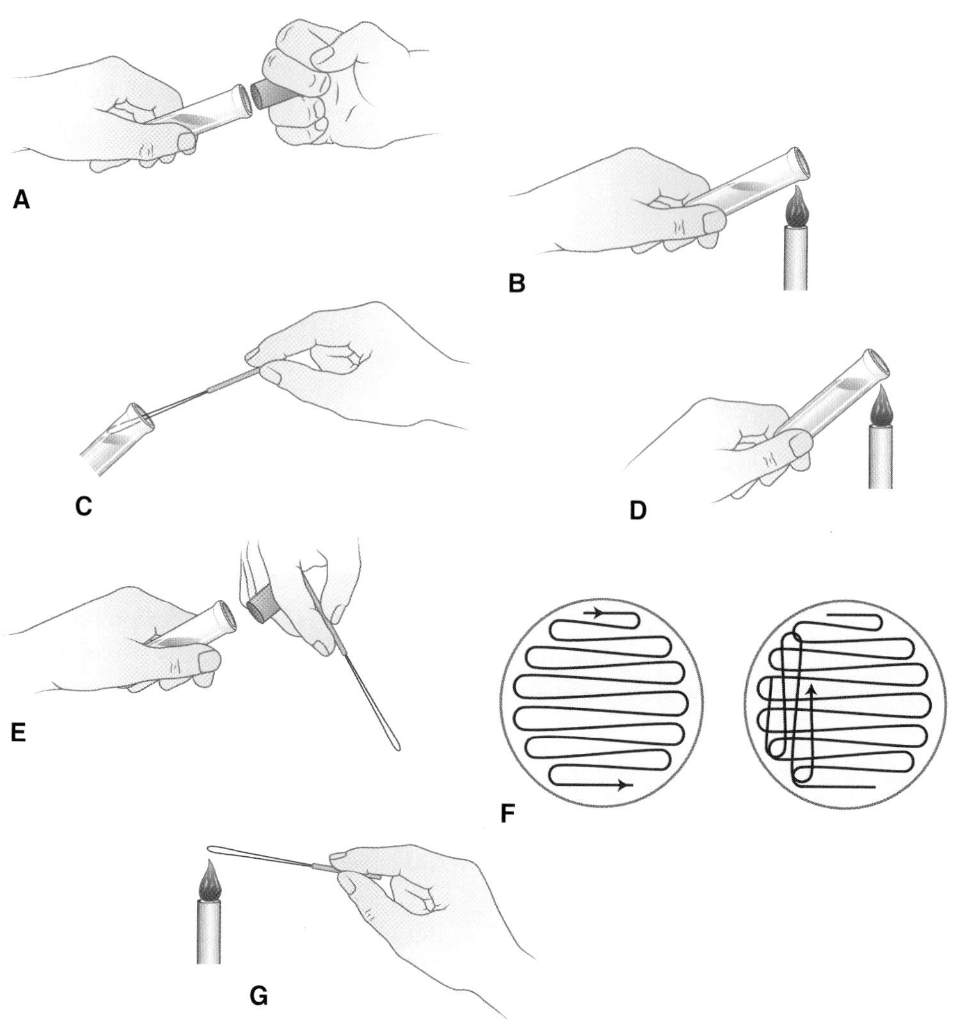

FIGURE 22-10 **A,** The cap is removed so that it can be held during the procedure to prevent contamination from a countertop. **B,** The lip of the test tube is flamed to kill any microorganisms that may be present on the outside of the test tube. **C,** The inoculating loop is inserted into the test tube to remove a specimen. **D,** The lip of the test tube is flamed again to kill any contaminants. **E,** The cap is replaced on the test tube without touching it to any surface. **F,** The plate is streaked in a pattern to promote even growth of the microorganism. **G,** The inoculating loop is flamed to kill all microorganisms before it is touched to any surface.

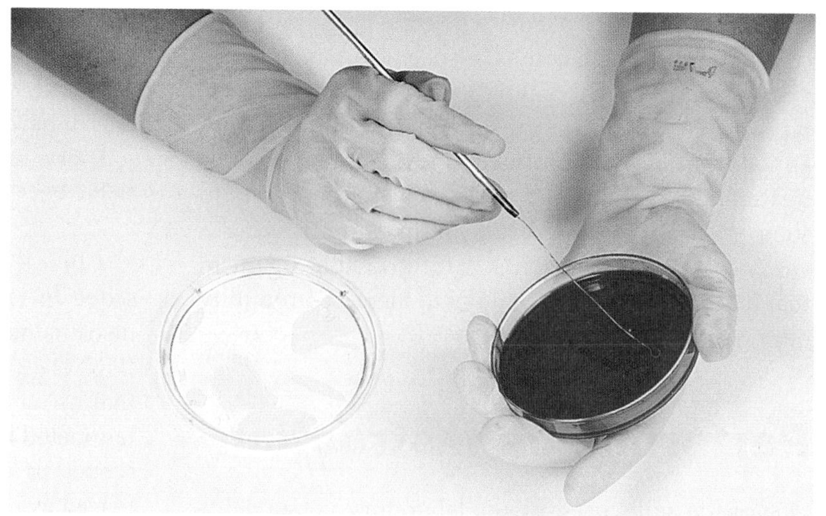

FIGURE 22-11 The microorganism is spread evenly over the surface of the agar without breaking it.

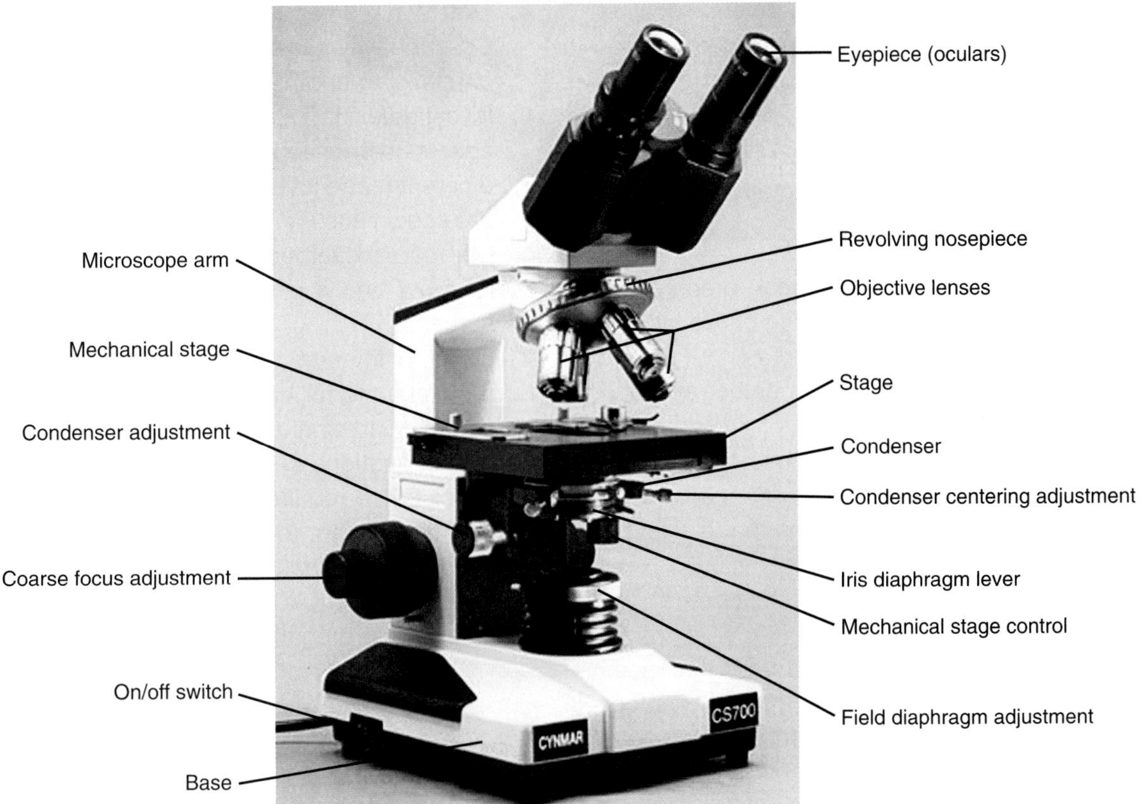

FIGURE 22-12 The microscope is a precise instrument made of several lenses to increase magnification. (From Klieger DM: *Saunders essentials of medical assisting*, ed 2, St. Louis, 2010, Saunders.)

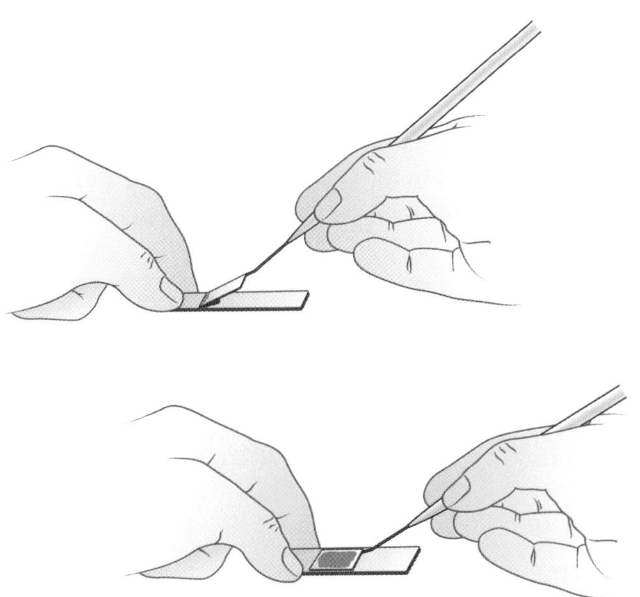

FIGURE 22-13 Air bubbles can be prevented on a wet mount microscope slide by placing the cover slip on it from one side to another.

worker may also be asked to perform venipuncture or draw blood after specialized training. This blood collected may then be used to determine the hematocrit, hemoglobin, erythrocyte sedimentation rate, or complete blood cell count. (See Skill List 22-4, Using a Microscope; and Skill List 22-5, Preparing a Wet Mount Slide, pp. 364-365)

Summary

- The role of the laboratory technologist includes testing and analyzing results, using independent judgment. This might include cross-matching blood for transfusion. Technologists usually complete a bachelor's degree and additional training.
- Pathogenic microorganisms cause disease, whereas nonpathogens do not.
- Six groups of organisms that may be pathogenic to humans are bacteria, fungi, protozoans, metazoans, viruses, and rickettsiae.
- Conditions that promote growth of microorganisms include warmth, darkness, moisture, and a source of food.

- Three ways that skin serves as a defense against infection are acidity, dryness, and barrier protection to prevent microorganisms from entering the body.

Review Questions

1. Describe the duties, educational preparation, lines of authority, and credentialing of five laboratory personnel.
2. Describe the difference between pathogenic and nonpathogenic organisms.
3. List four types of pathogenic microorganisms. Give an example of each.
4. List five environmental conditions that are favorable to the growth of microorganisms.
5. Describe the three methods of defense of the body against infection.
6. Use the following terms in one or more sentences that correctly relate their meaning: immunity, infection, microorganism, pathogen, and phagocyte.

Critical Thinking

1. Choose one career from Box 22-1. Use the Internet to research the cost of education and annual earnings in local institutions.
2. Compare the size of pathogenic organisms with methods used to prevent their spread.
3. Convert the measurements in Table 22-4 to make a model demonstrating the relative size of listed items using a scale of 100 m equals 0.1 mm.
4. Create a career ladder for laboratory careers. Describe why it is or is not possible to move from one level to another in the field.
5. Investigate the types of contrast media and reagents used in laboratory health care. Explain why different reagents are necessary to process different specimens.
6. Compare the temperature at which bacteria prefer to grow and the normal temperature range of humans.
7. Use the Internet to research and describe the requirements for vaccinations required to attend school, participate in the military, or for health care practitioners. Write a paragraph to support or reject the required vaccines.
8. Use the Internet to research and describe five of the diseases that are reportable to the CDC. Explain why it is important for these disease statistics to be gathered by a central agency.

Explore the Web

Career Information

Bureau of Labor Statistics
http://www.bls.gov/

Salary.com
http://salary.com

Professional Association

American Society for Clinical Laboratory Science
http://www.ascls.org/index.asp

SKILL LIST 22-1 Transferring Bacteria

1. Maintain medical asepsis by using the guidelines provided in the Standard and Transmission-Based Precautions, including good handwashing technique and use of gloves as needed.
2. Microorganisms may be nonpathogenic in certain areas of the body but pathogenic in others.
3. Hold the test tube so that the opening is not straight up to prevent dust from entering it while the cap is off.
4. Flame a wire loop by holding the wire in the center of the flame until red hot. Flaming the loop kills any microorganisms that are present.

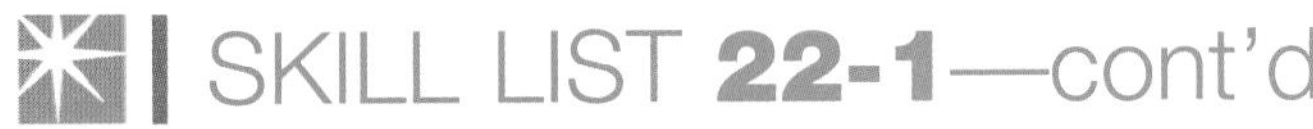

SKILL LIST 22-1—cont'd Transferring Bacteria

5. Remove the cap or lid. Hold the cap so that the inside edges do not touch anything. If the inside surface or edges of the lid touch anything that is not sterile, the specimen is contaminated.
6. Pass the opening of the test tube through the flame. Heat will kill any bacteria that might be present on the edges of the test tube.
7. Insert the wire loop into the test tube or onto the plate without touching any edges. Edges are considered to be contaminated.
8. Run the loop or applicator on the surface of the agar to remove or add bacteria to the surface. Do not break the surface of the agar. If the surface of the agar is broken, the microorganism will grow down and under the media.
9. Reflame and recap the tube or replace the lid on the agar plate. Immediately recapping the tube avoids contamination.
10. Flame the loop to kill all bacteria before putting it on any surface.
11. Label all containers with the date and type of bacteria.
12. Incubate bacterial cultures for growth. The best temperature for most bacteria is 35° to 36° C.

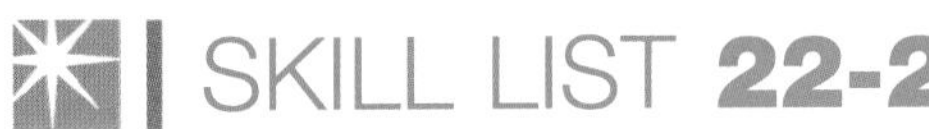

SKILL LIST 22-2 Preparing an Agar Plate

1. Maintain medical asepsis by using the guidelines provided in the Standard and Transmission-Based Precautions, including good handwashing technique and use of gloves as needed.
2. Prepare the agar mixture according to the manufacturer's instructions.
3. Using a funnel, pour warm agar into the clean test tubes or Petri dishes until they are half full. Agar will harden when cooled. If the tube is too full, the tube cannot be slanted and contamination may occur at the edge.
4. Allow the agar to cool and cap the tubes with cotton balls. Tubes may be cooled in a slanted position to provide more surface area for bacterial growth.
5. Sterilize the tubes or agar plates in an autoclave. Tubes and Petri dishes may be sterilized before adding sterile agar if sterile technique is used for the transfer.
6. Refrigerate the sterilized, hardened agar with the container closed until used. Store the Petri dishes in an inverted position to prevent condensation from forming on the inner surface. Once sterilized, the container must remain sealed to ensure sterility.

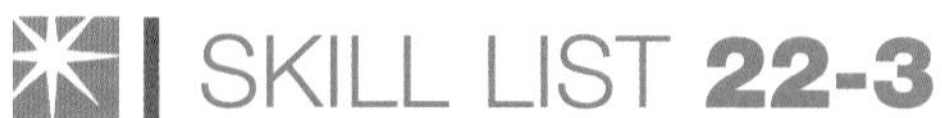

SKILL LIST 22-3 Making a Streak Plate

1. Maintain medical asepsis by using the guidelines provided in the Standard and Transmission-Based Precautions, including good handwashing technique and use of gloves as needed.
2. Follow the procedure given to remove bacteria from an agar plate or slant or to collect a culture swab.
3. Open sterile agar plate slightly. The less the plate is opened, the less chance for contamination by microorganisms carried on air droplets.
4. Touch the loop or swab carrying the inoculate microorganism (inoculum) on one spot of the Petri dish and spread it across the plate. Do not break the surface of the agar. Colonies will grow under the agar if the surface is broken.
5. Reflame the loop and allow it to cool. The swab is not resterilized. The loop must cool before retouching it to the agar because excessive heat may kill the microorganism.
6. Touch the loop to the area that has been streaked, and carry the inoculum across the plate in right angles to the first streak area.
7. Remove the loop and reflame it before placing it on any surface. Discard the swab in the designated location for biological waste. Flaming the loop prevents the undesired contamination of any surface.
8. Cover, label, and incubate the Petri dish. Store in an inverted position. Label the dish on the bottom side. Labeling the dish on the top may prevent viewing of the microorganisms when they grow.
9. Incubate the dish for 2 or 3 days before observing growth.
10. Use aseptic technique to dispose of plate and bacteria.
11. Clean and return equipment to designated location.

SKILL LIST 22-4 Using a Microscope

1. Maintain medical asepsis by using the guidelines provided in the Standard and Transmission-Based Precautions, including good handwashing technique and use of gloves as needed.
2. Place the microscope at least "thumb's length" from the edge of the table. Plug in the cord so that it is coiled away from the edge of the table. Fold and place the dust cover away from the working area. Microscopes are expensive and may be easily damaged if dropped.
3. Turn on the light. Adjust the diaphragm to the desired opening. The diaphragm allows different light intensities to better clarify objects.
4. Revolve or turn the nosepiece until the low or shortest objective is in place.
5. Use the coarse adjustment to move the objective away from the platform.
6. Center the slide on the stage carefully, touching only the edges of the slide and corner label if one is present. Carefully adjust the stage clips to hold the slide in place, and avoid chipping on the slide.
7. While looking at the slide from the side, lower the objective to the stage. The slide is viewed from the side anytime the stage and objective are being moved together to avoid cracking the slide or contaminating the objective by touching them together.
8. Focus the slide by moving the objective away from the stage.
9. While looking at the slide from the side, move the high-power lens into place.
10. Use the fine adjustment only to focus the object. If the microscope is "parfocal," it is designed to

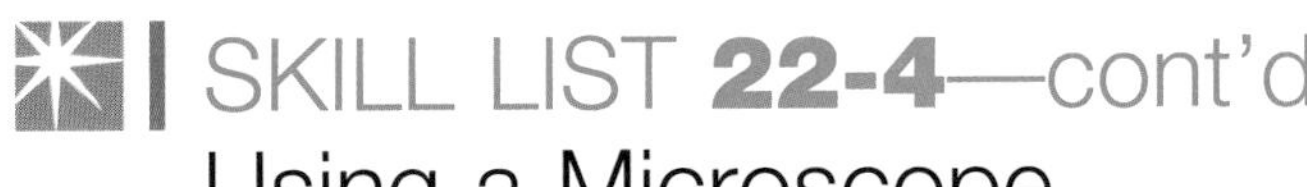

SKILL LIST 22-4—cont'd Using a Microscope

maintain the focus from one objective to the next.

11. Before removing the slide from the stage, move the objective away from it by raising the nosepiece.
12. Turn off the light, coil the cord, and replace the dust cover before returning the microscope to its designated location.
13. Clean and return the slides and materials to their designated location.

SKILL LIST 22-5 Preparing a Wet Mount Slide

1. Maintain medical asepsis by using the guidelines provided in the Standard and Transmission-Based Precautions, including good handwashing technique and use of gloves as needed.
2. Rinse a microscope slide and cover slip with water.
3. Use a soft cloth to dry the slide and cover slip.
4. Use a medicine dropper to place a drop of water on the center of the slide.
5. Place the specimen to be viewed in the drop of water.
6. Lower the cover slip from one side of the drop of water to the other to prevent air bubbles from forming on the slide.
7. Place the wet mount slide on the stage of the microscope, and position it so that the specimen is centered over the light source.
8. Using the coarse adjustment, lower the low-power objective as far as it will go without touching the slide. (Never lower an objective while looking through the eyepiece.)
9. While looking through the eyepiece, move the objective up until the specimen is in focus.
10. Using the fine adjustment knob, complete the focusing of the specimen.
11. Clean and return equipment to designated storage location.

CHAPTER 23

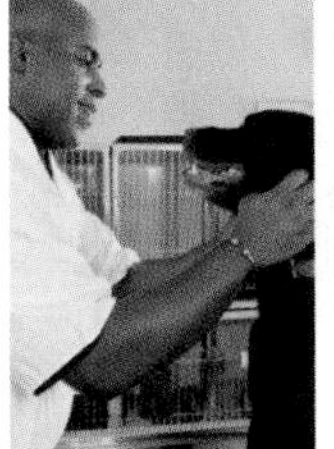
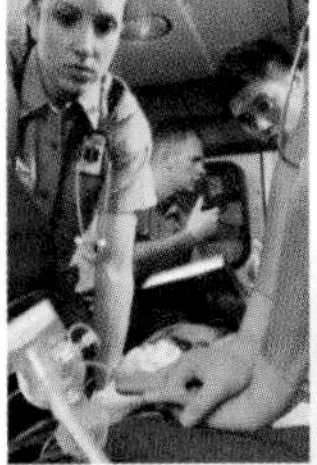
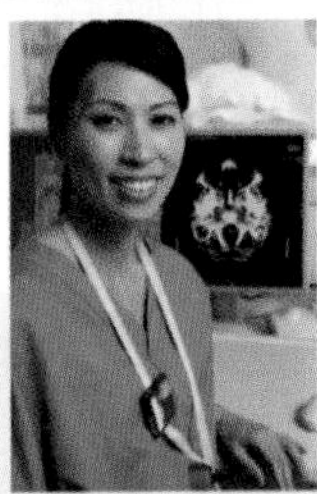

Imaging Careers

LEARNING OBJECTIVES

- Define at least seven terms relating to careers in medical imaging.
- Specify the role of selected diagnostic medical health care workers, including personal characteristics, levels of education, and credentialing requirements.
- Discuss three important developments in the field of diagnostic imaging.
- Identify one imaging technique that does not use radiation.

KEY TERMS

Echocardiography *(ek-o-kar-dee-OG-ruf-ee)* Recording the position and motion of the heart walls or its internal structures using ultrasonic waves

Fluoroscopy *(floor-OS-kuh-pee)* Immediate visualization of part of the body on a screen using radiography

Isotope *(ISE-uh-tope)* One or more forms of an atom with a difference in the number of neutrons

Polarity *(po-LARE-it-ee)* Distinction between positive and negative charges of particles

Radiographic contrast media *(ray-dee-uh-GRAF-ik KON-trast MEE-dee-uh)* A chemical that does not permit passage of roentgen rays (x-rays)

Radiography *(ray-dee-OG-ruf-ee)* Making film records of internal structures by passing radiographs or gamma rays through the body to make images on specially sensitized film; roentgenography

Tomography *(tom-OG-ruf-ee)* Radiograph producing a detailed cross section of tissue at a predetermined depth

Ultrasound *(uhl-truh-sound)* Visualization of deep structures of the body by recording reflections of sound waves directed into the tissues

Imaging Careers Terminology*

Term	Definition	Prefix	Root	Suffix
Angiogram	Record or image of a vessel		angi/o	gram
Echocardiograph	Record or image of the heart using sound	echo	cardi/o	graph
Fluoroscopy	Look with a fluorescent screen		fluor/o	scopy
Hemogram	Record or image of blood		hem/o	gram
Mammography	Making a record or image of a breast		mamm/o	graphy
Myelogram	Record or image of bone marrow		myel/o	gram
Radiologist	One who studies radiation (interprets radiographs)		radi/o	logist
Radiology	Study of radiation		radi/o	logy
Sonogram	Record or image made by using sound waves		son/o	gram
Tomography	Making a record or image of a plane of the body		tom/o	graphy

*A transition syllable or vowel may be added to or deleted from the word parts to make the combining form.

Abbreviations for Imaging Careers

Abbreviation	Meaning
BE	Barium enema
CAT	Computerized axial tomography
CT	Computed tomography
CXR	Chest x-ray
EEG	Electroencephalogram
ECG	Electrocardiogram
IVP	Intravenous pyelogram
MRI	Magnetic resonance imagery
NMT	Nuclear medical technician
PET	Positron emission tomography

BOX 23-1

Imaging Careers

Cardiac monitor technician
Cephalometric analyst
Electrocardiogram technician
Electroencephalogram technologist
Holter scanning technician
Medical dosimetrist
Nuclear medicine technologist
Pulmonary function technician
Radiologic technologist
Radiologist
Ultrasound technologist

Careers

The careers in diagnostic imaging include workers with a broad range of interests, abilities, and training (Box 23-1). The career opportunities in this area include **radiography** and related occupations (Table 23-1). The radiology department of most health care facilities provides additional radiography procedures, such as monitoring of the heart (electrocardiography) and the brain (electroencephalography).

Medical Imaging

Operators of radiographic machinery are called radiographers or radiologic technologists. Radiologic technologists work under the direction of a physician (radiologist) and may specialize in one area of diagnosis or treatment (Fig. 23-1). Responsibilities of the medical radiographer include transferring and positioning the patient and selecting the proper technical factors to ensure the quality of the radiographs. They also use safety equipment and administer opaque media (dye) to make the internal body parts visible. Radiopaque materials may be administered by mouth or rectum or intravenously. Radiographers may take portable films at the bedside or in an emergency department or operating room. The radiographer must use sterile technique, maintain records, and assist with special procedures such as arteriograms. Radiographers must be reliable, have mechanical aptitude, and possess good communication skills. Additionally, moving patients may require some lifting skills and ability.

Job opportunities in radiology are found in hospitals, privately owned facilities, and physician offices that provide radiologic services. The job involves some hazard of radiation exposure. Each worker wears a film badge that records the level of exposure to radiologic materials. The federal government

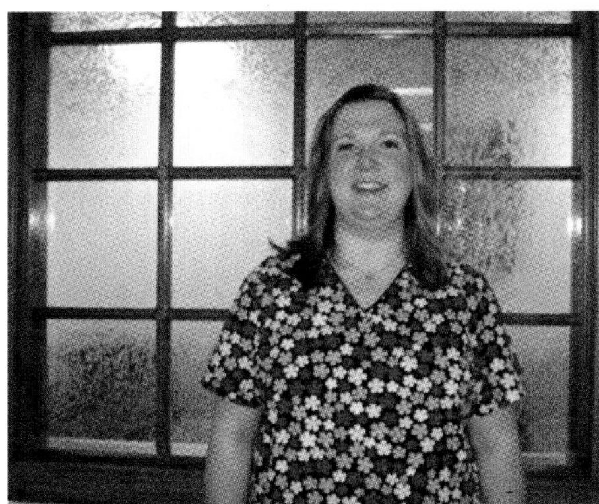

REBECCA VOLKMANN, RT (R)(M)

RADIOLOGIC SPECIALTY TECHNOLOGIST
UNIVERSITY OF MISSOURI, ELLIS FISCHEL CANCER CENTER

Educational background: Associate of applied sciences (2 years); also registered in mammography (required additional training and separate boards examination).

A typical day at work and job duties include:

- Daily and weekly quality control on all machines and equipment
- Checking the schedule and making sure the radiologist knows the schedule for the day
- Hanging outside films and images (hanging up films and images from other hospitals for comparison with images I took)
- Stocking examination rooms
- Seeing patients (performing mammograms and procedures)
- Charging examinations (entering computer codes for billing purposes)
- Checking on the progress of diagnostic exams with the radiologist and checking that reports are going out on time
- End of day duties include shutting down machines, laundry, any remaining paperwork to the radiologist for the next day, and taking down any outside films

The most gratifying part of my job: Knowing that not only have I touched someone's life but also helped save someone's life. Not a week goes by that I do not receive a "thank you" from a patient for delivering good news or a hug from a cancer survivor whose mammogram found her cancer at an early, treatable stage.

The biggest challenge(s) I face in doing my job: Gaining the patient's trust. I only have a few short minutes before I begin the mammogram to gain their trust. If I cannot form that connection, the patient's experience might be uncomfortable, which makes obtaining good images very difficult.

What drew me to my career? I have always loved helping people and always have been fascinated by medical issues, so being in the health care field seemed a good fit.

Something I learned in my early education that I currently use in my career or that caused me to be interested in my career is: When I was 15, I had to have many x-rays and an MRI; I was hooked from there.

Other comments: If you are not a people person, I would not suggest my job. Also, if you are uncomfortable with the naked human body and having to touch other people's bodies, I would definitely not recommend this career.

TABLE 23-1
Imaging Career Educational Cost and Earnings

Career	Educational Cost*	Earnings†
Radiologist assistant	Radiologist assistant; University of Arkansas for medical sciences (UAMS); Tuition (in state) $12,980 Books and supplies $732 Technology fee $176 Student health fee $374 Program fee $150 Graduation fee $58	Median annual salary: Little Rock, Ark.—$47,590

*(2009-2010) http://www.uams.edu/chrp/imaging/.
†http://data.bls.gov:8080/oes/datatype.do.

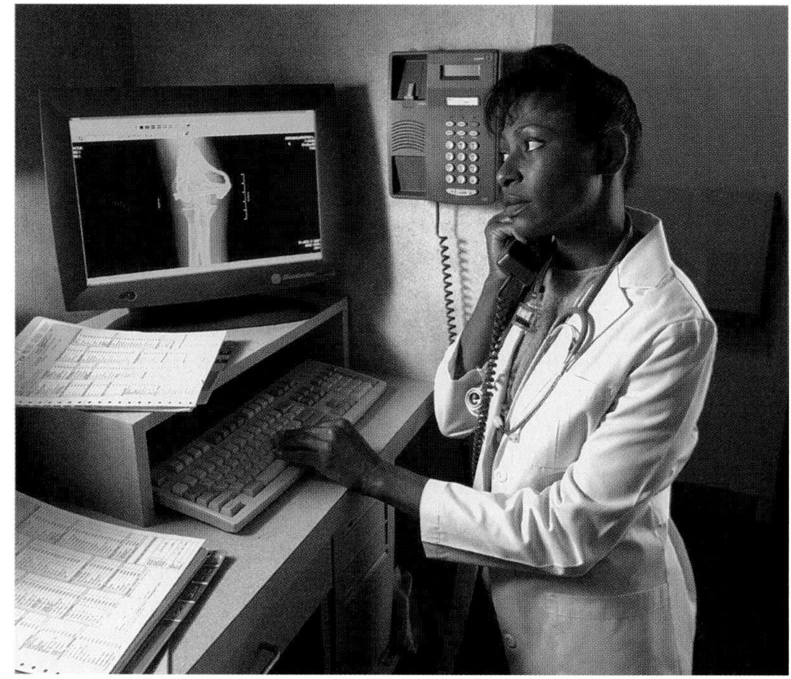

FIGURE 23-1 The radiologist is a physician who specializes in tests and treatments using radiographic materials. (Courtesy Swissray International Inc., Elmsford, N.Y.)

regulates the levels that are considered safe. Programs of study for radiographers range from 1 to 4 years; 2 years is the most common length. Radiographers need a strong background in human anatomy because identification of anatomic landmarks is important to obtain the best possible radiographs. To work as a technologist, a college or university degree may also be required. At least 38 states certify radiographers.

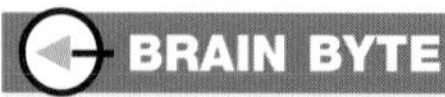

BRAIN BYTE

A plain chest x-ray or dental x-ray exposes a person to the same amount of radiation as the background radiation of daily exposure to the sun over 10 days (depending on the location).

One area of specialty for radiographers uses the properties of radioactive materials to make diagnostic evaluations and provide therapy. Along with other imaging technologists, the nuclear medicine, or radioisotope, technologist provides basic and emergency care, prepares and administers radioactive compounds, and participates in research activities. Radioactive compounds (radiopharmaceuticals) may be injected into the bloodstream, swallowed, or inhaled. The gamma ray emissions are traced through the body, and the length of time they remain in the body provides important diagnostic information. Some of the possible tests using nuclear medicine are blood volume, red blood cell survival, and fat absorption analysis. Brain, thyroid, lung, bone, and heart scans are also part of diagnostic nuclear medicine.

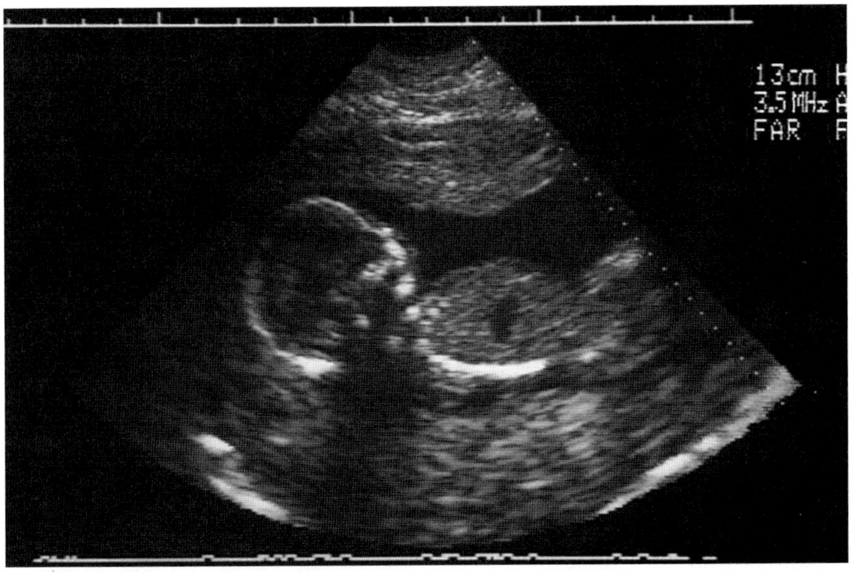

FIGURE 23-2 The sonogram produces a two-dimensional image of internal structures.

The diagnostic medical sonographer, or **ultrasound** technologist, produces two-dimensional images or sonographs of internal organs using sound waves at high frequency (Fig. 23-2). Ultrasonographers may specialize in obstetric and gynecologic, abdominal, or neurosonography. Echocardiography involves taking ultrasounds of the heart and blood vessels. The technologist positions the patient, explains the procedure, and adjusts the equipment to produce the images. The technologist also labels the images for identification. Certification, after completion of a 2-year community college program, is the minimum training requirement for an ultrasound technician.

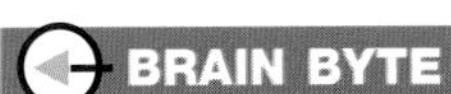

More than 150,000,000 chest x-rays are done yearly in the United States.

Related Imaging Personnel

Radiologic physics is concerned with the application of ionizing radiation to medical diagnosis and therapy. Physicists assist a physician with the care of patients, equipment selection, quality control, teaching, and radiation safety. Physicists may assist with selection of imaging or therapy equipment from technical and financial viewpoints and are responsible for developing and directing quality control programs for equipment and procedures. They may be responsible for establishing and supervising radiation safety programs, including monitoring personnel, handling radioactive materials, and advising radiation safety committees. Physicists may provide required in-service education to staff who are working with radiation. The preparation for becoming a radiologic physicist involves earning a master's degree (MS) or doctorate (PhD) in medical physics or a related discipline. Practical experience in a hospital is also required as part of a 2- to 3-year postgraduate program or clinical medical physics residency program. Physicists must pass a certification examination given by the American Board of Radiology.

Medical dosimetrists work under the supervision of the medical physicist. They calculate and plan radiation doses to treat cancer. Educational backgrounds of the medical dosimetrist vary but include mathematics and physics.

CASE STUDY 23-1 Your friend tells you that he would never work in radiology because he does not want to become sterile from exposure to radiation. What should you say?

Answers to Case Studies are available on the Evolve website: ***http://evolve.elsevier.com/Gerdin***

Electrocardiograph technicians, although not imaging personnel, may work in the radiology department or area. Electrocardiograph technicians attach electrode leads or pads on the patient to monitor or test the action of the heart. The results of the tests are edited and mounted for study by the cardiologist. The electrical impulse of the heart activity is monitored and recorded by the equipment. The patient may be asked to sit, lie down, or walk during the test.

Technicians may learn on the job or in community college or vocational programs. Specialized training qualifies the electrocardiograph technician to work in the areas of cardiac catheterization, echocardiography, continuous monitoring, and blood flow studies. Certification and registration are possible for the cardiology technologist with additional training. More information regarding electrocardiography is found in Chapter 25.

Electroencephalographic (EEG) technologists measure the electrical activity of the brain to aid in diagnosis of disorders. Although not using radiographic materials, they may be included in the radiology department of the health care facility. The responsibilities of the EEG technologist include placing the electrode instrument on the patient, adjusting the machine, and monitoring the patient during testing. The EEG technologist training may range from 1 to 2 years. EEG technologists may seek registration after completion of an accredited program.

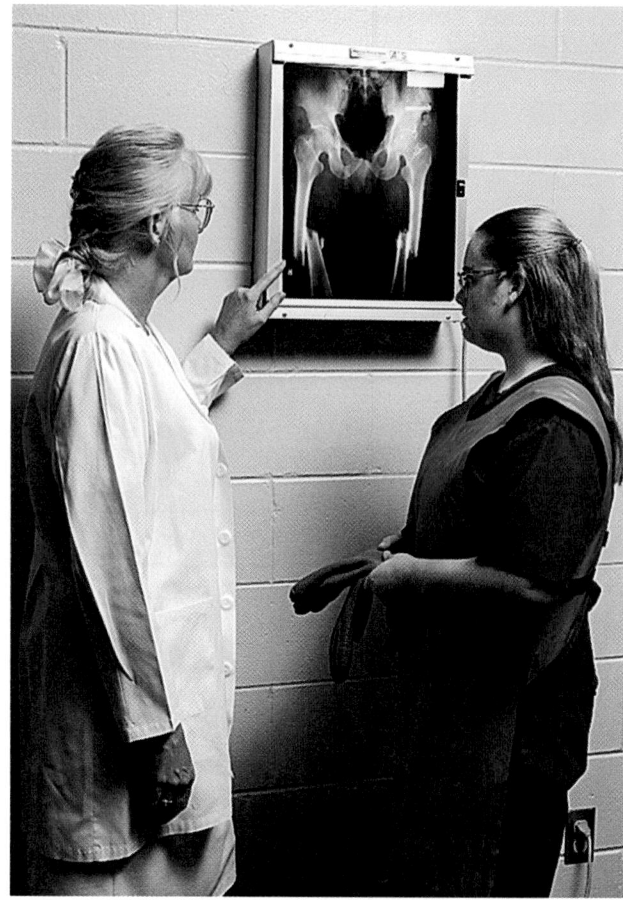

FIGURE 23-3 Radiographs are viewed using a light box to illuminate the film.

Content Instruction

Medical imaging became a reality when Wilhelm Conrad Roentgen discovered "x-rays" in 1895. He called the electromagnetic energy "X" because it was unknown. Contrast agents were developed by pharmacists to allow better visualization of the inside of the body by using this technique. By the 1950s, several other radioactive isotopes and other energy forms, such as sound waves, were being used for diagnosing disorders.

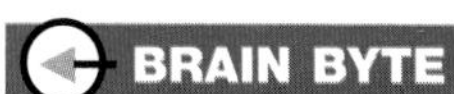

Radiographs are named after the discovery of x-rays by Wilhelm Conrad Röentgen.

CASE STUDY 23-2 Your patient tells you that she is having therapeutic radiation done for treatment of lung cancer. What should you do?

Answers to Case Studies are available on the Evolve website: *http://evolve.elsevier.com/Gerdin*

Most medical imaging of today continues to be diagnostic radiology using conventional radiographs. More than 100 tests use radiographs (Fig. 23-3). They include everything from examination of a simple fracture to angiography to visualize blood vessels. Fluoroscopy is a type of radiography that shows the internal organs in real time. Mammography is the fastest growing diagnostic procedure.

Radiographers may receive advance certification to perform mammography. A mammogram is a radiograph of the breast used to detect breast cancer. A mammogram makes it possible to detect a tumor that cannot be felt. The Mammography Quality Standards Act is a federal law designed to ensure that mammograms are safe and reliable. The U.S. Food and Drug Administration must accredit all mammography facilities in the United States. The radiograph may be taken by a technologist and is read or interpreted by a radiologist. Digital mammography, approved in January 2000, is a technique for recording radiograph images in computer code instead of on radiograph film. Digital technology reduces radiation exposures, allows correction of the image for underexposure or overexposure of the radiograph, and allows examination of all areas of a breast with varying tissue densities.

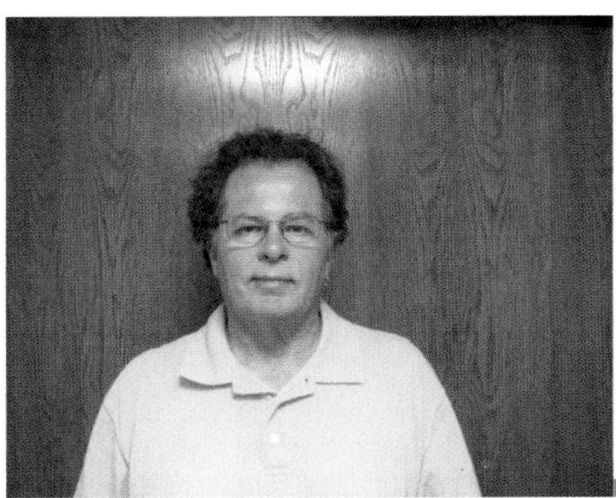

MICHAEL E. RICHARDS, MD

DIRECTOR, BREAST DIAGNOSIS, RADIOLOGY DEPARTMENT
UNIVERSITY OF MISSOURI-COLUMBIA
UNIVERSITY OF MISSOURI-COLUMBIA SCHOOL OF MEDICINE

Health Careers in Practice

Educational background: Undergraduate college degree (4 years), medical school (4 years), radiology residency and mammography fellowship (5 years total for residency and specialty training)

A typical day at work and job duties include:

- Interpreting breast images: ultrasound, mammography, MRI, cancer patient computed tomography (CT) scans
- Performing breast biopsies
- Teaching general radiology as well as how to interpret mammography images

The most gratifying part of my job: Helping patients and teaching.

The biggest challenge(s) I face in doing my job: Dealing with life-threatening situations and people with devastating disease.

What drew me to my career? The challenge and difficulty level as well as an opportunity to help people.

Something I learned in my early education that I currently use in my career or that caused me to be interested in my career is: Attending college.

CASE STUDY 23-3 Your friend tells you she is not going to have mammograms taken because she believes she will get cancer from the x-rays. What should you say?

Answers to Case Studies are available on the Evolve website: ***http://evolve.elsevier.com/Gerdin***

The field of radiography has expanded greatly as modern methods of imaging have combined the use of computers with radiographic procedures. Computed **tomography** (CT) revolutionized the field by linking the use of computers to radiographs. The images produced by "CT scans" provide cross-sectional views of the whole body instead of just one region (Fig. 23-4).

Positron emission tomography scans use computers and radiographic technique to visualize the metabolic activities of the body, as well as its structure. In this procedure, gamma rays are produced in the body when a radioactive biochemical, such as glucose or nitrogen, is inhaled or ingested. A computer produces colored images that are dependent on the amount of gamma rays produced. Because the radioactive materials used have a short period of activity, the patient is not exposed to much radiation. The biochemical activity of the brain in addition to blood flow in the heart and vessels are studied by using this technique. The location of higher brain functions such as speech,

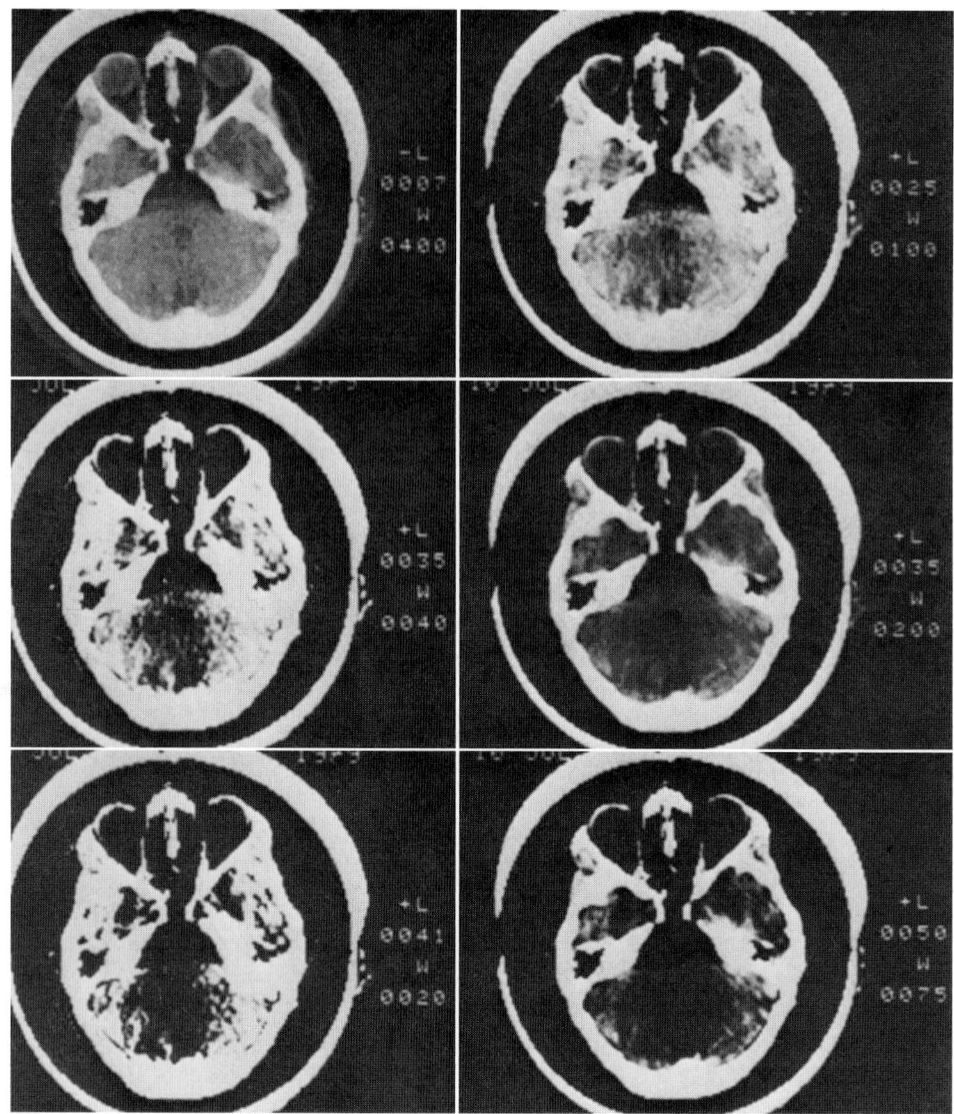

FIGURE 23-4 Computed axial tomography or computed tomography scan of the heart. (From Snopek A: *Fundamentals of special radiographic procedures*, ed 4, Philadelphia, 1999, Saunders. In Bonewit-West K, Hunt S, Applegate E: *Today's medical assistant: clinical & administrative procedures*, St. Louis, 2009, Saunders.)

memory, and emotion have been demonstrated by using this technique.

Magnetic resonance imaging (MRI) is a process that creates detailed image resolution and tissue contrast (Fig. 23-5). The contrast of different soft tissues is much better in an MRI than in a CT scan (Fig. 23-6). MRI is particularly useful in diagnosing problems of the brain and spine. It forms pictures by measuring the magnetic field produced by hydrogen ions in body cells. Radiofrequencies are used to change the electronic pulses of the hydrogen nucleus in cells to one **polarity**. The speed of realignment when the radio frequencies are changed determines the type of image that is produced to represent the tissue. No exposure to radiation occurs. The procedure may be done with a closed or open machine. The open machine has a larger opening and may not be used for all types of scans. As in many innovative health care practices, most technologists in this field began in another area of radiography and were trained for the new technology on the job. MRI may also be referred to as nuclear magnetic resonance imagery even though no radioactive materials are used.

BRAIN BYTE

Two scientists, Dr. Paul Lauterbur and Sir Peter Mansfield, received the Nobel Prize for Physiology or Medicine in 2003 for the discovery of MRI.

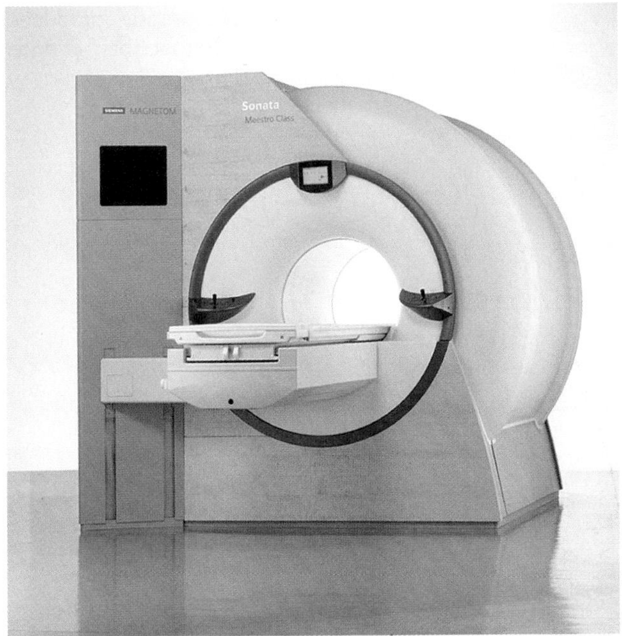

FIGURE 23-5 A magnetic resonance imaging machine. (Courtesy Siemens Medical Systems, Malvern, Pa.)

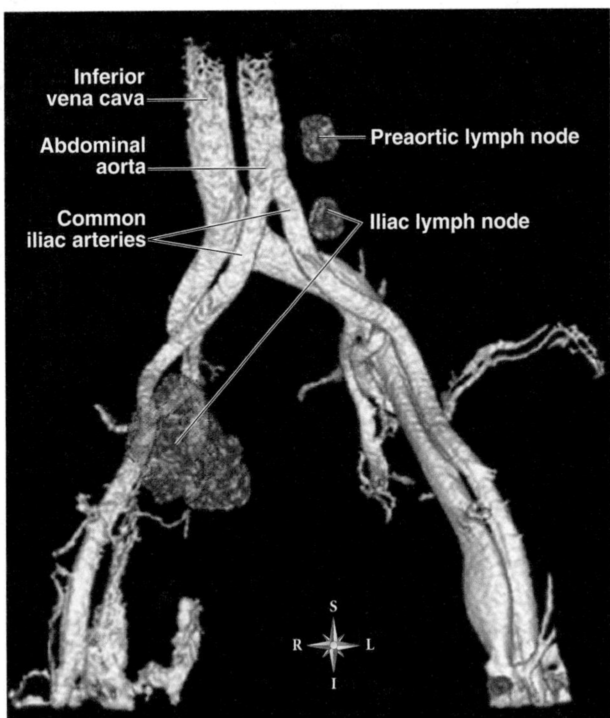

FIGURE 23-6 Three dimensional MRI of the lymph nodes. (From Patton KT, Thibodeau GA: *Anatomy & Physiology*, ed 7, St. Louis, 2010, Mosby.)

CASE STUDY 23-4 Your patient tells you she is scheduled for a bone density scan and wants to know whether she has to do anything special to prepare for it. What should you say?

Answers to Case Studies are available on the Evolve website: ***http://evolve.elsevier.com/Gerdin***

Near infrared spectroscopy is a new technique that allows noninvasive measuring of cerebral functions. Because near-infrared light passes through the human body easily, the light that penetrates the skull and brain can be detected by the spectrograph. In this region, oxyhemoglobin and deoxyhemoglobin have differing spectrums that can be individually measured. Blood flow change in the cerebral cortex and the change in the amount of oxygen saturation that accompany neural activity can be measured.

Digital radiography is an emerging technique that is being used to reduce the time needed for and the expense of processing film (Fig. 23-7). Although the time and expense of this procedure are reduced and the contrast is better than images taken with film, the amount of exposure to radiation is increased with this method.

Bone density scans or bone densitometry is an enhanced radiographic method used to detect bone loss. It is the standard for measuring bone mineral density. It is usually performed on the lower spine and hips and is most often used to diagnose and monitor osteoporosis and the risk of developing fractures.

Interventional radiology is another development in the imaging field. With this technique, small tubes or catheters are inserted into the blood vessels to correct abnormalities. An example of interventional radiology is the balloon angioplasty used to enlarge a vascular constriction by inflating a balloon in a narrowed portion of the vessel. Injecting small amounts of radiographic contrast media into diseased arteries to see vascular structures and narrowing determines the location for placement of the balloon. Interventional techniques have also been used to correct malformations of the brain's blood vessels, although this has been done only rarely.

Performance Instruction

Because imaging involves the use of radiation, exposure is monitored and regulated by the federal government. The entry-level worker does not usually participate directly in procedures that require radiation. However, the radiology assistant may assist with procedures in many ways, such as helping to move

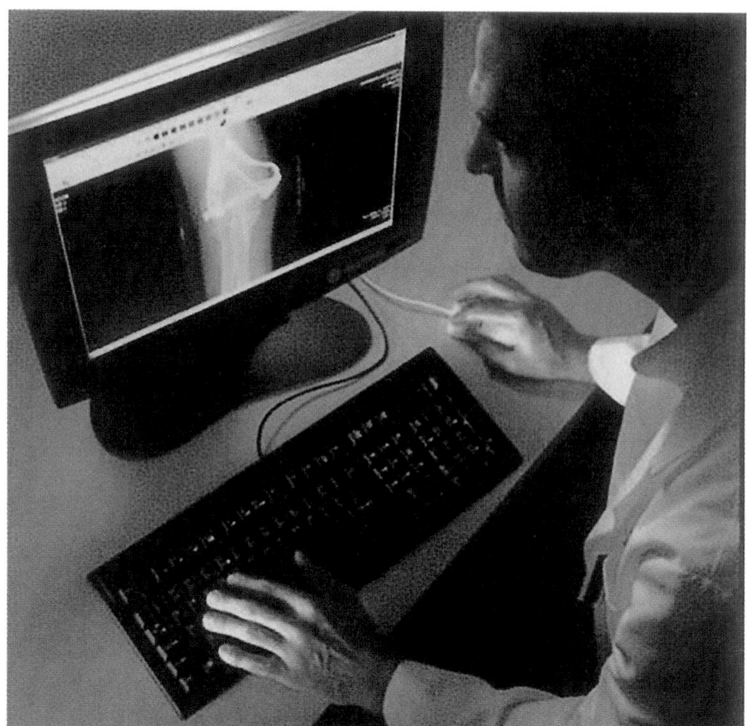

FIGURE 23-7 Digital radiography produces images that show better contrast than images produced by conventional methods. (Courtesy Swissray International Inc., Elmsford, N.Y.)

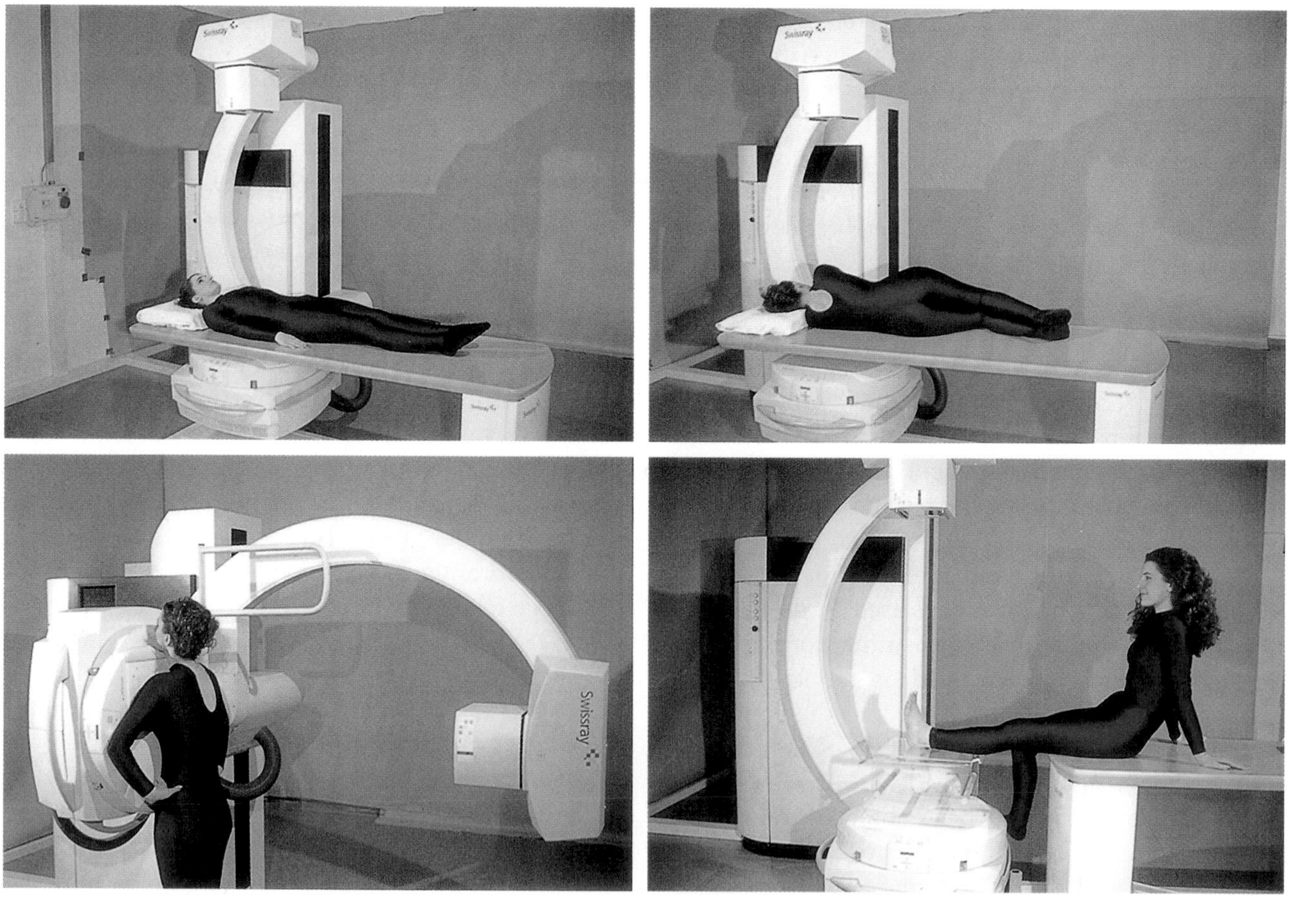

FIGURE 23-8 Correct positioning is important to ensure that radiographs provide the best image possible. **A**, Chest. **B**, Spine. **C**, Chest. **D**, Ankle. (Courtesy Swissray International Inc., Elmsford, N.Y.)

and position patients for examination or treatment (Fig. 23-8). An entry-level worker may also perform loading and processing of films used in radiology. (See Skill List 23-1, Loading and Unloading Film; and Skill List 23-2, Processing Film, p. 378)

Summary

- Medical imaging careers include the radiologist, nuclear medicine technologist, and sonographer. Workers in medical imaging must be reliable, have mechanical aptitude, and possess good communication skills.
- Developments in diagnostic imaging include near infrared spectroscopy, digital radiology, and interventional radiology.
- One imaging technique that does not use radiation is MRI.

Review Questions

1. Describe the duties, educational preparation, and credentialing of five careers in medical imaging.
2. Describe the history of developments in radiography.
3. Compare the uses of conventional radiograph and MRI.
4. Choose one career from Box 23-1. Use the Internet to research the cost of education and annual earnings in local institutions.
5. Use each of the following terms in one or more sentences that correctly relate their meaning: fluoroscopy, radiography, tomography, and ultrasonography.

Critical Thinking

1. Research and compare the cost of various types of imaging tests.
2. Explore and describe three common contrast media used in imaging.
3. Investigate and compare the cost of education and available programs for two health care careers in medical imaging.
4. Create a career ladder for imaging careers. Describe why it is or is not possible to move from one level to another in the field.

Explore the Web

Career Information

Bureau of Labor Statistics
http://www.bls.gov/

Salary.com
http://salary.com

Professional Associations

American Society of Radiologic Technologists
https://www.asrt.org/

American College of Radiology
http://www.acr.org/

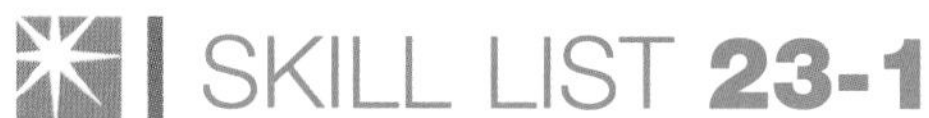

SKILL LIST 23-1 Loading and Unloading Film

1. Maintain medical asepsis by using the guidelines provided in the Standard and Transmission-Based Precautions, including good handwashing technique and use of gloves as needed.
2. Gather all supplies in a darkroom environment. White light will fog unexposed film.
3. Close the darkroom door and turn off the white light. Check for white light leaks.
4. Turn on safe light. Safe light illuminators will not fog unexposed film.
5. Use the fingertips to open the back panel of the film holder with the front side down placed on the work surface.
6. Open the unexposed film storage bin and select a film.
7. Touch the film on the edges with only the fingertips to place the unexposed film into the film holder.
8. Close the film holder. The film holder protects the unexposed film from exposure until it is used.
9. Turn off the safe light. Turn on the white light.
10. Place the film holder in the proper storage area.

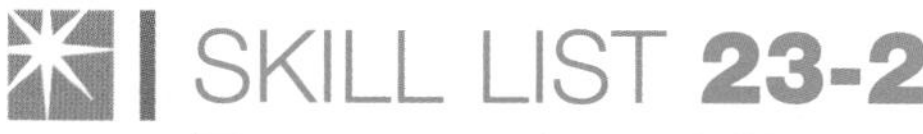

SKILL LIST 23-2 Processing Film

1. Maintain medical asepsis by using the guidelines provided in the Standard and Transmission-Based Precautions, including good handwashing technique and use of gloves as needed.
2. Gather all supplies in a darkroom environment. White light will fog exposed film.
3. Close the darkroom door and turn off the white light. Check for white light leaks.
4. Turn on the safe light. Safe light illuminators will not fog unexposed film.
5. Open the film holder (cassette or magazine).
6. Open the unexposed film storage bin and select film.
7. Touch only the edges to remove processed film. Touching the film will alter the image.
8. Place the film on the feed tray of an automatic processor.
9. Hold the edges of the film firmly and push it forward until caught on rollers. A bell will ring to indicate that the film has entered the processor completely.
10. Place unexposed film into the cassette.
11. Remove processed film when it is released by the processor.
12. Turn off the safe light. Turn on the white light.
13. Place the film in the proper storage area.

CHAPTER 24

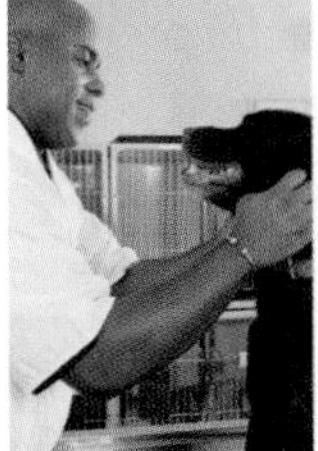

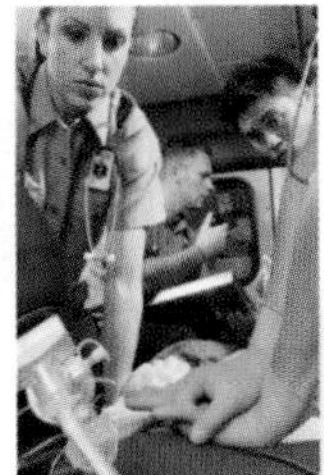

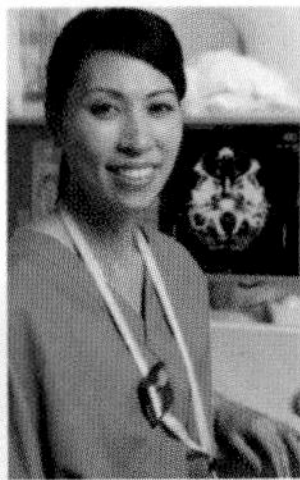

Nursing Careers

LEARNING OBJECTIVES

- Define at least eight terms relating to nursing careers.
- Specify the role of nurses and related providers, including personal qualities, levels of education, and required credentialing.
- Differentiate among the roles of the registered nurse, licensed practical nurse, and nurse assistant.
- Identify three items considered to be intake and three to be output.
- Identify three conditions that indicate the need to measure intake and output.
- Describe methods of maintaining a clean and safe facility or unit.

KEY TERMS

Apical *(AY-pik-ul)* Pertaining to, or located at, the apex of the heart

Asepsis *(ay-SEP-sis)* Process of removing pathogenic microorganisms or protecting against infection by such organisms

Emesis *(EM-e-sis)* Vomit

Intravenous *(in-truh-VENE-us)* Within a vein or veins

Perinatal *(pare-ih-NAY-tul)* Pertaining to the period shortly before and after birth

Pulse *(puls)* Heartbeat that can be felt, or palpated, on surface arteries as the artery walls expand with blood

Unit *(YOO-nit)* Part of a facility, including equipment and supplies organized to provide specific care

Vital *(VIE-tul)* Necessary to life

Nursing Careers Terminology*

Term	Definition	Prefix	Root	Suffix
Abduction	Move away from the center	ab	duction	
Atrophy	Without nutrition (waste away)	a	troph	y
Bradypnea	Slow breathing	brady	pnea	
Cyanoderm	Blue skin	cyan/o	derm	
Dyspnea	Painful breathing	dys	pnea	
Hematemesis	Vomiting blood	hem/at	emesis	
Hemiplegia	Pertaining to being half paralyzed (one side of the body)	hemi	pleg	ia
Insomnia	Pertaining to being without sleep	in	somn	ia
Intravenous	Inside a vein	intra	venous	
Sublingual	Below the tongue	sub	lingual	

*A transition syllable or vowel may be added to or deleted from the word parts make the combining form.

Abbreviations for Nursing Careers

Abbreviation	Meaning
AP	Apical
BSN	Bachelor's of science in nursing
HCA	Home care assistant
I&O	Intake and output
LPN	Licensed practical nurse
NA	Nurse assistant
RN	Registered nurse
PCA	Personal care attendant
PO	By mouth
ROM	Range of motion

BOX 24-1

Nursing Careers

Birth attendant
Child care attendant, school
Community health nurse
Counselor
Geriatric nurse assistant
Licensed practical nurse
Nurse aide
Nurse anesthetist
Nurse midwife
Nurse, office
Nurse practitioner
Nurse, private duty
Nurse, school
Occupational health nurse
Orderly
Practical nurse
Registered nurse

BRAIN BYTE

New England has the highest concentration of nurses relative to its population according to the ANA, with 1107 RNs per 100,000 people.

Careers

With more than two million jobs, nurses make up the largest group of health care workers (Box 24-1). Nursing is also among the 10 occupations projected to have the largest number of new jobs in the future (Table 24-1). In fact, the American Nurses Association (ANA) and Bureau of Labor Statistics project that employment for registered nurses will grow by 22% from 2008 to 2018. Levels of workers classified as the registered nurse (RN), licensed practical nurse (LPN), and nursing assistant (NA) give nursing care. Nurses and related caregivers work with their patients in a close, or primary, relationship. The function of the nurse is to promote optimal health and provide care during illness. The duties of the nurse focus on the patient's physical and mental needs.

Nurses must have the ability to get along with other people and communicate well. They must provide, without prejudice, the best care possible for all patients. Especially during critical moments, the nurse must be self-controlled and efficient and show problem-solving ability. Health care personnel, including student nurses, may be required to undergo a background check to work in a Joint Commission on

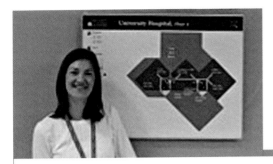

BRIJITH Y. DIAZ, CNA

PATIENT CARE ASSISTANT (PCA)
UNIVERSITY OF VIRGINIA MEDICAL CENTER

Health Careers in Practice

Educational background: High school degree; some college; I hold a CNA (certified nursing assistant) license.

A typical day at work and job duties include:

- Assigned a set of patients to oversee and monitor
- Take vital signs, blood sugars (accu-test), electrocardiograms
- Assist patients with everyday needs such as hygiene, shaving, cleaning, eating, phone calls
- Keep the room safe for patients
- Report to nurse any abnormalities seen in the patients

The most gratifying part of my job: When a patient who has been on the unit waiting for a heart transplant receives it and comes back in the future to tell us that they are living a normal life. Also, when I am able to do "little" things for patients they normally took for granted and then feeling their gratitude for making their day better.

The biggest challenge(s) I face in doing my job: When you do everything you can for a patient and he or she still does not feel better. Also when a patient is stable but dies unexpectedly.

What drew me to my career? I want to eventually become a nurse, and this position is a starting point for that goal. I like taking care of people and am comfortable working with people who are sick. I am a natural caretaker, which fits well with this job.

Something I learned in my early education that I currently use in my career or that caused me to be interested in my career is: I learned I wanted to work directly with people when I did volunteer work at a community center in high school. During high school biology class, I became interested in the how the body works. In the back of my mind, I wanted to be a nurse as long as I can remember.

TABLE 24-1
Nursing Career Educational Cost and Earnings

Career	Educational Cost*	Earnings†
Certified nursing assistant	American Red Cross, 171 hours, $1750 Tuition fee includes: Training books Uniforms and supplies Live scan fingerprinting State examination for certification Hands-on real life experience	Median annual salary: Los Angeles, Calif.—$26,060

*http://redcrossla.org/classes/nurse-assistant-training.
†http://data.bls.gov:8080/oes/datatype.do.

Accreditation of Health Care Organization (JCAHO) hospital or health care facility. Chapter 33 provides more information about background checks.

Registered Nurse

The RN may complete a 2-year community college program, 3-year hospital diploma program, or 4-year college or university program to qualify to take the licensing examination. However, the 3-year programs are being phased out in many locations. Registered nursing is the largest health care occupation, employing more than two million people. RNs may hold a bachelor's, master's, or doctorate degree. RNs supervise the nursing care of patients. Most nurses work under the supervision of a physician in a hospital, a long-term care facility, home health, or other health care agency.

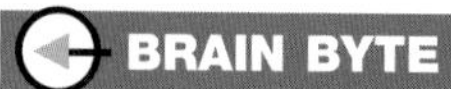

A study by the Health Resources and Services Administration found that 404,163 of the 3.1 million nurses in the United States in 2008 held a master's or doctoral degree.

Community health nursing is concerned with the care of the family and community. The primary focus of community or public health nursing is the prevention of disease and promotion of the highest possible level of health and well-being. The public health nurse identifies needs, determines the plan for care, mobilizes appropriate resources, and evaluates the services given to the patients. Professional public health nursing did not evolve until the twentieth century. Most public health nurses work for government health agencies. They visit people in their homes to provide care and evaluate the environmental conditions that may affect that care. A bachelor's degree in nursing is required for public health nursing.

Advanced preparation by the RN may lead to work as a nurse practitioner, clinical nurse specialist, nurse anesthetist, or nurse midwife. Nurse practitioners perform physical examinations, order and interpret tests, and may recommend or prescribe medication in some states. Nurse practitioners emerged as a profession to meet the needs of rural communities. They function independently from the physician in these settings and assume primary responsibility for care. Nurse practitioners commonly specialize in the areas of adult, pediatric, family, or geriatric practice. Nurse practitioners are certified by the state in which they practice. Nurse midwives provide **perinatal** care and deliver infants under the supervision of an obstetrician. Nurse anesthetists provide anesthesia during obstetric and surgical procedures under the supervision of an anesthesiologist.

Areas of specialization for the RN include **units**, such as the operating room, recovery room (postanesthesia), critical care, and emergency department, as well as practices, such as oncology, cardiovascular, and many others. Nursing opportunities are available all days of the week and all hours of the day.

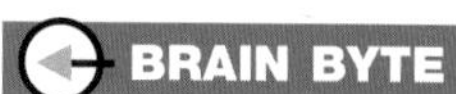

Only three of five RNs work in a hospital.

Licensed Practical Nurse

LPNs, or vocational nurses, complete a 1- to 2-year program and provide personal care under the direction of a physician, dentist, or RN. Many LPNs work in a hospital, making beds (Fig. 24-1), taking

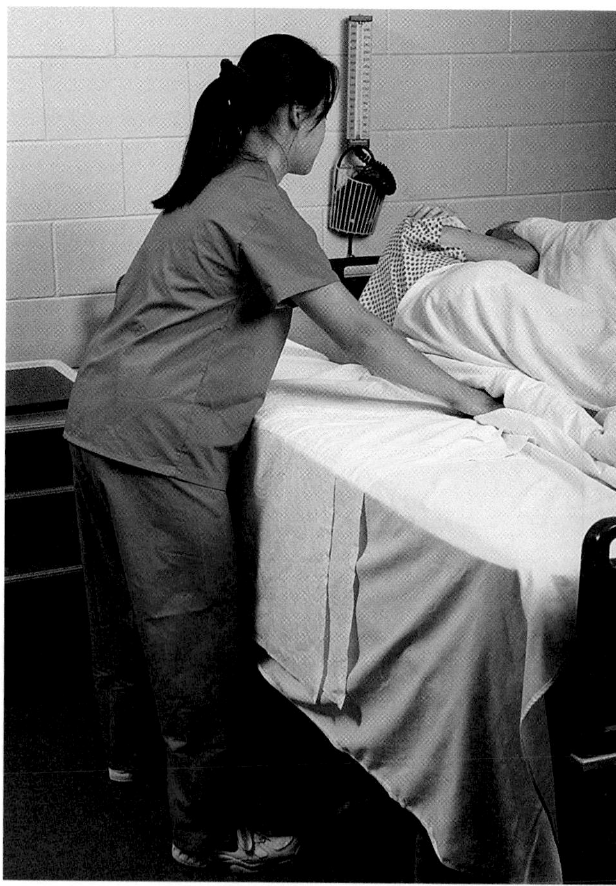

FIGURE 24-1 Making beds is just one way a nurse provides for a patient's comfort.

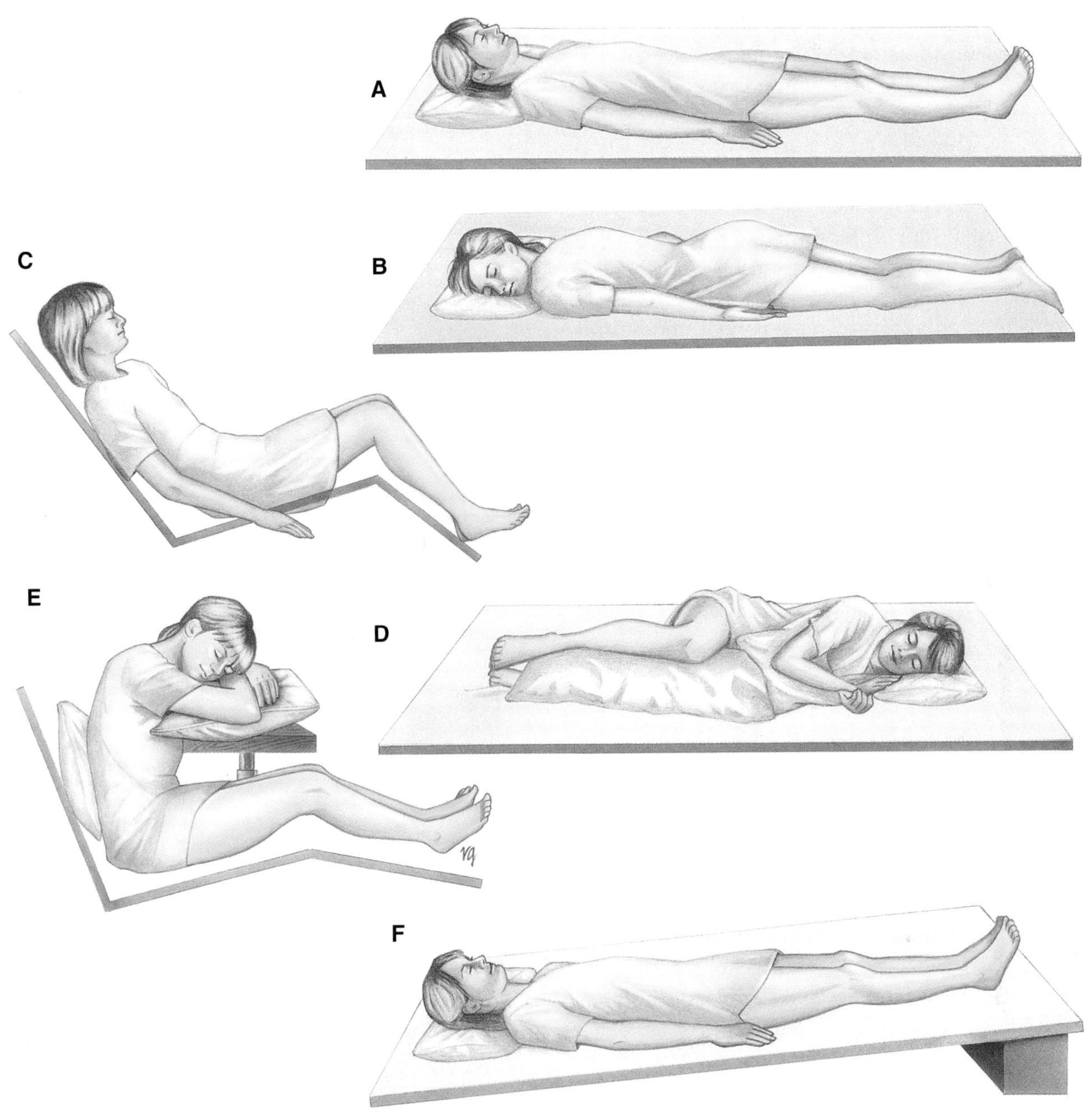

FIGURE 24-2 Body positions. **A,** The horizontal or supine position may be used for comfort or sleep. **B,** The prone position may be used for comfort or treatments to the back. **C,** Semi-Fowler's position may be used for comfort or to decrease pressure on the abdominal organs. **D,** The left Sims' position is used for taking a rectal temperature and for administering enemas. **E,** The orthopneic position may be assumed to ease respiratory distress. **F,** The Trendelenburg position, or a modified version that raises only the legs, may be used to treat conditions of lowered blood pressure such as shock.

vital signs, positioning (Fig. 24-2), and providing personal hygiene for patients. Other LPNs provide care in long-term care facilities. LPNs may legally administer certain medications, insert catheters, and dress wounds. In some states they may also take orders from the physician and input the orders in a computer for implementation. They may also assist physicians with procedures and train students at some levels.

Nurse Assistant

The nurse assistant (NA) works under the direction of the RN or LPN to provide basic care. NAs may be called orderlies, personal care assistants, personal care attendants, or patient care technicians. In most states, NAs must complete a certification program at least 75 hours long and complete a nationally approved written and skill examination.

Certified nursing assistants (CNAs) work under the supervision of a nurse to provide assistance to patients with activities of daily living. They are responsible for basic care such as bathing, grooming, and feeding. They also assist nurses with the use and security of medical equipment and assessment, such as the patient's vital signs. They also provide emotional and social support for the patient. The CNA can follow a career ladder to become an LPN or RN with additional education and training.

CNAs may provide care in the patient's home and are called *home care assistants*. Their role includes assistance with personal care, such as bathing, bed making, and meal preparation, as well as general maintenance of the home. Home care assistants usually work with a patient over an extended period. The home care assistant may be trained to perform all the functions of the NA.

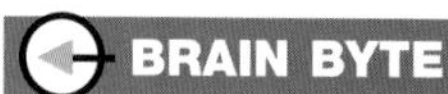

Travelling nurses may work in different facilities locally and internationally.

Content Instruction

Nursing Process

One model for delivery of care that is used by the nursing staff is called the "nursing process" (Box 24-2). It is a goal oriented framework for meeting the patient's needs. The five steps or phases of the nursing process include assessment, nursing diagnosis, planning, implementation or intervention, and evaluation (ADPIE). Data for assessment are gathered by interviewing the patient, physical examination, and observation. The information may be objective (signs) that can be heard, smelt, or felt. It may also be subjective (symptoms) or reported to the nurse by the patient (Fig. 24-3). The nursing process is cyclical (repeating) and ongoing.

BOX 24-2

Nursing Process

- Assessment (collect and analyze subjective and objective data to meet patient needs)
- Diagnosis (make clinical judgment about needs)
- Planning (set short- and long-term goals for patient care)
- Implementation (establish a care plan)
- Evaluation (continual reassessment of the effectiveness of the care plan and patient status)

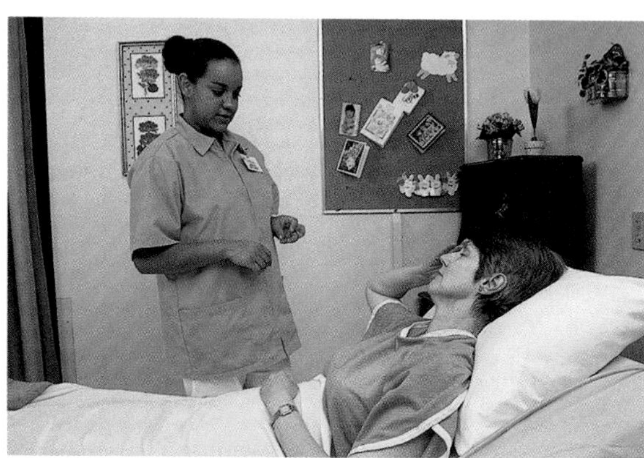

FIGURE 24-3 The patient may be asked to point to an area of pain to clarify subjective observations. (From Sorrentino SA: *Mosby's textbook for nursing assistants*, ed 7, St. Louis, 2008, Mosby.)

Fluid Balance

Within a 24-hour period, the fluid taken into the body and that eliminated from the body should be approximately equal in volume to maintain the balance of the electrolytes and fluid needed to perform body processes. When an individual is unable to eat, has severe diarrhea, or high fever, the output may be greater than intake. In some instances the patient may be unable to ingest adequate liquids because of physical limitations. The order may be given to "force fluids." Forcing fluids means to offer at least 100 mL of liquid each hour.

Oral intake is considered anything that is liquid at room temperature and taken by mouth (Fig. 24-4). This includes foods such as ice cream and Jell-O. The average adult takes in 32 qt (3.3 L) of fluid daily in food and beverages. **Intravenous** fluids and tube feeding are considered intake.

Administration and measurement of intravenous fluids is a function of the RN. All members of the nursing staff observe the site of insertion for any redness, swelling, and complaint of pain that may indicate problems with the treatment. When the fluid is nearly gone, this is reported to the RN or, in some cases, the LPN who changes the fluid.

Output includes urine, vomit (**emesis**), drainage from wounds, and liquid stool. The body also loses fluid that cannot be measured in the form of

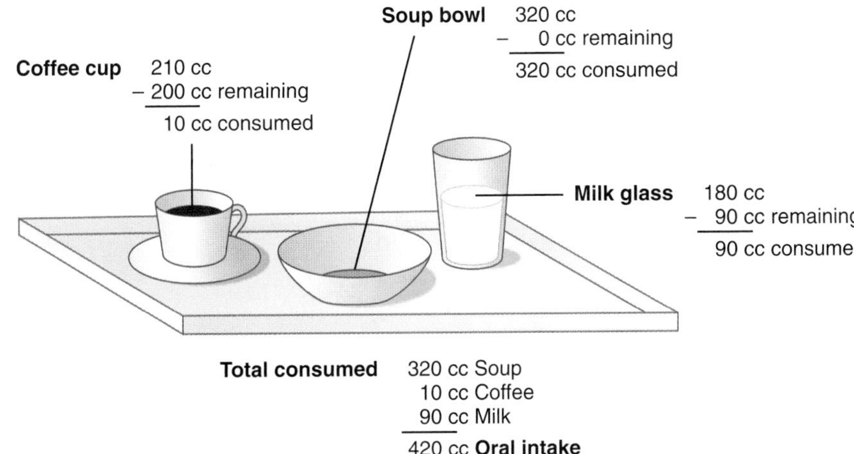

FIGURE 24-4 Oral intake is determined by estimating the amount of liquid that is not consumed when the meal is finished. To estimate the amount consumed, the amount remaining is subtracted from the total amount held by the container.

perspiration on the skin and through lungs during respiration.

Personal Care

Personal or direct care is usually necessary for the hospitalized patient. Assistance with activities of daily living, as well as treatments, may be necessary if the patient is weak or ill (Fig. 24-5). The manner in which the health care worker provides personal care often determines the patient's reaction to having someone assist with these activities or treatments. The health care worker should approach direct contact with the patient in a professional, calm, and caring manner. (See Skill List 24-1, Positioning the Patient, p. 392.)

Personal hygiene on a daily basis includes morning, afternoon, and evening care. Before eating in the morning, the patient is assisted to the bathroom or to use a bedpan or urinal. The patient is assisted to wash the hands and face and to brush the teeth before or after eating breakfast as desired. The bed linens and unit are straightened, and the patient is positioned for comfort in a sitting position when possible. After eating, the patient is assisted to bathe and shave as desired. (See Skill List 24-2, Assisting the Patient to Eat, p. 393.)

The linens and gown are changed. The hair is combed or brushed. A bed bath, backrub, and range-of-motion (ROM) exercises may be provided if the patient has limited movement (Fig. 24-6).

ROM exercises are designed to move the muscles and tendons of the joints for patients who are not able to move independently or have limited abilities. Movement of the joints may prevent contracture or reduction in the amount of movement possible. ROM

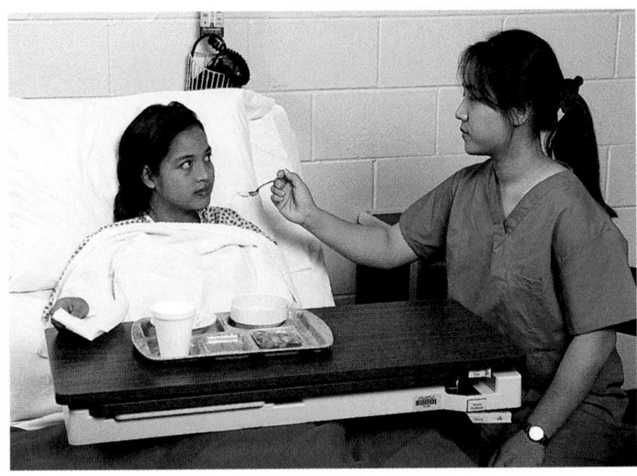

FIGURE 24-5 Creating an atmosphere of being unhurried and interested in assisting with the patient's daily activities is important.

exercises should be performed once every 8 hours when the patient is not mobile. (See Skill List 24-3, Range-of-Motion Exercises, pp. 393-394.)

CASE STUDY 24-1 Your patient's care plan calls for the patient to walk twice a day. When you suggest it is time for the walk, the patient tells you he does not want to do it. What should you say?

Answers to Case Studies are available on the Evolve website: ***http://evolve.elsevier.com/Gerdin***

Throughout the day the patient is assisted with hygiene needs of elimination, such as using the bathroom or bedpan. Also, assistance is given with washing of the hands and face as needed. The unit is straightened, including providing fresh water at the bedside periodically throughout the day. The patient

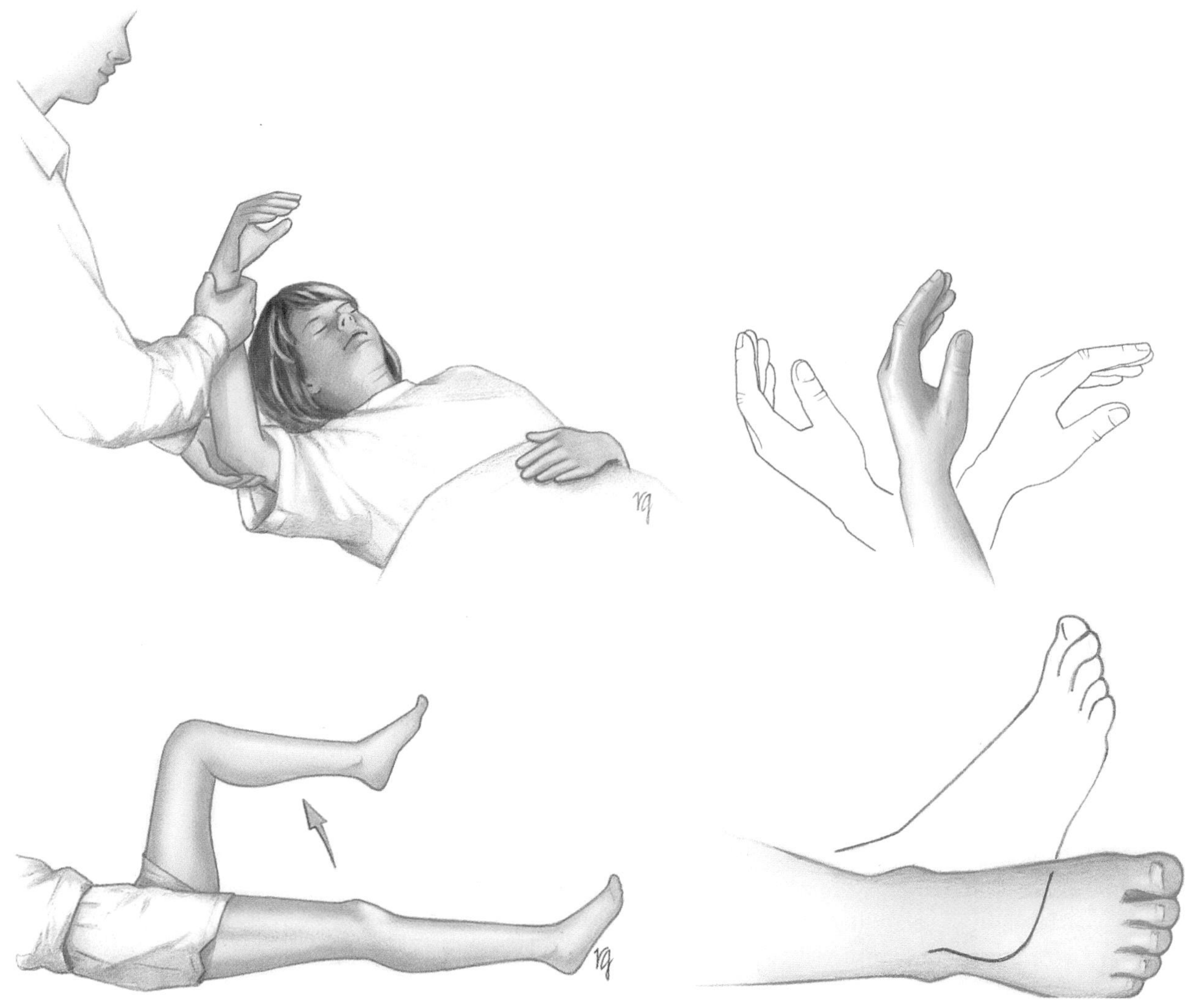

FIGURE 24-6 Range-of-motion exercises may be performed as part of the bed bath.

is also assisted as needed to change positions frequently to prevent the development of a pressure sore (decubitus ulcer). This includes repositioning a patient who is not able to move independently every 2 hours.

CASE STUDY 24-2 You are assigned daily care for a patient. While assisting with the bed bath, you notice the patient has an open wound on his back. What should you do?

Answers to Case Studies are available on the Evolve website: ***http://evolve.elsevier.com/Gerdin***

At bedtime the patient is assisted to use the bathroom, bedpan, or urinal as needed. Oral hygiene is provided, as well as changing damp or soiled linens and gown. The patient is given a backrub to promote sleep.

Postmortem Care

Care of the body after death is called *postmortem care*. Postmortem care is started when the patient is declared dead by a doctor and includes creating a good appearance of the body and gathering belongings for the family. The body is treated respectfully by providing dignity and privacy. Preparation is made for viewing by the family or removal of the body by the funeral services (Box 24-3). After the body is removed, the all linens are removed and the unit is thoroughly cleaned. Funeral rites differ with cultural and religious beliefs (Box 24-4).

Unit Maintenance

Maintaining an orderly and safe environment for care of the patient is the responsibility of all health care practitioners. Clean sheets and a tidy unit benefit

BOX 24-3

Postmortem Procedures*

- Wear gloves during care.
- Arrange the body in a supine position.
- Close the eyes and mouth of the body.
- Insert dentures if present.
- Remove jewelry.
- Remove drainage containers, tubes, and catheters.
- Bathe soiled areas with water.
- Remove soiled linens, and place a bed protector under the buttocks.
- Put clean linens and a gown on the body.
- Brush or comb the hair.
- Cover the body to the shoulders with a clean sheet for family viewing.
- Gather the patient's belongings in a labeled bag.
- Remove supplies, equipment, and soiled linens from room for family viewing.
- Complete and attach identification tags to the body.
- Apply shroud for funeral services pickup after family viewing.
- Provide privacy by pulling the curtain or closing the door.

*Postmortem care procedures may vary according to agency policy and cultural beliefs. Appropriate isolation precautions are used throughout the procedure.

BOX 24-4

Cultural Beliefs and Practices Regarding Death and Funerals*

- Buddhists believe life is an endless cycle and death leads to another state.
- Christians believe in one God and resurrection.
- East Indians usually cremate the body within 24 hours of death.
- Hindus believe in reincarnation.
- Humanists believe there is only one life and accept death as inevitable and natural.
- Jews believe there is only one life and bury the body within 24 hours of death.
- Muslims believe there is only one life and bury the dead before noon with minimum delay after death.
- Native Americans and Alaskan Natives believe death is a journey to another world, and death traditions reflect their reverence for nature.
- Roman Catholics believe in purgatory that is a state of purification before the soul enters heaven.
- Sikhs welcome death as opening a door to God and dress the body in symbols of faith.

*Responses to death and funeral rituals vary greatly within individual cultures and religious groups.

the patient and the health care team. Sheets may be changed with the patient out of the bed (unoccupied) or in the bed (occupied). Special bed-making skills may be necessary in the case of postsurgical patients (Fig. 24-7). Sheets should be changed regularly and when soiled. When changing linens, rules of medical asepsis are followed to keep the environment as clean as possible and prevent the spread of microorganisms. Sheets that are free of wrinkles are more comfortable and help prevent the formation of bedsores (decubitus ulcers), which are caused by pressure. (See Skill List 24-4, Maintaining the Unit, p. 394)

CASE STUDY 24-3 You are assisting the nurse to change a dressing and notice that the new gauze is no longer sterile because it touched the dirty bed linens. What should you do?

Answers to Case Studies are available on the Evolve website: ***http://evolve.elsevier.com/Gerdin***

The nursing team is also responsible for the security procedures for medical supplies and equipment. This includes correct use and care of equipment. It includes maintaining an accurate inventory of supplies. It also includes following ethical and legal guidelines when performing care or administering medications. One of the most basic and important safety practices used by nursing personnel is to check the identification of the patient before administering care (Fig. 24-8). Additionally, the nursing staff must be familiar with the emergency procedures such as "codes" used to signal various threats. For example, the facility may use a color (e.g., code red = fire) or numbers (e.g., code 32 = fire). The nursing staff must recognize the call signals used to indicate a cardiac arrest, fire, bomb threat, intruder (sniper), and other emergencies. The nursing policy and procedure manual is one resource used to guide staff members regarding security practices. Chapter 3 provides more information regarding emergency and disaster procedures.

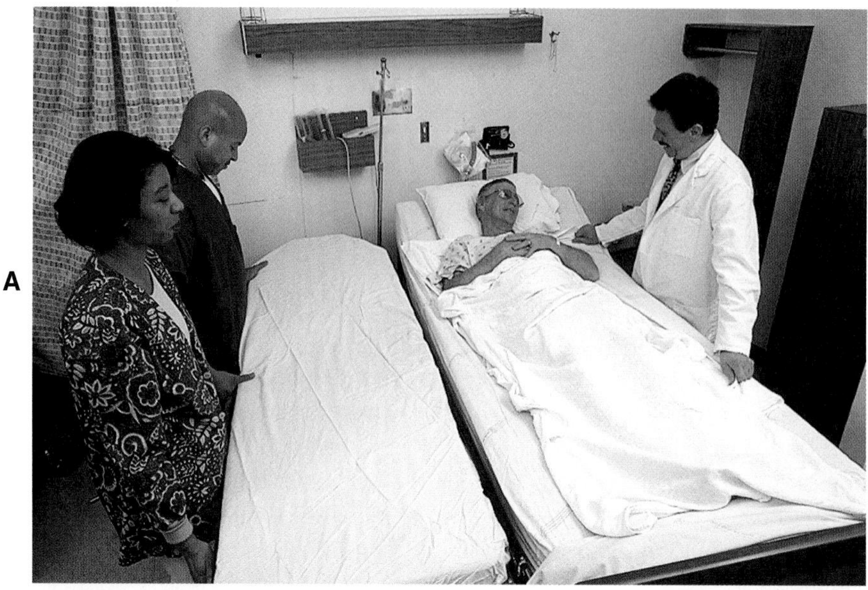

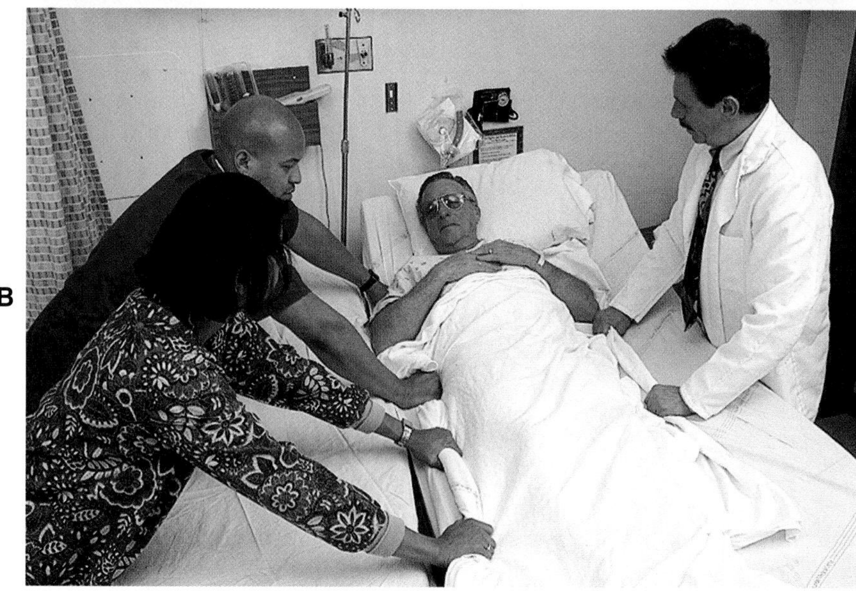

FIGURE 24-7 Transferring the person to a stretcher. **A,** The stretcher is against the bed and is held in place. **B,** A draw sheet is used to transfer the person from the bed to a stretcher.

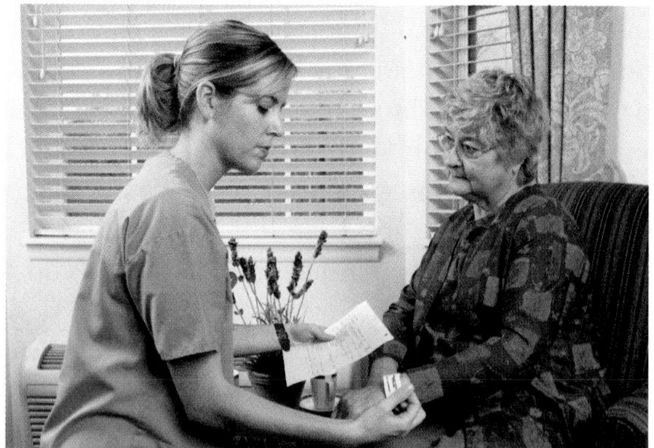

FIGURE 24-8 It is the responsibility of all staff members to check the patient's identification bracelet before giving care. (From Sorrentino SA: *Mosby's textbook for nursing assistants*, ed 7, St. Louis, 2008, Mosby.)

Performance Instruction

One of the duties that may be provided by nurses is the bed bath (Fig. 24-9). Patients who are unable to perform this task alone may need assistance with bathing (Fig. 24-10). The assistant uses standard isolation precautions such as wearing gloves to avoid the spread of microorganisms throughout this procedure. Patients are encouraged to perform as much of the care as possible independently. A routine is established for assisting with the bed bath, moving from the cleanest areas such as the eyes to dirtier areas such as the face, hands, back, and so forth. A backrub may be given at the same time as the bed bath to increase circulation and provide comfort (Fig. 24-11). (See Skill

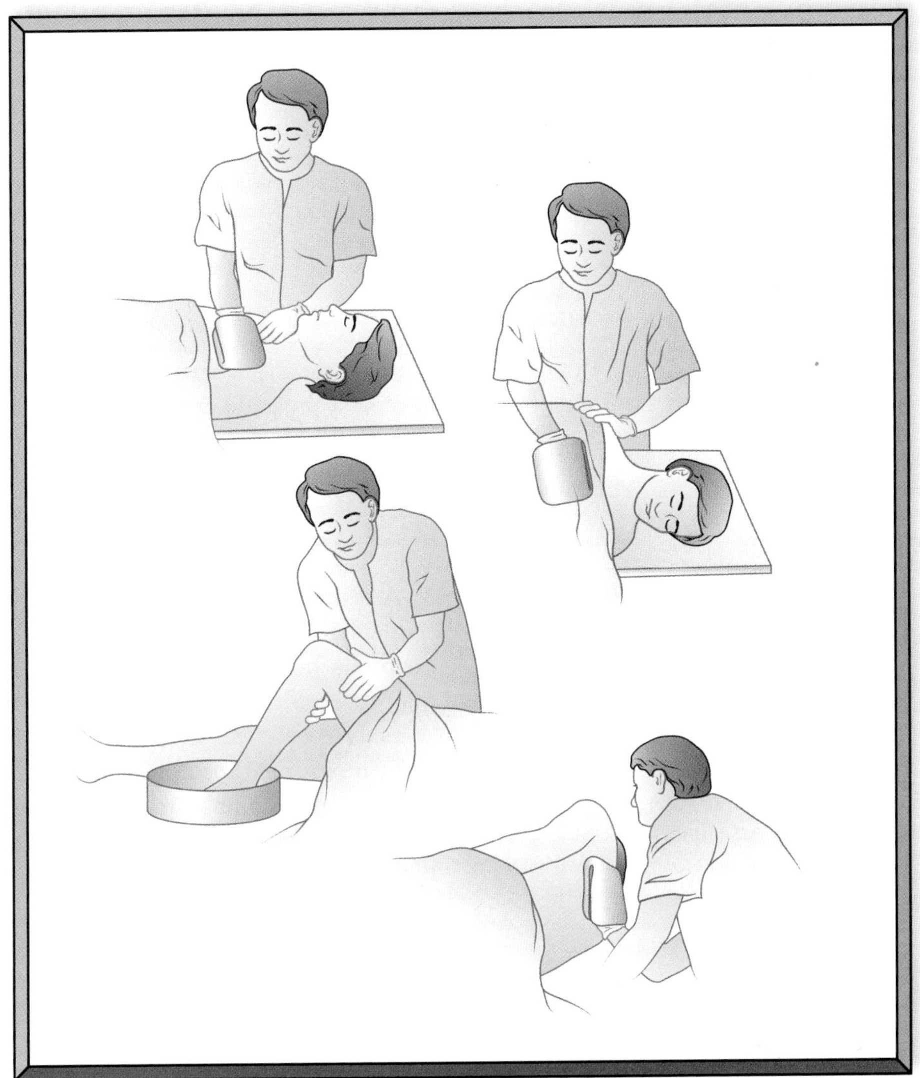

FIGURE 24-9 The bed bath provides comfort and cleanliness for the patient confined to a bed while protecting his or her dignity.

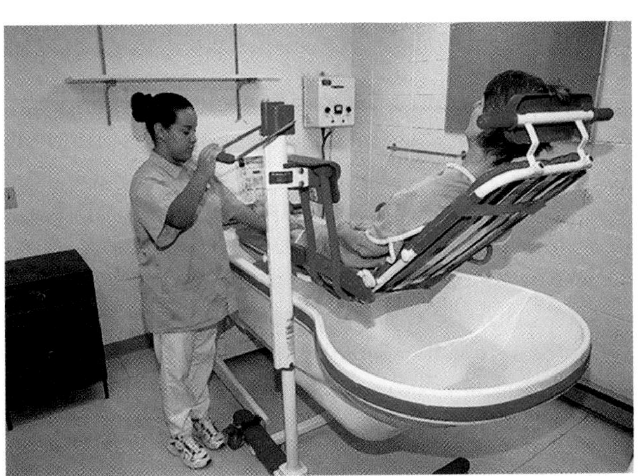

FIGURE 24-10 Patients who are unable to walk can be bathed using a stretcher and tub. (From Sorrentino SA: *Mosby's textbook for nursing assistants*, ed 7, St. Louis, 2008, Mosby.)

List 24-5, Giving a Backrub; and Skill List 24-6, Giving a Bed Bath, pp. 394-396.)

Some conditions of the heart and peripheral arteries may lead to a difference or deficit in the pulse rate at the heart and at the radial artery. In this instance the assistant must use the apical-radial method to assess the pulse. The procedure requires two people. One person counts the pulse rate by using a stethoscope over the heart while at the same time another counts it over the radial artery.

Oral intake may be recorded by estimating the amount of fluids consumed after a meal is finished. Additionally, all the liquid taken at other times of the day is counted. Some patients might not be able to move to the restroom to use the toilet. The patient may then use a urinal, bedpan, or catheter for elimination (Fig. 24-12). Privacy is provided for the patient as the

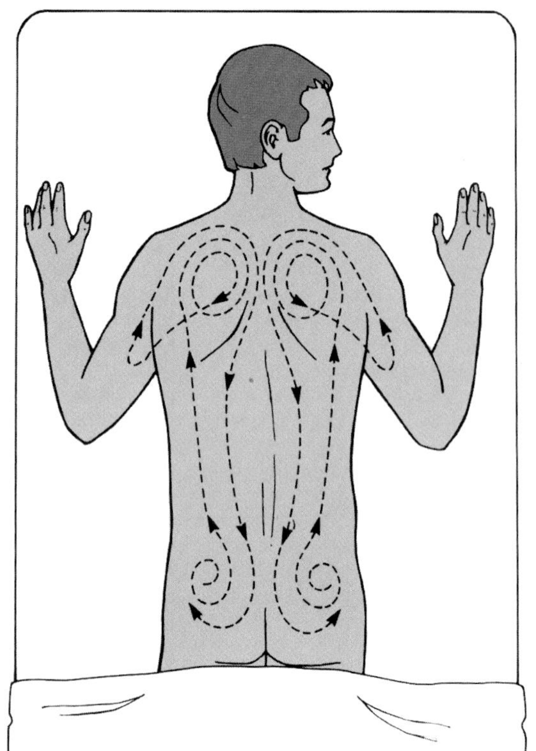

FIGURE 24-11 The backrub stimulates circulation to the tissues of the back and provides comfort. (From Sorrentino SA: *Mosby's textbook for nursing assistants*, ed 7, St. Louis, 2008, Mosby.)

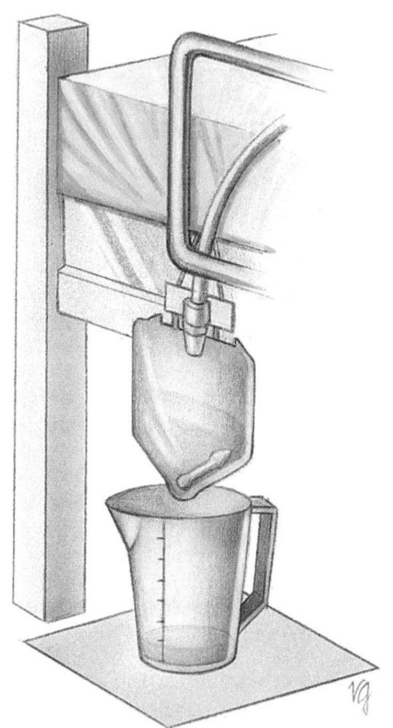

FIGURE 24-12 When a catheter is used, a paper towel is placed under the graduated cylinder to prevent any urine from contaminating the floor during emptying of the catheter bag.

bedpan is placed under the patient in a position that collects the waste material as it is eliminated. Urine output may be collected and measured by using a catheter, bedpan, or urinal. The amount of fluid intake and output should be fairly close over a 24-hour period. (See Skill List 24-7, Measuring Oral Intake; Skill List 24-8, Assisting with the Bedpan; and Skill List 24-9, Measuring Urine Output, pp. 396-397.)

CASE STUDY 24-4 When you start to chart notes for a patient, you notice that someone has already entered notes showing a later time than you gave the care you are charting. What should you do?

Answers to Case Studies are available on the Evolve website: ***http://evolve.elsevier.com/Gerdin***

Assistants also help the patient by making beds (Fig. 24-13). Bed linens are usually changed daily in hospitals but might need to be changed more frequently because of body secretions from a sick person.

Linens may be changed with the patient out of the bed (unoccupied) or in the bed (occupied). The assistant must use good body mechanics and safety guidelines to prevent injury to himself or the patient during the procedure. This includes raising the bed to a comfortable working height to maintain good body mechanics and keeping the bed rails in a raised position if the assistant is not directly at the bedside. The patient is made comfortable, and the bed is lowered to the lowest level when the bed is completed. (See Skill List 24-10, Making an Unoccupied and Surgical Bed; and Skill List 24-11, Making an Occupied Bed, pp. 398-399.)

Summary

- The role of nursing careers includes working with patients directly to provide care and promote health. The personal qualities of providers include the ability to get along with others, communicate well, and be self-controlled under pressure.
- The NA usually works under the supervision of an LPN, RN, or medical doctor. The LPN usually works under the supervision of the RN or medical doctor. The RN may work under the supervision of a medical doctor or independently.
- The items considered to be input include water, Jell-O, and intravenous fluids. Three types of output include urine, vomit, and drainage from wounds.

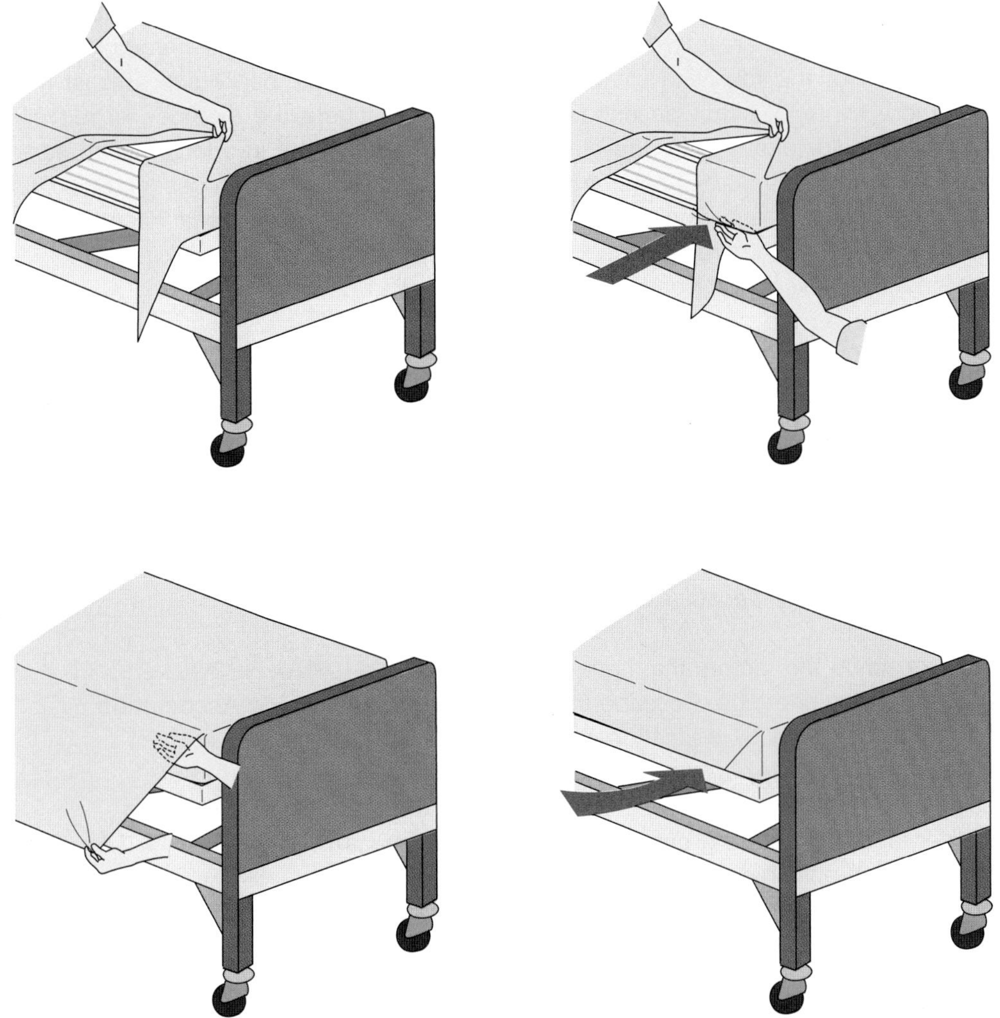

FIGURE 24-13 The unoccupied bed is made with mitered corners. (From Sorrentino SA: *Mosby's textbook for nursing assistants*, ed 7, St. Louis, 2008, Mosby.)

- Three situations that may indicate measurement of intake and output include the inability to eat, diarrhea, and fever.
- Methods of maintaining a clean and safe facility or unit include providing clean sheets, keeping a tidy room, and following procedures to prevent spread of pathogens.

Review Questions

1. Describe four nursing specialties.
2. Describe the education, role, and credentialing of three levels of nursing.
3. Describe the importance of assessing fluid balance in the body.
4. Describe the importance of a clean unit and bed.
5. List three types of intake and output.
6. List five conditions that indicate assessment of intake and output.
7. Describe the process of forcing fluids and indications for its use.
8. Choose one career from Box 24-1. Use the Internet to research the cost of education and annual earnings in local institutions.
9. Use each of the following terms in one or more sentences that correctly relate their meaning: apical, pulse, and vital.

Critical Thinking

1. Investigate the requirements and cost of education programs for three types of nurses.
2. Write a narrative paragraph describing to a patient the procedure for and importance of monitoring intake and output.

3. While nurses give direct care to patients, it is common for the patients to share information with the nurse. For each of the following situations, write one or more sentences that describe the action the nurse should take. Justify the action chosen for each of the situations. (Chapter 4 provides additional information regarding ethical and legal responsibilities of health care workers.)
   a. The nurse notices several old scars that are small and circular on the patient's back and chest while giving a bed bath.
   b. The nurse hears a patient arguing with someone on the phone indicating that no one is coming to give the patient a ride on discharge from the facility.
   c. The patient tells the nurse that he or she will never follow the physician's orders once discharged from the facility because the orders are too impractical.
4. Research and describe the factors that have led to the projected nursing shortage. Describe three actions that might be taken by educational and health facilities to recruit and keep more nurses in the profession.
5. Create a career ladder for nursing careers. Describe why it is or is not possible to move from one level to another in the field.
6. Use the Internet to investigate and summarize the funeral rites of two cultural or religious groups. Compare and contrast their cultural beliefs and how they are reflected in funeral services.
7. Use the Internet to investigate emergency "codes" used in health care workplaces. Compare and contrast the benefits of at least two systems.
8. Investigate the methods of recycling and waste management in a local health care facility. Write a paragraph that describes how the practices promote cost containment and environmental protection.

Explore the Web

Career Information

Bureau of Labor Statistics
http://www.bls.gov/

Salary.com
http://salary.com

Professional Associations

American Nursing Association
http://www.nursingworld.org//

National League for Nursing
http://www.nln.org/

National Student Nurses Association
http://www.nsna.org/

Nurses.info
http://www.nurses.info/

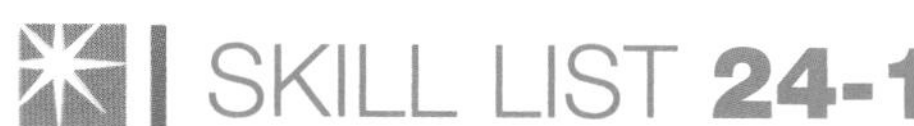

SKILL LIST 24-1 Positioning the Patient

1. Maintain medical asepsis by using the guidelines provided in the Standard and Transmission-Based Precautions, including good handwashing technique and use of gloves as needed.
2. Identify the patient and explain the procedure.
3. Determine the position to be assumed. The appropriate position is determined by the health care worker or ordered by the physician.
4. Keep all unattended side rails in the upright position for safety.
5. Move cranks or electrical adjustments to achieve desired position. Replace adjusting devices to their original position. Injury may occur to the patient or health care worker if devices protrude from the bed.
6. Cushion points of pressure with pillows or linens. Points of pressure include areas where bones are close to the surface of the skin, such as the elbows, heels, tail bone (coccygeal) area, and knees. Impaired circulation on pressure points may lead to formation of bedsores (decubitus ulcers).
7. Assess the body alignment of the patient. The body should be aligned as naturally and comfortably as possible to prevent points of pressure and contracting of limbs.

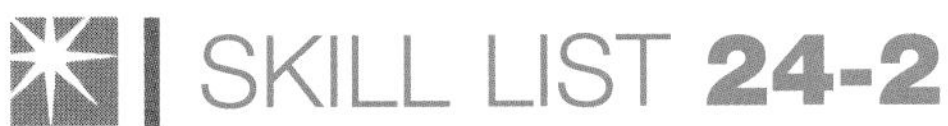

SKILL LIST 24-2
Assisting the Patient to Eat

1. Maintain medical asepsis by using the guidelines provided in the Standard and Transmission-Based Precautions, including good handwashing technique and use of gloves as needed.
2. Gather all necessary supplies and equipment including the patient's tray, a chair for the assistant, washcloth, and hand towel.
3. Prepare the tray according to the nutritional requirements. Dietary requirements may be limited by the patient's condition or ability to eat.
4. Assist the patient to assume an upright position. The upright position helps encourage eating and promotes digestion.
5. Assist the patient to use the restroom if desired.
6. Assist the patient to wash his or her face and hands.
7. Place the tray in front of the patient. Open containers and remove food covers.
8. Sit next to the patient during the meal. The assistant should be seated, relaxed, and not appear hurried to encourage the patient to eat.
9. Assist the patient with eating as needed. The patient should be allowed to do as much as possible without assistance to preserve independence and dignity. A hand towel may be used as a napkin under the chin to catch any food that is dropped.
10. Talk with the patient during the meal. Maintaining a conversation with the patient helps make the meal a pleasant experience and encourages eating.
11. Pause at times to allow the patient to rest. The patient needing assistance with the meal also needs time to rest during the meal.
12. Assist the patient to clean his or her face, hands, and teeth after eating.

SKILL LIST 24-3
Range-of-Motion Exercises

1. Maintain medical asepsis by using the guidelines provided in the Standard and Transmission-Based Precautions, including good handwashing technique and use of gloves as needed.
2. Identify the patient and explain the procedure. ROM exercises may be performed during the bed bath or at another time. The type of exercises that can be accomplished by the patient is determined by his or her condition. The patient should perform as much of the exercise as possible. If the patient cannot perform the movements, the health care worker can provide the same benefits by moving the parts of the body.
3. Provide for privacy. Position the patient comfortably in the supine position. The supine position allows movement of all body parts.
4. Ensure safety by keeping all unattended side rails in an upright position.
5. Exercise the neck 5 to 10 times. The neck can be hyperextended, rotated, flexed, and moved in a lateral flexion.
6. Exercise the shoulder 5 to 10 times. The shoulder can be flexed, extended, abducted, adducted, and rotated by grasping the hand and elbow to keep the arm straight.
7. Exercise the elbow 5 to 10 times. The elbow can be flexed and extended by grasping the hand and upper arm.
8. Exercise the forearm 5 to 10 times. The arm can be turned downward, or pronated, and turned upward, or supinated.
9. Exercise the wrist 5 to 10 times. The wrist can be flexed and extended by bending the wrist with the fingers.
10. Exercise the thumb and fingers. The fingers can be abducted, adducted, extended, and flexed. The thumb can also be rotated.

Continued

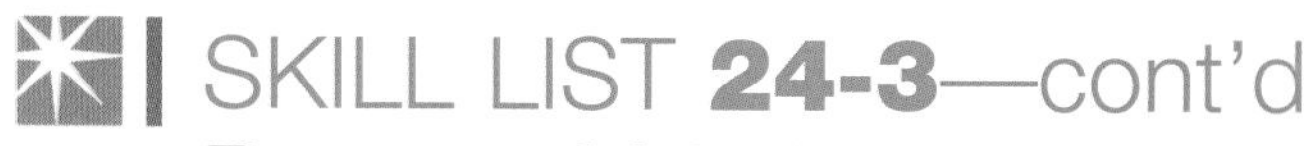

SKILL LIST 24-3—cont'd
Range-of-Motion Exercises

11. Exercise the hip 5 to 10 times. The hip can be flexed, extended, abducted, adducted, and rotated by grasping the knee and ankle to keep the leg straight.
12. Exercise the knee 5 to 10 times. The knee can be flexed and extended by supporting the upper leg and foot.
13. Exercise the ankle 5 to 10 times by flexing and extending it.
14. Exercise the toes 5 to 10 times. The toes can be flexed, extended, abducted, and adducted.
15. Repeat the exercises on the other side of the body.
16. Position the patient for comfort and safety.
17. Record the treatment. Any observations about the skin, complaint of pain, muscle spasm, and degree of assistance with the exercises should be recorded. The time of treatment and joints exercised are also recorded.

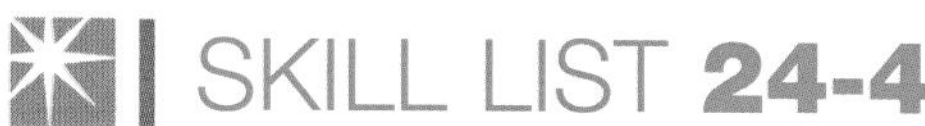

SKILL LIST 24-4
Maintaining the Unit

1. Maintain medical asepsis by using the guidelines provided in the Standard and Transmission-Based Precautions, including good handwashing technique and use of gloves as needed.
2. Change the sheets daily and when soiled. Remove soiled linens from the room frequently.
3. Replace equipment, supplies, and the patient's possessions to the designated location after each use.
4. Throw trash in the appropriate location and empty frequently.
5. Supply the patient with fresh water once a shift and as needed.
6. Clean surfaces of tables regularly and as soiled.
7. Keep the call bell within reach of the patient at all times.

SKILL LIST 24-5
Giving a Backrub

1. Maintain medical asepsis by using the guidelines provided in the Standard and Transmission-Based Precautions, including good handwashing technique and use of gloves as needed.
2. Identify the patient and explain the procedure. The backrub may be performed during the bed bath. Patients who are unable to leave their beds should have a massage at least every 8 hours. Bedsores may occur if circulation to an area has been decreased because of immobility. Backrubs increase circulation to the back area, as well as promote comfort.
3. Provide privacy by drawing curtains or closing the door.
4. Ensure safety by keeping all unattended bed rails in an upright position.

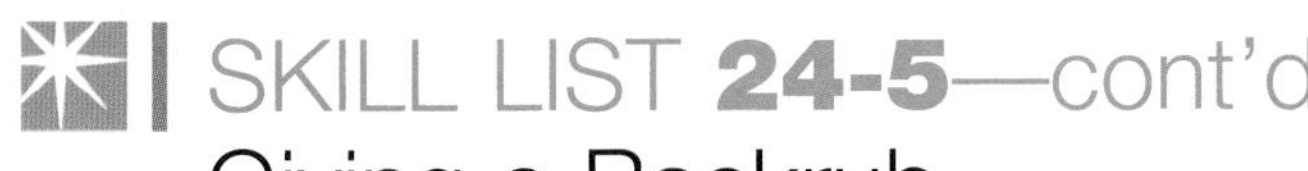

SKILL LIST 24-5—cont'd
Giving a Backrub

5. Assist the patient to turn to the far side.
6. Apply lotion to the hands and rub from the neck to the buttocks in circular motions. The strokes should be firm and smooth. To loosen muscles, knead them with the fingers. The patient may prefer a specific type of lotion or that no lotion be used.
7. Observe for reddened pressure areas on the bony prominences. Pressure areas that are noted and treated promptly may prevent bedsores.
8. Reposition the patient for safety.
9. Report any unusual findings immediately and record observations.

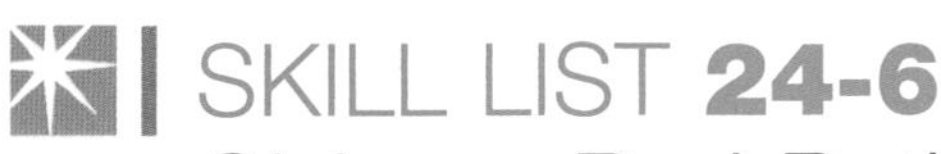

SKILL LIST 24-6
Giving a Bed Bath

1. Maintain medical asepsis by using the guidelines provided in the Standard and Transmission-Based Precautions, including good handwashing technique and use of gloves as needed.
2. Collect all necessary equipment, including clean bath towels, washcloths, bath blanket, gown, soap, and warm water. Water for bathing should be approximately 110° F (43° C).
3. Ensure safety throughout the procedure by keeping all unattended bed rails raised.
4. Identify the patient and explain the procedure. The type of bath given is determined by the patient's mobility and condition.
5. Provide privacy. A bath blanket is used to cover the patient before removing the gown and top bed linens. The patient should be covered at all times during the procedure to preserve his or her dignity.
6. Assist the patient to use the restroom or bedpan if necessary. Exposure to water stimulates the need for urination.
7. Assist the patient with oral hygiene. The male patient may need assistance with shaving.
8. Wash the eyes without using soap, which may irritate the eyes. The eyes should be wiped from the inner to the outer aspect, each with a separate part of the washcloth. A mitt can be made with the washcloth to provide better control.
9. Wash the face, ears, and neck with soap. Rinse and dry. Establishing a routine of washing head to toe and far side to near side ensures speed and complete coverage.
10. Place a towel under each area of the body as it is cleaned. The towel prevents water and soap from collecting in the bed linens under the patient.
11. Wash, rinse, and dry the patient in sections of the arms, chest, abdomen, legs, and feet. The body is washed and dried in parts to promote comfort. The skin should be washed with firm but gentle strokes. Patting the skin dry prevents damage to sensitive areas.
12. Change the water. The water becomes progressively soapy, dirty, and cool with use.
13. Turn the patient to the far side to wash, rinse, and dry the back from neck to buttocks. A back massage or rub may be done at this time to increase circulation and provide comfort.
14. Allow the patient to wash, rinse, and dry the genital area unless he or she needs assistance. The genital area should be washed thoroughly to prevent infection and odor.
15. Wash, rinse, and dry the perineal area from front to back. Microorganisms that normally live in the intestinal tract can cause infection when transmitted to the urinary tract.

Continued

SKILL LIST 24-6—cont'd
Giving a Bed Bath

16. Depending on patient preference, apply lotion and antiperspirants during the bath.
17. Assist the patient with dressing. The patient may need assistance to comb, brush, or arrange the hair.
18. Reposition the patient for comfort and safety.
19. Clean and replace equipment in the storage area. Place the soiled bath linens in the designated area.
20. Change the bed linens if necessary.
21. Record observations. Report any unusual findings to the supervisor immediately. The bed bath provides a time for the patient to voice opinions about care that is being given and for the health care worker to observe any problems with the patient's skin.

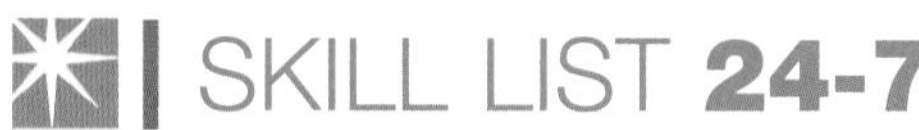

SKILL LIST 24-7
Measuring Oral Intake

1. Maintain medical asepsis by using the guidelines provided in the Standard and Transmission-Based Precautions, including good handwashing technique and use of gloves as needed.
2. Collect the food tray after the patient has finished eating. Compare the remains with the list of food and liquid served. Be alert to families and visitors who may eat what the patient does not want.
3. Estimate the amount of liquids consumed during the meal. Anything that is a liquid at room temperature is considered oral intake. Examples include ice, ice cream, and Jell-O. Oral intake is measured in cubic centimeters.
4. Record oral intake in designated area.
5. Replace the tray on the cart.

SKILL LIST 24-8
Assisting with the Bedpan

1. Maintain medical asepsis by using the guidelines provided in the Standard and Transmission-Based Precautions, including good handwashing technique and use of gloves as needed.
2. Collect the necessary equipment and supplies including a bedpan, washcloth, hand towel, toilet tissue, and disposable gloves. Urine and feces are body secretions, and care should be taken to prevent exposure to them.
3. Explain the procedure to the patient and provide for privacy.
4. Raise the bed to a comfortable working height, making sure that all unattended side rails are up. Side rails should be up when the bed is raised to prevent injury if the patient should attempt to move around or leave the bed.
5. Position the patient in the supine position with the head slightly raised.
6. Fold the top linens to the foot of the bed. Keep the lower body lightly covered with a gown or top sheet. Linens and other materials are moved to prevent contamination with urine or feces.

Continued

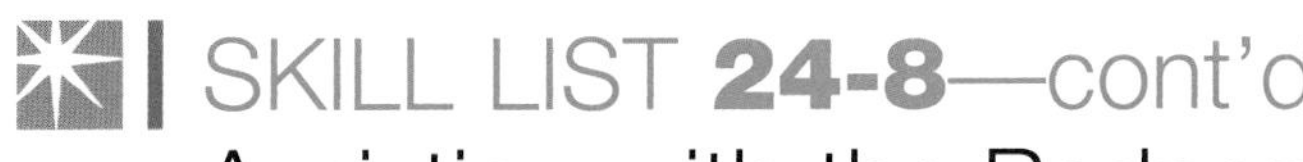

SKILL LIST 24-8—cont'd
Assisting with the Bedpan

7. Assist the patient with flexing the knees and raising the hips.
8. Place the bedpan under the patient's buttocks. The patient may be turned to the side and rolled onto the bedpan if unable to raise the buttocks.
9. Cover the patient with the top sheet.
10. Raise the head of the bed to a sitting position.
11. Check the positioning of the bedpan.
12. Raise the side rail and lower the bed. Place toilet paper and call bell within reach. Instruct the patient to call when finished using the bedpan.
13. If the patient is strong enough to sit unassisted, he or she may be left alone so as to provide some privacy. It may be difficult for a person to feel free to eliminate waste with someone present.
14. Knock or call to the patient before entering the curtained area.
15. Raise the bed, and lower the side rail and head of the bed.
16. Put on gloves to assist the patient in raising up off the bedpan in the same manner in which the bedpan was placed.
17. Cover the bedpan and place it aside.
18. Clean the perineal area if the patient is unable to do so.
19. Assist the patient to wash his or her hands.
20. Lower the bed, and reposition the patient for comfort and safety. Clean the call bell with disinfectant and place it within reach of the patient.
21. Take the bedpan to the bathroom or dirty utility room to empty. Measure the urine if the patient is on intake and output.
22. Rinse the bedpan and empty it into a toilet or proper receptacle. Clean it with disinfectant.
23. Discard gloves in appropriate container.
24. Lower the bed and position the patient for comfort and safety.

SKILL LIST 24-9
Measuring Urine Output

1. Maintain medical asepsis by using the guidelines provided in the Standard and Transmission-Based Precautions, including good handwashing technique and use of gloves as needed.
2. Gather all necessary equipment and supplies, including paper towel, alcohol pledget, graduated cylinder, paper, and pen.
3. Identify the patient, and explain the procedure.
4. Empty the catheter bag, urinal, or bedpan into a graduated cylinder. Paper tissue should not be placed in the bedpan because the tissue displaces the urine and makes the reading too high.
5. Clean the draining tube of the catheter bag with an alcohol pledget before reinserting it into the bag.
6. Place the graduated cylinder on a flat surface out of the patient's vision. Read it at eye level. The angle of the container will change the reading.
7. Record the amount, color, and consistency of the specimen. Report any unusual findings to the supervisor.
8. Rinse the graduated cylinder, urinal, or bedpan with cool water and empty the contaminated water into the toilet. Return the urinal or bedpan to a convenient location for the patient.
9. Dispose of the used paper toweling, disposable gloves, and alcohol pledget in the appropriate container.

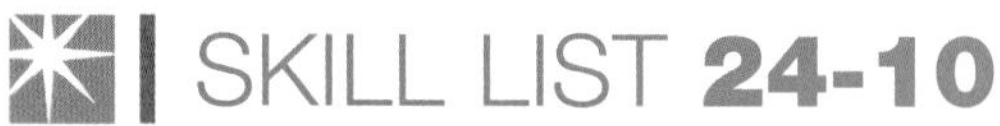

SKILL LIST 24-10
Making an Unoccupied and Surgical Bed

1. Maintain medical asepsis by using the guidelines provided in the Standard and Transmission-Based Precautions, including good handwashing technique and use of gloves as needed.
2. Collect clean linens in order of use: mattress pad, bottom sheet, draw sheet, top sheet, blanket, bedspread, and pillowcases. Do not allow the linens to touch the uniform. The linens are considered to be cleaner than the uniform and should be held away from it.
3. Place the linens on a clean surface in their order of use so that the mattress pad is on top. Once brought into a room, linens may not be returned to the linen cart. If not soiled, some linens may be reused on the same bed, depending on agency policy.
4. Raise the bed to a comfortable working height.
5. Remove dirty linens to an appropriate receptacle. To prevent the spread of microorganisms in the unit, dirty linens should be placed directly into the linen basket or bag, not on the other furniture or the floor.
6. Push the empty mattress to the head of the bed. The mattress slides to the foot of the bed when the head of the bed is raised.
7. Place the mattress pad on the mattress, extending it from the area of the shoulders to the knees.
8. Without shaking it, place the bottom sheet on the bed with the center fold in the middle of the bed and with the hem seams down. Place the sheet so that the bottom edge is even with the mattress at the foot of the bed. Shaking the sheets in the air increases the number of microorganisms on the linens.
9. Tuck in the top edge of one side of the bed to make a mitered corner. Tuck the sheet on the one side from the head to the foot of the bed.
10. Miter the other corners, and tuck the sheet tightly on the opposite side of the bed. Wrinkles are uncomfortable and can lead to skin irritation and bedsores, or decubitus ulcers.
11. Place the draw sheet on the bed so that it covers the area from the shoulders to the knees. Tuck each side tightly. The draw sheet may be used to move the patient because most of the weight of the patient is located in the trunk of the body.
12. Place the top sheet and blanket on the bed with the blanket 4 to 6 inches lower than the sheet to make a cuff.
13. Place the bedspread on the bed. A closed bed is made when the bedspread, blanket, and top sheet cover the bottom sheet completely. The top sheet, blanket, and bedspread may be folded back to the foot of the bed to make an open bed. In a surgical bed, the top linens are not tucked under the mattress to provide easy access to the bed and to make postsurgical assessment easier.
14. Place the pillowcase on the bed next to the pillow. Using the center of the closed end of the pillowcase, grasp the center of the pillow and pull the cover on. Place the pillow so that the open edge is away from the door. To prevent the spread of microorganisms, do not hold the pillow under the chin to assist in putting on the pillowcase.
15. Return the bed to its lowest level.

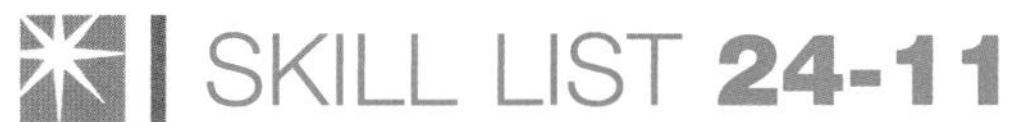

SKILL LIST 24-11 Making an Occupied Bed

1. Maintain medical asepsis by using the guidelines provided in the Standard and Transmission-Based Precautions, including good handwashing technique and use of gloves as needed.
2. Collect clean linens, following the same procedure as for the unoccupied bed.
3. Identify the patient and explain the procedure.
4. Provide for the privacy and safety of the patient. Place side rails in the upright position.
5. Raise the bed to a comfortable working height, and lower the head of the bed. Remove the pillows to make moving the patient easier. One pillow may be left under the patient's head for comfort.
6. Lower the side rail. Without exposing the patient, assist him or her to turn to one side.
7. Roll the soiled sheets toward the patient. The sheets are wrapped as tightly as possible because the patient will be asked later to roll over these linens to the clean side.
8. Make the unoccupied side of the bed, placing the clean sheets for the occupied half of the bed under the roll of soiled sheets. The bottom side of the soiled sheets is cleaner than the top.
9. Raise the side rail and assist the patient to roll across the sheets to the cleaner side.
10. Lower the side rail, and make the unoccupied side of the bed. Remove the soiled linens and immediately place them in an appropriate container.
11. Assist the patient to return to the center of the bed.
12. Place the clean top sheet over the soiled top sheet, and remove the soiled sheet. Do not expose the patient at any time during this procedure. Add the blanket to the top sheet.
13. Make the top sheet and blanket corners. Raise the side rail.
14. Change and replace the pillowcases.
15. Lower the bed to its lowest level.
16. Reposition the patient for comfort, privacy, and safety.

CHAPTER 25

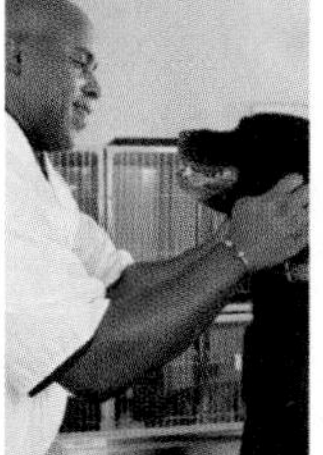

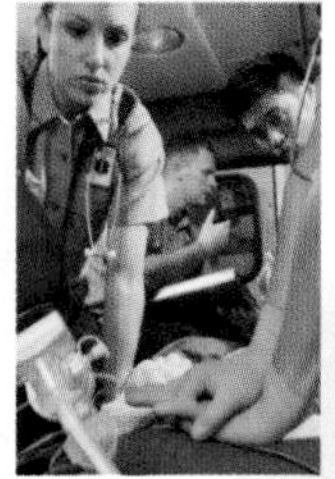

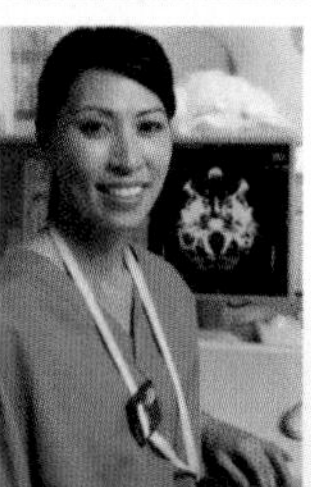

Medical Careers

LEARNING OBJECTIVES

- Define at least 10 terms relating to careers in medicine and related fields.
- Specify the role of selected medical care providers, including personal qualities, levels of education, and credentialing requirements.
- Define visual acuity, and describe at least two methods used to determine it.
- Describe two types of electrocardiography used by medical personnel.

KEY TERMS

Acuity *(uh-KYOO-it-ee)* Clearness or sharpness of perception

Allopathic *(al-o-PATH-ik)* Treatment of disease and injury with active intervention

Anesthesiology *(an-es-thee-zee-AHL-uh-jee)* Study of medicine to relieve pain during surgery

Biomechanics *(by-o-meh-KAN-iks)* Study of the mechanical laws and their application to living organisms, especially locomotion

Internship *(IN-tern-ship)* Period of initial training under the supervision of a qualified practitioner

Osteopathic *(os-tee-o-PATH-ik)* Treatment of disease and injury with an emphasis on the relationship between the body organs and musculoskeletal system

Residency *(REZ-ih-dent-see)* Period of training in a specific area under the supervision of a qualified health care practitioner

Vision *(VIZH-un)* Capacity for sight

Medical Careers Terminology*

Term	Definition	Prefix	Root	Suffix
Electrocardiogram	Record of the electrical activity of the heart	electro	cardio	gram
Gynecology	Study of women		gyne/c	ology
Oncology	Study of cancer		onc	ology
Ophthalmic	Pertaining to vision		ophthalm	ic
Orthoptics	Science of vision using both eyes	orth	opt	ics
Osteopathy	Therapeutic approach to medicine (literally, disease of bone)	osteo	path	y
Phlebotomy	Incision into a vessel		phleb	otomy
Podiatrist	One who treats the feet		pod/ia	trist
Psychiatry	Medicine dealing with mental, emotional, and behavioral disorders		psych/ia	try
Psychology	Study of the mind		psych	ology

*A transition syllable or vowel may be added to or deleted from the word parts to make the combining form.

Abbreviations for Medical Careers

Abbreviation	Meaning
AMA	American Medical Association
CMA	Certified medical assistant
DO	Doctor of osteopathy
DPM	Doctor of podiatry
ECG	Electrocardiogram
MA	Medical assistant
MD	Medical doctor
OB	Obstetrician, obstetrics
PA	Physician assistant
RMA	Registered medical assistant
CST	Certified surgical technologist

Careers

Physicians and other medical care personnel work with their patients in a close or primary relationship (Box 25-1). The function of medical care providers is to promote optimal health and provide care during illness. Physicians must complete one of the most demanding educational programs of all health careers. Acceptance in these programs is determined by excelling academically, as well as participating in leadership and extracurricular activities. Individuals in medical care must be self-motivated and able to work long hours under pressure (Table 25-1).

Physicians

Two types of medical doctors exist: the MD (doctor of medicine) and DO (doctor of osteopathic medicine). Although osteopathic doctors are also physicians, the largest group of physicians providing direct care is the MDs, or allopathic physicians. The education for the MD includes 4 years of medical school after completion of a college or university degree. Additional training under the supervision of a practicing doctor is necessary for specialization. The additional training may be a 1-year internship that includes general training. Most physicians complete a residency, or training of several years, in an area of specialty.

BRAIN BYTE

The first surgery that was performed using general anesthesia (ether) occurred in 1842.

MDs provide care through all phases of life. About one third of MDs and one half of DOs are primary care physicians. They are usually the first doctor to see the patient, and they see patients on a regular basis. Some of the many areas of specialization in medicine include anesthesiology, surgery, pediatrics, obstetrics, and urology. Information regarding the specialty of psychiatry is provided in Chapter 30. Information regarding careers in pathology is provided in Chapter 22. Most MDs work in private practice, although an increasing number work for health maintenance organizations or as hospital staff. MDs are licensed by the state after successful completion of medical school and passing a comprehensive board examination. The American Board of Medical Specialists certifies doctors in more than 145 specialties and subspecialties.

Health Careers in Practice

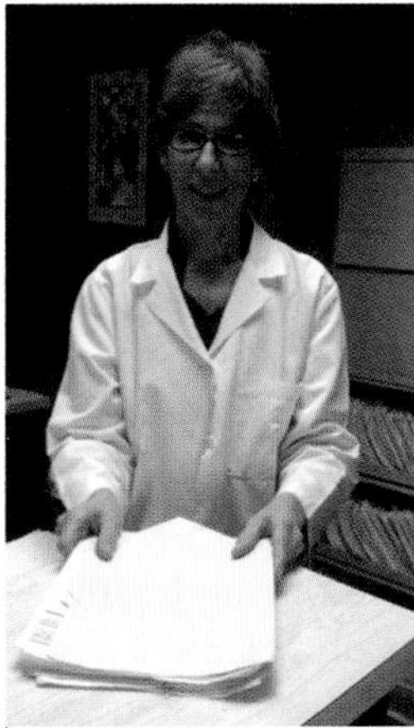

AMY

PHYSICIAN—GENERAL SURGEON SPECIALIZING IN BREAST SURGERY
PRIVATE PRACTICE—OFFICE AND HOSPITAL

Educational background: College, bachelor's degree; medical school, MD degree; 5 years of surgical residency

A typical day at work and job duties include:

- Seeing patients 3 days a week
- Operating room 2 days a week

The most gratifying part of my job: Helping patients feel better and understand their disease process, as well as how their surgical and medical treatment works.

The biggest challenge(s) I face in doing my job: Dealing with insurance companies and overall declining reimbursement.

What drew me to my career? I like science very much and also working with people.

Something I learned in my early education that I currently use in my career or that caused me to be interested in my career is: I became interested in medicine after studying biology in ninth grade.

Other comments: I believe that a physician is a great career choice, even with the challenges we face today. It gives us an opportunity to be at the forefront of scientific knowledge as well as integrating that knowledge with direct relationships with patients and being able to see the results.

BRAIN BYTE

There are 158 medical schools in the United States; 130 awarding an MD and 28 awarding DO degrees.

Hospitals may hire a physician, physician assistant (PA), or nurse practitioner to serve as a hospitalist. The hospitalist acts as a case manager to integrate the care when a patient is hospitalized. The hospitalist provides patient care, teaching, and leadership for the health care team.

Ophthalmologists are MDs who diagnose and treat diseases of and injuries to the eyes. The ophthalmologist may prescribe medication and perform surgery. Ophthalmologists write prescriptions for glasses and give instruction for corrective eye exercise. Ophthalmology requires a medical degree and license to practice medicine, as well as specialty education and experience.

Education for the DO emphasizes the overall body and the physiology of movement. The philosophy of osteopathic medicine is based on the belief that the human body is an integrated organism with a natural ability to resist disease and heal itself. In addition to using the modern tools of medicine, osteopaths are trained to perform manipulation. The moving or manipulation of muscles and bones is called **biomechanics**. The education for the DO is similar in length to that for the MD. After successful completion of an accredited program and a national examination, DOs are licensed by the state in which they practice. More

BOX 25-1

Medical Careers

Allergist-immunologist
Anesthesiologist
Cardiologist
Dermatologist
Dispensing optician
Family practitioner
General practitioner
Gynecologist
Hospitalist
Intern
Internist
Medical assistant
Medical officer
Neurologist
Obstetrician
Ophthalmologist
Optical engineer
Optometric assistant
Optometrist
Osteopathic physician
Otolaryngologist
Pediatrician
Physiatrist
Physician
Physician assistant
Physician extender
Podiatric assistant
Podiatrist
Proctologist
Surgeon
Urologist

than 14,000 osteopathic physicians work in the United States. To continue practice in many states, osteopathic physicians must complete at least 150 hours of continuing education every 3 years.

Other Medical Care Providers

Doctors of podiatric medicine, or podiatrists, treat common foot disorders by using corrective devices, orthopedic shoes, surgery, and medication. Podiatry school includes 4 years of classroom and clinical instruction following completion of at least 2 years of college. Podiatrists are licensed by the state and may be required to complete an internship to qualify. More than 10,000 podiatrists work in the United States.

The role of the PA is different from other health care professions in that it was not developed to meet the needs of advanced medical technology. It was developed to relieve some of the tasks performed by the MD to extend the availability of care. PAs, working under the direction of a physician, perform about 70% of the duties of the MD, including taking the patient history, conducting the physical examination, performing minor surgical procedures, and ordering diagnostic tests. The PA may be called a *physician extender*. In some states PAs may write prescriptions. New roles for the PA include serving as house staff in hospitals (hospitalist), emergency settings, and occupational health clinics. Most PA programs accept students with 2 years of college and prior experience in the health care industry. Education for the PA includes 2 years of classroom and clinical training. Three PA programs train surgeon assistants. Completion of the program may result in a certificate or academic degree.

TABLE 25-1

Medical Career Educational Cost and Earnings

Career	Educational Cost*	Earnings†
Medical assistant	Broward College: 9 mo (1156 clock hours), $4372.92 Fees include: Application Insurance Tuition Insurance Texts Background check and drug screening Physical examination and vaccines Uniforms Graduation fee	Median annual salary: Fort Lauderdale, Fla.—$29,180

*http://www.broward.edu/medicalassisting/MedicalAssisting/cost/page14834.html.
†http://data.bls.gov:8080/oes/datatype.do.

PAs may be registered or licensed by the state in which they practice. Every 6 years, they must be recertified on the basis of completing at least 100 hours of continuing education.

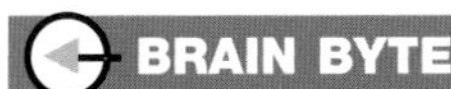

The most frequently consulted online medical resource is MEDLINE/PubMed.

Orthoptics is the clinical science of vision using both eyes (binocular). Orthoptists are eye muscle specialists who work under the direction of an ophthalmologist and who help the patient develop the ability to use both eyes together. Exercises may be used to improve vision. Most orthoptists complete 2 years of college and 24 months of specialized training. Certification is recommended for most employment opportunities.

Opticians (also called *ophthalmic dispensers*) design and fit lenses and frames using an optical prescription. The optician grinds lenses to fit the patient's needs. Training for opticians is available on the job, in vocational schools, and in 2-year colleges. Licensing of opticians is required in at least 22 states.

Optometrists examine and test eyes to evaluate vision and detect diseases of the eye for referral to an MD (Fig. 25-1). The optometrist may use lenses or therapy to improve vision. Optometry requires at least 2 years of college work followed by 4 years of professional study at an accredited optometric school. The degree earned is Doctor of Optometry (OD). Optometrists are licensed by the state.

Support Personnel

Surgical technologists (STs), also called *surgical* and *operating room technicians*, assist during surgical operation under the supervision of the surgeon and registered nurse (Fig. 25-2). STs help prepare the operating room. They assemble and sterilize the instruments, drapes, and solutions and may also prepare the patient by shaving and cleaning the incision site. STs assist the rest of the team to put on sterile gowns and gloves. During surgery, STs pass the instruments and materials needed for the procedure to the surgeon. STs receive training in community college, university, military, and vocational school programs. In 2008 there were 450 accredited programs; these programs last 9 to 24 months. STs may achieve voluntary certification after completing an accredited program and a national examination. Some certified STs specialize and may become certified as a first assistant or surgical assistant.

The medical assistant (MA) is expected to be one of the fastest growing occupations through the year 2010. The MA performs both clerical and clinical functions under the supervision of a physician. Clerical duties that may be performed by the MA include answering the telephone, filling out insurance forms, handling correspondence, and scheduling appointments, hospital admissions, and laboratory services. (See Skill List 25-1, Answering the Telephone, pp. 412-413.) The MA prepares the treatment room, drapes and positions patients, sterilizes equipment, and maintains and inventory supplies and equipment (Fig. 25-3). (See Skill List 25-2, Opening Sterile Packages, p. 413.) MAs who have a specialty may make

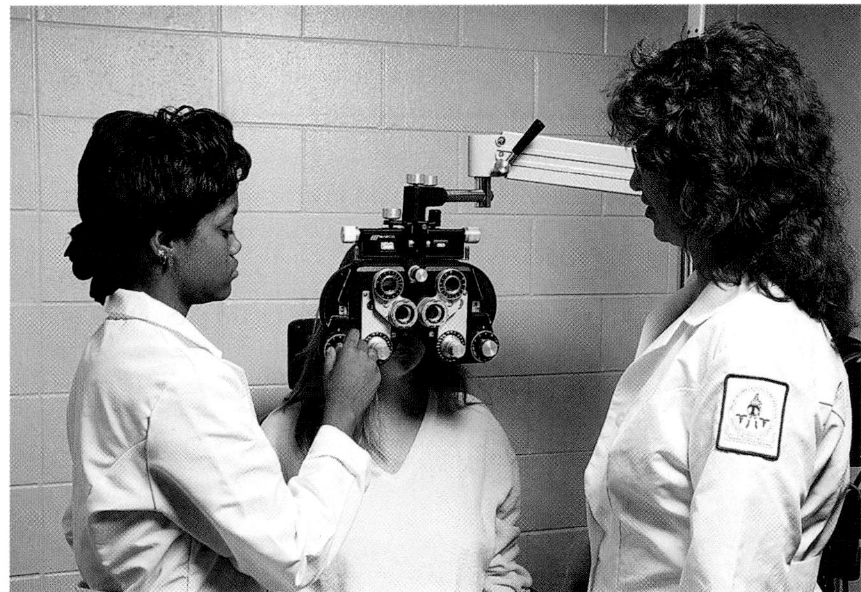

FIGURE 25-1 The optometrist uses an ophthalmoscope to view the interior eye and detect ocular diseases.

Health Careers in Practice

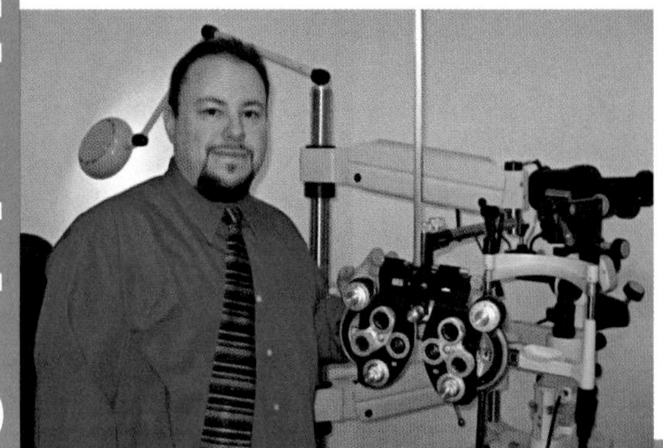

MATTHEW J. SCHROEDER, OD

OPTOMETRIST
TOM SOWASH OD AND ASSOCIATES, PC
(LOCATED INSIDE ARIZONA EYEMASTERS)

Educational background: Bachelor of arts, psychology (4 years); Doctor of optometry (4 years)

A typical day at work and job duties include:

- Ten to 20 full eye examinations plus a half dozen or so shorter visits, including contact lens follow-up appointments and patients with a specific medical complaint, such as eye infections, injuries, or visual disturbances
- Examinations include:
  - Basic assessment of the status of the visual system, including acuity, eye movements, and neurologic activity associated with the eyes
  - Refraction or determination of the spectacle prescription
  - Complete assessment of the external and internal ocular health
- Write prescriptions for vision correction and any ocular disease or systemic disease
- Address any ocular complications via direct treatment, referral to a specialist, or communication with the patient's primary care doctor

The most gratifying part of my job: I love my job because of the daily interactions with patients of all ages and backgrounds and the opportunity to help each of them solve the visual issues that might otherwise constrict the activities in his or her life. No two patients are exactly alike, and that makes every day at the office interesting.

The biggest challenge(s) I face in doing my job: Diseases and the various ocular problems present differently in each patient, which can make my determination of treatment difficult. What I learn in a textbook is not always how a disease presents in a particular patient. I have to make treatment and follow-up care decisions very carefully, knowing that what I learned in school or in my resource books might not be the right choice for a particular patient.

What drew me to my career? Optometry provides a unique combination of opportunities within the health care field. There are many settings and areas of specialization, the largest amount of my time is spent in direct patient care, the cost of malpractice coverage is minimal, and there is significant clinical independence (I get to make my own decisions).

Something I learned in my early education that I currently use in my career or that caused me to be interested in my career is: I have always been interested in biology and was drawn to a career in health care. In school I learned that the eye is the only place on the body where blood vessels and nerves can be directly viewed without first using a scalpel, which I found fascinating.

Other comments: To find the job you want or need, you may have to be willing to move to a different state after acquiring your degree.

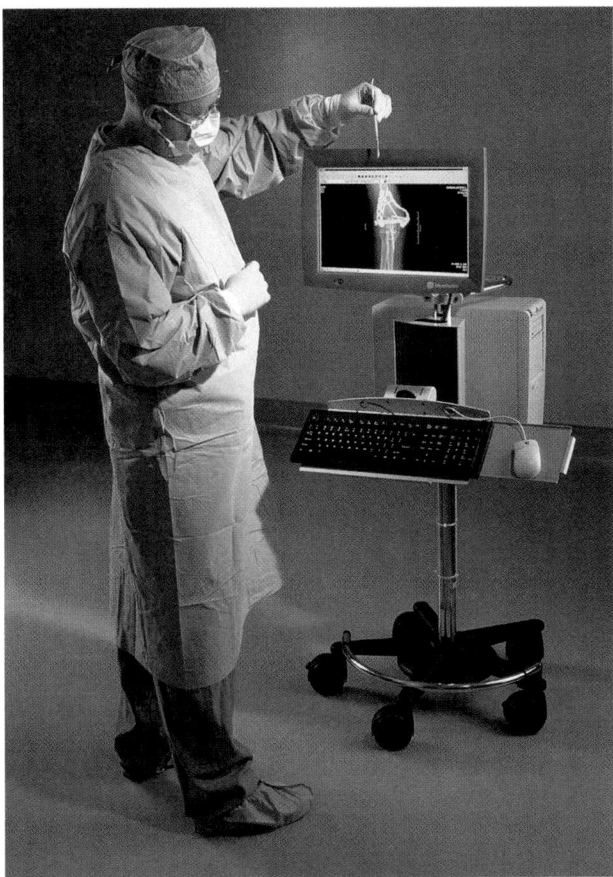

FIGURE 25-2 Radiographs allow the surgery team to prepare for procedures. (Courtesy Swissray International, Inc., Elmsford, N.Y.)

casts or take radiographs and electrocardiographs. The MA may also greet and interview patients and assess vital signs. Training for the MA ranges from 1 to 2 years in a vocational or community college program. Some MAs are trained on the job by the doctor. Medical assistants may become certified (CMA) through the American Association of Medical Assistants. The American Medical Technologists organization grants a certification called Registered Medical Assistant to those who have 5 years of service and have completed an approved course. The American Registry of Medical Assistants also awards the Registered Medical Assistant certification to those who have completed an approved course, have 1 year of experience and have a letter of recommendation from an employer.

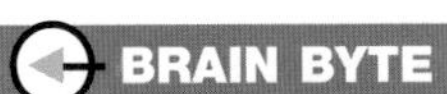

BRAIN BYTE

There are about 670 accredited medical assistant programs in the United States.

CASE STUDY 25-1 You are acting as the receptionist as well as the MA in a doctor's office because someone called in sick. You notice that one of the patients has been waiting a long time and acting agitated and talking loudly. What should you do?

Answers to Case Studies are available on the Evolve website: ***http://evolve.elsevier.com/Gerdin***

The podiatric assistant performs routine procedures such as patient preparation, equipment sterilization, development of radiographs, and general office duties. Podiatric assistants may be trained on the job or attend vocational school.

Ophthalmic assistants and technicians provide care to the patient of the ophthalmologist by measuring vision, changing dressings, administering eye and oral medications, applying contact lenses, and assisting with specialized ocular tests. Ophthalmic assistants maintain equipment and supplies. Assistants may learn on the job or complete a home-study course offered by the American Association of Ophthalmology. Technicians perform all of the tasks of the assistant and may be trained to prepare specimens for examination and to assist with ocular surgery. Ophthalmic technicians complete a 2-year certificate program.

Paraoptometric personnel extend the optometrist's capability by performing the routine tasks of vision care. Paraoptometric personnel work under the supervision of an OD. Optometric technicians complete an associate or 2-year degree. They perform tests such as vision screening, measuring pressure on the cornea (tonometry), and recording patient histories (Fig. 25-4). Technicians may also determine the power of existing lenses and assist with frame selection and fitting. Technicians instruct patients on the care and proper method of contact wear. They assist the optometrist during examinations and may work with children who have disabilities such as wandering eyes (amblyopia). Optometric assistants may be trained on the job or in 1-year programs.

CASE STUDY 25-2 You find a used blood collection tube in the trash basket after another CMA has used the examination room. What should you do?

Answers to Case Studies are available on the Evolve website: ***http://evolve.elsevier.com/Gerdin***

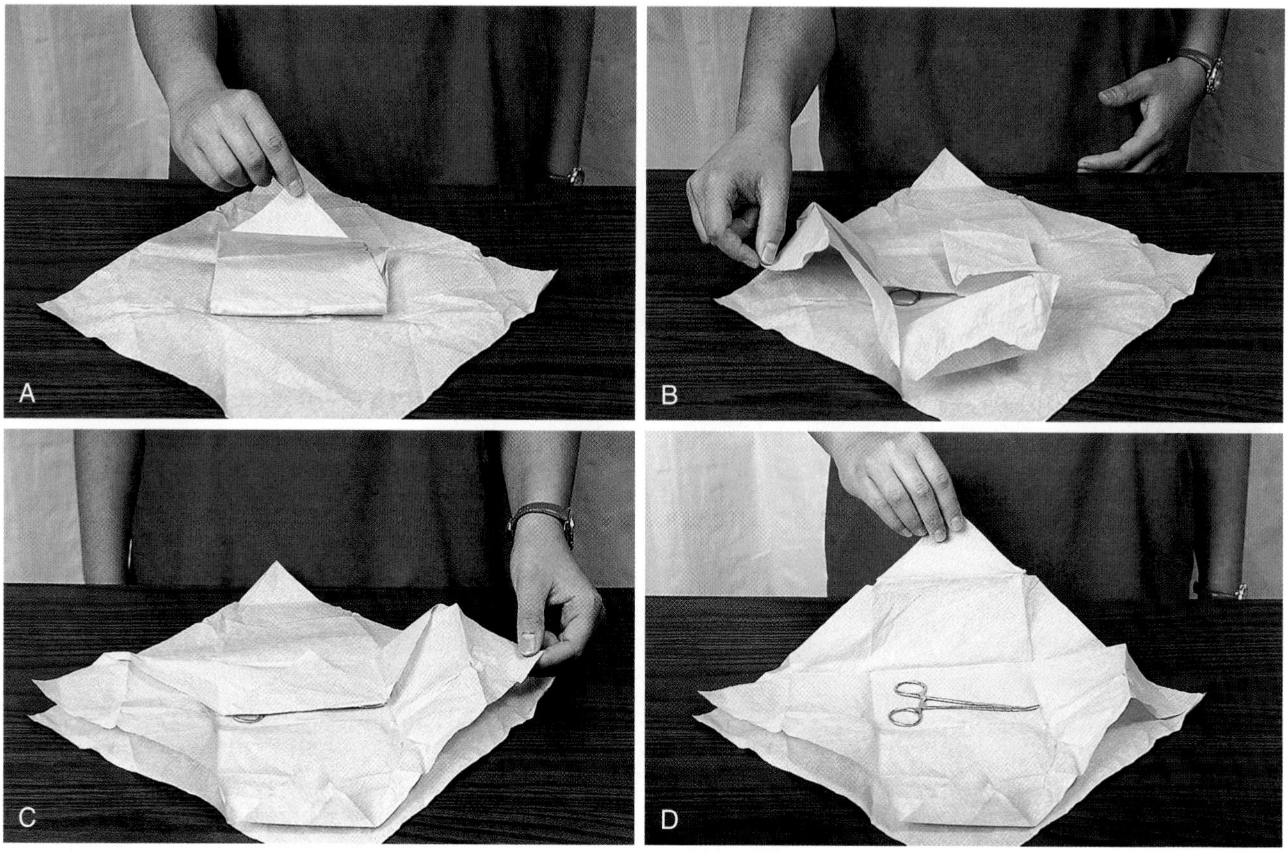

FIGURE 25-3 Opening a sterile package.

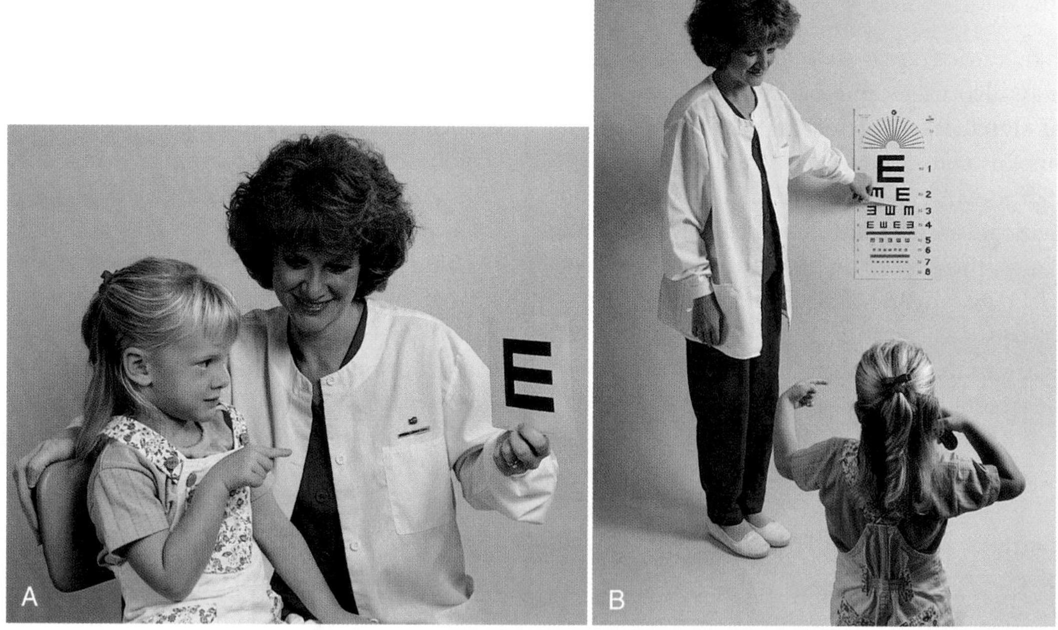

FIGURE 25-4 A preschool child can point the direction of a letter to assess visual acuity. (From Bonewitt-West K: *Clinical procedures for medical assistants*, ed 7, St. Louis, 2008, Saunders. In Bonewit-West K, Hunt S, Applegate E: *Today's medical assistant: clinical & administrative procedures*, St. Louis, 2009, Saunders.)

Content Instruction

Vision

Visual acuity is the ability to differentiate shapes and color to interpret their meaning. The ophthalmoscope is used to view the interior of the eye to examine its structures. Another assessment method is the field vision test, which measures how wide the field of vision reaches around each eye.

Comprehensive eye examination includes testing for visual acuity for distance and near objects. It also measures focusing, tracking, and fixation skills. The ability to use both eyes together at the same time (binocular vision) is assessed, as well as depth perception (stereopsis). (See Skill List 25-3, Measuring Visual Acuity, p. 414.)

Electrocardiogram

Electrical currents in the heart are measured by using electrocardiography. This may be done with 3 to 12 leads (or electrodes) or more attached to the person being tested (Fig. 25-5). The electrocardiograph is a strip of graph paper that is produced as the heart's electrical activity is recorded. More information regarding electrocardiographs and the function of the heart may be found in Chapter 11.

Performance Instruction

Physical Examination and Treatment

The MA may assist with a physical examination or simple medical procedure (Box 25-2). Preparation of the examination room includes providing the needed equipment, supplies, and linens for the procedure to be completed (Fig. 25-6). The assistant greets the

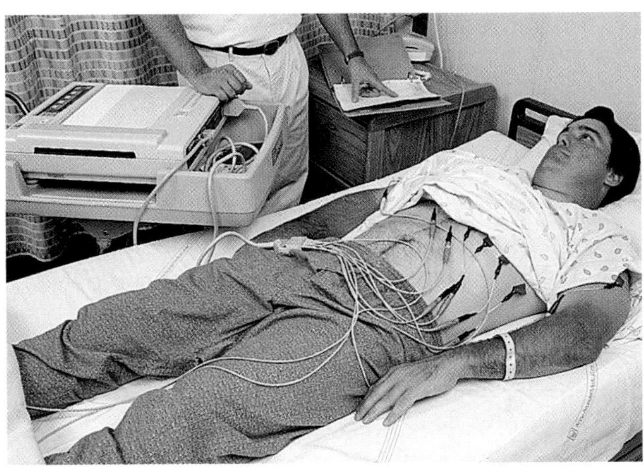

FIGURE 25-5 Cables are connected from the electrocardiogram machine to the electrodes. (From Sorrentino SA: *Mosby's textbook for nursing assistants*, ed 7, St. Louis, 2008, Mosby.)

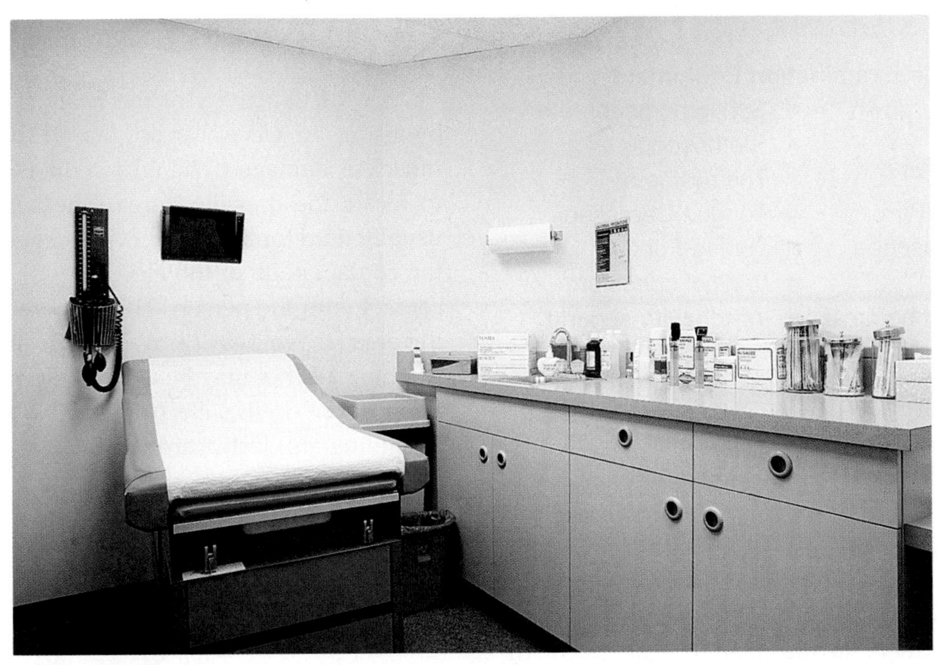

FIGURE 25-6 Preparing the examination room is an important duty of the medical assistant.

BOX 25-2

Types of Physical Examinations

Vital Signs
- Temperature
- Pulse rate
- Respiratory rate
- Pain

Biometrics
- Height
- Weight

Physical Examination: Positions
- Sitting—examine head, neck, chest, and upper extremities; take vital signs
- Supine—examine head, chest, abdomen, and extremities
- Prone—examine back and extension of hip joint
- Dorsal recumbent (horizontal recumbent)—examine breasts, vaginal and rectal areas
- Lithotomy—examine vaginal, rectal and pelvic areas
- Sims' (left lateral)—examine vaginal and rectal areas, assess rectal temperature, administer enema
- Knee-chest—examine rectum, perform proctoscopic examination
- Fowler's—examine upper body

Laboratory Tests
- Blood analysis
- Urinalysis
- Other body secretion and tissue analysis

Sample Examination Equipment
- Disposable gown and linens
- Gloves
- Laryngeal mirror
- Ophthalmoscope
- Otoscope
- Percussion hammer
- Specimen containers/labels
- Sphygmomanometer
- Stethoscope
- Thermometer
- Tongue Depressor
- Tuning Fork
- Vaginal speculum
- Watch with second hand

patient, takes him or her to the examination room, and takes vital signs. If necessary for the procedure, the assistant explains the use of an examination gown and provides the patient with privacy to change into it. The assistant then assists the physician in positioning and giving treatment to the patient (Fig. 25-7). All specimens are labeled at the time that they are collected with the patient's name, identification number, date and time of collection, and the name of the physician. The patient is provided with privacy to redress when the procedure is completed. The assistant then cleans and prepares the room for the next procedure. (See Skill List 25-4, Assisting with the Physical Examination, and Skill List 25-5, Assisting with Suture Removal, pp. 414-415.)

CASE STUDY 25-3 Your employing physician asks you to draw blood for a patient. You have never performed the procedure before although you did learn how to do it in school. What should you do?

Answers to Case Studies are available on the Evolve website: ***http://evolve.elsevier.com/Gerdin***

Vision Assessment

Vision may be tested by the medical or optometric assistant using a Snellen chart, which measures the ability to see symbols from a specified distance (Fig. 25-8). The patient is asked to sit or stand 20 feet from the chart and identify the characters on the chart with each eye separately and then together. The height of the characters on the chart that can be seen is used to describe the patient's vision. For example, a measurement of 20/30 means that the patient can see characters that are 30 mm high when the patient is 20 feet from the chart. A reading of 20/20 is considered normal vision.

Electrocardiogram

The electrical activity of the heart may be measured by using an electrocardiogram (ECG). If the heart muscle is damaged, changes in the ECG may be used to locate the damaged area. The supine position is usually used for taking an ECG. To get a clear reading, the contact pads of the electrodes should have good contact with the person. This may require shaving of the area, as well as removal of oils and perspiration. Rubbing alcohol may be used to clean the skin before application of the electrodes. (See Skill List 25-6, Obtaining an Electrocardiogram, pp. 415-416.)

CASE STUDY 25-4 You are asked to give a medication to a patient before a procedure is started in the office. You are not familiar with the medication. What should you do?

Answers to Case Studies are available on the Evolve website: ***http://evolve.elsevier.com/Gerdin***

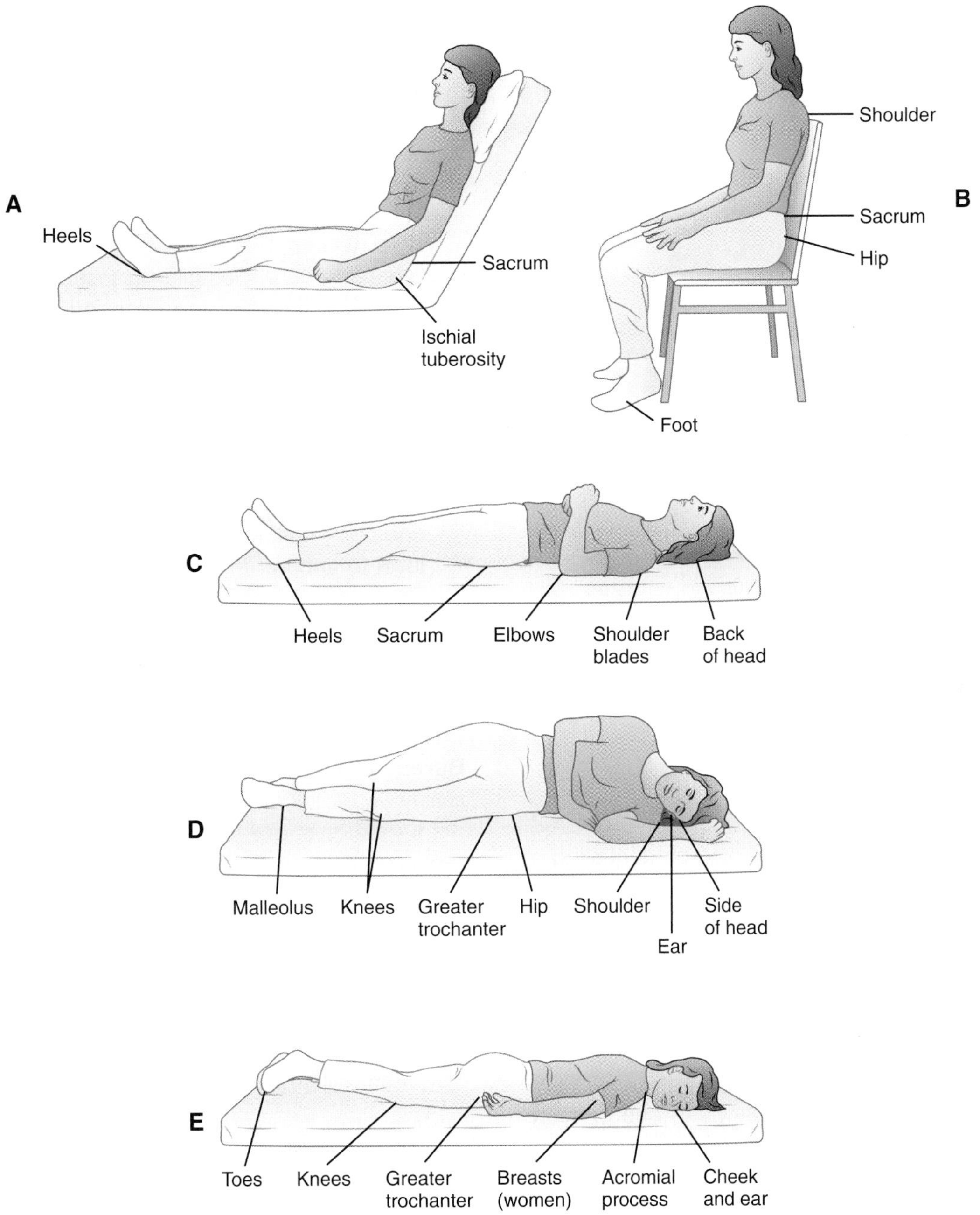

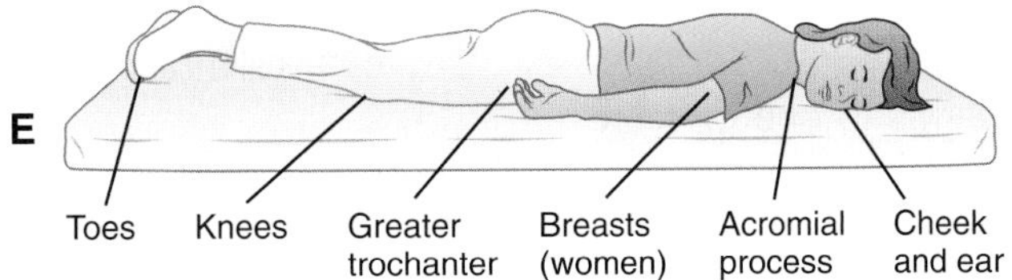

FIGURE 25-7 The best position is determined by the health care worker or ordered by the physician. **A,** Modified semi-Fowler's position. **B,** Sitting position. **C,** Horizontal or supine position. **D,** Left Sims' position. **E,** Prone position.

Summary

- The role of medical care providers is to promote optimal health and provide care during illness. Personal qualities that are necessary include leadership skills, ability to work under pressure, and self-motivation.
- Visual acuity is the ability to differentiate shape and color and to interpret their meaning. Two methods used to assess it include using a Snellen chart and a field-vision test to determine the width of the field vision.
- ECG may be completed by using 3 or 12 electrodes.

Review Questions

1. Describe the function of the medical health care providers.

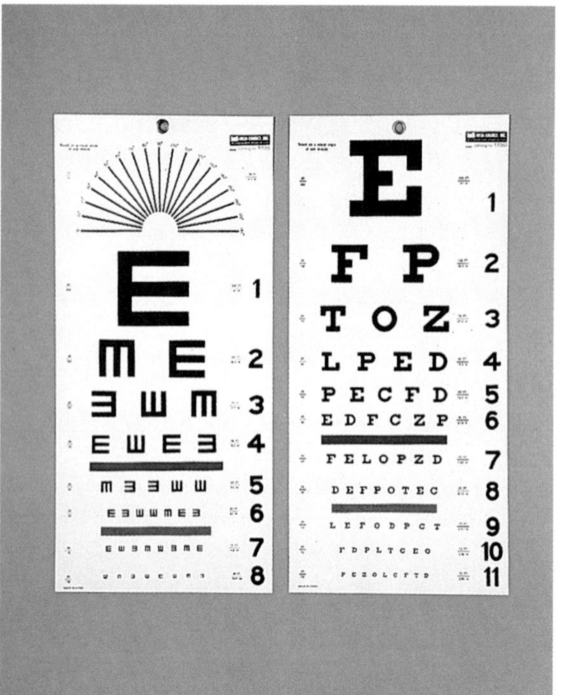

FIGURE 25-8 Snellen and Jaeger charts are used to measure visual acuity.

2. Describe the education, role, and credentialing of three medical health care providers.
3. Describe two methods of assessment of vision.
4. Choose one career from Box 25-1. Research the cost of education and annual earnings in local institutions. Write a paragraph describing the factors that might explain why the local and national economic figures vary.
5. Use each of the following terms in one or more sentences that correctly relate their meaning: allopathic, biomechanics, and osteopathic.

Critical Thinking

1. Investigate the requirements and cost of education programs for five types of medical health care providers.
2. Describe a normal and abnormal pattern for an ECG. (Chapter 11 provides additional information regarding cardiovascular assessments).
3. Use Fig. 25-7 and the information learned from the anatomy and physiology chapters to determine what position would be used for the following procedures: chest radiograph, ECG, injection, lumbar puncture, phlebotomy, suture of hand wound.
4. Create a career ladder for medical careers. Describe why it is or is not possible to move from one level to another in the field.

Explore the Web

Career Information

Bureau of Labor Statistics
http://www.bls.gov/

Salary.com
http://salary.com

Professional Associations

American Medical Association
http://www.ama-assn.org/ama/pub/education-careers/careers-health-care.shtml

The American Association of Medical Assistants
http://www.aama-ntl.org/

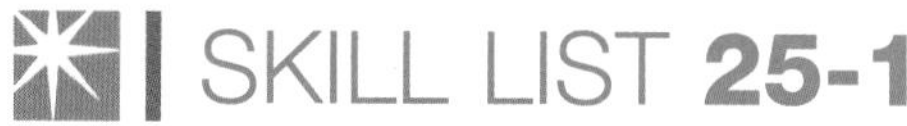

SKILL LIST 25-1 Answering the Telephone

1. Maintain medical asepsis by using the guidelines provided in the Standard and Transmission-Based Precautions, including good handwashing technique and use of gloves as needed.
2. Answer the telephone promptly.
3. Speak in a polite, clear, and well-modulated voice.
4. Determine who is calling, the person for whom the call is intended, and the nature of the business.

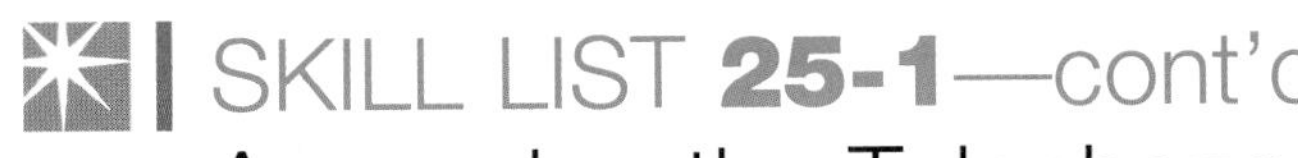

SKILL LIST 25-1—cont'd
Answering the Telephone

5. Do not give out any information about patients or other personnel unless directed to do so by the supervising personnel.
6. In a designated location, write the name of the caller, to whom the message is directed, the time and date of the call, the telephone number of the caller, and any information that is given by the caller.
7. Repeat the name of the caller, the telephone number, and information to verify its accuracy with the caller.
8. Deliver the message to the person for whom it is intended as directed by supervising personnel.

SKILL LIST 25-2
Opening Sterile Packages

1. Maintain medical asepsis by using the guidelines provided in the Standard and Transmission-Based Precautions, including good handwashing technique and use of gloves as needed. The hands are never sterile. If a clean hand touches a sterile object or surface, the object or surface is contaminated.
2. Place the sterile package on a clean, dry surface, or hold the package above the level of the waist. The edges and parts of sterile packaging that fall below the level of the waist are considered to be contaminated. The surface must be dry because moisture allows microorganisms to move through the wrapping material by capillary action, called the *wicking effect*.
3. Check the color of the sterilization tape. The tape changes color when the temperature and pressure of the autoclave reach sufficient levels to destroy all microorganisms and endospores. Remove the tape if the color has changed.
4. Open the far side of the package first. If any part of the arm or hand passes over the sterile area, the item is then considered contaminated because particles of dead skin and microorganisms may fall into the sterile area.
5. Open one side, and carefully avoid crossing over the sterile field. When holding the package, the free hand is passed under it to avoid contamination.
6. Open the near corner last. If the sterile object is being held, secure the ends of the package before passing the contents to the sterile field. If the unsterile parts of the draping cross over the edge of the sterile field, the area is contaminated.

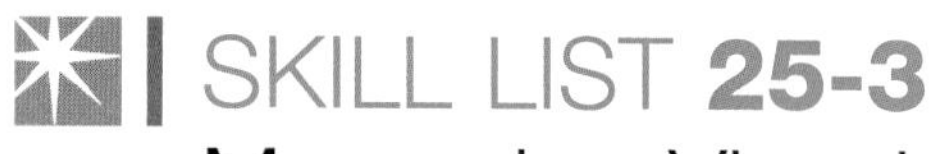

SKILL LIST 25-3 Measuring Visual Acuity

1. Maintain medical asepsis by using the guidelines provided in the Standard and Transmission-Based Precautions, including good handwashing technique and use of gloves as needed.
2. Identify the patient and explain the procedure.
3. Hang the Snellen chart on a light-colored wall at eye level 20 feet from the location of the patient. Make sure there is no glare and the chart is completely illuminated. The patient might not be able to read the chart accurately if the light is placed incorrectly.
4. Place the patient's heels on a line 20 feet from the chart. If the patient is sitting, the back of the chair should be 20 feet from the chart. The chart is designed to measure the height of the letters that can be read correctly from a distance of 20 feet.
5. Cover the patient's left eye when testing the right eye. Have the patient read the letters on each line, beginning with the 100 line and descending to the smallest line that can be read. If the patient wears glasses, have the patient complete the test first with the glasses on, and then repeat the procedure with the glasses removed for comparison. The comparison of vision with and without the glasses indicates the effectiveness of the corrective lenses.
6. Repeat the procedure to test the left eye and then both eyes together.
7. Record the visual acuity as a proportional value. The numerator is the distance from the chart (20 feet). The denominator is the height of the letters of the smallest line that is read accurately. Normal vision is considered to be 20/20.

SKILL LIST 25-4 Assisting with the Physical Examination

1. Maintain medical asepsis by using the guidelines provided in the Standard and Transmission-Based Precautions, including good handwashing technique and use of gloves as needed.
2. Prepare the examination room with necessary linens, equipment, and supplies for the procedures to be completed.
3. Assist the patient to the room, and take vital signs.
4. Instruct the patient to undress and put on an examination gown.
5. Leave the room briefly to provide the patient with privacy.
6. Knock before reentering the room.
7. Position and drape the patient for examination.
8. Hand supplies and equipment to the examiner as they are needed.
9. Label all specimen containers with appropriate information, including date, time, type of specimen, the patient's name, and name of person collecting the sample. Place specimens in designated areas for examination.
10. Instruct the patient regarding procedures to follow before leaving the office.
11. Provide the patient with privacy to dress when the examination is completed.
12. Clean and restock the examination room.

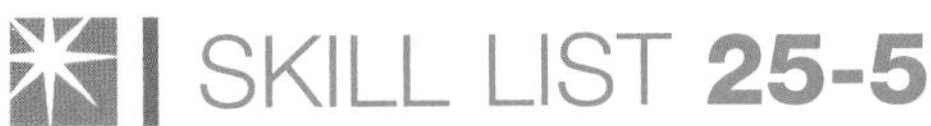

SKILL LIST 25-5 Assisting with Suture Removal

1. Sutures may be removed by trained personnel under the supervision of the physician.
2. Maintain medical asepsis by using the guidelines provided in the Standard and Transmission-Based Precautions, including good handwashing technique and use of gloves as needed.
3. Position the patient and remove clothing as needed to expose the sutured area. Provide privacy as needed.
4. Put on examination or nonsterile gloves to remove dressings. Gloves prevent the spread of microorganisms from body fluids contained in the dressing to the health care worker.
5. Remove the dressing gently, and retain it or dispose of it in the appropriate container. The tape may be loosened using hydrogen peroxide to prevent reopening of the wound.
6. Clean the suture line and skin around it with an antiseptic.
7. Use aseptic technique to open a sterile suture removal kit. The opened tray is considered the sterile field for this procedure. Only the handles of the forceps and suture scissors are touched by the health care worker so that the tips that touch the patient remain sterile.
8. Grasp the knot of the suture and pull it away from the skin.
9. Slip the curved cutting edge of the scissors under the short end of the suture and cut as close to the skin as possible. Cutting the suture close to the skin decreases the chance of infection because less of the exposed suture is pulled through the tissue.
10. Slowly and steadily pull the knot of the suture straight up from the skin. A slow, steady pull prevents tissue damage and pain.
11. Remove every other suture first to assess healing of the suture line. If gaps in the wound occur, the physician may want to resuture the wound.
12. If no gaps occur, remove all remaining sutures.
13. Clean the site again with antiseptic. Leave the wound area exposed unless directed to use a dressing.
14. Inform the patient of any restrictions in movement that might be necessary.
15. Dispose of used items appropriately in the biohazard waste receptacle.

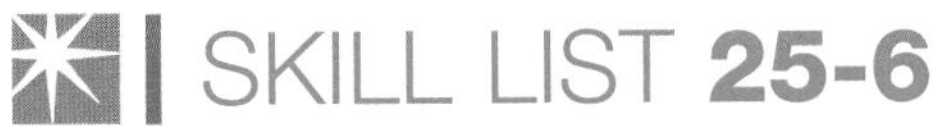

SKILL LIST 25-6 Obtaining an Electrocardiogram*

1. Maintain medical asepsis by using the guidelines provided in the Standard and Transmission-Based Precautions, including good handwashing technique and use of gloves as needed.
2. Review the procedure with the supervising personnel and patient.
3. Provide for privacy. Assist the patient with elimination needs.
4. Raise the bed to a comfortable working height.
5. Measure and record vital signs.
6. Expose the chest, arms, or legs as needed for electrode placement.
7. Wear gloves to wash and shave designated electrode sites.
8. Clean electrode sites with alcohol.
9. Apply electrodes to chest, arms, and legs.
10. Connect cables from the ECG machine to the electrodes.
11. Plug in ECG machine.

*Medical assistants may perform this procedure when specially trained, if it is allowed by the state, and if the medical assistant is supervised by licensed personnel.

Continued

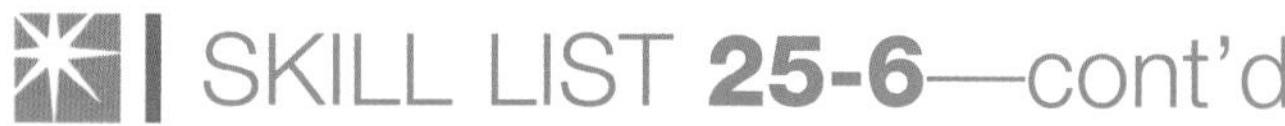

Obtaining an Electrocardiogram

12. Instruct the patient to lie still without talking during the test.
13. Obtain 8 to 12 inches of heart tracing for each lead. Notify the supervising personnel if any unusual patterns are seen.
14. Turn off the ECG machine.
15. Remove the tracing from the machine.
16. Return the patient to a comfortable bed level and position.
17. Return all equipment to the designated location.

CHAPTER 26

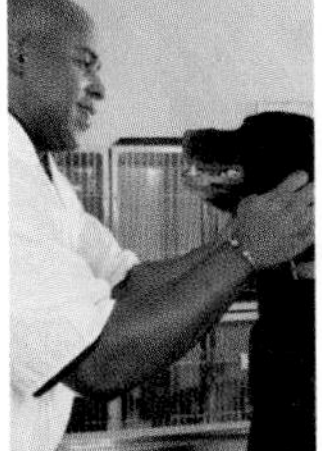
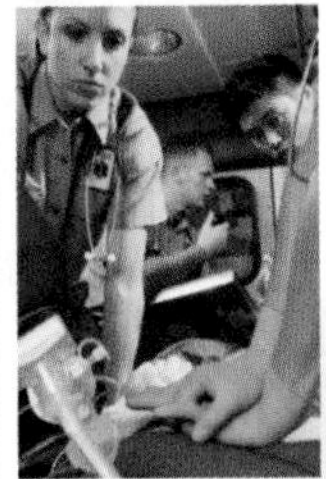
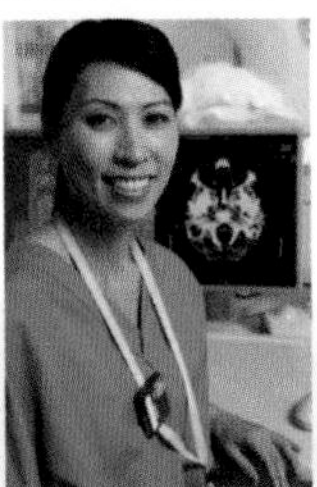

Dental Careers

LEARNING OBJECTIVES

- Define at least 10 terms relating to dental health care.
- Specify the role of the dentist, dental hygienist, dental assistant, and dental laboratory technician, including personal qualities, levels of education, and credentialing requirements.
- Identify the difference between the dentition of the child and that of the adult.
- Identify at least five structures of the oral cavity.
- Describe the location, structure, and function of four types of teeth.
- Chart at least three types of dental variations using a selected method of charting.
- Describe methods of prevention and detection of caries and periodontal disease.
- Describe techniques of brushing and flossing to promote dental health.

KEY TERMS

Abscess *(AB-ses)* Localized collection of pus in a cavity formed by destruction of tissue

Alloy *(AL-oy)* Solid mixture of two or more metals

Alveoli *(al-VEE-o-lie)* Bony cavities in maxilla and mandible in which the roots of the teeth are attached

Calculus *(KAL-kyoo-lus)* Calcium phosphate and carbonate with organic matter deposited on the surfaces of teeth; tartar

Caries *(KARE-eez)* Decalcification of the surface of the tooth followed by disintegration of the inner part of the tooth; cavity

Deciduous *(de-SID-yoo-us)* The teeth that erupt first and are replaced by permanent dentition; primary teeth

Dentition *(den-TISH-un)* Used to designate natural teeth in the mouth

Gingiva *(JIN-jiv-uh)* Gum of the mouth; mucous membrane with supporting fibrous tissue

KEY TERMS cont'd

Halitosis *(hal-ih-TOE-sis)* Offensive or bad breath

Hygiene *(HI-jeen)* Proper care of the mouth and teeth for maintenance of health and the prevention of disease

Mandible *(MAN-dih-bul)* Bone of the lower jaw

Maxilla *(mak-SIL-uh)* Irregularly shaped bone that forms the upper jaw

Periodontal *(pare-ee-o-DON-tul)* Situated or occurring around a tooth

Permanent *(PER-muh-nent)* The teeth that erupt and take the place of deciduous dentition; secondary teeth

Plaque *(plak)* Mass adhering to the enamel surface of a tooth; composed of mixed bacterial colonies and organic material

Restoration *(res-tore-AY-shun)* Replacement of part of a tooth, usually with silver alloy, gold, or aesthetic composite material

Dental Careers Terminology*

Term	Definition	Prefix	Root	Suffix
Buccal	Pertaining to the cheek		bucc	al
Endodontic	Pertaining to treatment of disease of the inside of the tooth	endo	dont	ic
Gingivitis	Inflammation of the gums		gingiv	itis
Mandibular	Pertaining to the lower jaw		mandibul	ar
Maxillofacial	Pertaining to the upper jaw and face	maxillo	faci	al
Mesial	Pertaining to the middle		mesi	al
Odontology	Study of the tooth		odont	ology
Orthodontics	Pertaining to correcting tooth placement	ortho	dont	ics
Pedodontics	Pertaining to teeth of children	ped/o	dont	ics
Prosthodontist	One who places artificial appliances on teeth	prosth/o	dont	ist

*A transition syllable or vowel may be added to or deleted from the word parts to make the combining form.

Abbreviations for Dental Careers

Abbreviation	Meaning
ADA	American Dental Association
amal	Amalgam
ant	Anterior
DA	Dental assistant
DDS	Doctor of dental surgery
DH	Dental hygienist
DLT	Dental laboratory technician
DMD	Doctor of medical dentistry
ext	Extract, extraction
post	Posterior

Careers

The dental team includes the dentist, dental hygienist, dental assistant, and dental laboratory technician (Box 26-1). The goal of the dental team is to provide optimal care of the oral cavity for all patients. Dental team members work in a variety of settings, including group practice, specialty practice, schools, government or community clinics, and dental insurance and supply companies (Table 26-1).

Dentist

The role of the dentist has changed greatly because improved methods of dental care and nutrition have reduced the number of caries. Dentists now perform a variety of services, including public education

TABLE 26-1
Dental Career Educational Cost and Earnings

Career	Educational Cost*	Earnings†
Dental hygienist	Community College of Denver, 2-year program Fees include: Tuition $5044.70 Books $1050 Equipment $8550 Fees including background check, drug testing, and clinic use $1263 Board fees $1200	Median annual salary: Denver, Colo.—$76,540

*http://www.ccd.edu/DentalHygiene/Expenses.aspx.
†http://data.bls.gov:8080/oes/datatype.do.

BOX 26-1

Dental Careers

Dental assistant
Dental health director
Dental hygienist
Dental laboratory technician
Dentist
Endodontist
Oral pathologist
Oral surgeon
Orthodontic technician
Orthodontist
Pedodontist
Periodontist
Prosthodontist

directed to prevent tooth decay, detection of disease such as cancer, cosmetic improvement of appearance, and correction of oral problems such as misaligned teeth and jaws (Fig. 26-1). Some dentists perform surgery to correct facial and dental deformities caused by accidents or birth defects. Pain control and anesthesia in dentistry have become two of the roles of the professional, because many people become anxious and even phobic when needing dental care. Types of anesthesia that may be administered include local anesthesia, sedation, and general anesthesia. Some sedation may even cause retrograde amnesia or the inability to remember the treatment.

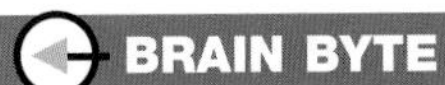

BRAIN BYTE

Water supply fluoridation to prevent dental caries began in Grand Rapids, Michigan, in 1945.

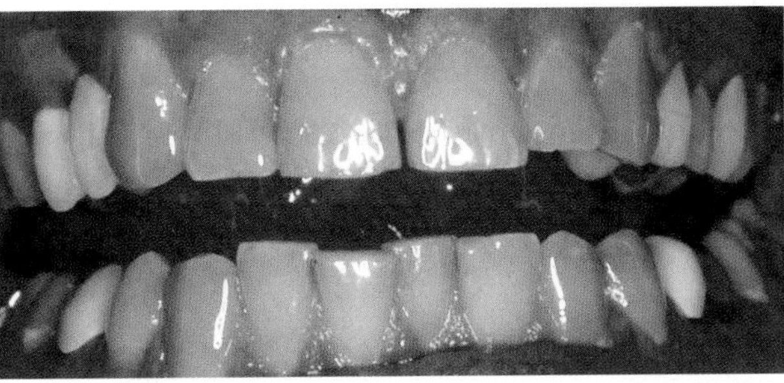

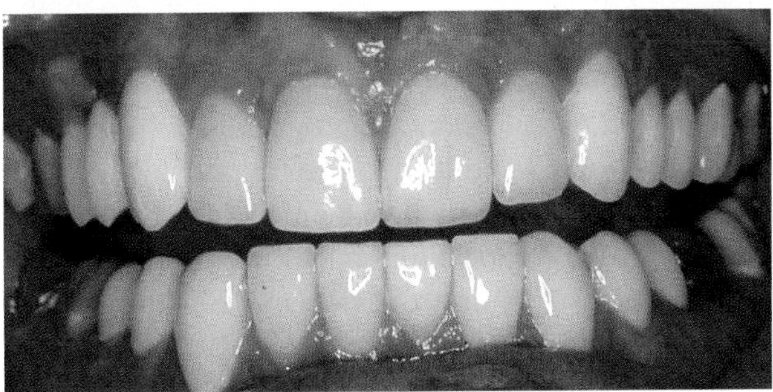

FIGURE 26-1 Bonded veneers improve the appearance, change the shape of, and restore the function of teeth. (Courtesy Joyce Bassett, DDS, FAGD, Scottsdale, Ariz.)

Dentists are highly respected professionals. Dentistry offers a great deal of flexibility and independence. Private practitioners can choose to work either full or part time. Many dentists now choose to work in a group practice to share the cost of maintaining an office. All types of communities need dentists.

Dentistry offers nine specialties that allow practice in specific areas:

- Endodontics: treatment of disease of the dental pulp, usually with root canal
- Oral and maxillofacial surgery: extraction and treatment of injury, disease, and deformity of the mouth, such as cleft palate

- Oral pathology: laboratory testing and biopsy to diagnose oral conditions
- Orthodontics: prescription and fitting of braces to correct misaligned teeth or jaws
- Pedodontics: prevention of disease and decay and therapeutic care of children's teeth from birth through adolescence
- Periodontics: treatment of gum disease and education for prevention
- Prosthodontics: design and fitting of bridgework and dentures, as well as substitutes for missing teeth or tissue
- Public health dentistry: promotion of prevention and treatment of dental disease
- Oral and maxillofacial radiology: includes the diagnosis and treatment of oral and maxillofacial disorders by using radiation

Dentists work with people of all ages and personalities. They must possess leadership ability and good interpersonal skills. The work requires creativity and decision-making ability. Much of dentistry involves precise work by hand, so manual dexterity is necessary.

The educational requirement for a dentist includes at least 2 years of college classes before entering dental school. More than 90% of students entering dental school have completed a 4-year degree at a college or university. Dental school training ranges from 3 to 4 years and offers either a doctor of dental surgery (DDS) or a doctor of medical dentistry (DMD) degree. Two additional years of training are necessary to practice in one of the nine areas of specialization. After successful completion of an accredited dental program and a national examination, dentists are licensed by the state.

Dental Hygienist

With the purpose of providing preventive oral health, dentists developed dental **hygiene** as a career in the early 1900s. Jobs for dental hygienists are projected to grow 36% through 2018. Dental hygienists work in a variety of settings that range from private practice to corporate clinics located in foreign countries. Some areas in which the dental hygienist may specialize include clinical work, education, administration, research, consumer advocacy, or veterinary dental practice. Hygienists may work flexible hours, depending on the type of practice.

The scope of practice of dental hygienists varies from state to state. The role of the hygienist is influenced by the level of education and type of practice.

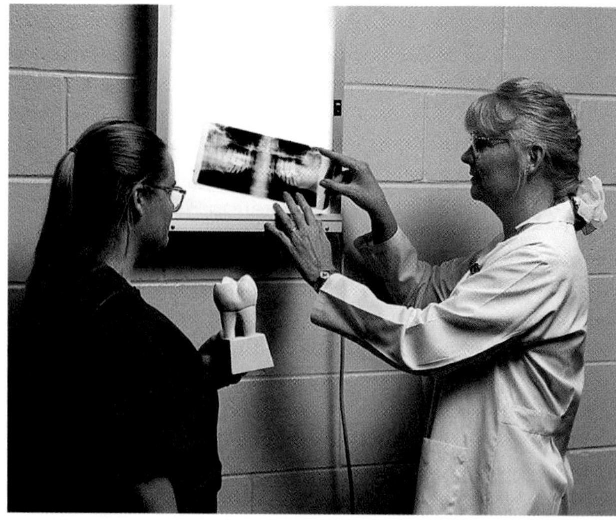

FIGURE 26-2 The use of dental radiographs is regulated by law to protect the patient and caregiver from unnecessary exposure to radiation.

It may include recording the patient's health history, removing **calculus** and **plaque** from above and below the gum line, examining the teeth and oral structures, and screening for oral cancer and blood pressure abnormalities. Hygienists expose, process, and may interpret dental radiographs (Fig. 26-2). In addition to removing plaque from the teeth surfaces, dental hygienists also polish and floss the teeth as part of the cleaning procedure. In some practices hygienists apply a fluoride treatment to the teeth. Dental hygienists instruct patients on the procedures for home care, including making dietary recommendations. Hygienists may be responsible for the recall system to alert patients of the next appointment. They may also place temporary fillings and apply cavity-preventive agents such as fluoride and sealants. Expanded functions of dental hygienists may include administration of local anesthesia.

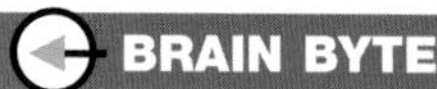

One state, Colorado, has independent practice laws that allow registered dental hygienists to practice without the supervision of a dentist in all settings.

The practice of hygiene requires manual dexterity to use dental instruments in the small area of a mouth. Good health and personal cleanliness are also important characteristics of hygienists. The education for hygienists ranges from a 2-year community college to a 4-year college or university program. The community college program usually includes 2

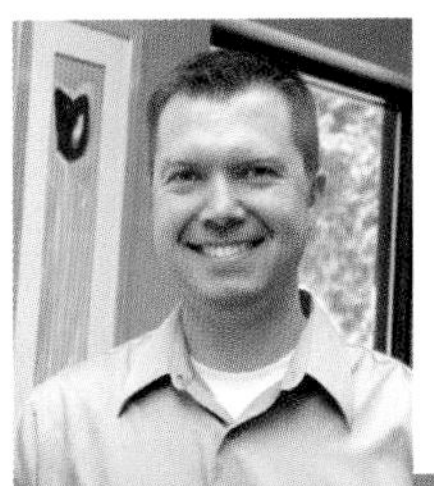

RICHARD JASON WHITE, DDS, MS

ORTHODONTIST
OLSON & WHITE ORTHODONTICS

Educational background: College degree, bachelor's of science (4 years); dental school, DDS (4 years); orthodontic specialty certificate and master's degree (2 years)

A typical day at work and job duties include: A typical week for me involves seeing about 60 to 75 patients. I perform various tasks from the initial consultation with a new patient, to placing, adjusting, or removal of braces and other orthodontic appliances, interpretation of radiographs, and cosmetic adjustment of people's smiles.

The most gratifying part of my job: The most gratifying part of my job is right after a patient has their braces removed, they look at themselves in the mirror and they cannot stop smiling. I can tell that they are so happy and excited to see their new smile! They cannot wait to show their parents and friends.

The biggest challenge(s) I face in doing my job: One of my biggest challenges is convincing patients about the need for good oral hygiene during their treatment. Without good oral hygiene, the end result can be severely compromised with cavities, white-spot lesions, swollen gum tissue, and tooth sensitivity.

What drew me to my career? I was drawn to this career because it allows me to use both my mind and my hand skills to improve people's lives. A great smile has many benefits. Not only are straight teeth easier to brush and floss, but a great smile improves people's self-esteem and makes them more attractive to others. It has been proven that people with nice smiles get better paying jobs and are more likely to be hired and promoted.

Something I learned in my early education that I currently use in my career or that caused me to be interested in my career is: I discovered in high school that I was very good at fixing things with my hands and therefore pursued a career that would allow me to use this talent. Find what you are particularly good at, and that which interests you, and look for careers that will allow you to use these skills, which will not only make your career rewarding but also fun.

Other comments: A mentor of mine once told me when I was in college, "Find a job that you enjoy so much that you would do it for free. Then when you get paid for it, it is just icing on the cake!" I truly feel this way about my career and would encourage others to follow this advice.

Health Careers in Practice

years of prerequisite work in addition to dental training.

Dental hygienists are licensed by the state in which they practice after they have successfully completed an accredited program and a national examination. Hygienists are registered with the National Board of Registered Dental Hygienists.

Dental Assistant

The role of the dental assistant varies greatly with the size and type of practice in which the assistant works. The job responsibilities may include answering the telephone, making appointments, and working with billing accounts. Assistants are responsible for maintaining infection control. They clean and sterilize instruments, prepare the treatment room and dental materials, and assist with procedures (Fig. 26-3). Exposing radiographs, taking and recording dental histories, and assessing vital signs are also responsibilities of the dental assistant. The dental assistant must work under the supervision of a dentist.

Personal qualities that are important for a dental assistant include the ability to work well with others.

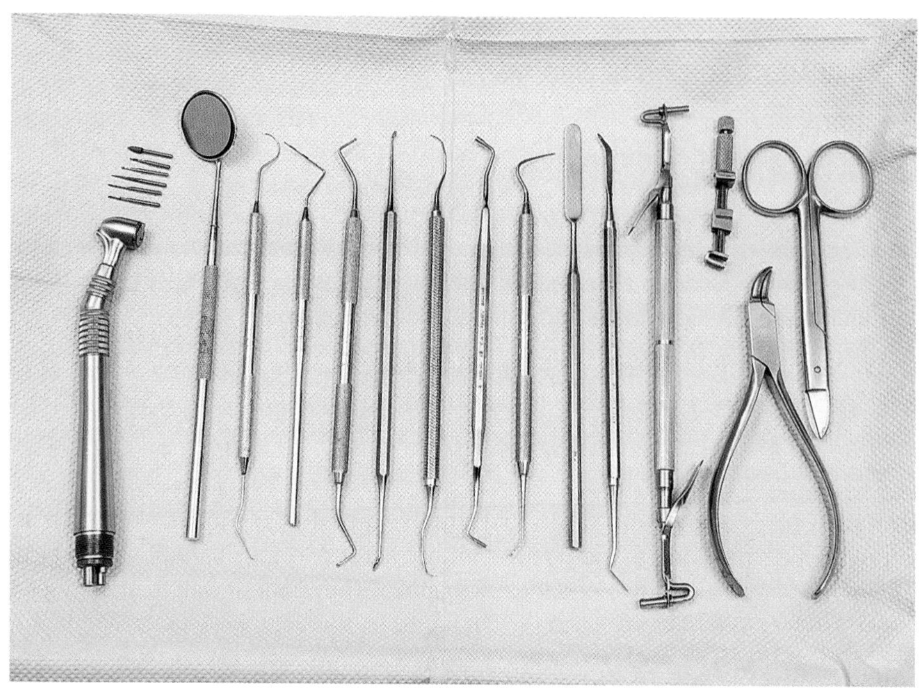

FIGURE 26-3 Cleaning and sterilizing dental instruments are part of the dental assistant's role.

Good physical and psychosocial health is also necessary. No educational standards are required by all states for a dental assistant, and some tasks can be learned with on-the-job training. Accredited programs for dental assistants run 1 to 2 years. Certification is available through the Dental Assisting National Board. Some states require licensure or registration.

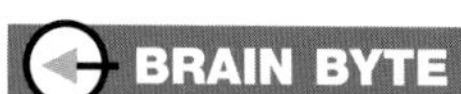

Chewing gum can help eliminate food particles caught between teeth after a meal and also helps prevent plaque build-up by stimulating saliva production.

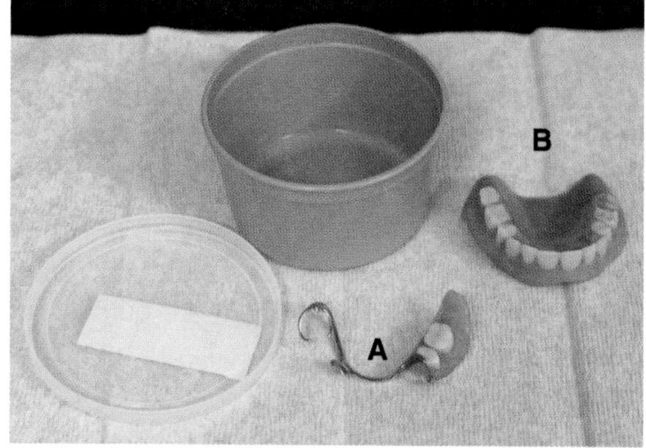

FIGURE 26-4 Dentures. **A,** Partial denture. **B,** Full denture. (From Sorrentino SA: *Mosby's textbook for nursing assistants*, ed 7, St. Louis, 2008, Mosby.)

Dental Laboratory Technician

Dental laboratory technicians are the only members of the dental health care team who do not work directly with patients. Technicians make prostheses following the orders of a dentist. These prostheses include bridges, dentures, crowns, inlays, space maintainers, and corrective orthodontic appliances (Fig. 26-4). Dental laboratory technicians work with a variety of materials, including gold alloy, nonprecious metal, porcelain, wax, acrylic, and wires. Most dental technicians work in commercial laboratories and receive a salary for a standard 40-hour week.

The work of the dental laboratory technician involves minute detail and requires excellent manual dexterity. An awareness of detail, accuracy, and patience are necessary, as well as artistic ability. Most dental laboratory technicians learn their work on the job. However, 20 programs in dental laboratory technology were approved by the Commission on Dental Accreditation in 2008. Certification for dental laboratory technicians (CDT) is available through the National Association of Dental Laboratories (NADL). Three states require dental laboratories to have one CDT to operate.

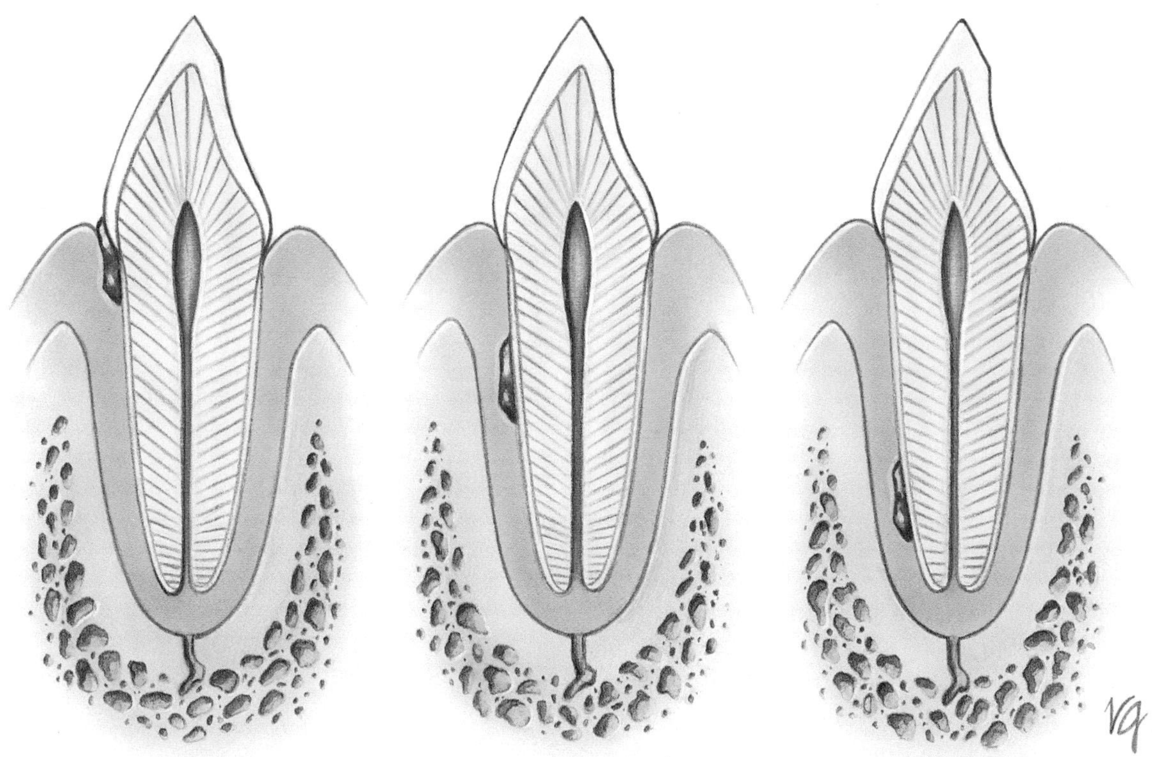

FIGURE 26-5 Dental caries and gingivitis develop as plaque is pushed into the soft tissues that support the mouth.

Content Instruction

Maintaining Dental Health

Neglect or improper care of the teeth can lead to formation of cavities (caries) or periodontal disease (pyorrhea) with resulting tooth loss. Cavities, or caries, are inflammation or disease of the inner tooth. They result from the destruction of the enamel that protects the tooth.

CASE STUDY 26-1 Your friend tells you she wants to get her teeth whitened to help prevent cavities. What should you say?

Answers to Case Studies are available on the Evolve website: ***http://evolve.elsevier.com/Gerdin***

Periodontal disease is caused by infection in the supporting structures of teeth such as the gingiva and bones. Periodontal disease affects one of every two people in the United States. It can be acute or chronic. Most periodontal disease begins in the mouth by age 13. It may be asymptomatic for 20 to 30 years. Eventually bleeding gums may result. The major cause of periodontal disease is formation of bacterial plaque. Plaque is composed of 75% bacterial colonies and 20% organic material that stick to the surface of the tooth. Plaque is usually colorless and forms in 12 to 24 hours. Bacteria normally found in the mouth produce lactic and formic acids, which irritate the gum and cause tenderness and inflammation. The gingiva then pulls away from the irritant, allowing more plaque to form. Acids also dissolve the protective enamel on the surface of the tooth. Plaque may harden and discolor and become tartar (calculus). Plaque can reach the root of the tooth and the bone supporting the tooth (Fig. 26-5). The tooth eventually falls out. The most common types of periodontal disease are gingivitis and periodontitis. Gingivitis is the early stage of the disease. Periodontitis may result in formation of pockets of pus called abscesses.

BRAIN BYTE

A toothbrush should be replaced at least every 3 months, when bristles wear out and after illness.

Only 60% of people in the United States brush and 25% floss their teeth regularly. Brushing removes plaque and prevents bad breath (halitosis). Flossing

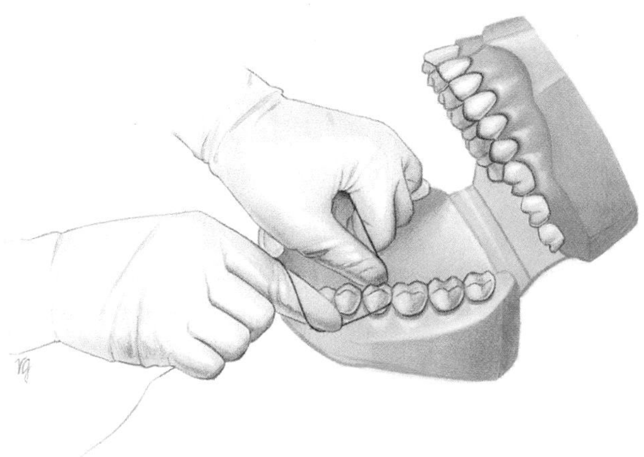

FIGURE 26-6 Flossing instruction is made easier with an enlarged model of teeth.

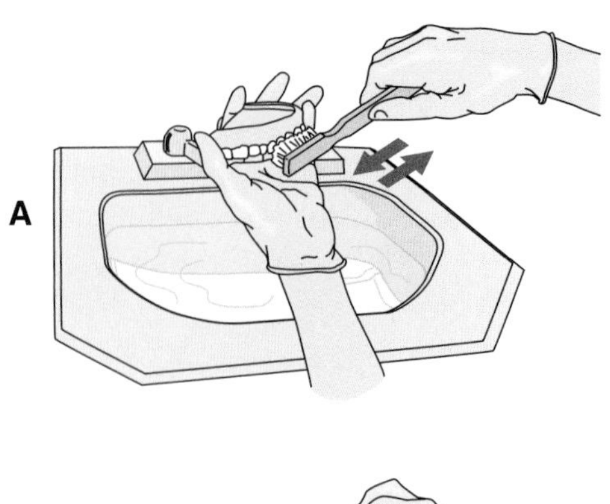

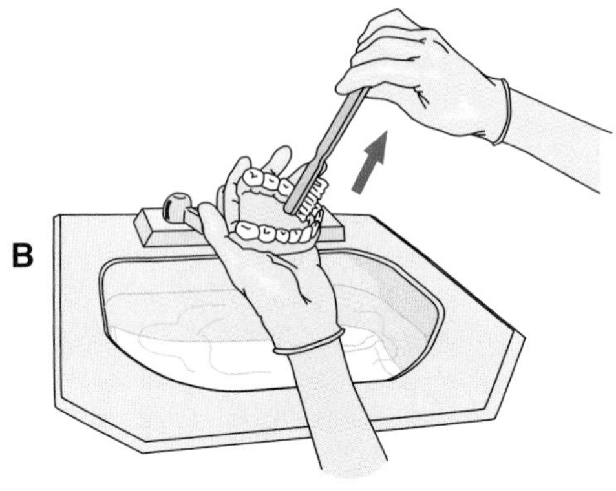

FIGURE 26-7 Dentures are cleaned over a sink of water to prevent breakage. (From Sorrentino SA: *Mosby's textbook for nursing assistants*, ed 7, St. Louis, 2008, Mosby.)

removes plaque from areas the toothbrush cannot reach (Fig. 26-6). Sugar and sticky foods increase the chance of plaque formation. Local irritants that inflame the gums include smoking and chewing tobacco products. Poorly aligned teeth (malocclusion) and grinding of the teeth (bruxism) also increase the chance of periodontal disease. Medications, such as oral contraceptives, steroids, and chemotherapeutic agents, affect the gingiva by making it more susceptible to gingivitis and periodontitis. Systemic conditions also contribute to formation of caries and periodontal disease. They include hormonal imbalances such as in pregnancy, diabetes, and immunologic deficiency. A balanced diet provides the proper nutrients necessary to maintain dental health. (See Skill List 26-1, Assisting with Oral Hygiene Instruction; and Skill List 26-2, Teaching Patients to Floss Teeth, p. 430.)

CASE STUDY 26-2 Your friend asks you if scraping your tongue helps prevent bad breath. What should you say?

Answers to Case Studies are available on the Evolve website: ***http://evolve.elsevier.com/Gerdin***

In 2006 the Centers for Disease Control and Prevention (CDC) reported that 25% of adults 60 years old or older were toothless (edentulous). Dentures are replacement prostheses for total tooth loss. Dentures function to chew food, present a normal facial appearance, and allow clear speech. Dentures wear out and must be replaced. It is important that denture wearers continue to maintain dental health routines to prevent destruction of gum tissues. The gums should be brushed daily. Dentures should be cleaned daily by brushing, soaking in cleaning solution, or placing in an ultrasonic cleaner (Fig. 26-7).

Structures of the Oral Cavity

Functions of the teeth include the mechanical portion of digestion, shape of the face, and aid in the production of speech. **Dentition** is the natural teeth in their normal position in the mouth.

The teeth are located in sockets (**alveoli**) of the mandible and maxilla. The areas of the **mandible** and **maxilla** in which the teeth are located are called the *mandibulary* and *maxillary arches*. The mandible is the longest and strongest bone of the face. It is the only movable bone of the skull. The sinuses are air cavities, lined with mucous membrane, that decrease the weight of the skull and also warm air during respiration. The frontal and maxillary sinuses connect with the maxillary bicuspid teeth.

The mouth, or oral cavity, is covered with mucous membrane (Fig. 26-8). The roof of the mouth is divided into two portions. The anterior portion, or hard palate, is attached to the bones of the skull by the membranous tissue that covers it. The membrane of the posterior portion hangs loosely and is called the *soft palate*. The mandible and maxilla are surrounded by the inner surface of the lips. The lips are connected to the midline of the mandible and maxilla by a fold of mucous membrane called the frenulum. The tongue (lingua) lies on the floor of the mouth.

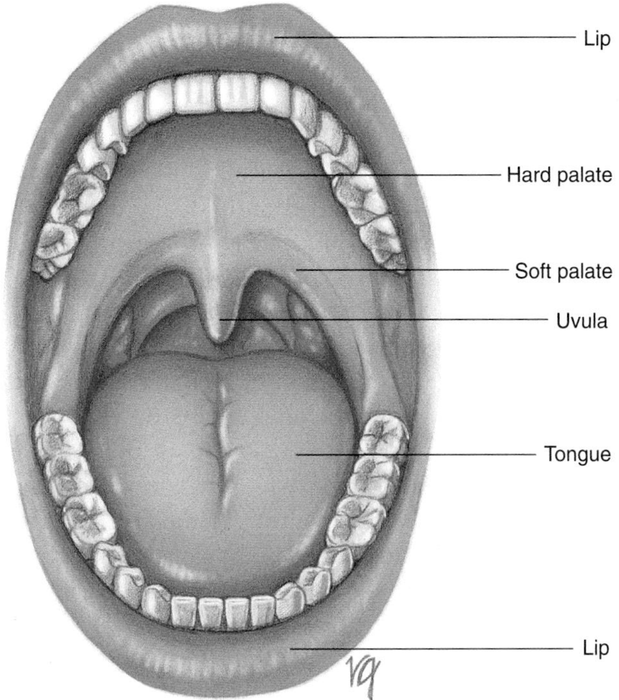

FIGURE 26-8 Structures of the oral cavity (the frenulum cannot be seen below the tongue).

Tooth Formation

Tooth formation begins during the second month of gestation. At birth the neonate has 44 tooth buds at various stages of development in the gums (**gingiva**). Twenty primary or **deciduous** teeth begin to erupt at about 6 months of age. Most deciduous teeth erupt by the age of 2 to 3 years, although the rate of tooth development varies greatly among individuals. Twenty-four of the buds are permanent teeth. The **permanent** teeth replace the deciduous teeth by about the twelfth year, but they might not completely appear until age 20 (Fig. 26-9).

CASE STUDY 26-3 The mother of a newborn tells you she heard that she should not give her newborn a bottle in bed. What should you say?

Answers to Case Studies are available on the Evolve website: ***http://evolve.elsevier.com/Gerdin***

Structures of the Tooth

The tooth is divided into two sections: the *crown* and *root* (Fig. 26-10). The crown is covered with shiny, white enamel, which is the hardest substance in the body. Enamel is composed mostly of calcium and phosphorus. The middle layer of the crown is composed of dentin. It forms the bulk of the tooth. Dentin

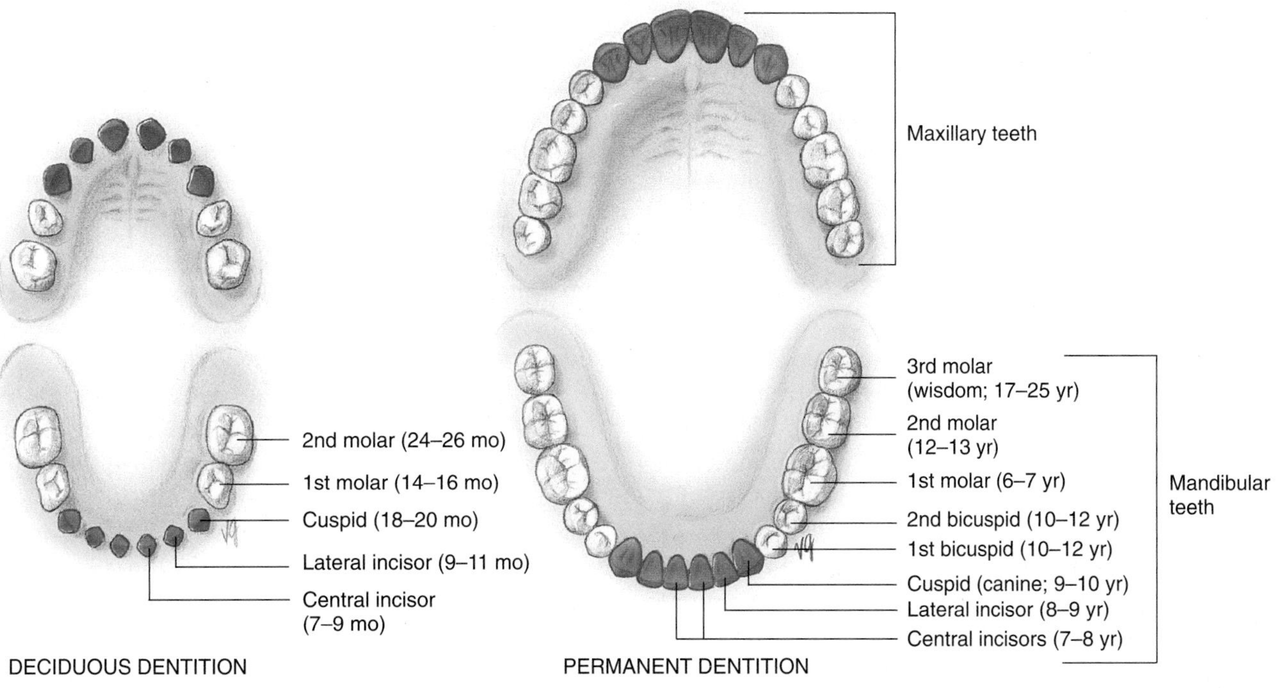

FIGURE 26-9 Identification of teeth with eruption times (anterior teeth are shaded).

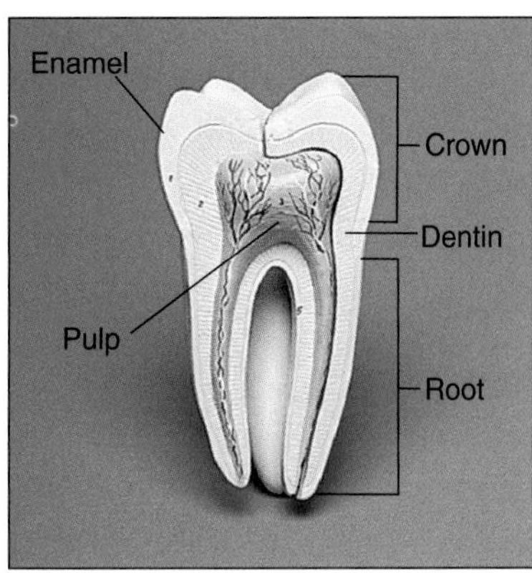

FIGURE 26-10 Structure of a molar tooth.

is harder than bone but softer than enamel. Although it does not have nerves, dentin reacts to tactile (touch), thermal (temperature), and chemical stimulation. The inside layer of the crown and root is made of soft tissue called *pulp*. Pulp contains the nerves and blood vessels of the tooth. It forms and nourishes the dentin of the tooth.

CASE STUDY 26-4 You friend tells you he does not want to drink a soda with you because it hurts his teeth. What should you say?

Answers to Case Studies are available on the Evolve website: ***http://evolve.elsevier.com/Gerdin***

Cementum, a hard, bonelike substance on the outside surface of the root, anchors the tooth. The neck (cervix) of the tooth is the narrowed area where the enamel of the crown and the cementum of the root join. The periodontal ligament is located between the alveolar bone and cementum. It holds the tooth in place. The gum tissue around the root of the tooth is the gingiva.

Types of Teeth

Descriptive anatomy of the tooth is called *odontology*. Teeth can be divided into four main types. They are the incisors (8), cuspids (4), bicuspids (8), and molars (12). The incisors, located in the front of the mouth, help to cut food. The cuspids, also called *canines* or *eyeteeth*, are the longest teeth in the mouth and they tear food. Bicuspids, or premolar teeth, are not present in the deciduous teeth. Bicuspid teeth tear and crush food. The molars are located in the back of the mouth. The largest and strongest teeth, the molars, grind the food. The third molars are commonly called *wisdom teeth*, but they do not appear in all people. They may be removed if the space in the jaw is insufficient for the new teeth.

Identification of Teeth

Teeth in the upper jaw are called *maxillary teeth*. Those in the lower jaw are referred to as *mandibular teeth*. The teeth in the front of the mouth (incisors and cuspids) are identified as being anterior. The bicuspids and molars are considered to be located posteriorly.

Each tooth can be named individually by its type and location. Location of a defect or structure of the crown of the tooth can also be identified by using five surfaces of the crown (Fig. 26-11). The Universal System for numbering teeth was adopted by the American Dental Association in 1968. It numbers the adult teeth from 1 to 16 beginning with the right maxillary third molar to the left maxillary third molar. Numbering the mandibulary teeth begins with the left third molar as 17 to the right third molar as number 32. Primary teeth are lettered in the same manner from A to T (Fig. 26-12). Other systems used for charting include the Federation Dentaire International System and the Palmer System. The type of cavity (caries) or restoration can be charted by using the five classes developed by G.V. Black.

Performance Instruction

Dental health care personnel use radiographs to visualize the teeth in the gums. Both intraoral and extraoral films may be used. The standards for safety and limits of exposure to radiation are regulated by the U.S. National Council on Radiation Protection. Dental care workers wear a film badge that records the amount of exposure to radiation.

New technology has changed dental practice. Computerized probes measure and record the depth of a pocket or recession of the gum. Lasers are used to soften calculus and seal some applications. Intraoral camera systems enlarge and visualize the inside of the mouth for the patient and dentist (Fig. 26-13). Digital images have reduced the use of radiation for some images. Another innovation is the use of electronic dental anesthesia, which blocks the pain caused by dental work with electronic impulses.

One of the duties performed by the dental assistant is charting of dental conditions at the direction of the

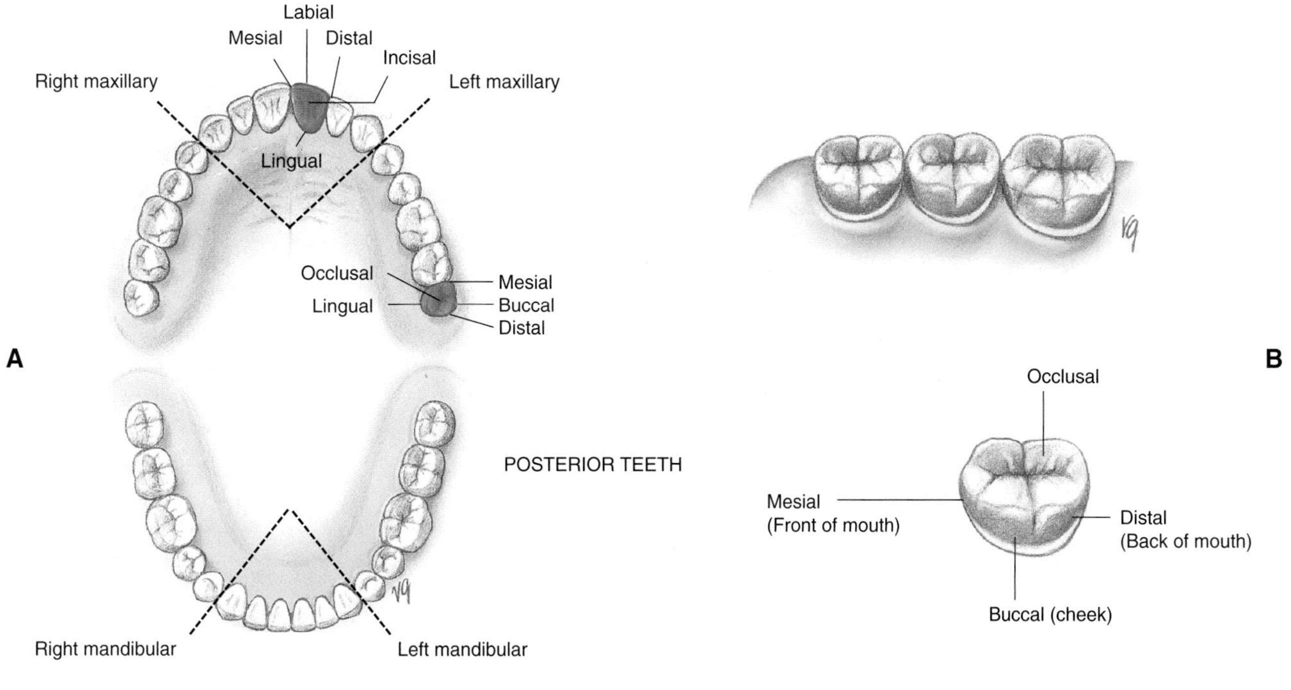

FIGURE 26-11 **A,** Five surfaces of the crown. **B,** Surface of a posterior crown (lingual side is not visible).

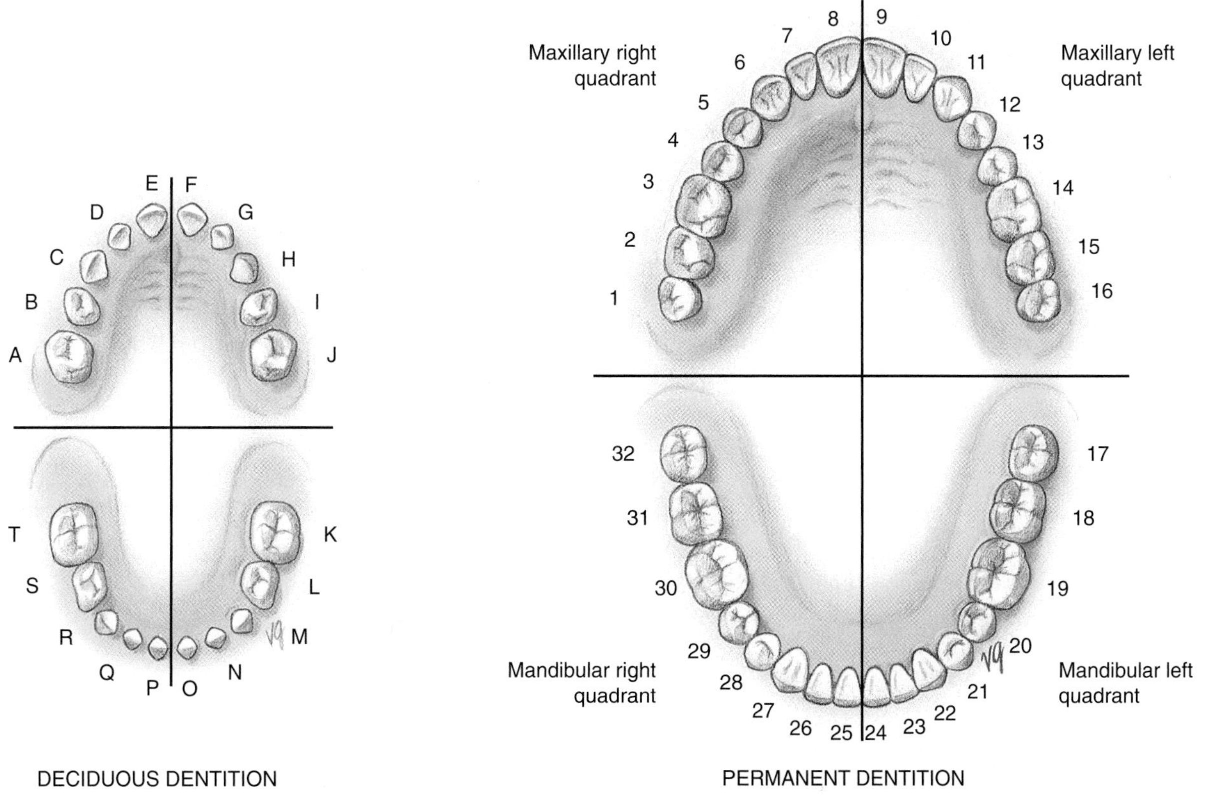

FIGURE 26-12 Universal system of tooth identification.

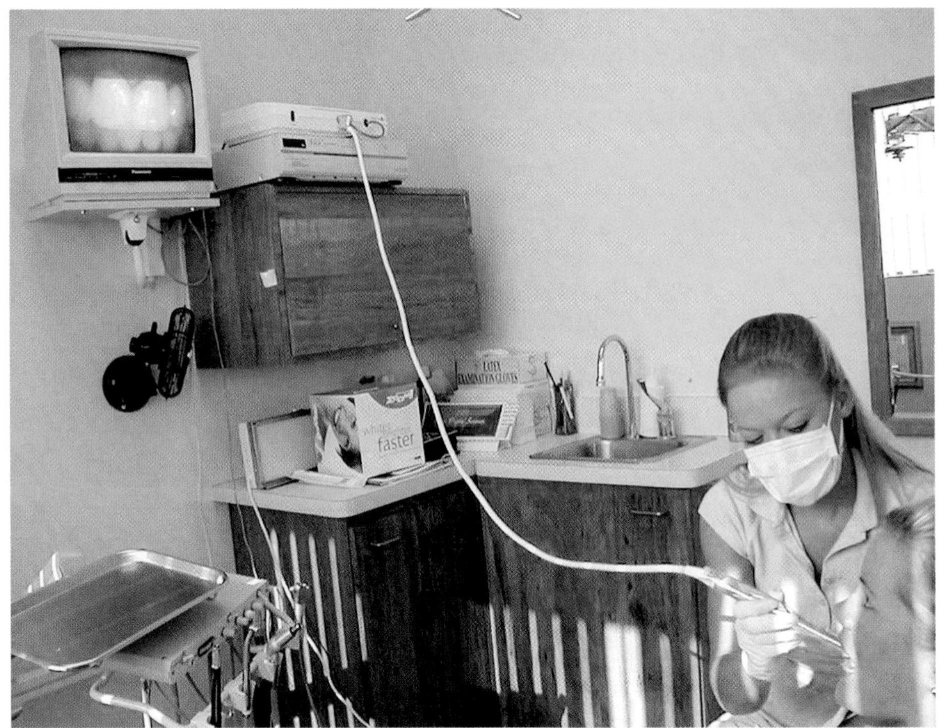

FIGURE 26-13 The intraoral camera allows the dental health worker and patient to see the tooth structure on a larger scale. (Courtesy Joyce Bassett, DDS, FAGD, Scottsdale, Ariz.)

dentist (see Fig. II-5, *A* and *B* in Appendix II). The assistant must be familiar with the structures of the individual teeth and their location in the mouth. The assistant also prepares the dental operatory and equipment for procedures (Fig. 26-14). (See Skill List 26-3, Maintaining and Preparing the Dental Operatory, p. 431.) This includes adjusting the height of the chairs and placement of the lights, disinfecting surface areas, and sterilizing dental instruments after use. When necessary, the assistant prepares restorative materials such as amalgam or cement (Fig. 26-15). Amalgam (amal) is an alloy of silver and mercury that may be used to fill teeth. The assistant also prepares gels or alginate materials to make impressions of the teeth in the mouth. These models are then filled with plaster to make molds. (See Skill List 26-4, Making a Dental Impression and Mold, p. 431.)

Summary

- The role of the dentist is to give care and supervise the dental hygienist, assistant, and laboratory technician to provide optimal oral care for the patient. Dental personnel must possess leadership ability, creativity, and good interpersonal skills.
- Dentition of the adult and that of the child differ in the number and size.
- Five structures of the oral cavity include the tongue, teeth, maxilla, mandible, and mucous membrane.
- Three types of dental variations are crowns, cavities, and fillings.
- Methods to prevent caries and periodontal disease include brushing and flossing the teeth regularly.
- Techniques for brushing teeth include using a soft brush, holding the brush at a 45-degree angle to the gum, and moving the brush in the direction of the tooth growth. Flossing should be performed at least once daily. The floss should be moved in a C-shape motion around the tooth.

Review Questions

1. List the four members of the dental health care team.
2. Describe the purpose of the dental health care team.
3. Describe the role of four dental specialties.
4. List each of the four types of teeth and the purpose and number of each in the adult mouth.
5. Draw and label the five surfaces of a molar tooth.
6. Describe the formation of plaque and calculus.

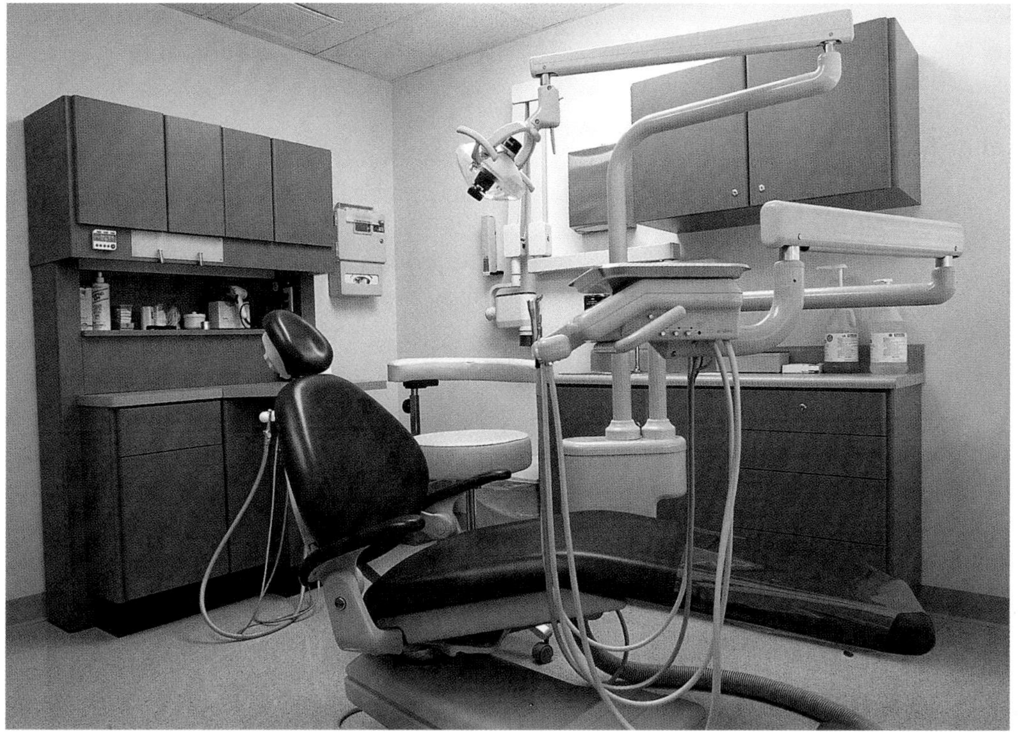

FIGURE 26-14 The dental operatory is arranged for convenience and comfort.

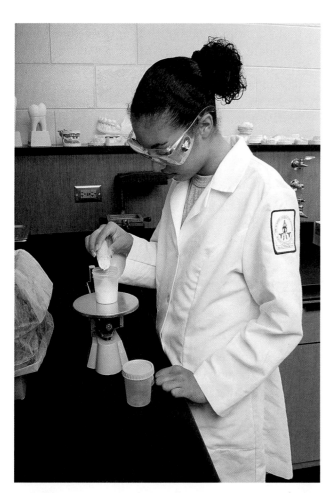

FIGURE 26-15 The dental assistant must know how to prepare a variety of dental materials.

7. List three factors that contribute to the formation of plaque.
8. Describe the correct technique for brushing and flossing teeth.
9. Choose one career from Box 26-1. Research the cost of education and annual earnings in local institutions. Write a paragraph describing the factors that might explain why the local and national economic figures vary.
10. Use each of the following terms in one or more sentences that correctly relate their meaning: calculus, gingival, halitosis, hygiene, and plaque.

Critical Thinking

1. Investigate and compare the cost of various types of dental treatments and procedures.
2. Investigate five common medications used in dental health care.
3. Investigate and compare the cost of education for the dental assistant, dental hygienist, and dentist.
4. Investigate the relative number of private and corporate practices for dentists.
5. Create a career ladder for dental careers. Describe why it is or is not possible to move from one level to another in the field.

Explore the Web

Career Information

Bureau of Labor Statistics
http://www.bls.gov/

Salary.com
http://salary.com

Professional Associations

American Dental Association
http://www.ada.org/

American Dental Hygienists' Association
http://www.adha.org/

American Dental Assistant Association
http://www.dentalassistant.org/

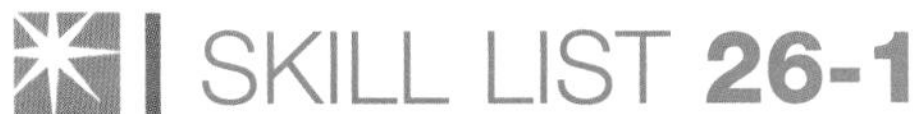

SKILL LIST 26-1 Assisting with Oral Hygiene Instruction

1. Maintain medical asepsis by using the guidelines provided in the Standard and Transmission-Based Precautions, including good handwashing technique and use of gloves as needed.
2. The teeth should be brushed for at least 5 minutes, twice daily. Regular brushing removes organic material and prevents bad breath (halitosis).
3. Use a soft brush with rounded bristles and a small head. Soft bristles prevent injury to the gum tissues, and a small head allows all areas of the mouth to be reached. Replacing worn brushes ensures effectiveness.
4. Use a toothpaste of individual choice. Toothpastes contain a foaming agent and mild abrasive. Some toothpastes contain fluoride, which helps to strengthen teeth. Tartar-softening agents have been added to some varieties.
5. With the brush held at a 45-degree angle to the gum line, move the brush in the direction of the tooth growth. Thoroughness in brushing is more important than technique to remove debris.
6. The back side of the front teeth is cleaned by tilting the brush upward.
7. Brush the gums and the tongue. Brushing the soft tissues of the mouth removes debris and increases circulation to the area.

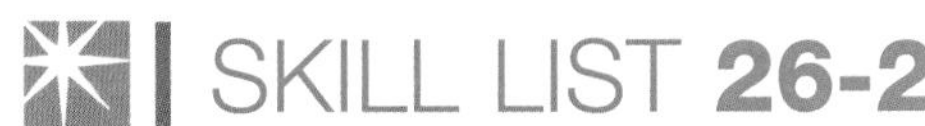

SKILL LIST 26-2 Teaching Patients to Floss Teeth

1. Maintain medical asepsis by using the guidelines provided in the Standard and Transmission-Based Precautions, including good handwashing technique and use of gloves as needed.
2. Floss at least once daily. Plaque forms within 24 hours on teeth. Flossing reaches areas of the teeth that are missed by a toothbrush.
3. Use a 12- to 18-inch length of waxed or unwaxed floss supported between two fingers. Used properly, waxed and unwaxed floss are both effective. Supporting the floss between the fingers prevents cutting injury to the gums.
4. Move floss back and forth in a C-shape motion on the side of each tooth. The floss should reach below the gum line without cutting the tissue.

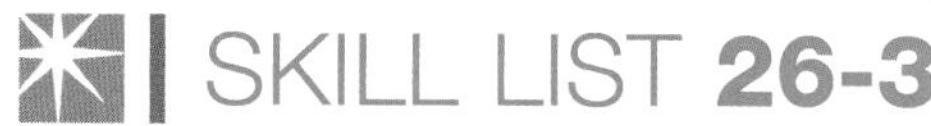

SKILL LIST **26-3**
Maintaining and Preparing the Dental Operatory

1. Maintain medical asepsis by using the guidelines provided in the Standard and Transmission-Based Precautions, including good handwashing technique and use of gloves as needed.
2. Remove all evidence of prior visits, and position the dental chair in an upright position before escorting the patient to the treatment room. Make sure the light is out of the way while entering and exiting the room. Height of the chair and armrests can be adjusted to fit any size of person comfortably.
3. Make sure the chair is in an upright position when escorting the patient from the operatory.
4. Clean the operatory surfaces and chair with disinfectant daily, according to the manufacturer's directions. Cleanliness of equipment and supplies reduces the spread of microorganisms that can cause infection.

SKILL LIST **26-4**
Making a Dental Impression and Mold*

1. Maintain medical asepsis by using the guidelines provided in the Standard and Transmission-Based Precautions, including good handwashing technique and use of gloves as needed.
2. Fit the empty impression tray into the mouth to gage fit.
3. Mix alginate with a stick (putty by hand) for designated time.
4. Place putty into the impression tray, making sure it completely fills and is even with the edges of the tray.
5. Gently place impression tray deeply into the mouth, making sure the teeth go all the way to the bottom of the tray.
6. Allow the impression to set for manufacturer's designated time.
7. Gently remove impression from mouth.
8. Mix and spoon plaster into the impression with a stick or tongue depressor.
9. Remove any air bubbles by tapping the mold.
10. When dried, remove the plaster cast from the mold.
11. Clean equipment with disinfectant according to the manufacturer's directions, and return it to the designated location.

*Instructions may vary with different impression products.

CHAPTER 27

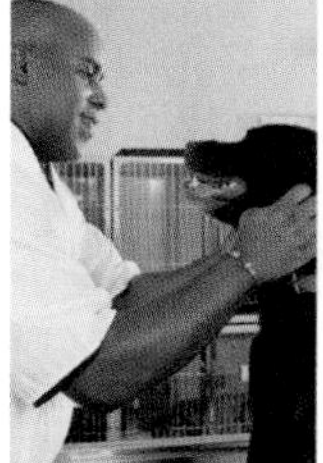
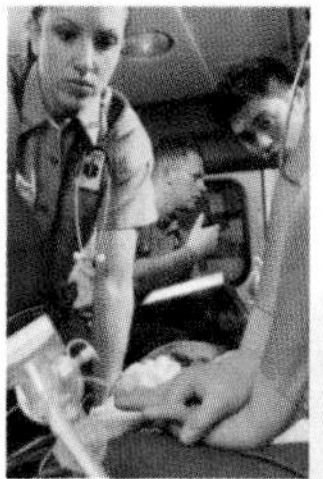
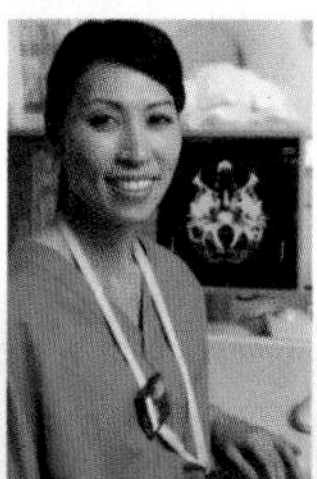

Complementary and Alternative Careers

LEARNING OBJECTIVES

- Define at least eight terms relating to careers in complementary and alternative medicine (CAM).
- Specify the role of selected CAM providers, including personal qualities, levels of education, and credentialing requirements.
- Describe the methods used in allopathic, holistic, and homeopathic health care.
- List five domains of complementary and alternative health care as described by the National Institutes of Health.

KEY TERMS

Allopathic *(al-o-PATH-ik)* System of medical practice that uses remedies designed to produce effects that are different from those caused by the disease being treated

Biofeedback *(bie-o-FEED-bak)* Conscious control of biological functions normally controlled involuntarily

Chiropractic *(kie-ro-PRAK-tik)* System of therapy based on the theory that health is determined by the condition of the nervous system

Holistic *(ho-LIS-tik)* Practice of medicine that considers the person as a whole unit, not as individual parts

Homeopathic *(ho-me-o-PATH-ik)* System of medical practice that uses remedies designed to produce similar effects to those caused by the disease being treated

Hydrotherapy *(hie-dro-THER-uh-pee)* External use of water to treat disease

Megavitamin *(MEG-e-vi-te-men)* Dose of a vitamin much greater than required amount to maintain health

Subluxation *(sub-luk-SAY-shun)* Incomplete dislocation of a joint

Complementary and Alternative Terminology*

Term	Definition	Prefix	Root	Suffix
Aromatherapy	Treatment with odors	aroma	therapy	
Chiropractic	Pertaining to adjustment of the spine by hand		chiro/pract	ic
Homeopathic	Treatment with similar disease	homeo	path	ic
Hydrotherapy	Treatment with water	hydro	therapy	
Hypnotherapy	Treatment using hypnosis	hypno	therapy	
Neuromuscular	Pertaining to the nerves and muscles	neuro	muscul	ar
Orthopedic	Pertaining to correction of bones	ortho	ped	ic
Osteoarthritis	Inflammation of the bones and joints	osteo	arthr	itis
Radiography	Picture taken using radiation	radi/o	graph	y
Thermography	Picture taken showing heat	therm/o	graph	y

*A transition syllable or vowel may be added to or deleted from the word parts to make the combining form.

Abbreviations for Complementary and Alternative Medicine

Abbreviation	Meaning
ADHD	Attention deficit hyperactivity disorder
BCIA	Biofeedback Certification Institute of America
CAM	Complementary and alternative medicine
DC	Doctor of chiropractic
EEG	Electroencephalogram
EMG	Electromyogram
GSR	Galvanic skin response
ND	Doctor of naturopathy
NIH	National Institutes of Health
TMJ	Temporomandibular joint dysfunction

BOX 27-1

2009 Alternative Therapies Studies*

- Arthritis and Traditional Chinese Medicine
- Chinese Herbal Therapy for Asthma
- Dosing Study of Massage for Neck Pain
- Herbal Research on Colorectal Cancer
- Metabolic and Immunologic Effects of Meditation
- Omics and Variable Responses to Placebo and Acupuncture in Irritable Bowel Syndrome
- Restorative Yoga for Therapy of the Metabolic Syndrome
- Roles of Grape-Derived Polyphenols in Alzheimer Disease
- Soy and Estrogen Interactions in the Breast
- Z Joint Changes in Low Back Pain Following Adjusting

*http://nccam.nih.gov/research/extramural/awards/

Careers

Complementary medicine, alternative medicine, and **holistic** health are therapies based on wellness and natural treatment. Complementary and holistic health practices are used at the same time as conventional medical techniques. Alternative health care is used in place of conventional methods. Integrative medicine incorporates alternative practices that have been shown to be effective by research.

In a 2007 survey, the National Institutes of Health (NIH) reported that more than 38% of Americans use complementary and alternative therapies. If **megavitamin** therapy and prayer are included in the definition, the total rises to at least 62%. Nonvitamin, nonmineral, and natural products were the most commonly used CAM therapy. Practices that have increased significantly between 2002 and 2007 include deep breathing, meditation, massage, and yoga.

The National Center for Complementary and Alternative Medicine (NCCAM) provides grants for research and training to determine the effectiveness of their treatments (Box 27-1). More than 20 states have laws that allow the practice of CAM. Some of the conditions that draw consumers to complementary health care include chronic pain, arthritis, addiction,

BOX 27-2

Complementary and Alternative Methods

Whole Medical Systems
Acupuncture
Ayurveda
Counseling
Herbal medicine
Homeopathy
Hydrotherapy
Naturopathy
Oriental massage

Mind-Body Interventions
Aromatherapy
Art therapy
Counseling
Hypnotherapy
Meditation
Mental healing
Music therapy

Biological-Based Therapies
Biological therapies
Dietary therapy
Herbal therapy
Orthomolecular therapy

Manipulative and Body-Based Methods
Alexander technique
Chiropractic
Massage therapy
Osteopathy
Reflexology

Energy Therapies
Crystal therapy
Electrical therapy
Magnet therapy
Qi gong
Reiki
Therapeutic touch

TABLE 27-1
Complementary and Alternative Career Educational Cost and Earnings

Career	Educational Cost*	Earnings†
Chiropractor	Northwestern College of Chiropractic, three-trimester program Fees include tuition, books, fees, parking, etc. $24,015	Median annual salary: Bloomington, Minn.—$92,920

*Costs assume starting with a bachelor of science degree in biology. http://www.nwhealth.edu/admit/tuition/tuitchir.html.
†http://data.bls.gov:8080/oes/datatype.do.

headache, anxiety, chronic fatigue, sprains, and muscles strains.

The NIH organizes CAM practices into five domains (Box 27-2). These five domains or categories include whole medical systems, mind-body interventions, biological-based treatments, manipulative and body-based methods, and energy therapies.

Many of the health care workers specializing in CAM have education and training in other health careers (Table 27-1). For example, holistic practitioners include nurses, physicians, veterinarians, pharmacists, and many other professionals. Two CAM professions that have specific educational requirements include the chiropractor and naturopath.

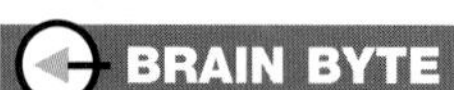

St. John's wort is named after St. John the Baptist and has been shown to help mild depression.

CASE STUDY 27-1 You ask a patient what medications she is taking. She says only aspirin for an occasional headache. She then asks whether you want to know about her supplements, such as St. John's wort. What should you say?

Answers to Case Studies are available on the Evolve website: ***http://evolve.elsevier.com/Gerdin***

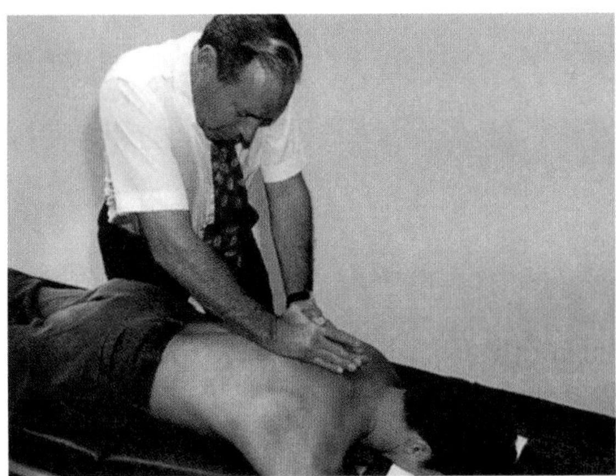

FIGURE 27-1 Chiropractic physicians adjust the spinal column and other body joints. (From Bonewit-West: *Today's medical assistant*, ed 1, Philadelphia, 2009, Saunders.)

BOX 27-3

Areas of Diplomate Certification for Chiropractors

- Chiropractic Acupuncture
- Chiropractic Pediatrics
- Chiropractic Physiological Therapeutics and Rehabilitation
- Diagnosis and Internal Disorders
- Diagnostic Imaging (Radiology)
- Neurology
- Nutrition
- Occupational Health
- Orthopedics
- Sports Physician

Chiropractor

Chiropractors, or doctors of chiropractic, treat health problems associated with the muscular, skeletal, and nervous system. Chiropractors adjust the spinal column and other body joints to correct subluxations (Fig. 27-1). Subluxations are incomplete or partial dislocations of the spine.

The chiropractor uses radiography and other tests to diagnose and assess progress in the adjustment. Chiropractors use a holistic approach to treatment emphasizing health and wellness. Treatments are drugless and nonsurgical. When appropriate, the chiropractor may refer a patient to an allopathic practitioner.

Education for the chiropractor includes a minimum of 2 years of college and completion of a 4- or 5-year chiropractic program. In 2009, 16 programs were accredited by the Council on Chiropractic Education in the United States. Licensure by the state is required for chiropractic practice. Certification (diplomate) in 10 clinical specialties is granted the American Chiropractic Association (Box 27-3).

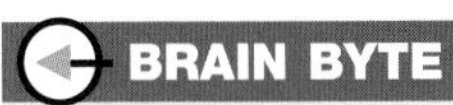

BRAIN BYTE

Peppermint is a cross between spearmint and watermint and has been used to soothe stomach cramping.

Naturopath

Licensed naturopathic doctors are primary care physicians who focus on treatment of the whole person with emphasis on wellness and disease prevention. They perform all of the routine medical examinations, laboratory tests, and office procedures, such as minor surgery, used by the allopathic doctor. They do not use synthetic medication, nor do they perform major surgeries. Naturopathic doctors may refer patients to allopathic practitioners for specialized treatment or major surgery.

Naturopathic physicians attend a 4-year graduate medical school. In addition to the standard curriculum of medical school, naturopathic doctors study nutrition, homeopathy, botanical medicine, and hydrotherapy. The degree earned is called a doctor of naturopathy. Four accredited schools of naturopathic medicine exist in the United States. At least 12 states license naturopathic doctors.

CASE STUDY 27-2 Your friend tells you that she does not believe that any CAM therapies are useful. What should you say?

Answers to Case Studies are available on the Evolve website: ***http://evolve.elsevier.com/Gerdin***

Other Complementary and Alternative Practitioners

Massage therapists (also known as masseuses or masseurs) use skillful touch to loosen muscles and relieve pain (Fig. 27-2). In addition to working with the manipulation of muscle, skin, tendon, and ligaments, massage therapists may also apply light, water, or

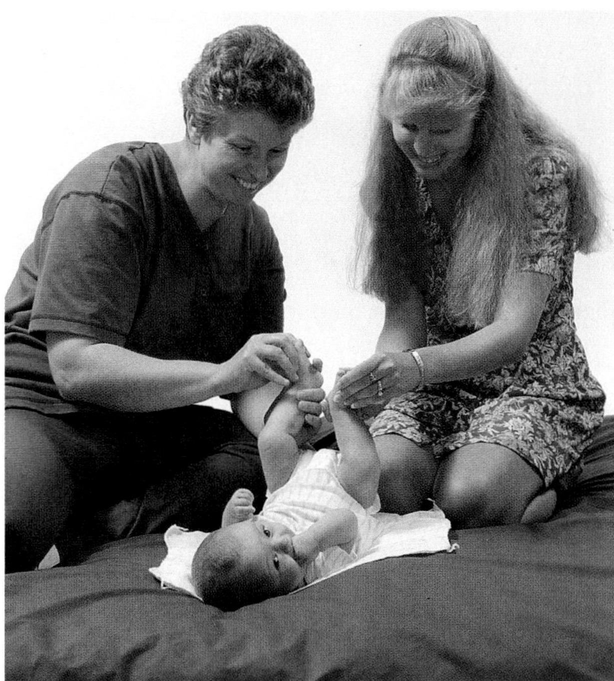

FIGURE 27-2 A massage therapist teaches a new mother how to massage her infant. (From Fritz S: *Mosby's fundamentals of therapeutic massage*, ed 2, St. Louis, 2000, Mosby.)

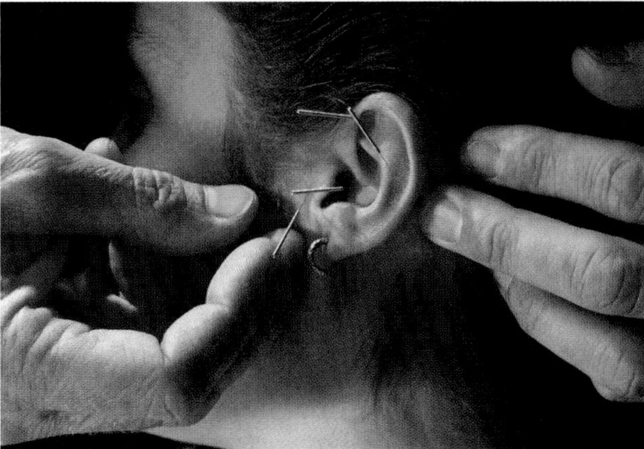

FIGURE 27-3 Acupuncture has been in use for 5000 years. (From Bonewit-West: *Today's medical assistant*, ed 1, Philadelphia, 2009, Saunders.)

BOX 27-4

Applications for Biofeedback

- Anxiety and panic disorders
- Asthma
- Attention deficit hyperactivity disorder
- Epilepsy
- Headache
- Hypertension
- Irritable bowel syndrome
- Neck and shoulder pain
- Neuromuscular disorders
- Raynaud syndrome
- Rheumatoid arthritis
- Temporomandibular joint dysfunction
- Urinary and fecal incontinence

vibration devices. Forms of massage include Swedish, polarity, sports, infant, facial, and scalp. Education and training for massage therapists vary from state to state. The American Massage Therapy Association has approved 55 schools. Thirteen states require licensure.

Hypnotherapists help clients to overcome bad habits and treat emotional problems by using hypnosis. The method of hypnosis may differ greatly from one practitioner to another. Many hypnotherapists are licensed in a related field, such as medicine, nursing, or psychology. Licensure is not required, although a permit to practice may be necessary.

Acupuncturists insert needles into peripheral or surface nerves to control pain, provide anesthesia, relieve symptoms, and modify psychosomatic (mind-caused) disorders. Acupuncture has been in use for 5000 years. It originated with the Chinese. The practitioners of today usually hold credentials in another health care field and are trained in the application of needles (Fig. 27-3).

Acupuncture is believed to release endorphins and other mood-elevators when the appropriate meridian points, or "mens," are stimulated. The training for acupuncture varies greatly and may include up to 2 or 3 years of study after completion of a minimum of 2 years of college. Ten schools are approved by the National Accreditation Commission for Schools and Colleges of Acupuncture and Oriental Medicine in the United States. Only 20 states regulate the practice of acupuncture. A national board examination for acupuncturists is available on a voluntary basis. Acupressure is a similar treatment that applies pressure, instead of needles, to the points.

Biofeedback is a technique used to change normally involuntary reactions of the body by using conscious control, such as lowering heart rate or changing the size of blood vessels (Box 27-4). For example, a person may raise the temperature of one hand higher than the other. Raising the temperature of both hands by using biofeedback has been demonstrated to

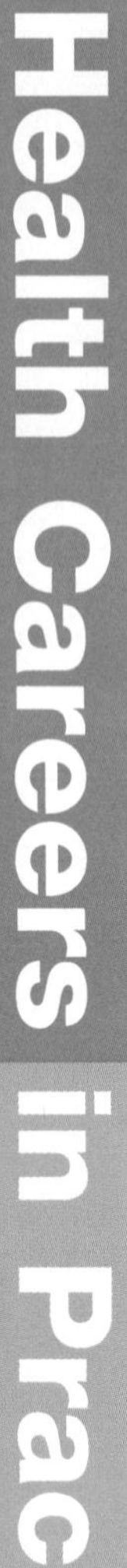

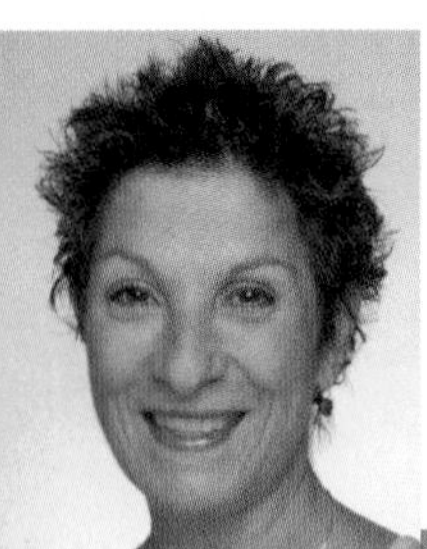

ELAINE STILLERMAN, LMT

MASSAGE THERAPIST, TEACHER, AUTHOR

I am self-employed and work out of my home office. My classes are taught at massage schools, spas, and resorts across the country.

Educational background: Bachelor of arts degree; massage therapy license from the Swedish Institute, New York, New York

A typical day at work and job duties include: I sold my massage practice in 2003, but I continue writing and teaching. My course is a professional seminar that runs 3 days, 24 hours, so those days are spent teaching, lecturing, and demonstrating massage techniques and modalities for pregnancy, labor, and postpartum recovery.

The most gratifying part of my job: Connecting with students and imparting the passion I feel for the subject to them. I am honored and gratified when students continue their studies because of my influence.

The biggest challenge(s) I face in doing my job: Students come from various educational backgrounds and personal experiences, so individualizing the training can prove difficult at times.

What drew me to my career? In 1980 no one was massaging pregnant women when one of my clients became pregnant. She did not want to stop her massages, so we continued working together during her entire pregnancy. Because there was little information available to me for reference, I had to study the appropriate modalities on my own. I researched traditional Chinese medical texts; sociologic and anthropologic texts; and finally nursing, midwifery, and obstetric texts to develop the MotherMassage technique I use(d) and teach.

Something I learned in my early education that I currently use in my career or that caused me to be interested in my career is: Even earlier than that, I remember being in day camp as an 8-year-old and having my counselors sit in front of me on the bus so I could massage their shoulders.

Other comments: I am proud of how the general public is educated about the beneficial effects of prenatal massage, labor support, and postpartum recovery. These services should be made available to all childbearing women who want them.

reduce the blood flow to the brain and relieve headache symptoms. Biofeedback practitioners may practice other areas of health care, such as nursing or medicine. Certification for biofeedback is possible through the Biofeedback Certification Institute of America, which requires that the applicant is licensed or working under the supervision of a licensed health care practitioner.

BRAIN BYTE

Most people pay for CAM products and services themselves without insurance coverage.

Content Instruction

Whole Medical Systems

Many of the alternative medical systems were developed before the conventional biomedical approach. Some are still practiced by cultures throughout the world. For example, traditional Oriental medicine emphasizes proper balance of a person's *qi* (pronounced "chee"), or vital energy. Some of the practices that are part of the alternative medical systems domain include acupuncture, herbal medicine, and Oriental massage.

India's traditional system of medicine is called *Ayurveda* and places equal emphasis on the body, mind, and spirit. The treatments are designed to restore harmony and include such things as diet, exercise, meditation, massage, sun exposure, herbs, and controlled breathing. Other systems have been developed by the Native Americans, Africans, and Central and South Americans.

Homeopathic medicine is a Western system based on the concept that "like cures like." Practitioners believe that small dosages of plant extracts and minerals that produce the same symptoms of a disease cure it by stimulating the body's defense and health mechanisms.

Naturopathic medicine emphasizes restoration of health and sees disease as a change in the body's natural process. It is based on the medical philosophy called *vitalism* that sees a person as a combination of body, spirit, and mind. Some examples of techniques used by naturopaths include nutrition, acupuncture, herbal medicine, hydrotherapy, spinal manipulation, electrical therapy, ultrasound and light therapy, counseling, and pharmacology.

CASE STUDY 27-3 Your patient tells you that she has been using only complementary and alternative care for her baby since birth. What should you say?

Answers to Case Studies are available on the Evolve website: ***http://evolve.elsevier.com/Gerdin***

Mind-Body Intervention

Mind-body interventions are not all recognized by the NIH to be CAM therapy. The NIH recognizes interventions such as hypnosis, meditation, prayer, dance, music, art therapy, and mental healing. The mind-body interventions that are considered to be part of mainstream medicine are educational or behavioral in nature. All these techniques are designed to help the mind treat the body.

Biological-Based Therapy

Many of the biologically based therapies that are considered to be CAM overlap with conventional medicine and involve special dietary supplements or programs. Herbal therapy uses plants that act on the body. Special diet programs that are considered to be CAM include those proposed by Drs. Atkins, Pritikin, and Weil. Use of chemicals such as magnesium, melatonin, and vitamins in megadoses is called orthomolecular therapy. Biological therapies that are used to treat cancer include laetrile and shark cartilage. Bee pollen is used to treat autoimmune and inflammatory diseases.

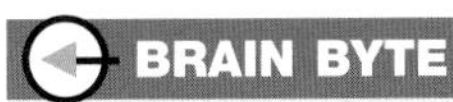

Echinacea has been used to reduce the risk of a common cold.

Energy Therapy

Energy therapies are divided into two types. Bioelectromagnetic-based therapies use energy fields that come from an external source, and biofield therapies come from the body (biofields). Biofields have not been experimentally proven to exist. These therapies may involve pressure and manipulation of the body. They include Qi gong, Reiki, and therapeutic touch. External sources of therapy include pulsed fields, magnets, and alternating or direct electrical current devices.

Reiki originated in Japan. Practitioners place their hands lightly on or above the skin of the person to facilitate the person's own healing ability. Reiki is based on the idea that there is a universal source of energy that allows the body to heal. It can be received from someone else or as a form of self-care. According to the 2007 National Health Interview Survey, more than 1.2 million adults had used an energy healing therapy like Reiki in the previous year. Training and certification for Reiki are not regulated. Traditionally Reiki has three degrees or levels of training. The NCCAM is currently conducting several studies involving Reiki.

CASE STUDY 27-4 Your friend tells you he has heard about an herbal cancer treatment on the Internet and wants your opinion about it. What should you say?

Answers to Case Studies are available on the Evolve website: ***http://evolve.elsevier.com/Gerdin***

Performance Instruction

Biofeedback techniques are designed to change blood pressure, muscle tension, heart rate, and other bodily

TABLE 27-2
Relaxation Response

Technique	Oxygen Consumption	Respiratory Rate	Heart Rate	Alpha Waves	Blood Pressure	Muscle Tension
Transcendental meditation	Decreases	Decreases	Decreases	Increases	Decreases*	Not measured
Zen and yoga	Decreases	Decreases	Decreases	Increases	Decreases	Not measured
Autogenic training	Not measured	Decreases	Decreases	Increases	Inconclusive	Decreases
Progressive relaxation	Not measured	Not measured	Not measured	Not measured	Inconclusive	Decreases
Hypnosis with suggested deep relaxation	Decreases	Decreases	Decreases	Not measured	Inconclusive	Not measured

*In patients with elevated blood pressure.

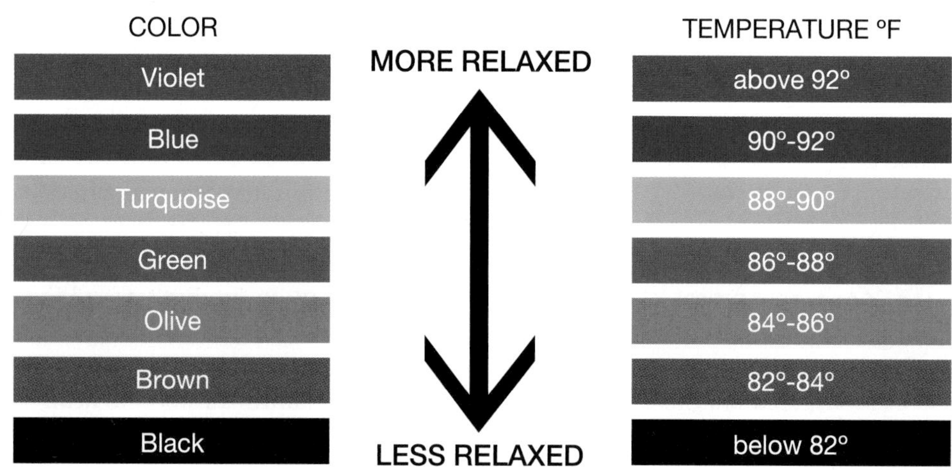

COLOR
Violet
Blue
Turquoise
Green
Olive
Brown
Black
MORE RELAXED
LESS RELAXED
TEMPERATURE °F
above 92°
90°-92°
88°-90°
86°-88°
84°-86°
82°-84°
below 82°

FIGURE 27-4 The Biodot color chart shows how temperature corresponds with relaxation.

functions that are not normally under voluntary control. (See Skill List 27-1, Using Biofeedback, p. 441.) The technique allows people to use signals from their own bodies to change their health (Table 27-2). Biofeedback machines or techniques include electromyograms to measure muscle tension, galvanic skin response monitors to measure sweat production, skin temperature sensors, and electroencephalograms to measure brain wave activity. Other techniques include measuring vital signs. Stress dots made of liquid crystal were developed as a way to measure the change in temperature of the skin. When the temperature of the hand becomes warmer, that indicates a more relaxed state (Fig. 27-4). Through conscious thought, a person may learn to adjust to a more relaxed state.

Summary

- Many CAM providers have education, credentials, and characteristics of other health professions. Chiropractors manipulate the spine. Naturopathic physicians are doctors that focus on treatment of the whole patient.
- Allopathic health care is treatment designed to produce effects that are different from a disease. Holistic health care is treatment of the whole person. Homeopathic health care uses treatments designed to produce effects similar to those caused by a disease.
- The five domains of complementary and alternative health care are whole medical systems, mind-body intervention, biological-based therapy,

manipulative and body-based methods, and energy therapies.

Review Questions

1. List three health professions that might practice allopathic and alternative therapies.
2. Describe two differences between the practice of medical and naturopathic doctors.
3. Describe each of the five domains into which the NIH places complementary and alternative therapies.
4. Choose one career from Box 27-3. Research the cost of education and annual earnings in local institutions. Write a paragraph describing the factors that might explain why the local and national economic figures vary.
5. Use the following terms in one or more sentences that correctly relate their meaning: allopathic, holistic, and homeopathic.

Critical Thinking

1. A group of practitioners in the United States call themselves certified naturopaths. They have not completed the training and education of the licensed naturopathic physician. Explain how this situation has occurred, how a consumer can be confident about the training of a practitioner, and what could be done to remedy the confusion.
2. Research one of the CAMs listed in Box 27-2, including its use, effectiveness, and credentialing of practitioners.
3. Create a career ladder for CAM careers. Describe why it is or is not possible to move from one level to another in the field.

Explore the Web

Career Information

Bureau of Labor Statistics
http://www.bls.gov/

Salary.com
http://salary.com

Professional Associations

American Chiropractic Association
http://www.acatoday.org/

American Association of Naturopathic Physicians (AANP)
http://www.naturopathic.org/

National Center for Complementary and Alternative Medicine (NCCAM)
http://nccam.nih.gov/

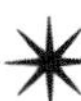

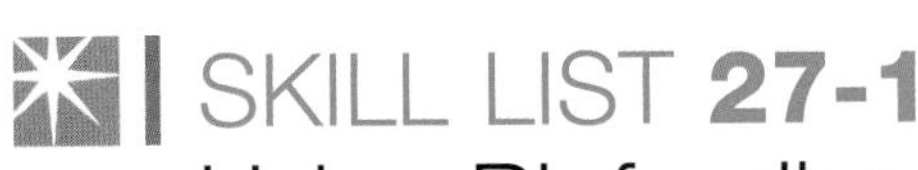

SKILL LIST 27-1 Using Biofeedback*

1. Maintain medical asepsis by using the guidelines provided in the Standard and Transmission-Based Precautions, including good handwashing technique and use of gloves as needed.
2. Apply a stress dot to the back of the hand between the thumb and index finger.
3. Match the color of the dot to the stress dot color chart.
4. Increase the level of relaxation by breathing evenly and deeply.
5. Relax the muscles of the hand by holding a fist for 5 seconds and then releasing it. Repeat with the other hand.
6. Compare the color of the stress dot with the chart.

*Procedures vary with the type of device used to measure physiologic changes.

CHAPTER 28

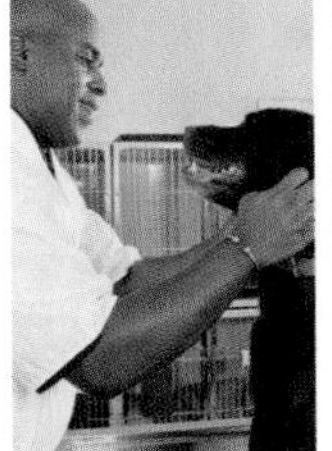
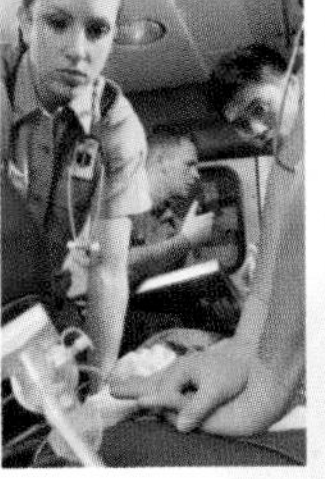
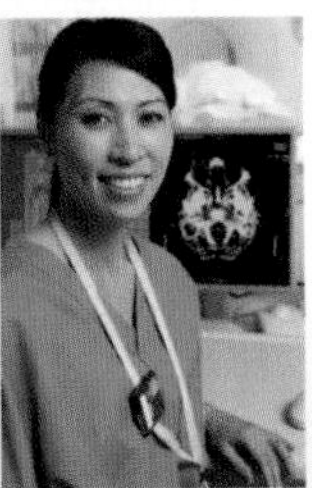

Veterinary Careers

LEARNING OBJECTIVES

- Define at least 10 terms relating to veterinary care.
- Specify the role of selected veterinary workers, including personal qualities, levels of education, and credentialing requirements.
- Describe the function of the veterinary team.
- Identify the functions that animals serve in the daily life of humans.
- Identify at least three characteristics of a healthy animal.
- Identify at least five signs of disorders in animals.
- Identify at least five methods of restraint for care or examination of animals.
- Describe at least five disorders affecting animals.
- Identify at least three methods of assessment of disorders in animals.

KEY TERMS

Bovine *(BOH-vine)* Pertaining to cattle

Canine *(KAY-nine)* Pertaining to dogs

Carcass *(KAR-kus)* Dead body of an animal

Equine *(EE-kwine)* Pertaining to horses

Feline *(FEE-line)* Pertaining to cats

Immunize *(IM-yoo-nize)* Secure against a particular disease

Parasite *(PARE-uh-site)* Plant or animal that lives on or within another living organism at the expense of the host organism

Quarantine *(KWAR-an-teen)* Period of detention or isolation as a result of a disease suspected to be communicable

Theriogenology *(thee-ree-o-gen-OL-o-gee)* Branch of veterinary medicine dealing with reproduction

Vaccination *(vak-sin-AY-shun)* Introduction of a microorganism that has been made harmless into a human or animal for the purpose of developing immunity

Veterinary *(VET-er-in-air-ee)* Pertaining to animals and their diseases

Veterinary Careers Terminology*

Term	Definition	Prefix	Root	Suffix
Cutaneous	Pertaining to the skin		cut/an	eous
Encephalitis	Inflammation on the inside of the brain	en	ceph/al	itis
Hepatitis	Inflammation of the liver		hepat	itis
Intravenous	Inside the vessel	intra	ven	ous
Pathology	Study of disease		path	ology
Rhinotracheitis	Inflammation of the nose and windpipe	rhino	trache	itis
Toxicology	Study of poison		toxic	ology
Tracheobronchitis	Inflammation of the windpipe and bronchus	tracheo	bronch	itis
Urologic	Pertaining to urine		urolog	ic
Zoology	Study of animals		zoo	ology

*A transition syllable or vowel may be added to or deleted from the word parts to make the combining form.

Abbreviations for Veterinary Careers

Abbreviation	Meaning
CENSHARE	Center for the Study of Human-Animal Relationships
CPV	Canine parvovirus
CVT	Certified veterinary technician
DVM	Doctor of veterinary medicine
EE	Equine encephalomyelitis
FP	Feline panleukopenia
FUS	Feline urologic syndrome
FVR	Feline viral rhinotracheitis
RVT	Registered veterinary technician
VMD	Veterinary medical doctor

Careers

Veterinary care personnel work in a variety of settings, including private practice, public health, research, zoos, circuses, and racetracks (Box 28-1). Those interested in aquatic animals may work in the area of marine biology (Table 28-1). The purpose of animal health care is to prevent illness and provide care for sick and injured animals. Animal health care providers also prevent the spread of disease carried by animals to humans (zoonosis).

Good physical health is necessary for those who work with animals. The work may involve lifting and manipulating heavy animals and supplies for their care. Veterinary personnel may be exposed to disease and injury by unrestrained animals. They must work well with others and with the animals receiving care.

BOX 28-1

Veterinary Careers

- Animal breeder
- Animal health technician
- Animal keeper
- Animal maintenance supervisor
- Animal-nursery worker
- Dog groomer
- Feed-research aide
- Horseshoer (farrier)
- Marine biologist
- Stable attendant
- Veterinarian
- Veterinarian, laboratory animal care
- Veterinarian, poultry
- Veterinary hospital attendant
- Veterinary laboratory technician
- Veterinary livestock inspector
- Veterinary meat inspector
- Veterinary pharmacologist
- Veterinary virus-serum inspector
- Zoo laboratory assistant
- Zoo veterinarian

Veterinarian

Veterinarians constitute the largest group of animal health care providers. Their professional oath describes the use of their knowledge and skills "for the benefit of society, for the protection of animal health, the relief of animal suffering, the conservation of livestock resources, the promotion of public health, and the advancement of medical knowledge."

TABLE 28-1
Veterinary Career Educational Cost and Earnings

Career	Educational Cost*	Earnings†
Veterinary Technician	Texas A&M University (Blinn College), 2-yr program Fees include: Tuition & fees $5500 Books $1400-1800 Uniforms & supplies $400-600 Misc. $800-1000	Median annual salary: College Station, Tex.— $26,370

*http://www.cvm.tamu.edu/vettech/appreq.shtml.
†http://data.bls.gov:8080/oes/datatype.do.

According to the U.S. Food and Drug Administration, there are more than 99.5 million cattle (**bovine**), 59.9 million hogs (swine), and 7.6 million sheep in the livestock industry. More than 5.3 million horses (**equine**), 93.6 million cats (**feline**), and 77.5 million dogs (**canine**) are kept as domestic pets. More than 8.8 billion chickens are raised annually in the United States. Veterinarians are instrumental in artificial insemination procedures to produce selected types of stock. Methods used for this selective breeding include embryo transplants and freezing.

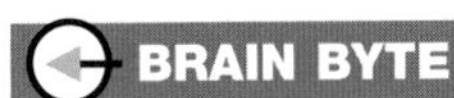
BRAIN BYTE

Thirty-nine percent of U.S. households have at least one dog.

Veterinarians are licensed by the state in which they practice. The veterinarian must first obtain a college or university degree followed by the completion of study at a 4-year accredited veterinary college. The degree earned is a doctor of veterinary medicine (DVM). One college awards a degree called a veterinarian medical degree (VMD). Passing a written and oral examination is necessary for licensure. The United States has 28 colleges of veterinary medicine in 26 states that are accredited by the American Veterinary Medical Association (AVMA). About 75% of the 8500 students enrolled are women. Veterinarians who work in research may have an additional doctoral degree in pathology, toxicology, or laboratory animal medicine.

Veterinary medicine has 39 recognized specialties. These include anesthesiology, dentistry, dermatology, internal medicine, laboratory animal medicine, microbiology, neurology, ophthalmology, pathology, preventive medicine, radiology, surgery, reproduction (**theriogenology**), toxicology, veterinary practice, zoo medicine, poultry, behaviorism, pharmacology, nutrition, and emergency care.

Veterinarians must work well with both people and animals. The profession requires good hearing, vision, and manual dexterity. Veterinarians may work long hours, and in rural areas a great deal of travel may be required. Care of animals may result in injury or exposure to disease.

More than 80% of veterinarians work in private practice. Many veterinarians work exclusively with either large or small animals, although some, especially those in rural areas, work in a mixed practice. Animal care veterinarians diagnose, perform surgery, and provide treatments and medication for sick and injured animals. They also **immunize** animals against disease and advise owners about ways to keep pets healthy. Veterinarians who care for companion animals usually work in hospitals or clinics. In rural areas large animal care may be provided using a van equipped as a clinic.

CASE STUDY 28-1 Your friend tells you she wants to be a veterinarian but cannot afford the out-of-state tuition that would be needed because there is no in-state veterinary college. What should you say?

Answers to Case Studies are available on the Evolve website: *http://evolve.elsevier.com/Gerdin*

Veterinarians may also specialize in fields such as wildlife and international economics. Wildlife veterinarians may travel to treat animals affected by oil spills and natural disasters. Economic veterinarians may travel throughout the world to help set policies and procedures to deal with international food and agriculture.

Health Careers in Practice

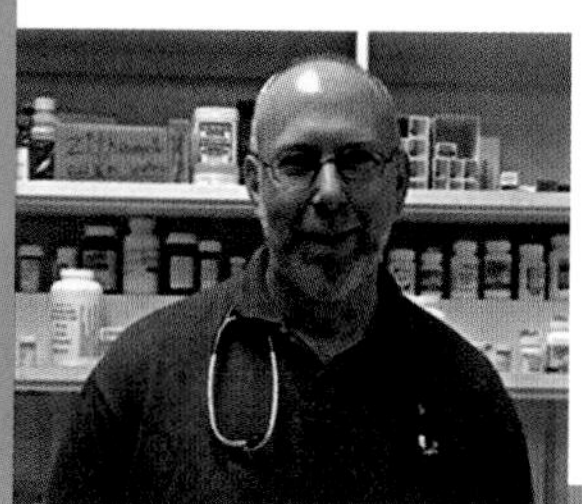

KEN GONSIER, DVM

ASSOCIATE/STAFF VETERINARIAN
ANTIOCH VETERINARY CLINIC

Educational background: Bachelor of arts, psychology, Dartmouth College (4 years); San Francisco State University (3 years additional college classes); doctor of veterinary medicine, University of California Davis School of Veterinary Medicine (4 years)

A typical day at work and job duties include:

- I am a small animal clinical veterinarian, meaning that I see patients in a clinic or hospital setting.
- I perform examinations, dental procedures, surgeries, and imaging, including radiographs and ultrasound examinations, in addition to ordering and evaluating laboratory tests.
- I diagnose and treat a myriad of diseases in primarily dogs and cats but also occasionally in the rabbit, guinea pig, rat, hamster, and mouse.

The most gratifying part of my job: I enjoy problem solving and helping my patients get well and stay healthy, and for the most part, I like working with the clients and owners.

The biggest challenge(s) I face in doing my job: The primary difficulty in veterinary medicine is the economic decision the owner has to make to pursue appropriate veterinary care. The fun challenge is continuing to learn to improve my level of practice and keep up with the latest information and techniques.

What drew me to my career? I always enjoyed being with and working with animals. Also, I became interested in medicine when my older sister pursued a career as a medical doctor.

Something I learned in my early education that I currently use in my career or that caused me to be interested in my career is: Learning the scientific method as a way to think rationally and logically about problems in the physical world is of the utmost importance, as are basic math skills.

Research veterinarians work to find better methods to prevent and cure animal disorders. Many of these methods have been a direct benefit to treatment of human disorders. Veterinary research has led to the development of many modern drugs and treatments. Some animals commonly used for research include dogs, cats, guinea pigs, mice, rats, rabbits, gerbils, and monkeys. Laboratory animals are usually bred specifically for the purpose of research to have healthy and similar specimens. Small animals are preferable to larger animals because the generations and life cycles are shorter.

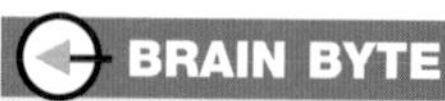

It cost $155,000 to clone a Labrador retriever in 2009.

Veterinarians specializing in toxicology and pathology protect humans from diseases transmitted by animals. They also work to control and eliminate disease in livestock. The federal government employs veterinarians in the Department of Agriculture and in the Public Health Service. In public health a veterinarian may work as an epidemiologist to prevent the spread of disease transmitted by animals.

Veterinary Technician

Veterinary technicians (VTs) may work in research settings, private clinics, food inspection, and laboratories or perform research under the supervision of a veterinarian, scientist, or senior technologist. The research technician prepares and tests serums (vaccinations)

BOX 28-2

Duties of the Certified or Licensed Veterinary Technician

Obtain and record animal case histories from and communicate with the animal's owner
Maintain the examination and kenneling facilities
Prepare animals for examination, treatment, or surgery
Assist with examination, treatment, or surgery
Monitor animal's condition after examination, treatment, or surgery
Collect specimens
Perform laboratory tests
Expose and develop radiographs
Train and supervise animal or kennel caretakers
Clean teeth, administer medication, and perform other extended duties after advance training

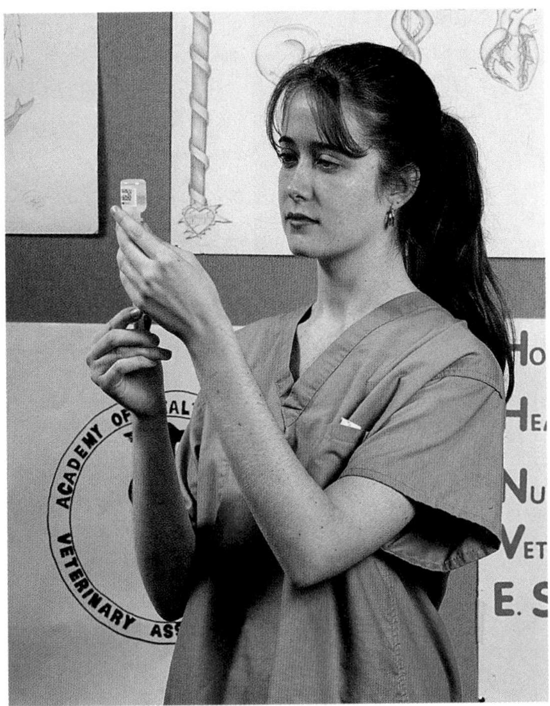

FIGURE 28-1 Injections are given only by trained personnel under the supervision of a licensed health care worker.

used to prevent animal diseases. Meat and dairy products are inspected for quality and purity by animal technicians. VTs in private practice assist the veterinarian by performing a variety of duties, including obtaining information, preparing animals and equipment, collecting specimens, and assisting with procedures. VTs may also administer medications, prepare laboratory samples, and apply bandages or dressings to wounds (Box 28-2).

VTs may be trained to perform extended duties such as teeth cleaning, removal of sutures, and administration of intravenous fluids. One method that the technician may use to administer medications is injection (Fig. 28-1). Medical asepsis is maintained throughout the procedure to prevent the spread of microorganisms. The correct dosage, medication, and route must be determined before giving an injection. The injection sites for animals are determined by the route of administration and type of animal.

The technician completes a minimum of 2 years of college-level vocational training for this occupation. Some colleges offer an associate degree in veterinary technology. More than 125 programs are accredited by the AVMA. Continuing education is necessary as the role of the technician expands. Animal technologists work in a more expanded role and must complete a 4-year baccalaureate degree program. Sixteen programs offer a 4-year degree in veterinary technology. In most states the veterinary technician and technologist must be certified (CVT), registered (RVT), or licensed (LVT).

Veterinary Assistant

Veterinary assistants provide a variety of services for animals as part of the care given in a clinic or animal hospital. The duties of the assistant include maintaining a clean and safe environment, observing behavior, preparing animals for examination or treatment, and maintaining daily records. Many animals show unusual behavior in an unfamiliar setting, so the assistant must show understanding and patience. Assistants may learn their training on the job or in a vocational program.

One of the duties of the veterinary assistant is to maintain the kennel or cage (Fig. 28-2). (See Skill List 28-1, Maintaining the Cage or Kennel, p. 459.) Living quarters for animals such as dogs and cats are cleaned and disinfected at least once daily to prevent the spread of microorganisms from one animal to another. The living area should be well ventilated and kept at a comfortable temperature. Animals need fresh food, water, and exercise on a daily basis. When necessary the assistant may bathe and groom the animals (Fig. 28-3). (See Skill List 28-2, Bathing and Grooming, p. 459.) Restraint may be necessary during bathing and grooming if the animal is uncooperative. The skin and coat are observed during bathing, and any unusual findings are reported to the veterinarian. The

Health Careers in Practice

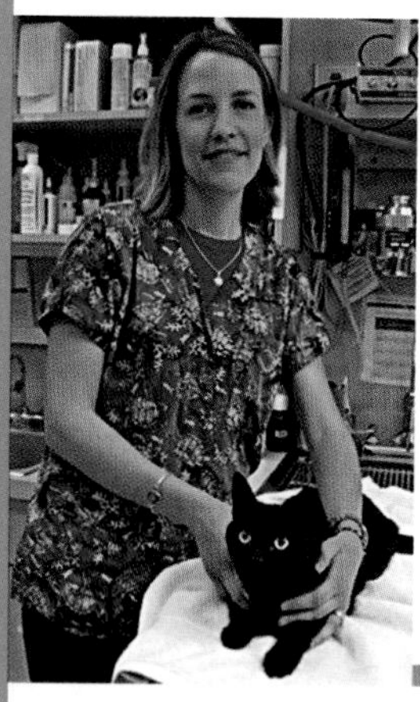

JULIE ELLIS

UNREGISTERED VETERINARY TECHNICIAN
VETERINARY HOSPITAL, PHOENIX, ARIZONA

Educational background: Bachelor of arts, elementary education, Arizona State University (5 years)

A typical day at work and job duties include:

- Monitoring hospitalized animals
- Administering medications
- Assisting the doctor with procedures
- Obtaining samples for testing
- Performing dental cleanings
- In addition to the medical tasks and procedures, I am required to communicate with and educate pet owners, perform general maintenance, cleaning, and animal care.

The most gratifying part of my job: I find that helping animals in need and educating pet owners is very rewarding.

The biggest challenge(s) I face in doing my job: The most difficult part of working in the veterinary field is the pain and suffering of animals.

What drew me to my career? A longtime love of animal companionship and animal medicine.

Something I learned in my early education that I currently use in my career or that caused me to be interested in my career is: I use my general knowledge of anatomy, biology, and science gained during high school while working in the veterinary medical field.

Other comments: Even though I am not a registered technician, I am still able to perform all duties required in my job. I gained the skills through hands-on job training. I do plan to become a registered technician in the near future, but juggling family life and my career has been challenging.

animal is wetted thoroughly with lukewarm water before the soap is applied. Care is taken to prevent the soap from entering the animal's eyes. The animal is rinsed thoroughly and dried before returning it to the cage or kennel. The nails may be clipped during the procedure if necessary.

Animal Caretaker

Animal caretakers may be called by a variety of titles depending on the job responsibilities. Some examples of animal caretakers include kennel, stable, shelter, pet shop, wildlife, and grooming attendants such as a farrier (one who shoes horses) assistant. The animal caretaker performs routine tasks of daily care and assessment for domestic and exotic animals under the supervision of the facility supervisor or a veterinarian. The animal caretaker may be trained on the job or complete a home study program for kennel technicians offered by the American Boarding Kennel Association. No special education or experience is required for many entry-level jobs in animal care.

Animal Breeder

Animal breeders raise animals using selective breeding to maintain or improve the traits of existing breeds, as well as to develop new breeds. Breeders use

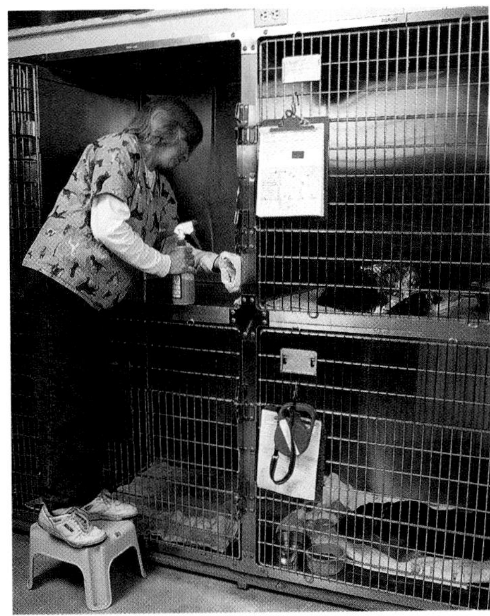

FIGURE 28-2 Kennel cleanliness prevents the spread of disease.

BOX 28-3

Sample Veterinary Examination Equipment

- Air freshener
- Antibacterial soap
- Bandages
- Centrifuge
- Disposable drapes
- Gloves
- Hemacytometer
- Lighting
- Ophthalmoscope
- Otoscope
- Pulse oximeter
- Scale
- Stethoscope
- Surgical instruments
- Thermometer
- X-ray machine

selection of genetic traits to meet the needs of the owners. For example, they breed cows to produce better and more milk. Some breeders produce small animals for ownership as pets or use in research. They provide all care for the animals until a buyer takes them. In addition to on-the-job training, many breeders have a 4-year university degree in animal science because knowledge of the animal and genetics is important.

Marine Biologist

Aquatic or marine biologists study plant and animal life in saltwater environments. Marine biology is also known as *marine ecology* or *biological oceanography*.

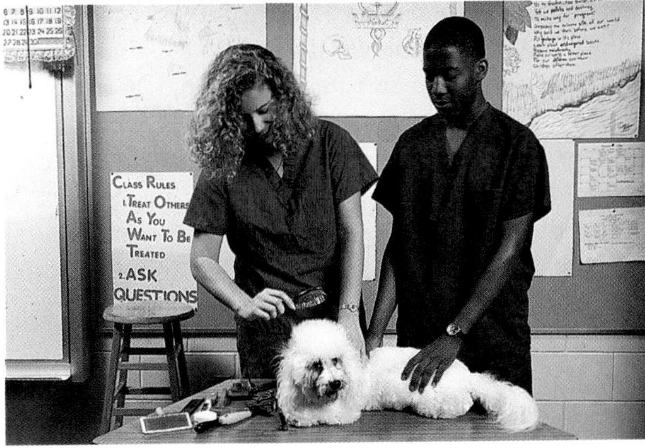

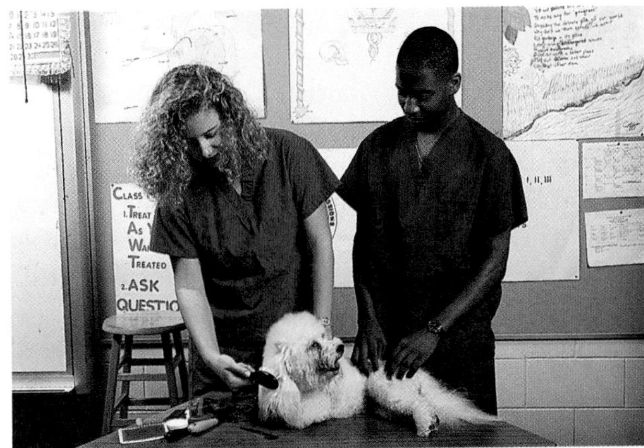

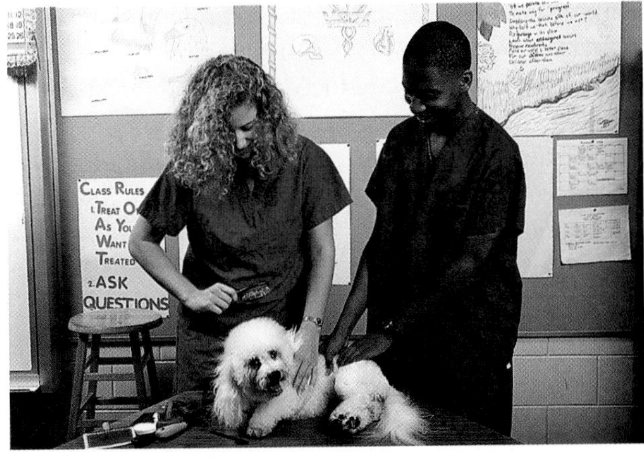

FIGURE 28-3 Grooming requires patience and confidence in handling methods.

The environmental conditions that affect marine life include the water salinity, temperature, acidity, light, and oxygen content. An example of the work completed by a marine biologist might include using research data to make a mathematical model to demonstrate changes in numbers of marine creatures. Marine biologists may study one species or the effect of environmental influences on a specific ecological area. Education for the marine biologist includes a master's or doctoral degree from a university. Employment may be available for those with a 4-year college or university degree in botany or zoology as a marine biology technician. Other professionals working as marine biologists include physiologists and ecologists. Marine biologists are employed in colleges or universities, by private industry, and by the federal government. Most marine biologists work in large marine laboratories.

Content Instruction

Animals as Pets

Animals serve many functions for humans. They provide a source of food in meat and milk products. The skins and coats of animals are used to make clothing and jewelry. Some animals are kept for observation, enjoyment, and preservation in zoos. Animals can also be trained to live with people (domesticated) for companionship, service, and protection.

Animals kept for companionship are called *pets*. About 62% of all households in the United States have at least one pet. Common pets include dogs, cats, turtles, birds, fish, small rodents, horses, and snakes (Fig. 28-4). Cats are more common than dogs as pets. Several research studies have indicated that people with pets have reduced stress and lower blood pressure during interaction with their companions. Some animals, such as guide dogs for the visually impaired, are used for service. Watchdogs are used for protection.

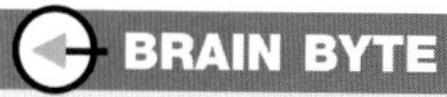

Thirty-three percent of U.S. households have at least one cat.

The birth rate of domestic animals is a serious problem in the United States. Neutering is the process of surgical sterilization to prevent unwanted births. In female animals the procedure is called *spaying*. In males the procedure involves the removal of the testes (orchiectomy). Each year more than four million unwanted or homeless domestic animals are destroyed.

Induction of death in a sick, severely injured, or unwanted animal is called *euthanasia*. The decision to end the life of a pet rests with the owner, who has assumed the responsibility for the care and accepted the companionship of the animal. Often the decision is difficult and is based on the owner's understanding of the quality of life. Euthanasia may also be necessary if an animal becomes vicious, dangerous, or unmanageable. Euthanasia is usually accomplished by injection of an anesthetic drug. The death is quick and painless. The owner and family of an animal that dies face the same process of grief felt with the death of a person. In addition, the person who chooses euthanasia for a pet may feel a sense of responsibility for the death. The dead animal is disposed of in a sanitary manner to prevent infestation of the carcass with microorganisms. The animal is placed in a plastic bag and disposed of in a city disposal, buried, or incinerated. If the animal carcass must be kept for any length of time, it is refrigerated or frozen until disposal is possible.

Animals in Health Care

Pet therapy for physically and mentally ill people is rapidly becoming an accepted treatment method in many health care settings. Involvement with pets has been shown to improve both physical and psychological health. For example, stroking the coat of a pet has been demonstrated to lower blood pressure and heart rate. At least 30 colleges and universities have research programs in the area of human and companion-animal bonding. The Center for the Study of Human-Animal Relationships (CENSHARE) is located at the University of Minnesota.

Most scientists agree that using animals for research is essential. Animal advocates believe that animal research is overused and could be replaced with other methods. Animals are used to test cosmetics and other products before human use is approved. One example of a controversial test is the Draize test, in which chemicals are sprayed into an animal's eyes to determine any possible damage that might occur.

Surgical transplant of animal organs or tissues has also been attempted. In 1984 a baboon heart was transplanted into a human infant whose heart was underdeveloped. Baby Fae lived 20 days with the baboon heart. Transplant into an adult was attempted in 1993. Other species have been used for heart valves and tissue grafts. More than 20 million animals are in use by research laboratories throughout the country. Many of these laboratories are regulated by the National Institutes of Health, which finances their research. The U.S. Department of Agriculture supervises the standard of care in other locations for animals, such as zoos and places where animals are sold.

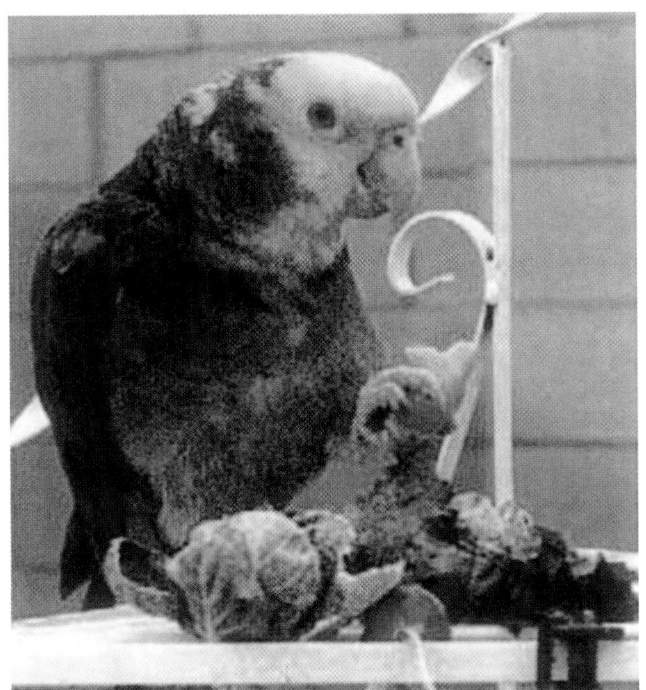
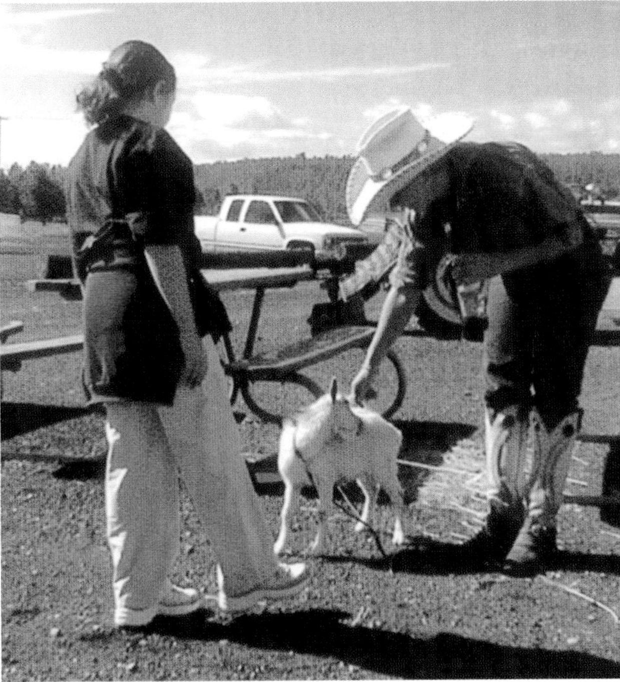
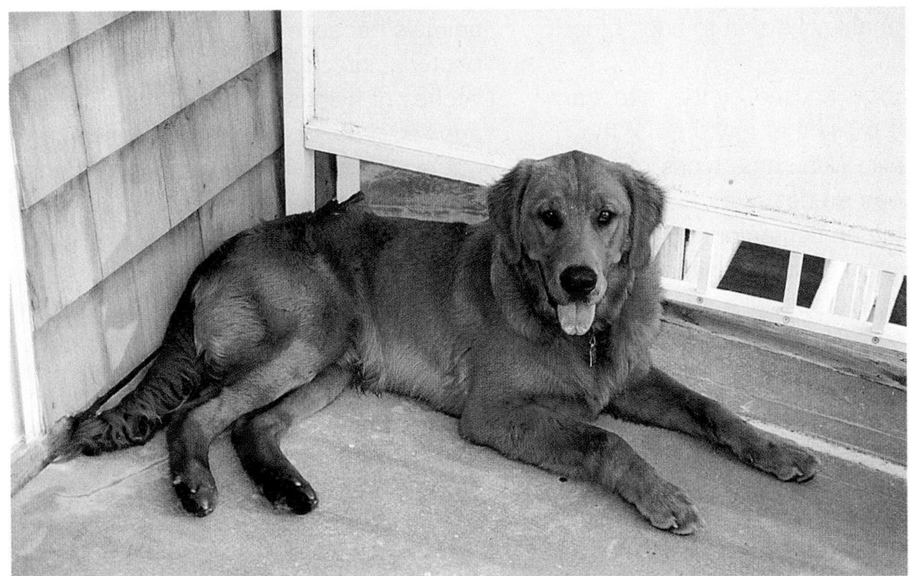

FIGURE 28-4 Pets come in all shapes and sizes.

Dogs and other animals assist people in many careers, including law and drug enforcement. They help people with disabilities to perform activities of daily living. Recently dogs have been trained to locate bedbugs by their smell in hotels, long-term care facilities, and hospitals. Bed bug-sniffing dogs have located the pests with 95% accuracy.

Animal Disorders

More than 150 diseases (zoonoses) can be transmitted from animals to humans. Some of these include anthrax, rabies, leptospirosis, cat scratch fever, ringworm, tapeworm, toxoplasmosis, and Rocky Mountain spotted fever. Most disorders that affect animals harm only their own species and do not harm humans (see the Animal Disorders table at end of chapter, pp. 457–458). Animals, like humans, are affected by both infectious and noninfectious diseases. Animal parasites are one of the most common and deadly of infections. **Parasites** are small organisms that live in or on a host, causing it harm (Table 28-2). The infested animal may need to be isolated or **quarantined** to prevent the spread of infectious organisms.

TABLE 28-2
External Parasites

Parasite	Description	Effects	Treatment
Ear mite	Ear mites are crablike parasites commonly found in dogs and cats.	Severe itching; scratching may lead to bacterial infection; bacterial infection in the ear may penetrate the brain and cause convulsions or death; scratching may lead to bleeding sores	Includes medication
Flea	Fleas have eggs that lie dormant during the winter and emerge in warm weather. They hatch into wormlike larvae, which eventually become fleas. Fleas may jump from one location to another. They can live in carpeting and on clothing.	Itching	Includes sprays, dips, powders, specially treated collars, and tablets
Louse	Lice are small and may penetrate the animal's skin to suck blood.	Itching; dangerous to small animals because of bacterial infection	Includes medication
Mite	Mange, caused by the mite, can be present at any time of the year. With some types of mange, dogs do not scratch. Mange may be contagious to people, as well as to other animals.	Patches of hairlessness and red, irritated skin	Includes shaving the hair, medicated baths, and oral or injected medication
Tick	The tick looks like a small wart or seed. Ticks embed themselves into the skin of the animal. Ticks can live in carpeting and on household items.	Possibly itching; may carry disease to animals and humans	Includes medicated shampoo and removal

Some indications that an animal is sick include abnormal behavior, especially sudden viciousness or listlessness (lethargy), abnormal discharge from any body opening, lumps, limping, or difficulty moving. Loss of appetite, large weight gain or loss, and excessive water consumption are also indications of illness. Difficult, abnormal, or uncontrolled waste elimination are other signs. Redness, swelling, or discharge from the eyes or ears; abnormal stance; foul odor; loss of hair; and twitching or scratching may also indicate a problem.

CASE STUDY 28-2 Your dog scratches and licks his feet all day. What should you do?

Answers to Case Studies are available on the Evolve website: ***http://evolve.elsevier.com/Gerdin***

Performance Instruction

Daily Care and Assessment

The procedures for the daily care of animals provide for the basic needs of the animal. Each animal should be fed regularly with the correct amount and type of food for the species. Fresh water should be available to animals at all times. The living space of a pet should be clean and dry. Bedding, appropriate for the climate, should be provided. Animals that are pets also need human companionship and exercise. The animal caretaker must observe the behavior of an animal to determine any change indicating illness. Observation is made about the intake of food, level of activity, attitude, and pattern of waste elimination (urination and defecation). The healthy animal should be alert and responsive. The animal should eat regularly and have a full, glossy coat. The nose is moist and cool in most animals with normal temperature. Vital signs may be assessed to determine more specific observations.

CASE STUDY 28-3 Your dog has bad breath. What should you do?

Answers to Case Studies are available on the Evolve website: *http://evolve.elsevier.com/Gerdin*

The method used to assess an animal's health is determined by the species. Medical asepsis is maintained while handling animals because some diseases in animals can be transmitted to humans. For dogs and cats, the animal's alertness, appetite, and condition of the coat are some indicators of health. The eyes and ears should be clear and clean in appearance. The nose, membranes of the mouth, posture, and vital signs are also indicators of the animal's health. (See Skill List 28-3, Assisting with an Assessment of a Dog or Cat, p. 460.)

Animal caretakers may need to help with delivery of the young, called *whelping* in dogs. Signs of the beginning of labor in animals may appear as restlessness, panting, scratching, or tearing 4 to 24 hours before delivery. In dogs, the first puppy should appear within 3 hours of the onset of true labor. Each puppy is born in a separate amniotic sac, which should be removed after birth. This may be done with a clean towel if the mother does not do it. The nose and mouth of the newborn must be kept clear of mucus, and the umbilicus must be tied. Respiration must be stimulated, and cardiac massage should be performed if the heartbeat is absent. Abnormal labor (dystocia) should be reported to a veterinarian immediately. The newborn should nurse or drink milk from the mother within the first 12 hours of life.

When an animal becomes ill, one of the duties of the veterinary care worker is to prepare the room for examinations and treatments (Fig. 28-5). (See Skill List 28-4, Preparing the Examination Room, p. 460.) This includes cleaning and disinfecting the room and equipment to prevent the spread of microorganisms. Supplies are gathered before the procedure to minimize the stress for the animal and owner. After completion of surgical procedures, the veterinary care worker may clean and sterilize instruments. Medical asepsis is maintained during handling of all specimens and contaminated instruments. Gloves may be worn during these procedures. Instruments are rinsed in cold water and scrubbed with a soapy brush before autoclaving for sterilization. Some may need to be oiled or sharpened according to the manufacturer's directions. Instruments may be arranged in advance in prepared sets for surgical procedures. The life of many animals can be saved by using the same advanced procedures such as surgery and cardiopulmonary resuscitation (CPR) that are used to treat humans (Fig. 28-6). (See Skill List 28-5, CPR for Cats and Dogs, p. 461.)

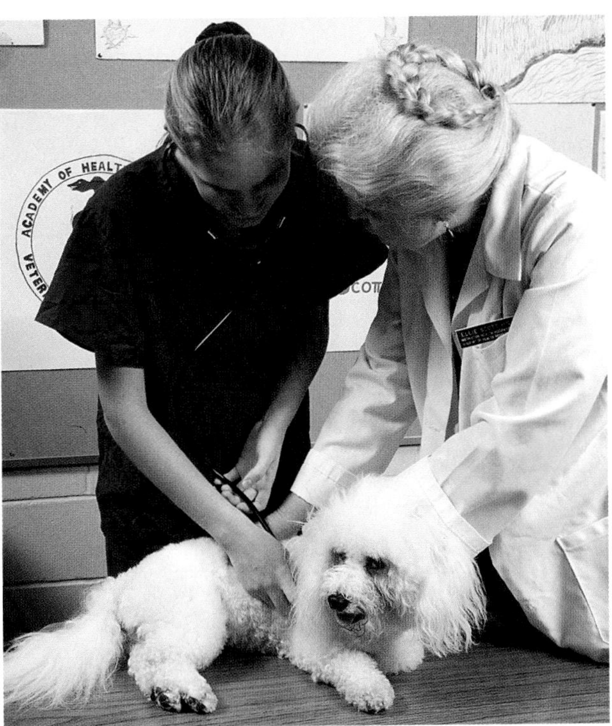

FIGURE 28-5 The examination room is arranged to provide easy access to materials and to limit the animal's movement.

Treatment Techniques

Restraint may be necessary to examine or treat an animal. Each animal responds differently to being handled by a stranger and should be observed before approach. The handler should always have a means to exit the area if necessary. To avoid accidents, the work area should be clean, quiet, and free from clutter. If the use of restraint is necessary, it should not impair

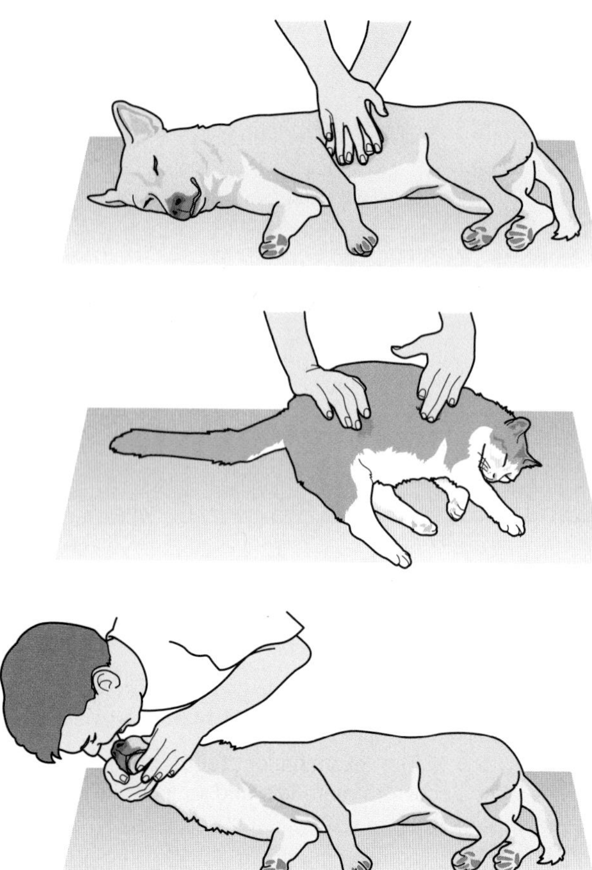

FIGURE 28-6 Cardiopulmonary resuscitation (CPR) and other advanced medical techniques can be used to treat animals.

the animal's circulation or respiration. Some methods of restraint include the use of gloves, boxes, nets, bags, muzzles, snares, and leashes (Fig. 28-7). Horses can be restrained by using a nose twitch, stanchion, halter, rope, or hobble. Cattle are restrained in a similar method with nose tongs, headgates, squeeze chutes, halters, hobbles, nose rings, bull staffs, or electric stock prods. Swine can be restrained by using hog snares, hog hurdles, ropes, and headgates.

Collection of blood samples may be accomplished in a variety of locations on animals. The site that is used depends on the amount of blood needed and type of animal. Some veins that might be used to collect blood from domestic animals, such as the dog and cat, include the jugular, cephalic, saphenous, sublingual, anterior vena cava, and the ear (Fig. 28-8).

Fecal specimens may be collected to look for internal parasite infestation. Flotation, which is the mixing of fecal material with solutions, may be used to find the eggs (ova) of parasites. Viewing feces by microscope (direct smear) provides another method. Fecal solutions can also be centrifuged, or separated by spinning, to reveal parasites.

CASE STUDY 28-4 Your friend tells you her dog ate a box of chocolate, and she wants to know what she should do. What should you say?

Answers to Case Studies are available on the Evolve website: ***http://evolve.elsevier.com/Gerdin***

Urine samples may be collected from some animals by placing a collecting receptacle under the animal as it voids. Catheterization may be necessary to collect the specimen. Urine may also be obtained by surgical puncture of the urinary bladder with a sterile needle (cystocentesis). Urine can be obtained from an unconscious animal by continuous, gentle pressure on the bladder. Bacterial or fungal cultures may be obtained by using a variety of collection methods and supplies such as culture tubes and tissue samples.

Summary

- The role of the veterinary assistant and technician is to provide services under the supervision of the veterinarian. Good physical health and interpersonal skills are necessary to work with animals.
- The function of the veterinary team is to prevent illness and provide care for sick and injured animals.
- Some of the functions that animals serve in human life include providing food, companionship, and service.
- The healthy animal should be alert and responsive. The animal should eat regularly and have a full, glossy coat. The nose should be moist and cool in most animals with normal temperature.
- Five signs of a disorder in an animal are abnormal behavior, discharge from a body opening, loss of appetite, difficulty with movement, and difficulty with elimination.
- Five methods of restraint for care and examination of animals are muzzles, twitches, chutes, bags, and snares.
- Five disorders that affect animals are heartworm, hepatitis, kennel cough, feline leukemia, and distemper.
- Three methods used to assess disorders in animals are palpation, taking vital signs, and testing blood specimens.

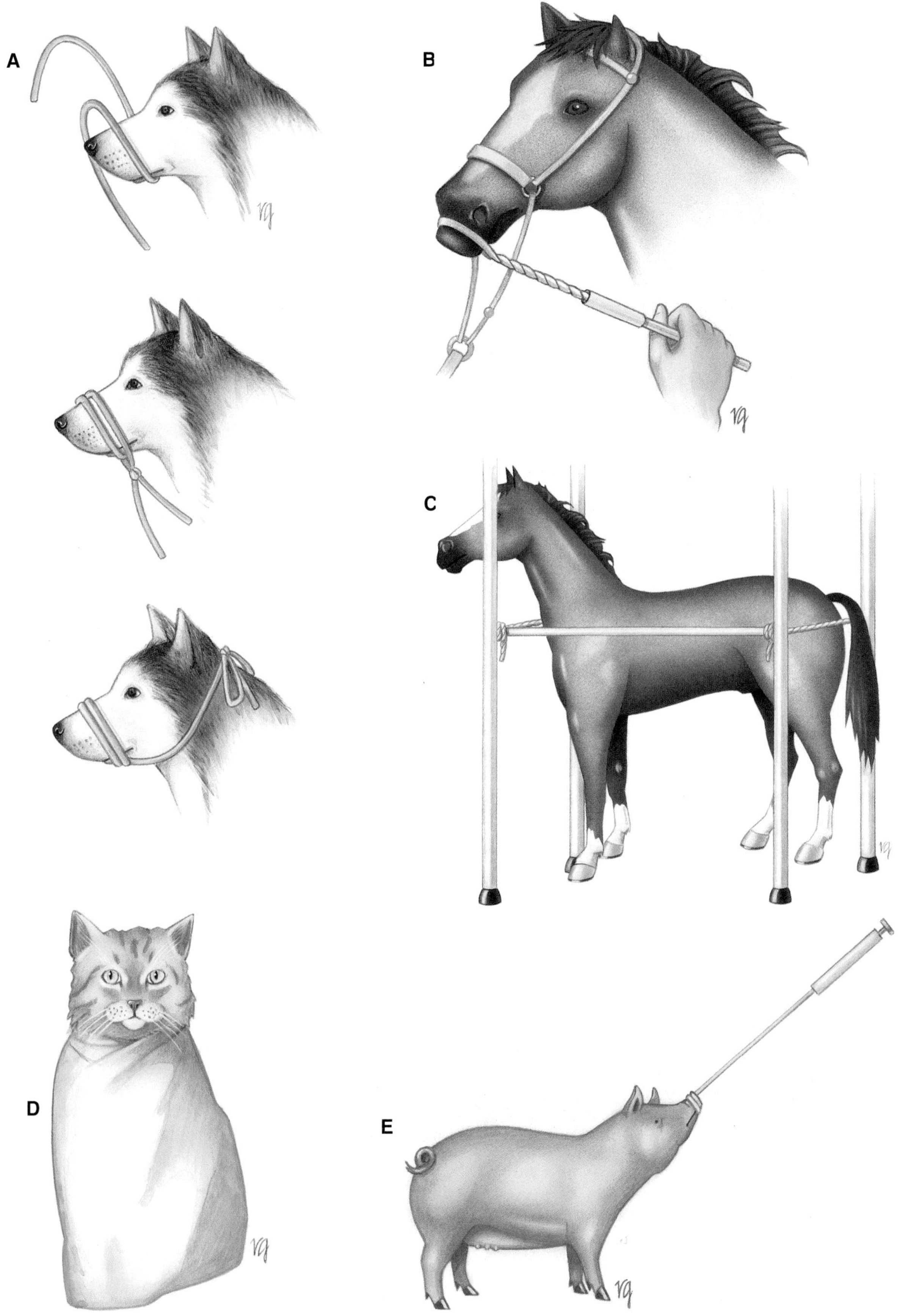

FIGURE 28-7 Methods of restraint. **A,** Muzzle. **B,** Twitch. **C,** Chute. **D,** Bag. **E,** Snare.

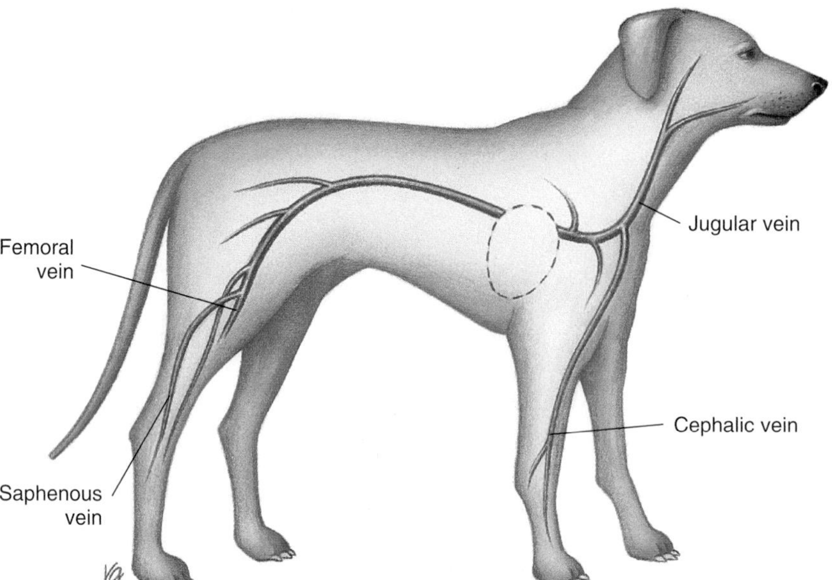

FIGURE 28-8 Venous blood collection sites.

Review Questions

1. Describe the function of the veterinary team.
2. Describe the function of the veterinary technician.
3. Describe the functions that animals serve in the daily life of humans.
4. Describe five methods of restraint used for animal treatment and care.
5. Identify six signs of illness in animals.
6. Describe six common disorders that affect animals.
7. Describe five methods of assessment of disorders in animals.
8. Choose one career from Box 28-1. Research the cost of education and annual earnings in local institutions. Write a paragraph describing the factors that might explain why the local and national economic figures vary.
9. Use each of the following terms in one or more sentences that correctly relate their meaning: canine, feline, quarantine, vaccination, and veterinary.

Critical Thinking

1. Investigate and compare the cost of various types of treatments related to veterinary care.
2. Investigate five common medications used in veterinary care.
3. Investigate the use of pets as therapeutic members of the health care team.
4. Create a career ladder for veterinary careers. Describe why it is or is not possible to move from one level to another in the field.

Explore the Web

Career Information

Bureau of Labor Statistics
http://www.bls.gov/

Salary.com
http://salary.com

Professional Associations

American Veterinary Medical Association
http://www.avma.org/

National Association of Veterinary Technicians in America (NAVTA)
http://www.navta.net/

Animal Disorders

Class	Condition or Disease	Cause	Method of Transfer	Signs and Symptoms	Prevention, Treatment, and Outcome
Bovine (cattle)	Brucellosis	Unknown	Unknown	May be asymptomatic; reproductive problems	Unknown
	Scours (calf enteritis)	Bacteria	Soiled environment	Diarrhea, dehydration, weight loss, depression, death	Replace fluids, electrolytes; quarantine; antibiotics
	Mastitis	Microorganisms	Dairy equipment	Loss of milk production; swelling of udder; milk clotted or watery; fever, death	Prevent injury to udders; antibiotics
	Bovine leptospirosis	Bacteria	Urine shed in water or soil or splashed in eyes or feed; rats, rodents	Decreased milk production; milk contaminated; fever	Vaccination*; antibiotics
Canine (dogs)	Canine heartworm (dirofilariasis)	Worm	Mosquitoes	Worms in heart 14 in. (35 cm) long; impaired circulation, difficulty breathing, cough, listlessness, weight loss	Drugs to prevent infections, kill worms
	Canine parvovirus (CPV)	Virus	Fecal waste	Depression, loss of appetite, fever, diarrhea, feces light or yellow-gray with blood	Vaccination*; replace lost body fluids; antibiotics for secondary infections
	Rabies	Virus	Saliva	Irritability, viciousness, drowsiness, paralysis of lower jaw	Vaccination†; supportive treatment, usually fatal
	Canine distemper	Virus	Secretions of nose and eyes, urine and feces; air droplets; inanimate objects	Damage to nervous system; discharge from eyes, nose; intestinal upset, weight loss, paralysis, convulsions	Vaccination*; supportive treatment; death in 50% of dogs affected
	Infectious canine hepatitis	Virus	Unknown	Fever, depression, loss of appetite, vomiting, abnormal thirst, diarrhea, death	Unknown
	Kennel cough (infectious tracheobronchitis)	Unknown	Unknown	Fever, cough, gagging, loss of appetite	Usually self-limiting; may become bronchopneumonia and be treated with antibiotics

Continued

Animal Disorders—cont'd

Class	Condition or Disease	Cause	Method of Transfer	Signs and Symptoms	Prevention, Treatment, and Outcome
Equine (horses)	Colic	Feeding, mismanagement, worms	Unknown	Severe abdominal pain, distention; frequent urination	Walking, preventing horse from rolling
	Distemper (strangles)	Bacteria	Direct contact, air droplets, contact with contaminated objects	Fever, loss of appetite, cough, enlarged lymph glands, yellow nasal discharge	Vaccination reduces severity; quarantine; antibiotics; hot compresses on lymph glands; rest
	Sleeping sickness (equine encephalomyelitis [EE])	Virus	Birds, as carriers, reservoir; mosquitoes	Fever, difficulty swallowing, teeth grinding, staggering, paralysis	Vaccination*; 80% to 90% die; those that recover have neural damage
	Swamp fever (equine infectious anemia)	Unknown	Unknown	Fever, depression, weight loss, weakness, leg swelling, death	Unknown
	Internal parasites	Bots-flies, strongyli, ascarides, pinworms	Licked from hair, grass blades, contaminated water	Diarrhea, weight loss, anemia	Dewormers/unknown
Feline (cats)	Feline panleukopenia (FP)	Virus	Direct contact with blood, urine, fecal material, fleas	Vary greatly; decrease in WBC, depression, loss of appetite, dehydration, vomiting	Vaccination*; supportive measures to counteract signs, symptoms; quarantine; death in hours or days if untreated
	Feline viral rhinotracheitis (FVR)	Virus	Unknown	Fever, conjunctivitis, nasal discharge, sneezing, death	Unknown
	Feline infectious peritonitis (FIP)	Unknown	Unknown	Fever, loss of appetite, depression fluid accumulation, death	Unknown
	Feline leukemia	Unknown	Unknown	Weight loss, anemia, depression, death	Unknown
	Feline urologic syndrome (FUS)	Unknown	Unknown	Painful, frequent urination; blood in urine; depression, death	Antibiotics, surgery
Porcine (swine)	Clostridial diarrhea	Bacteria	Unknown	Listlessness, diarrhea, bloody stool, death	Unknown

*Can prevent the disease.
†Required by law for most domestic pets.
WBC, White blood cell.

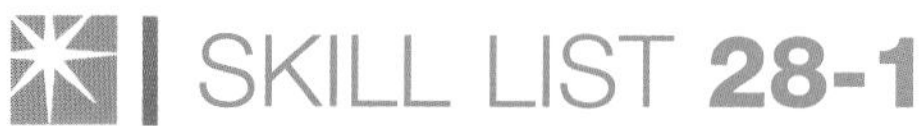

SKILL LIST 28-1 Maintaining the Cage or Kennel

1. Maintain medical asepsis by using the guidelines provided in the Standard and Transmission-Based Precautions, including good handwashing technique and use of gloves as needed.
2. Clean and disinfect the animal's living quarters daily. Microorganisms, present in the waste of infected animals, must be removed to prevent the spread to other animals.
3. Remove waste material on a regular basis during the day. Waste that is left may be spread to other cages by movement of the animal.
4. Check the area for appropriate ventilation, proper temperature, and shaded areas. A restrained animal cannot move to a more comfortable area in the cage or kennel. Dogs and cats cannot sweat to lower the body temperature, and they may become ill if left in an environment that is too hot.
5. Supply fresh food and water daily. The amount of food and number of feedings required depend on the breed. Nutritional requirements vary for different species and breeds of animals. Like humans, animals need all the nutrient groups each day.
6. Exercise kenneled animals at least twice daily for 30 to 45 minutes. Animals that are kept as pets need human companionship and exercise to remain emotionally and physically healthy.

SKILL LIST 28-2 Bathing and Grooming

1. Maintain medical asepsis by using the guidelines provided in the Standard and Transmission-Based Precautions, including good handwashing technique and use of gloves as needed.
2. Observe the condition of the skin and coat. Report any unusual findings to the veterinarian.
3. Select the proper shampoo or dip. Shampoos may be specific for the type of animal and type of condition. Shampoos may be designed for animals that are being bathed to remove parasites or debris or for those being prepared for sale or show.
4. Dilute the shampoo or dip according to the manufacturer's instructions.
5. Prepare the water or solution at a lukewarm temperature (100° to 115° F).
6. Place the animal into a half-full tub. Restrain the animal if necessary. Protect the animal's ears with cotton and the eyes with a lubricating ointment made for that purpose.
7. Wet the animal thoroughly. Rub the soap into the skin, and avoid getting soap in the eyes.
8. The soap or solution may have directions that specify the length of time of application to be effective. Rinse the soap off completely, and remove the animal from the tub. Soap that is left on the animal may cause skin irritation.
9. Dry the animal completely. Brush and comb hair as needed. Loose and matted hair should be removed.
10. Clean the ears and teeth. Clip nails if needed. Some animals may need to be anesthetized to clean their teeth and clip their nails.
11. Reward the animal with affection before returning it to the cage or pen. The animal might not like to be bathed, so the procedure should be made as pleasant as possible to avoid behavior problems at the next bath.
12. Record observations. Immediately report any unusual findings to the veterinarian or owner.
13. Clean any used equipment and return it to the designated area.

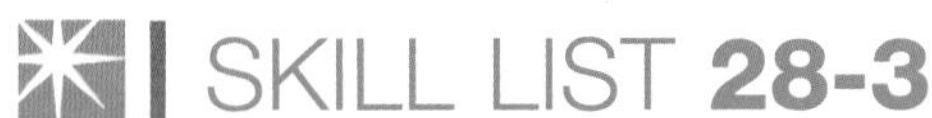

SKILL LIST 28-3
Assisting with an Assessment of a Dog or Cat

1. Maintain medical asepsis by using the guidelines provided in the Standard and Transmission-Based Precautions, including good handwashing technique and use of gloves as needed. Some animal disease may cause illness in humans. Also, the hands of the assistant may transfer many pathogens from one animal to another.
2. Restrain the animal if necessary.
3. Observe the animal's alertness and appetite for water and food.
4. Observe the condition of the animal's coat. The coat should be glossy and full. A dull or shedding coat may indicate inadequate nutrition or the presence of parasites.
5. Observe and describe the condition of the eyes and ears. Swelling, redness, or discharge may indicate infection or the presence of a parasite.
6. Observe and describe the condition of the nose. The nose should be cool and moist.
7. Observe and describe the condition of the mucous membranes of the mouth. The membranes should be pink and moist.
8. Observe and describe the condition of the stool and urine. The color, amount, odor, and consistency should be noted.
9. Observe the animal's stance and posture for normalcy.
10. Assess the vital signs. The pulse can be counted by using the femoral artery in many animals. In the horse, the submaxillary artery can be felt under the jaw bone. Temperature is taken rectally for 3 minutes. Normal values for vital signs differ according to the species. The vital signs provide a specific determination of the animal's condition. Abnormal vital signs indicate illness or infection.
11. Release and reward the animal with affection. The animal may feel more positive about the assessment procedure when rewarded.

SKILL LIST 28-4
Preparing the Examination Room

1. Maintain medical asepsis by using the guidelines provided in the Standard and Transmission-Based Precautions, including good handwashing technique and use of gloves as needed.
2. Check the records to determine the necessary equipment and supplies for the visit. Advance preparation for anticipated needs makes the treatment procedures more efficient and less traumatic for the animal.
3. Clean and disinfect the room and equipment. Many disease-causing organisms live outside the animal's body for long periods. Organisms or inanimate objects can be transmitted from one animal to another.
4. Restock the disposable items. Supplies should be available during a procedure to prevent delay.
5. Escort the animal to the examination room. Some veterinarians prefer that the animal's owner not be present. The pet may sense and react to the owner's anxiety about the treatment.
6. Assist with examination or treatment as needed. The animal may need to be restrained, or supplies may need to be opened for the veterinarian.
7. When the procedure is completed, return the animal to the cage or kennel as directed by the veterinarian. The animal may need observation or monitoring of vital signs after some procedures.

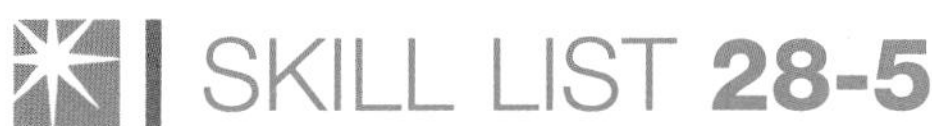

SKILL LIST 28-5 Cardiopulmonary Resuscitation (CPR) for Cats and Dogs*

1. Maintain medical asepsis by using the guidelines provided in the Standard and Transmission-Based Precautions, including good handwashing technique and use of gloves as needed.
2. Make sure the animal is arrested and unconscious by talking and gently shaking it.
3. Open the animal's mouth and make sure the air passage is clear. If not, remove any object obstructing the air passage. Sweep the airway if necessary to remove saliva or vomitus.
4. Pull the head back to open the airway and extend the tongue. Give two breaths (the chest should rise). For large animals, close the jaw and breathe through the nose. For small animals cover both the nose and mouth.
5. Perform chest compressions. Large animals can be positioned on their backs like humans. Small animals can be placed on their side or positioned on their backs.
6. Alternate compressions and breaths at a 30:2 ratio.
7. The rate of compression varies with the size of the animal:
   Over 60 lbs, 60 per minute
   11-60 lbs, 80-100 per minute
   10 lbs or less, 120 per minute

*CPR may also be called CPCR (cardiopulmonary cerebral resuscitation).

CHAPTER 29

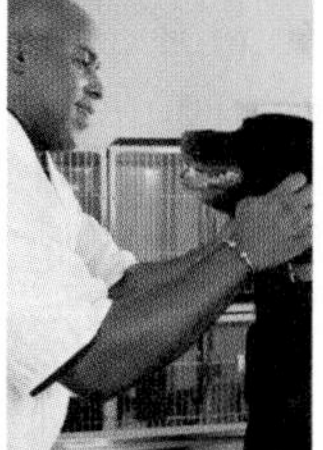
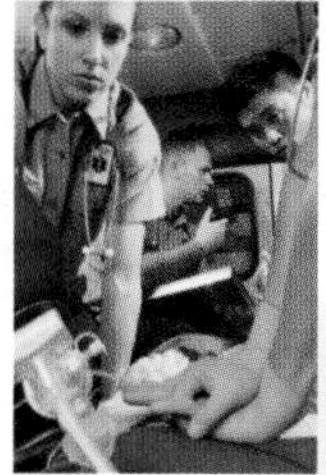
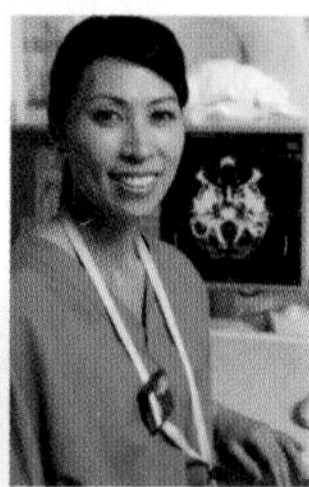

Community and Social Careers

LEARNING OBJECTIVES

- Define at least eight terms relating to community and social health care.
- Describe the function of the community and social health care team.
- Specify the role of the community and social health care team members, including personal qualities, educational requirements, responsibilities, and credentialing requirements.
- Identify at least six services provided by community health care agencies.
- Specify the difference between physical and psychological drug dependency.
- Identify at least four signs and symptoms of withdrawal from an addictive substance.

KEY TERMS

Communicable *(kum-YOO-nik-uh-bul)* Capable of being transmitted from one person or animal to another

Demographic *(dem-o-GRAF-ik)* Pertaining to the study of people as a group, especially of statistical groupings according to age, gender, and environmental factors

Dependence *(dee-PEN-dents)* Addiction to drugs or alcohol

Hallucination *(huh-loo-sin-AY-shun)* Sensory perception that occurs in waking state but does not have external stimulus

Immunization *(im-yoo-niz-AY-shun)* Process of becoming secure against a particular disease or pathogen

Pollution *(puh-LOO-shun)* Condition of being defiled or impure

Vector *(VEK-tur)* Carrier that transfers an infective agent from one host to another

Withdrawal *(with-DRAW-ul)* Unpleasant symptoms resulting with stoppage of drugs or substances on which a person is dependent; symptoms include anxiety, insomnia, irritability, impaired attention, and physical illness

Community and Social Careers Terminology*

Term	Definition	Prefix	Root	Suffix
Anesthetic	Pertaining to a lack of feeling	an	esthet	ic
Arthritis	Inflammation of the joints		arthr	itis
Chronic	Pertaining to time		chron	ic
Disable	Opposite of fitness	dis	able	
Euphoria	State of feeling well	eu	phor	ia
Gerontology	Study of aging		geront	ology
Hypertrophy	Increase in nourishment (size)	hyper	troph	y
Hypnotic	Pertaining to a state of sleep		hypnot	ic
Narcolepsy	Condition of uncontrolled sleep		narco	lepsy
Sociologist	One who works with society		sociol	ogist

*A transition syllable or vowel may be added to or deleted from the word parts to make the combining form.

Abbreviations for Community and Social Careers

Abbreviation	Meaning
ACSW	Academy of Certified Social Workers
DHHS	Department of Health and Human Services
DSW	Doctorate of social work
FDA	Food and Drug Administration
GHB	Gamma hydroxybutyrate
MSW	Master of social work
NIH	National Institutes of Health
PhD	Doctor of philosophy
THC	Tetrahydrocannabinol
WHO	World Health Organization

Careers

Community and social health care has broad goals and focuses on the health needs of a population (Fig. 29-1). The primary goals of community and social health care workers are prevention of illness and injury and provision of care to a population (Table 29-1). The community and social health care worker is involved in the search for the source of disease and the use of technical and regulatory means to protect the population from environmental, social, and behavioral hazards. Health problems addressed by community and social health care workers are often related to environmental hazards, sanitation, and work and living conditions. Other health problems may originate because of population growth and social and behavioral aspects of life.

Employees in community and social health careers may be trained as physicians, social workers, dentists, nurses, and counselors, as well as other health care providers (Box 29-1). These health care providers usually work for the government or volunteer agencies. They must develop the ability to consider many aspects of a problem or condition and analyze the many options that are provided by or limited by public health agencies. Community and social health care workers must also be able to function well in an environment that involves many regulations and agencies. Community and social workers may be required by law to document and report incidents of domestic violence or abuse as well as providing care for the victim (Box 29-2).

CASE STUDY 29-1 You notice some bruising on your friend's forearms and think her makeup might be covering a bruise on her face. What should you do?

Answers to Case Studies are available on the Evolve website: ***http://evolve.elsevier.com/Gerdin***

Community Health Providers

Community nutrition workers provide food and nutrition education through public health clinics and programs (Fig. 29-2). They screen patients to determine eligibility, based on health risk and income, for the program. Other job duties may include testing blood, taking dietary histories, assessing vital signs, and counseling on basic nutrition. The minimum qualification is a high school education and experience working with the public or training in nutrition education.

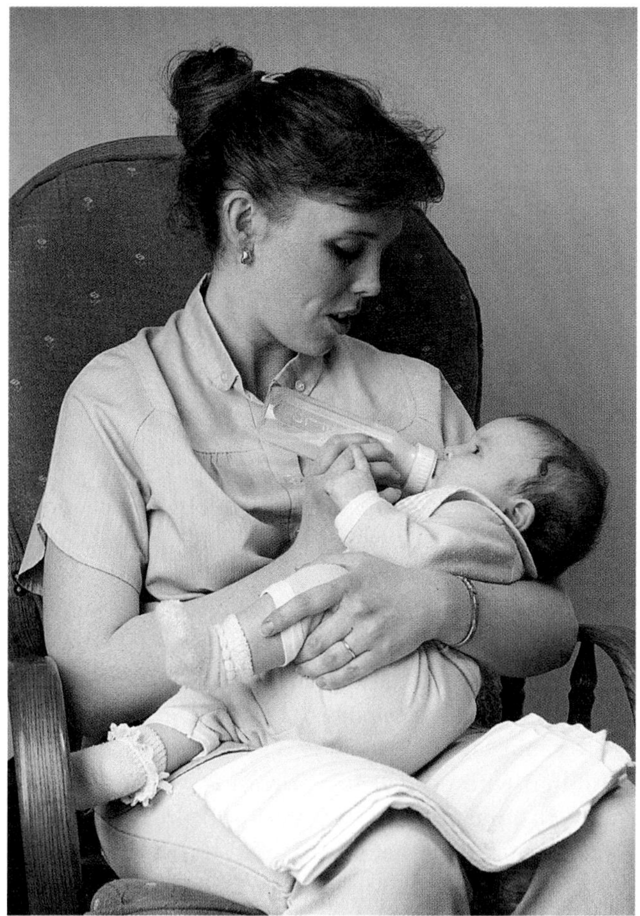

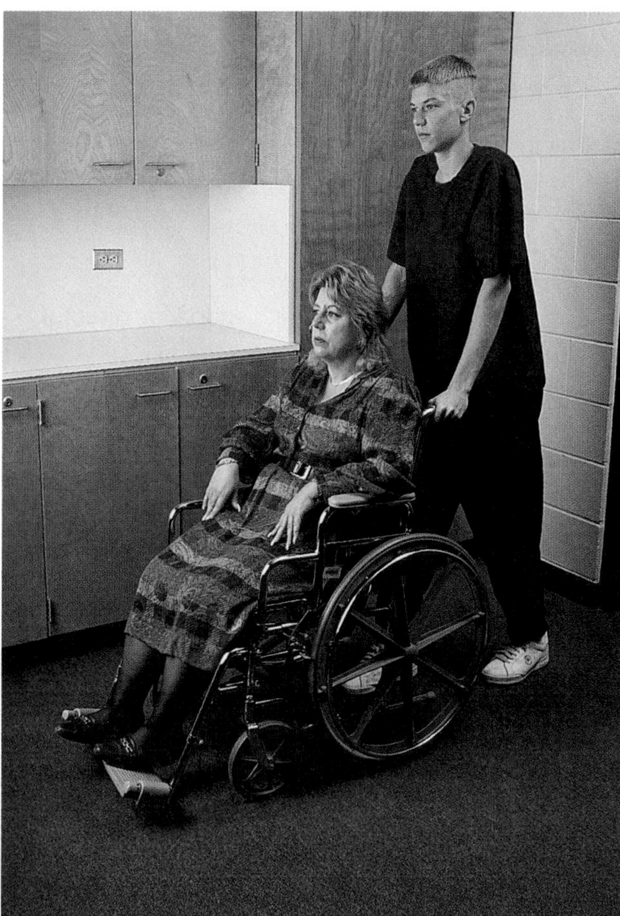

FIGURE 29-1 Community and social health care workers may work in many areas, ranging from maternal and child care to advocacy for people with physical challenges.

TABLE 29-1
Community and Social Career Educational Cost and Earnings

Career	Educational Cost*	Earnings†
Occupational health nurse	University of Michigan 2-year program, weekends on job/on campus; master's degree Fees include: Tuition & fees $35,050 Books $2384 Personal & miscellaneous $8184	Median annual salary: Ann Arbor, Mich.—$61,870

*http://www.finaid.umich.edu/financial_aid_basics/cost.asp.
†http://data.bls.gov:8080/oes/datatype.do.

CASE STUDY 29-2 Your neighbor is a single mom of three children and has lost her job. You notice that the children are not getting three meals a day. What should you do?

Answers to Case Studies are available on the Evolve website: ***http://evolve.elsevier.com/Gerdin***

Supervisors of caseworkers coordinate the activities of agency staff, volunteers, and students working in child welfare. The supervisor assigns the cases and assists with services. Graduate-level preparation plus social work experience is usually required. Caseworkers may investigate physical and psychological home conditions to determine the need for intervention of the agency workers. Caseworkers provide

BOX 29-1

Community and Social Health Careers

Child life specialist
Child welfare caseworker
Community dietitian
Community health nurse
Community organization director
Community service and health education director
Counselor
Counselor, residence
Counselor, vocational-rehabilitation
Director of counseling
Funeral director
Geriatric social worker
Mental health aide
Occupational health nurse
Red Cross executive director
Sheltered works director
Social group worker
Social services aide
Social worker, delinquency
Social worker, medical
Sociologist, clinical

BOX 29-2

Resources and Services for Domestic Violence Victims*

- Shelters
- Hotlines
- Foster care
- Police protection
- Protective court order
- Cosmetic and reconstructive support

*The National Coalition Against Domestic Violence provides links to many resources. http://www.ncadv.org/.

counseling for children, parents, and foster parents. The caseworker determines the suitability of foster homes and adoption applicants and places children in appropriate settings. Bachelor-level preparation in social work is the minimal level for employment, but a master's degree is preferred.

Under the supervision of the caseworker, case assistants perform such tasks as completing forms and explaining the services of the agency. Duties may include assisting patients to complete applications for unemployment compensation, food stamps, medical

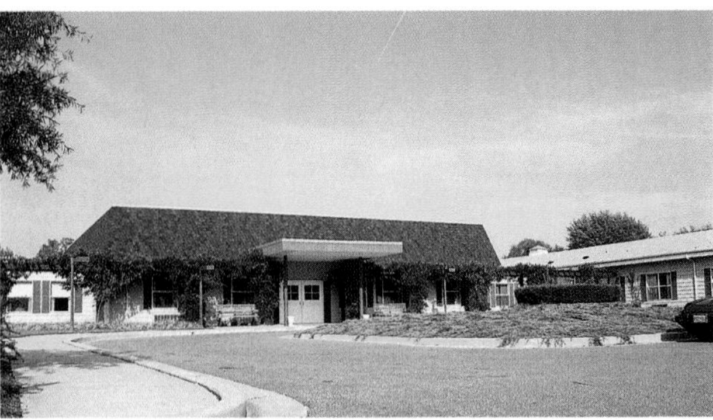

FIGURE 29-2 Community nutrition workers often present programs in public health clinics.

care, and other services. On-the-job or vocational school training for case assistants may be adequate for employment.

Under the supervision of the director, attendants for children's institutions provide care for children who are housed in city, county, private, or other institutions such as orphanages, child care homes, and day care centers. Duties include waking and assisting the children who need help in dressing. Responsibilities may also include assistance with feeding, schooling, and recreational activities. The attendant may be responsible for discipline when children misbehave. Attendants with high school diplomas are preferred. Little advancement is possible without additional education and training.

Disabled children may be assigned to a child care attendant while attending school. The attendant helps the student perform tasks needed to attend classes. Duties may include transporting the child, replacing braces or slings, and helping with participation in activities (Fig. 29-3). Most school attendants are employed by the school system, and a high school diploma is required for employment.

Social Care Providers

Health sociologists identify and explain the social factors affecting the care of patients. They specialize in the study of the effect of social factors on the incidence and course of disease. By gathering and interpreting data about the community, the health sociologist can advise the community and health care workers about the response to a new technology or service that may be expected. Health sociologists (medical sociologists) work in universities or for the government. Most health sociologists have a doctoral (PhD) degree. Neither certification nor licensure is required for the health sociologist.

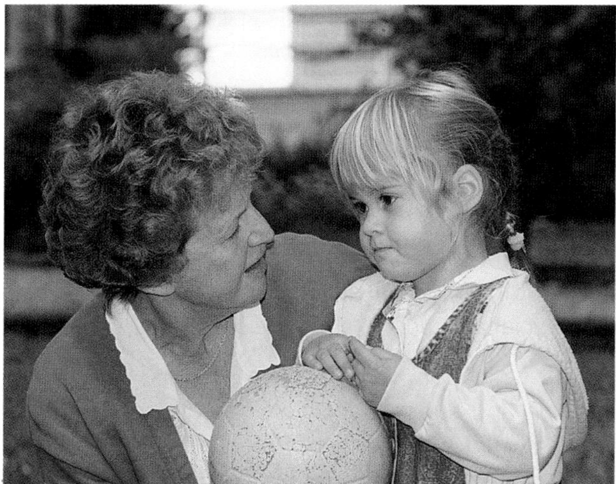

FIGURE 29-3 A child care attendant assists with recreational activities.

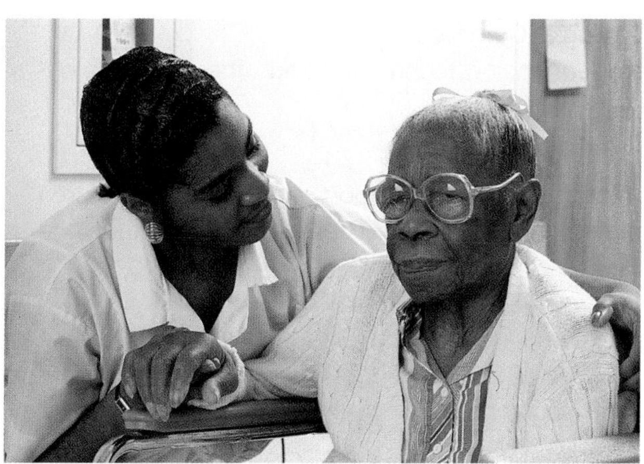

FIGURE 29-4 Geriatric social workers help to improve quality of life for the elderly.

Geriatric social workers specialize in providing assistance to older persons (Fig. 29-4). Some examples of positions for geriatric social workers include evaluation of patients for social services, working in a hospital to provide treatment for older patients, working in group homes or senior centers or hospices, and working in long-term care facilities. Most states require geriatric social workers to be licensed or registered. A master's degree in social work allows geriatric social workers to advance beyond entry-level positions.

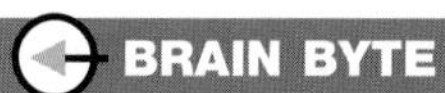

BRAIN BYTE

In 2004 the Centers for Disease Control and Prevention (CDC) reported there were 16,100 nursing homes with 1.5 million residents in the United States.

BOX 29-3

Areas of Specialization for Social Workers

- Administration
- Child welfare and family services
- Clinical practice (psychotherapy)
- Criminal justice
- Gerontology
- Health care
- Mental health practice
- Occupational services
- Planning and policymaking
- School
- Substance abuse

CASE STUDY 29-3 You pass by an older patient's room and hear her daughter yelling at her, calling her names, and saying how useless and costly the patient has become. What should you do?

Answers to Case Studies are available on the Evolve website: ***http://evolve.elsevier.com/Gerdin***

Three levels of education are available for professional social workers. These are the bachelor's degree (BSW), the master's degree (MSW), and the doctoral degree (DSW). Certification is available through the Academy of Certified Social Workers. A master's or doctoral degree is usually required for social workers employed in mental health and medical environments. Most social workers specialize in one area of practice (Box 29-3). Professional social workers use counseling, referral, and advocacy to help patients deal with their problems. Areas of specialization include child welfare, family counseling, corrections, aging, medical, and psychiatric care.

When a patient dies, the social worker may be asked to help with funeral preparations. Funeral directors and staff remove the deceased, prepare the remains, help to arrange the services, and dispose of the body according to the family's wishes. Funeral directors may also be called *morticians* or *undertakers*. Most funeral directors are also licensed embalmers and prepare the body for burial or cremation. All states, except Colorado, require licensure for funeral directors, and most have completed an associate or bachelor's degree. Chapter 24 provides more information about postmortem care and cultural practices regarding funeral rites.

Health Careers in Practice

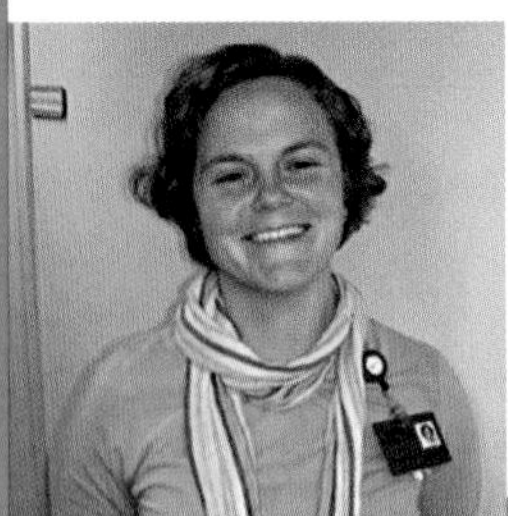

TERESA MCNAMEE, MSW, LCSW

SOCIAL WORKER
ST. LOUIS CHILDREN'S HOSPITAL

Educational background: Bachelor of social work with a minor in business administration (3½ years); master of social work with a concentration in social and economic development (2 years).

A typical day at work and job duties include: My typical day is difficult to describe because the tasks and responsibilities range from administrative and supervisory duties to direct practice with children and families. In any given week, I may have 1 to 3 days full of meetings with 1 to 3 days of direct casework tasks. My meetings may include the following:

- Team meetings for our asthma program (social services team, leadership team, and general asthma program team)
- Care conference meetings for the services I supervise
- Committee meetings for our department and the hospital in general (Employee Resource Allocation Committee, Going Green Committee, Social Committee, etc.)
- Administrative meetings that involve improving or enhancing technology and other methods of data collection or service provision
- One-on-one meetings and consultation with staff I supervise

I perform direct practice duties by providing case management and support services to the children and families on my caseload (which is approximately 100 children). These services include the following:

- Assessment
- Referrals to outside agencies
- Information about programs and services
- General social support to deal with behavioral and social barriers to appropriate medical care

I also spend a good deal of time developing the social services side of our program by:

- Researching best practices
- Developing goals and objectives
- Creating policies and procedures

Continued

Counselors help their patients solve problems of personal, social, career, and educational development. They work in a variety of settings, such as schools, rehabilitation agencies, mental health or correctional facilities, and colleges, or they may have a private practice. They may specialize in marriage, family, career selection, grief, or other types of guidance practice.

Counseling positions usually require a master's degree for entry-level work. An internship or supervised field experience is necessary for certification or licensure by the state. Most states require counselors to be licensed, certified, or registered.

Vocational and rehabilitation counselors assist disabled individuals and students to identify career opportunities and to learn a trade. They help the disabled individual adjust during training and find employment when the program is completed. Vocational counselors must complete a bachelor's degree for entry-level employment, but a master's degree may be required. Most vocational counselors work for state or local rehabilitation agencies and schools.

Some counselors specialize in treatment of drug or substance abuse. Duties of the substance abuse counselor include providing help for abusers and implementing preventive programs. Substance abuse counselors may be educated as psychologists, nurses, social workers, or in related occupational fields, as well as counseling.

The most gratifying part of my job: The most gratifying part of my job is working with families who are really struggling to find resources that help to support their child's asthma treatment and finding services to provide ongoing support for them. When barriers are reduced and people "get" the connection between increased barriers and decreased health outcomes, then I feel like my work is successful. When I am able to work with families to address these barriers and when my fellow team members understand the impact of the reduced barriers on the family's environment, I feel like I am really making a difference in people's lives. Making this kind of difference is rewarding and is one of the reasons I became a social worker.

The biggest challenge(s) I face in doing my job: When I first started working in the health care setting, I was surprised about how social workers were viewed. In the hospital, social workers have a different role from that in a community-based organization. I work in the outreach department of the hospital. We do a lot of things differently than what they practice in the hospital. It was challenging at first to get people to understand the depth and breadth of the work social workers can do. Also, it is very challenging for me to tell a family that there are few or no resources available to them. Hearing that some parents are faced with the choice of buying medicines for their child or putting food on the table is difficult to hear. It is a challenge not to be able to help everyone.

What drew me to my career? At a young age, I knew I wanted to help people when I got older. The profession of social work fit with that desire.

Something I learned in my early education that I currently use in my career or that caused me to be interested in my career is: When I was a junior in high school, I volunteered with an afterschool mentoring program in an elementary school. A social worker coordinated the program. I learned about what she did in the school, and I became interested in pursuing social work as a career.

Other comments: I believe social workers have a place in the health care field, particularly now, as barriers to medical care are increasing. Advocating and educating about that role are what social workers must continue to do.

Health Careers in Practice

BRAIN BYTE

In a 2009 National Institutes of Health (NIH) study, cigarette smoking was at its lowest point in the history of the survey in students in grades 8, 10, and 12. Daily use of smokeless tobacco increased significantly among tenth graders.

The child life specialist works in health care settings and focuses on the emotional and developmental needs of children. These specialists use play therapy, activities, and communication to reduce the stress of illness and improve the child's understanding of health care treatments and the environment. Children do not have the emotional maturity to understand confinement, the lack of privacy, separation from family, and pain resulting from tests and treatments during treatment for illness.

Educational programs in child life care are available at the baccalaureate and graduate level. Supervised field training in a hospital or clinic may be part of the program. Individuals with training in education, recreation, and child development may also qualify for this occupation. Voluntary certification for child life professionals is available through the Child Life Council. Child life specialists may have assistants who hold a 2-year community college degree. At present, child life specialists are not required to be licensed or certified.

The social and human service assistant field includes workers in many areas, including social work assistant, case management aide, and community outreach worker. Employment opportunities for this position are projected to grow by about 23% between 2008 and 2018. The social and human service assistant may give care directly to the patient or indirectly by helping a professional responsible for the care. Job duties of the social and human service assistant vary with the type of employment. Examples may include assessing patient needs for benefits, arranging transportation, organizing group activities, and keeping records of care given. There are no specific educational or certification requirements for the social and human service assistant.

Content Instruction

Substance Abuse

Drug **dependence** or addiction is the physical or psychological need to continue taking a drug or other substance. Psychological dependence is a state of mind that needs the substance to achieve a desired feeling. Physical dependence results when the body develops a need for the substance to function. **Withdrawal** occurs when the substance is not taken. Withdrawal causes extreme nervousness, uncontrollable trembling, excessive sweating, and painful cramps. Other symptoms may include nausea and imaginary visions (**hallucinations**). A person may develop tolerance to the substance and require a larger dose of the drug to achieve the same effect.

People use or abuse mind-altering substances for many different reasons. These include the desire to experience new sensations, relax, gain acceptance from others, or escape boredom. Some users state that these substances provide a temporary sense of control over the body or relieve a bad feeling or personal problem. As with any mind-altering substance, the problem or feeling remains when the effects of the drug wear off. Substance abuse is the misuse of drugs, including alcohol. Abuse may result from use of legal or illegal drugs (Table 29-2). Stimulants may be used to increase the activity of the central nervous system. Depressants have the opposite effect. Narcotics depress the central nervous system, but they also result in a "pleasurable" feeling followed by drowsiness, sleep, or unconsciousness. Some household cleaning and paint products are used to produce a change in mental status. Teenagers are increasingly abusing inhalants (Box 29-4). In 2008, the CDC Youth Risk Behavior Surveillance System reported that 13.3% of high school students had used inhalants. These are dangerous and have been the cause of death in many young people.

Alcohol is the most commonly abused substance in the United States, and alcoholism is a major medical problem. Treatment of alcoholism includes detoxification and therapy to prevent drinking. Most drug programs teach that not drinking (abstinence) is the only reasonable goal for the addicted individual.

Treatment of the symptoms of substance abuse is usually the first step after diagnosis. Once the person's addiction is controlled, treatment of the mental disorder can be started. Although many factors—such as age, values, culture, gender, family relationships, and other disorders—influence the type of treatment, most treatments have similar components. Medication may be used to control mood and behavior. Psychotherapy, group therapy, behavior modification, and cognitive therapy may also be used.

BOX 29-4

Warning Signs of Inhalant Abuse

- Empty lighters
- Empty plastic bags
- Fingernails painted with inhalants such as Liquid Paper
- Hair bands wrapped around wrists or upper arm (soaked in inhalant)
- Loss of appetite
- Nausea
- Persistent cough
- Runny nose or nosebleed
- Sores or rashes around the mouth
- Stains on skin or clothing

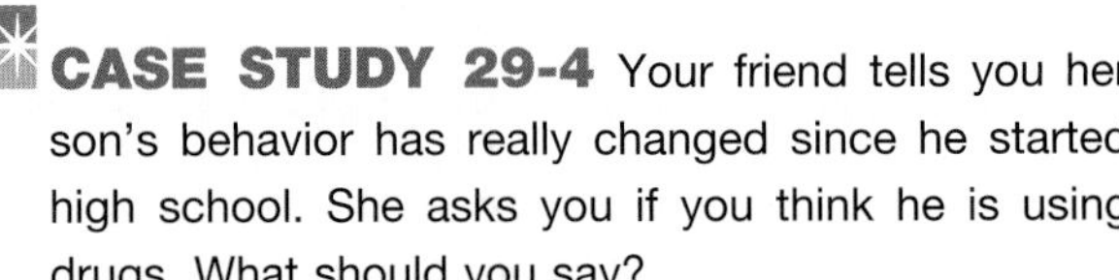

CASE STUDY 29-4 Your friend tells you her son's behavior has really changed since he started high school. She asks you if you think he is using drugs. What should you say?

Answers to Case Studies are available on the Evolve website: ***http://evolve.elsevier.com/Gerdin***

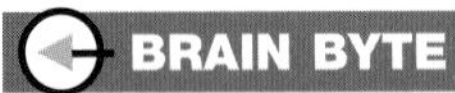

BRAIN BYTE

The NIH reports that about 40 million serious illnesses or injuries result from drug abuse each year.

Public Health Resources

Public health care agencies are concerned with maternal and child health, dental care, tuberculosis control,

TABLE 29-2
Commonly Abused Chemicals

Category	Chemical	Commercial and Street Names
Cannabinoid	Hashish	Boom, chronic, gangster, hash, hash oil, hemp
	Marijuana	Blunt, dope, ganja, grass, herb, joints, Mary Jane, pot, reefer, sinsemilla, skunk, weed
Depressants	Barbiturates	Amytal, Nembutal, Seconal; phenobarbital, barbs, reds, red birds, phennies, tooies, yellows, yellow jackets
	Benzodiazepines (other than flunitrazepam)	Ativan, Halcion, Librium, Valium, Xanax; candy, downers, sleeping pills, tranks
	Flunitrazepam*	Rohypnol; forget-me pill, Mexican Valium, R2, Roche, roofies, roofinol, rope, rophies
	Gamma hydroxybutyrate	GHB*; G, Georgia home boy, grievous bodily harm, liquid ecstasy
	Methaqualone	Quaalude, Sopor, Parest; ludes, mandrex, quad, quay
Dissociative anesthetics	Ketamine	Ketalar SV; cat Valiums, K, Special K, vitamin K
	Phencyclidine and analogs	PCP; angel dust, boat, hog, love boat, peace pill
Hallucinogens	Lysergic acid diethylamide	LSD; acid, blotter, boomers, cubes, microdot, yellow sunshines
	Mescaline	Buttons, cactus, mesc, peyote
	Psilocybin	Magic mushroom, purple passion, shrooms
Opioids and morphine derivatives	Codeine	Empirin with Codeine, Fiorinal with Codeine, Robitussin A-C, Tylenol with Codeine; Captain Cody, Cody, schoolboy; (with glutethimide) doors & fours, loads, pancakes and syrup
	Fentanyl	Actiq, Duragesic, Sublimaze; Apache, China girl, China white, dance fever, friend, goodfella, jackpot, murder 8, TNT, Tango and Cash
	Heroin	Diacetylmorphine; brown sugar, dope, H, horse, junk, skag, skunk, smack, white horse
	Morphine	Roxanol, Duramorph; M, Miss Emma, monkey, white stuff
	Opium	Laudanum, paregoric; big O, black stuff, block, gum, hop
Stimulants	Amphetamine	Adderall, Biphetamine, Dexedrine; bennies, black beauties, crosses, hearts, LA turnaround, speed, truck drivers, uppers
	Cocaine	Cocaine hydrochloride; blow, bump, C, candy, Charlie, coke, crack, flake, rock, snow, toot
	MDMA	DOB, DOM, MDA; Adam, clarity, ecstasy, Eve, lover's speed, peace, STP, X, XTC
	Methamphetamine	Desoxyn; chalk, crank, crystal, fire, glass, go fast, ice, meth, speed
	Methylphenidate	Ritalin; JIF, MPH, R-ball, Skippy, the smart drug, vitamin R
	Nicotine	Bidis, chew, cigars, cigarettes, smokeless tobacco, snuff, spit tobacco, tolerance, addiction
Other compounds	Anabolic steroids	Anadrol, Oxandrin, Durabolin, Depo-Testosterone, Equipoise; roids, juice
	Inhalants	Solvents (paint thinners, gasoline, glues), gases (butane, propane, aerosol propellants, nitrous oxide), nitrites (isoamyl, isobutyl, cyclohexyl); laughing gas, poppers, snappers, whippets

GHB, Gamma hydroxybutyrate; LSD, lysergic acid diethylamide; MDMA, methylenedioxy-methamphetamine; PCP, phencyclidine.
*Associated with sexual assaults.
Modified from "Commonly Abused Drugs." http://www.nida.nih.gov/DrugPages/DrugsofAbuse.html.

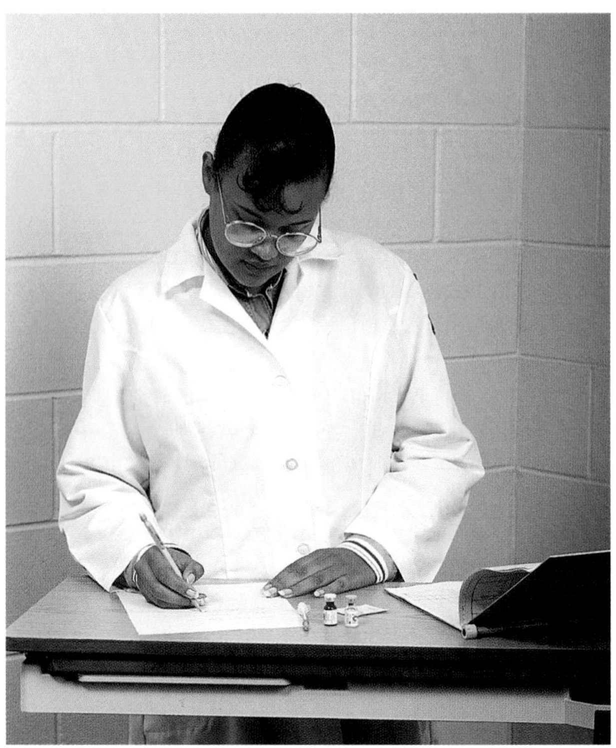

FIGURE 29-5 A health care worker prepares for immunizations.

sexually transmitted disease control, mental illness, care of the aged, addiction, and chronic and communicable diseases. State services include immunization, sanitation, animal control, vital statistics, public health nursing services, referral services, air and water pollution control, vector control, food and drug control, and community-sponsored blood testing (Fig. 29-5). Health needs are determined by surveying the community needs.

Each country in the world has a department that determines the health policies and protection plans for the citizens. The World Health Organization (WHO) is a nongovernmental agency that is organized to protect the health of the world community. In the United States, health agencies are organized on local, state, and federal levels.

The federal health agencies provide regulation of and protection against hazards that affect all the states. They collect and distribute demographic health statistics, support local and state agencies, and organize and support disaster relief programs. The U.S. Department of Health and Human Services (DHHS) is the main organization for public health care at the federal level.

The CDC is one branch of the Public Health Service department. It provides programs that prevent and control communicable, vector-borne, and chronic illnesses. The U.S. FDA regulates foods, drugs, medical devices, and cosmetics. The NIH deals with research in determining the cause, treatment, and methods of prevention of diseases. Other departments of the Public Health Service include the Health Resources Administration and Health Services Administration.

State and local agencies enforce state health laws and provide care for residents. These agencies are involved in preventive, environmental, and community health care services. Community health care provides services for individuals who do not use private health care because of economic, cultural, or similar reasons (Fig. 29-6). Immunization and education programs of the community health services are directed to provide care for the entire community. Eligibility for community health services is determined by state and federal regulations.

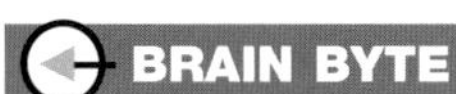

In 2009 1.6 million homeless people were in shelters.

Performance Instruction

Licensed personnel perform most of the duties that are performed as part of the health care treatment in mental and community settings. This is due to the legal and privacy rights of the people seeking care in this setting. Entry-level workers may provide assistance in these duties when supervised by licensed personnel.

Research has shown that hospital and medical experiences can be upsetting to children and their families. The certified child life specialist and related personnel help to meet the social and mental needs of the hospitalized child. Some examples of activities that may reduce anxiety for the child are tours of surgery, radiology, and other departments that may be visited during the hospital stay. Explanation and demonstration of equipment and supplies to be used are also helpful.

Summary

- The functions of the community and social health care team are to prevent illness and provide care to a population.

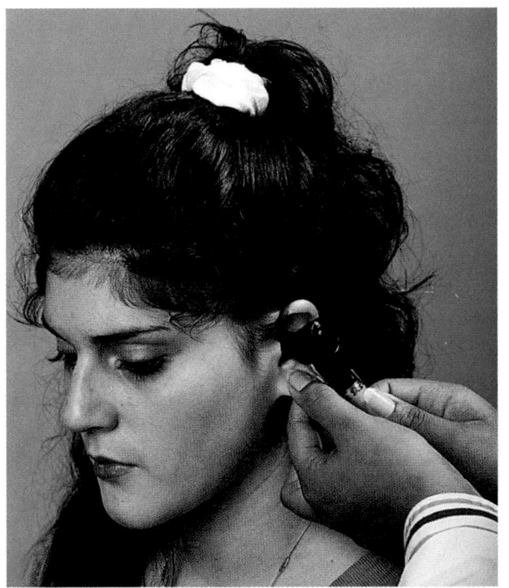

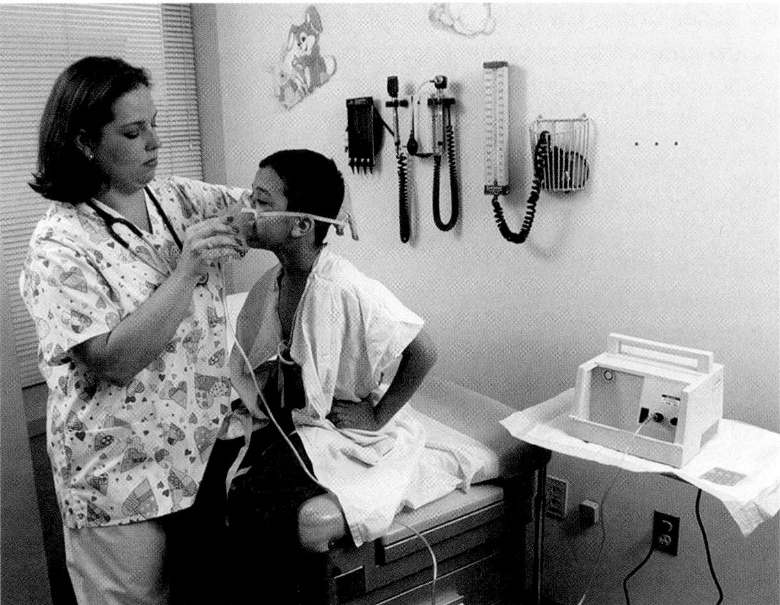

FIGURE 29-6 Community health care centers often provide care for those who cannot afford private health care.

- The roles of community and social health care workers are to search for the origin of disease and regulate potential sources of illness and injury.
- Services provided by community health care agencies include providing food, counseling, screening, examination, testing, and placement.
- The difference between physical and psychological drug dependency is that physical dependence results from the body needing a substance, whereas psychological dependence is a state of mind.
- Signs and symptoms of withdrawal from an addictive substance include nervousness, trembling, sweating, cramps, and hallucination.

Review Questions

1. Describe the role of three members of the community and social health care team.
2. List six services provided by community and social health care agencies.
3. Differentiate between physical and psychological dependence.
4. List four signs and symptoms of withdrawal.
5. Choose one career from Box 29-1. Research the cost of education and annual earnings in local institutions. Write a paragraph describing the factors that might explain why the local and national economic figures vary.
6. Use the following terms in one or more sentences that correctly relate their meaning: dependence, hallucination, and withdrawal.

Critical Thinking

1. Investigate and compare the cost of various types of community and social health care services.
2. Research and identify the types of immunizations required for school attendance.
3. Discuss situations that might lead to substance abuse and alternative coping mechanisms.
4. Research and write a paragraph describing one chemical from Table 29-2. Describe the intoxicating effects and potential health consequences of its use. Include a summary of one recent news story that involves the substance.
5. Plan a health fair on the basis of studying the needs of the community. Investigate the community resources, publicity, and other factors needed to produce the fair.
6. Research the local agencies and programs that provide assistance with housing or food for children and families without income. Make a brochure that provides information for the services available.
7. Create a career ladder for community and social careers. Describe why it is or is not possible to move from one level to another in the field.

8. Research and write a paragraph describing one example of the global impact of disease prevention and cost containment.

Explore the Web

Career Information

Bureau of Labor Statistics
http://www.bls.gov/

Salary.com
http://salary.com

Professional Associations

American Association of Occupational Health Nursing (AAOHN)
https://www.aaohn.org/

National Association of Social Workers (NASW)
http://www.socialworkers.org/

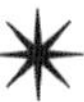

CHAPTER 30

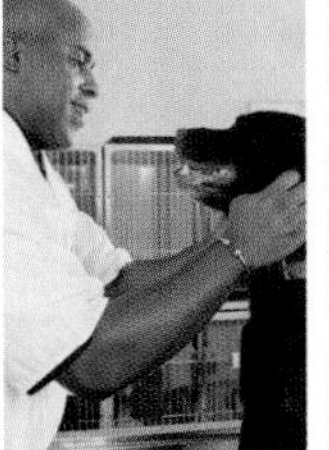
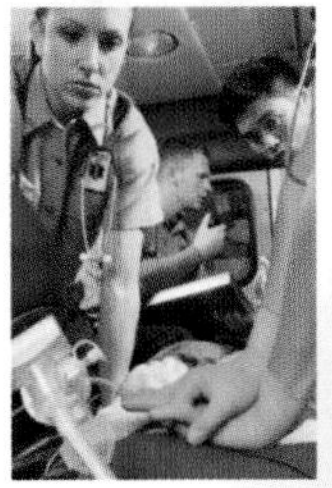
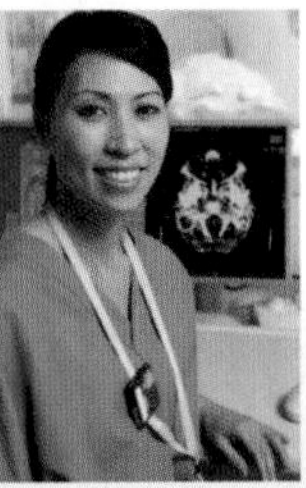

Mental Health Careers

LEARNING OBJECTIVES

- Define at least eight terms relating to mental health care.
- Describe the function of the mental health care team.
- Specify the role of selected members of the mental health care team, including the personal qualities, levels of education, and credentialing requirements.
- Define mental health and mental hygiene.
- Describe at least four psychoneurotic disorders.
- Describe at least two types of psychosis.
- Describe procedures for use of physical restraint.
- Identify at least three techniques of reality orientation.

KEY TERMS

Behavior *(bee-HAYV-yur)* Conduct, actions that can be observed

Phobia *(FOE-bee-uh)* Persistent abnormal dread or fear

Psychology *(sie-KOL-uh-jee)* Study of human and animal behavior, normal and abnormal

Psychoneurosis *(sie-ko-noo-RO-sis)* Functional disturbance of the mind in which the individual is aware that reactions are not normal

Psychosis *(sie-KO-sis)* Major mental disorder in which the individual loses contact with reality

Psychotherapy *(sie-ko-THARE-uh-pee)* Treatment of discomfort, dysfunction, or diseases by methods designed to understand and cope with problems

Reality orientation *(ree-AL-it-ee o-ree-en-TAY-shun)* Awareness of position in relation to time, space, and person

Restraint *(reh-STRAYNT)* Physical confinement

Mental Careers Terminology*

Term	Definition	Prefix	Root	Suffix
Anorexia	Condition of being without appetite	an	orex	ia
Bipolar	Having two extremes	bi	polar	
Hydrophobia	Condition of being afraid of water	hydro	phob	ia
Insomnia	Condition of lacking sleep	in	somn	ia
Neurotic	Pertaining to a functional disorder or disease of the nerves		neuro/t	ic
Phobia	Pertaining to fear		phob	ia
Photophobia	Fear of light	photo	phob	ia
Psychology	Study of the mind		psych	ology
Psychopathology	Study of disease of the mind	psych/o	path	ology
Psychosis	Condition of the mind		psych/o	sis

*A transition syllable or vowel may be added to or deleted from the word parts to make the combining form.

Abbreviations for Mental Careers

Abbreviation	Meaning
ECT	Electroconvulsive therapy
EdD	Doctor of education
EEG	Electroencephalogram
LOC	Level of consciousness
NCHSW	National Commission for Human Services Workers
Neuro	Neurology
NIMH	National Institute of Mental Health
PhD	Doctor of philosophy
PsyD	Doctor of psychology
RO	Reality orientation

BOX 30-1

Mental Health Careers

- Psychiatric aide
- Psychiatric technician
- Psychiatrist
- Psychologist, chief
- Psychologist, clinical
- Psychologist, counseling
- Psychologist, developmental
- Psychologist, educational
- Psychologist, engineering
- Psychologist, experimental
- Psychologist, industrial
- Psychologist, school
- Psychologist, social

Careers

The function of the mental health care team is to provide care and treatment for individuals with disorders of the mind, emotion, or behavior (Box 30-1). Mental health care workers must have an interest in **behavior** and the ability to communicate well. The work is challenging and requires the worker to be creative in finding unusual solutions to problems. Mental health care workers must be emotionally stable and mature. They must be able to lead and inspire others while demonstrating patience and perseverance.

The field of mental health care is constantly growing (Table 30-1). With the increasing age of the population in general and the higher cost of care, many of the mental health care services have moved into the homes of the patients, residential facilities, and neighborhood clinics. Additionally, more allied and support staff personnel are providing care and treatments that were done by professionals in the past.

It is now commonly accepted that a person's emotional and mental state may cause or have some effect on all physical disorders. According to testimony given by physicians to the Congress of the United States, more than half of all physician office visits do not result from physical illness. Disorders of the mind (psyche) may be caused by mental illness, loss of contact with reality, the inability to understand the environment, isolation, depression, or destructive life events.

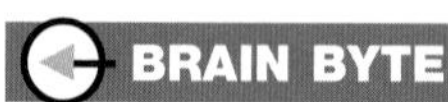

The National Institute of Mental Health reports that about one in four adults in the United States has a diagnosable mental disorder every year.

TABLE 30-1
Mental Health Career Educational Cost and Earnings

Career	Educational Cost*	Earnings†
Psychologist	Middle Tennessee State University master's degree (41 credit hours) Fees include: Tuition & fees $8,887 Books $350-$500	Median annual salary: Nashville, Tenn.—$74,340

*http://www.mtsu.edu/bursar/rates_main.shtml.
†http://data.bls.gov:8080/oes/datatype.do.

Psychiatrist

Psychiatrists are licensed physicians specializing in the treatment of mental, emotional, and behavioral disorders. Psychiatrists determine the type and severity of the disorder and plan the necessary therapy, which may include medication to treat the problem. Psychiatrists must complete at least a 4-year residency after earning a medical degree. Specialties in psychiatry include psychotherapy, child practice, psychoanalysis, behavior therapy, forensics, and industrial or organizational practice. About half of all psychiatrists work in private practice, with the remainder working in hospitals, clinics, research, and educational centers.

CASE STUDY 30-1 You are assigned to a patient who is confused and thinks you are her daughter. What should you do?

Answers to Case Studies are available on the Evolve website: ***http://evolve.elsevier.com/Gerdin***

Psychologist

Psychologists are professionals who specialize in treatment of mental and emotional disorders. They study human behavior and mental processes to understand and explain human actions. Methods of treatment include personal interviews, intelligence and aptitude testing, and observation. Most psychologists earn a doctoral (PhD, EdD, or PsyD) degree and complete an internship before obtaining the licensure or certification required to practice independently. The doctor of psychology degree is offered by professional schools that emphasize training for clinical practice. Psychologists may specialize in the area of educational, social, clinical, cross-cultural, quantitative, consumer, environmental, developmental, rehabilitative, or organizational behavior (Box 30-2). More than 40% of psychologists are self-employed.

Master's degree preparation in psychology allows an individual to work in a limited variety of settings, including schools, businesses, and mental health centers. Many individuals with master's degrees work under the supervision of a doctor of psychology. Certification or licensing is required in all states.

BOX 30-2

Areas of Specialty for Psychologists

- Childcare counseling
- Clinical psychology
- Community psychology
- Consumer psychology
- Counseling psychology
- Developmental psychology
- Educational psychology
- Engineering psychology
- Family therapy
- Forensic psychology
- Health psychology
- Hospital practice
- Human relations
- Industrial or organizational psychology
- Marriage therapy
- Military practice
- Neuropsychology
- Private practice
- Quantitative and measurement psychology
- Rehabilitation psychology
- Research psychology
- School psychology
- Social psychology
- Sports psychology
- Substance abuse therapy

Health Careers in Practice

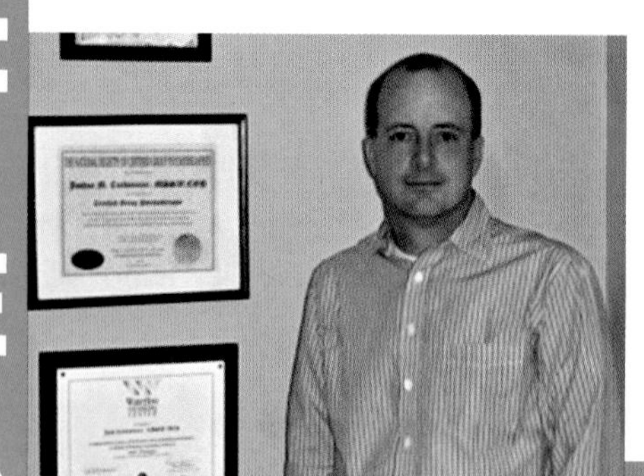

JOSHUA M. CORDONNIER, LCSW

PSYCHOTHERAPIST OR LICENSED CLINICAL SOCIAL WORKER
SELF-EMPLOYED AND PARTNER IN CHARLOTTESVILLE PSYCHOLOGICAL ASSOCIATES (wsw.cpatherapy.com)

Educational background: Bachelor of social work (BSW) from University of Missouri; master's of science in social work (MSSW) from University of Texas Austin

Note: You must have a master's degree to be a psychotherapist (psychology, social work, counseling); however, I received my MSSW in 1 year because of having a BSW.

A typical day at work and job duties include: I set and keep my own appointments and meet with people in my office. We discuss a myriad of issues that bring someone to therapy: depression, anxiety, relationships, social skills, obsessive thoughts, trauma history, occupational distress, etc. Other duties include the following:

- Routine note taking
- Consulting with doctors, teachers, parents as needed
- Completing treatment plans, insurance authorizations and billing forms as needed

The most gratifying part of my job: To assist someone in changing themselves and being able to be with someone in their most difficult moments and help that person get to a better place in his or her life. Knowing I am useful and can help people with my skills is also very gratifying.

The biggest challenge(s) I face in doing my job: Paperwork and insurance filing is the worst part of the job. Also, it can be difficult to hear the amount of pain and trauma some people have had to face in their life.

What drew me to my career? I went into social work to help people and to make the world a more livable place. I then specialized in psychotherapy because I get to directly work with patients in an intellectual and emotional way.

Something I learned in my early education that I currently use in my career or that caused me to be interested in my career is: I worked at a camp for inner-city kids in Denver, Colorado, which forever changed my view of the world. I realized there are so many people struggling to get by in life and being affected by the way it is shaped.

Support Personnel

Psychiatric technicians take an active part in the treatment of patients. They may interview, lead group sessions, give daily care, or make home visits. In some cases they may administer medications. Education for the psychiatric technician includes a 2-year associate degree. Many states require the psychiatric technician to be licensed. Psychiatric technicians may also be known as mental health technicians, human service workers, or mental health associates. Certification for mental health technicians is available from the National Commission for Human Service Workers.

Psychiatric assistants help patients with problems of mental health under the direction of nurses and physicians. The responsibilities of the psychiatric assistant include helping the patient with activities of daily living, such as dressing and eating. The assistant also socializes with the patients and may play games or lead recreational activities. The psychiatric assistant observes patients for unusual behavior and reports the observations to the professional staff. Some psychiatric hospitals and community colleges offer on-the-job training programs to prepare psychiatric assistants. These training programs usually last 4 to 6 months.

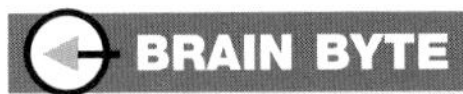

Autism and other autism spectrum disorders are generally diagnosed by age three and are four times more common in boys than girls.

Content Instruction

Mental Health

In the past, people with mental or developmental problems were placed in institutions called *asylums* or *sanatoriums*. Most people with mental illness in the United States now live in the community, not in institutions. Society believes that people with mental illness and developmental disabilities have the potential to improve and the right to try to live an independent life. The living environment for those with mental impairments must provide protection, opportunities for development, and support for daily tasks. Most experts feel that living at home is the optimal arrangement for individuals with mental or developmental disabilities. Assisted living centers and nursing homes may provide care for some people with mental disorders. Other alternatives include foster care, day care centers, halfway houses, and small group homes that provide supervised assistance (Fig. 30-1).

Mental health is a state of mind in which a person can cope with problems and maintain emotional balance and satisfaction in living. Mental disorders may be classified as organic or functional. Organic disorders are caused by injury to the brain, such as by high fever, tumor, or toxic substances such as drugs. Functional disorders have no known brain injury. Functional disorders include psychoneuroses, psychoses, and personality disorders. The severity of mental illness ranges from minor anxiety to a condition that prevents an individual from relating to other people. More than 16 million Americans seek some form of mental health care each year.

Psychoneuroses are functional disturbances of the mind. The individual with neuroses does not lose touch with reality and often knows that the reactions experienced are not appropriate. Anxiety and depression are two emotions experienced by everyone (Fig. 30-2). Anxiety is a feeling of fear or apprehension. Depression is a feeling of sadness. In some people these emotions are experienced without cause or in an overwhelming manner.

Panic disorder is a condition of feeling an unreasonable fear with no known cause. **Phobias** are specific, unrealistic fears. For example, agoraphobia is

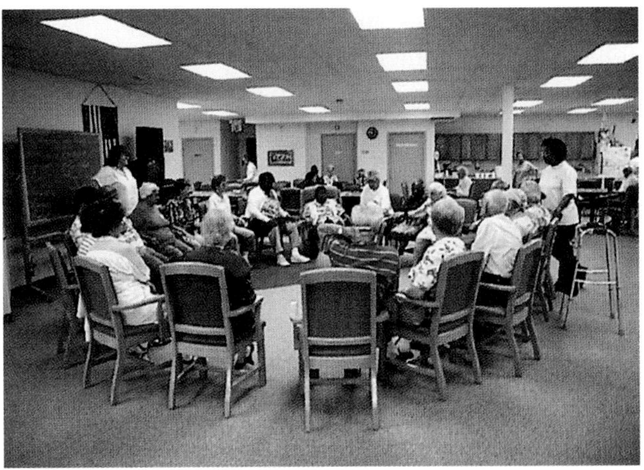

FIGURE 30-1 An adult day care center for patients with Alzheimer disease is an alternative to a long-term care environment.

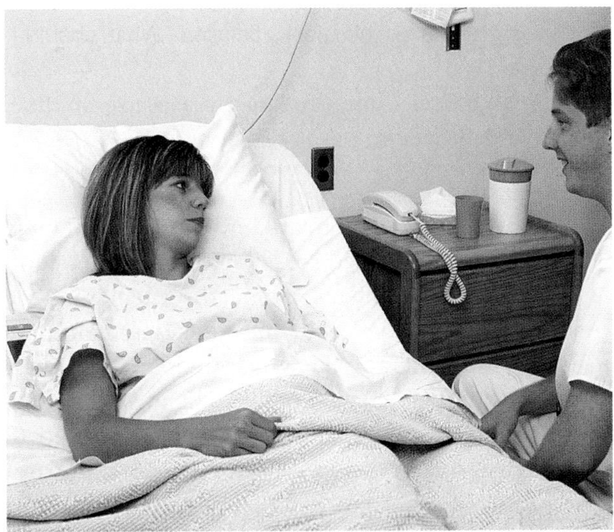

FIGURE 30-2 Anxiety and depression may affect anyone at any time of life.

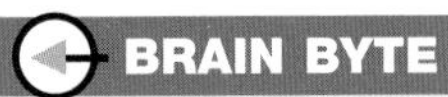

Anxiety disorders are the most common mental health or mental hygiene problem in the United States.

fear of being in a place where escape might not be possible, and it may cause a person to refuse or not want to leave the home. Another neurosis is hypochondria, or the belief in imaginary illness.

Psychoses are severe or major mental disorders in which the individual is not in contact with reality. The individual with a psychosis does not know that the behavior and thoughts are abnormal. Several types of schizophrenia result in a separation from the real world and in fixed ideas or obsessions. Manic-depressive or bipolar **psychosis** is a condition of repeating cycles in which severe depression is followed by extremely elated or excited behavior. In a condition of paranoia, the person feels persecuted and plotted against by others.

Deprivation syndrome is a condition in children resulting from inadequate nutrition and an environment unsuited for normal growth and development. These children develop an intellectual slowing (retardation) and difficulty fitting into society. Other mental disorders may result from the abuse of drugs and alcohol. Dissociative disorders are those in which the person loses or changes identity. An example of a dissociative disorder is an individual with multiple personalities.

CASE STUDY 30-2 Your patient tells you he is going to quit taking his medication for depression because it makes him feel confused. What should you say?

Answers to Case Studies are available on the Evolve website: ***http://evolve.elsevier.com/Gerdin***

Mental disorders are treated in many ways (Table 30-2). Psychotherapy is discussion to help understand and cope with problems. Some disorders may be treated or controlled with medication. Treatment may include group therapy, in which people share their thoughts and feelings with others who have the same problem. Electroconvulsive therapy may be used to treat depression by using electric shock to interrupt temporarily the normal function of the brain. Some disorders may be treated with behavioral modification to change the individual's lifestyle.

When a mental disorder is severe, suicide may occur (Box 30-3). Other risk factors include alcohol and substance abuse and a major stressing event. In 2006, suicide was the leading cause of death in people aged 15 to 24. Psychotherapy and medication are some of the methods used to prevent suicide.

BRAIN BYTE

In 2006 the Centers for Disease Control and Prevention reported suicide to be the eleventh leading cause of death among Americans.

CASE STUDY 30-3 Your friend has been giving her things away, saying goodbye to you and others, and talking about suicide. What should you do?

Answers to Case Studies are available on the Evolve website: ***http://evolve.elsevier.com/Gerdin***

TABLE 30-2
Forms of Therapy

Type of Therapy	Description
Behavioral	Focus is on symptoms and managing specific complaints, such as phobias
Cognitive	Focus is on patient's thinking and logic regarding dysfunctional behavior
Desensitization	Form of behavioral therapy that removes phobias by progressively exposing the patient to the source of fear
Family	Focus is on unhealthy patterns of interaction and inappropriate demands and expectations between family members
Gestalt	Focus is on challenging patient's defenses to strive for wholeness
Group	Focus is on interaction with others in a controlled setting
Humanistic	Focus is on helping the patient remove emotional barriers; nondirective
Interpersonal	Focus is on improving social skills
Play	Focus is on the patient's (child's) expression of problems through the use of play
Psychoanalytic	Focus is on continued, intensive treatment with one practitioner
Psychodynamic	Focus is on personal relationships
Short-term	Focus is on specific problems

Research is being conducted on the relationship of the function of the brain to psychological behavior. This field is called *neurobiology*. One example of the result of neurobiological research is the demonstration of "right-brain" and "left-brain" control. It is now known that the right hemisphere of the brain controls creative and nonverbal thinking, whereas the left hemisphere controls logical and verbal thought (Fig. 30-3). One new concept that is being researched by neurobiologists hypothesizes that there are periods of

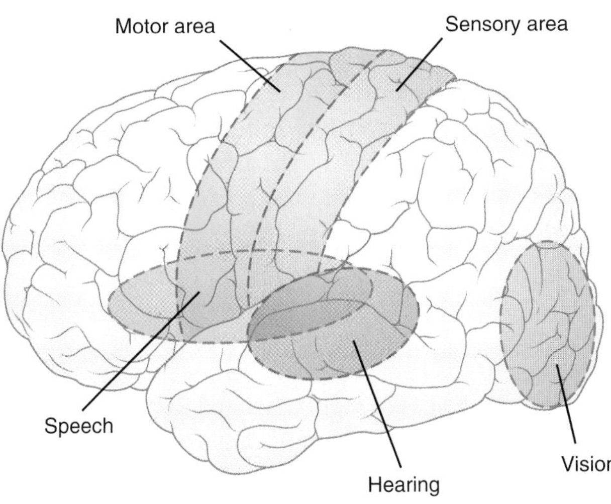

FIGURE 30-3 Functional areas of the brain. (From Milliken ME, Campbell G: *Essential competencies for patient care*, St. Louis, 1995, Mosby.)

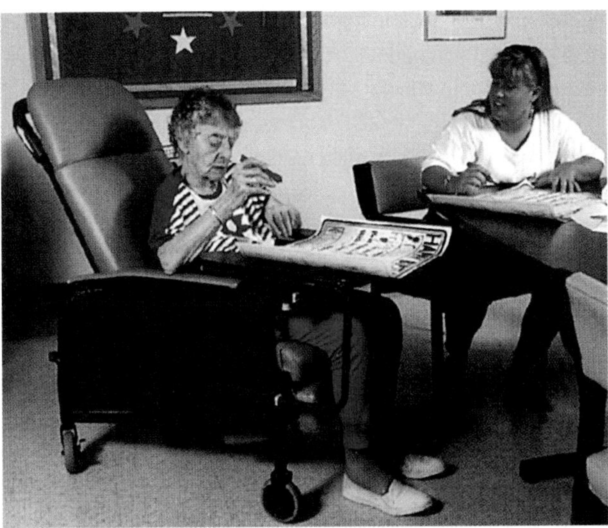

FIGURE 30-4 The geriatric chair is also a physical restraint. Restraints are used only with a physician's order so that the patient is protected from injury. (From Sorrentino S: *Mosby's textbook for long-term care assistants*, ed 3, St. Louis, 1999, Mosby.)

BOX 30-3

Common Warning Signs of Suicide

- Change in behavior
- Change in eating habits
- Change in personality
- Change in sleep patterns
- Clinical depression
- Fear of losing control
- Hopeless
- Low self-esteem
- Putting "affairs in order"
- Recent loss or major stress
- Reduced sexual interest
- Substance abuse
- Talk about dying, suicide
- Tempting fate by risky behavior
- Visiting or calling people to say goodbye

"neuroplasticity," or specific developmental times during which the brain needs certain experiences for optimal development to occur.

Other research has led to the theory that genes influence a person's personality and mental behavior. Studies conducted by the Minnesota Center for Twin and Adoption Research using identical twins that were separated at birth often reveal that the twins display the same mannerisms, pursue the same interests and careers, and even marry the same type (in appearance and personality) of individual. This field of study is often called *sociobiology*.

Mental Hygiene

Mental hygiene includes the methods used to preserve and promote mental health. Mentally healthy people can learn stress reduction techniques and adopt changes in lifestyle. The individual with mental disorders may need special treatment techniques to live safely and in the best manner possible. Examples of these techniques include the use of protective **restraints** and **reality orientation**.

Restraints, or protective devices, are used to protect patients from harming themselves or others (Fig. 30-4). Confinement may be to a bed or chair. Restraints may be made of cloth or leather. In many states a written order from a physician is required for use of restraints. Without a doctor's order, the use of restraints is considered false imprisonment. Restraints must be applied correctly to avoid injury to the patient and are used for as short a time as possible. In addition to meeting the physical needs of the restrained patient, the health care worker must also make sure that the patient's mental needs are met. Anxiety resulting from confinement may be reduced by visiting with the patient frequently and providing other distractions, such as activities.

Loss of orientation (confusion) may result in many situations. Loss of hearing, sight, or confinement may lead to temporary confusion. Confusion may result from a reduced blood supply to the brain. Confusion is frightening and frustrating for the person experiencing it. Reality orientation is a form of rehabilitation that promotes or maintains awareness of person, place, and time by reinforcing the correct information.

One of the methods used to help patients maintain their sense of reality is a systematic approach to orientation. Calendars, clocks, and a routine for daily activities help keep the patient oriented to place and time. Several times daily, the health care workers talk with and address the patient by name to help maintain the patient's orientation to person.

CASE STUDY 30-4 You observe that your friend has a lot of relationships that do not last very long. When you talk about it, she says that she feels that all the men she meets want to control her. She says she hates herself for that feeling. What should you say?

Answers to Case Studies are available on the Evolve website: *http://evolve.elsevier.com/Gerdin*

Performance Instruction

Restraint

Use of restraints must be ordered by a physician and only after proper instruction is given for its use. The least restrictive type of restraint is preferred. Safe restraints should not have tears, frayed edges, or other damage. Towels, bed sheets, tape, and other improvised restraints are not safe for use. The restraint should be applied according to manufacturer's instructions. They should be snug but allow some movement and blood circulation in the restrained area. Circulation in the restrained area should be checked every 15 minutes. Restraints should not be secured to moving parts of the bed or chair that might change the movement in the restrained area. Proper body alignment should be observed and maintained during restraint.

Reality Orientation

Confusion may result from many disorders or displacement to a health care facility. Care for a confused person should include stating of the caregiver's name and role with each visit to the room, as well as clarifying and repeating procedures as often as needed for the person to understand. The patient's name should also be called by name with each contact. Speaking slowly and clearly is one method to improve understanding. Instructions should be short and simple. A calm, relaxed environment and a routine may help reduce anxiety caused by confusion. Clocks, calendars, newspapers, and other articles may help the person remain oriented to the present. (See Skill List 30-1, Reality Orientation, p. 483.)

Summary

- The function of the mental health team is to provide care and treatment for individuals with disorders of the mind, emotion, or behavior.
- The role of the psychiatrist is to determine the type and severity of a mental disorder and provide treatment. Psychologists use interviews, testing, and observation to treat mental and emotional disorders. The work is challenging and requires the worker to be creative in finding unusual solutions to problems. Mental health care workers must be emotionally stable and mature. They must be able to lead and inspire others while demonstrating patience and perseverance.
- Mental health is a state of mind in which a person can cope with problems and maintain emotional balance and satisfaction in living. Mental hygiene includes the methods used to preserve and promote mental health.
- Four types of psychoneuroses are anxiety, depression, panic disorder, and phobias.
- Two types of psychosis are schizophrenia and bipolar disorder.
- The procedures for use of physical restraint include obtaining a written order from a physician, using the least restraint necessary to provide for safety, and checking that restraints are applied properly.
- Three techniques of reality orientation are displaying clocks and calendars, addressing the patient by name, and placing articles in the same place.

Review Questions

1. Describe the function of the mental health care team.
2. Specify the role of the members of the mental health care team.
3. Define mental health and mental hygiene.
4. Define psychoneurosis. Describe four types of psychoneuroses.

5. Define psychosis. Describe two types of psychoses.
6. Specify the need for physical restraint and two precautions that may be used to avoid injury.
7. Describe three techniques that can be used to promote orientation to reality in a confused patient.
8. Choose one career from Box 30-1. Research the cost of education and annual earnings in local institutions. Write a paragraph describing the factors that might explain why the local and national economic figures vary.
9. Use each of the following terms in one or more sentences that correctly relate their meaning: behavior, phobia, psychoneurosis, and psychology.

Critical Thinking

1. Investigate and compare the cost of various types of mental health care treatments and tests.
2. Investigate five common medications used in mental health care treatments.
3. Investigate the local availability of mental health care facilities and services in the area.
4. Use the Internet to research the risk and protective factors associated with suicide. Compare and contrast the following terms: suicidal ideation, suicide attempt, and suicide.
5. Create a career ladder for mental health careers. Describe why it is or is not possible to move from one level to another in the field.
6. Describe and evaluate how mental health and healthy relationships influence career goals.

Explore the Web

Career Information

Bureau of Labor Statistics
http://www.bls.gov/

Salary.com
http://salary.com

Professional Associations

American Psychology Association (APA)
http://www.apa.org/

American Psychiatric Nurses Association (APNA)
http://www.apna.org/i4a/pages/index.cfm?pageid=1

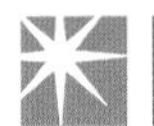

SKILL LIST 30-1
Reality Orientation

1. Maintain medical asepsis by using the guidelines provided in the Standard and Transmission-Based Precautions, including good handwashing technique and use of gloves as needed.
2. Identify the patient and explain the procedure.
3. Face the individual and speak clearly and slowly. Speaking in this manner helps the patient process the information.
4. Call the individual by name or title (Mr., Mrs., Ms., or Miss) according to his or her preference. It is not appropriate to call adults by their first name without permission.
5. Identify yourself to the patient by name and role.
6. Tell the individual the date and time of day.
7. Give simple and clear instructions or answers to any questions.
8. Allow enough time for a response. Older people require more time to process new information.
9. Keep calendars and clocks with large numbers in clear view.
10. Assist the patient to use glasses and hearing aids if needed.
11. Provide items of current information, such as newspapers, and place familiar objects and pictures in view. Remind the patient of special events such as holidays.
12. Maintain a cycle of day and night activities. Street clothes should be worn during the day and pajamas or nightgowns at night.
13. Be consistent with the procedure. Routine helps the patient to retain information.

CHAPTER 31

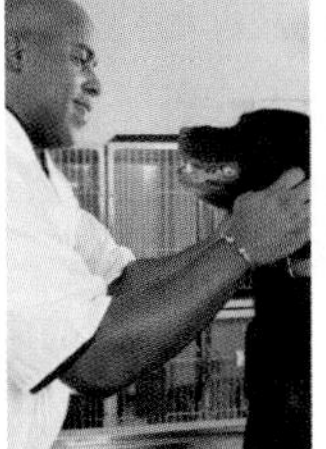
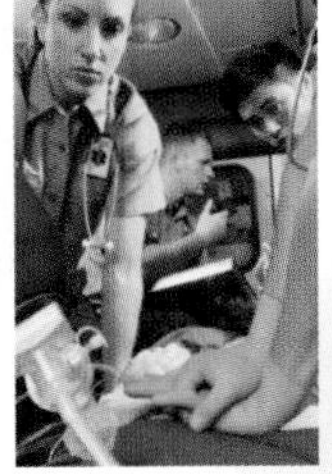
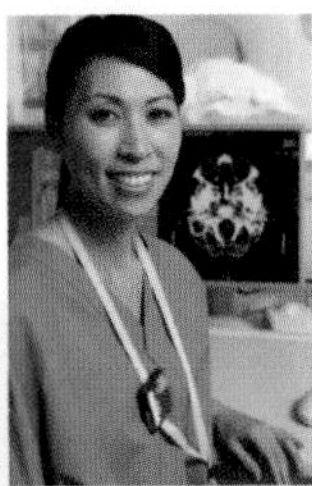

Rehabilitative Careers

LEARNING OBJECTIVES

- Define at least 10 terms relating to rehabilitative health care.
- Identify the function of the rehabilitative health care team.
- Describe the role of at least five of the rehabilitative health care team members, including personal qualities, levels of education, and credentialing requirements.
- Identify at least five methods or devices used to improve activities of daily living for the disabled.
- Describe two types of hearing loss and two methods of assessing defects in hearing.
- Identify at least five common drug types and the expected action of each.
- Identify the necessary components of a legal drug prescription, including the personnel qualified to write one.
- Describe three other types of rehabilitative treatments.

KEY TERMS

Articulation *(ar-tik-yoo-LAY-shun)* Enunciation of words and syllables, how sounds are spoken

Audiology *(aw-dee-OL-uh-jee)* Science of hearing

Disability *(dis-uh-BIL-uh-tee)* Lack of ability to function in the manner that most people function physically or mentally

Dispense *(dis-PENTS)* Prepare, package, compound, or label for delivery according to a lawful order of a qualified practitioner

Dosage *(DOSE-age)* Regulation of size, frequency, and amount of medication

Frequency *(FREE-kwen-see)* Number of times an event occurs in a given period; measured in cycles per second (hertz [Hz]) in hearing

Hydrotherapy *(hie-dro-THAIR-uh-pee)* Application of water

Nebulizer *(NEB-yoo-lie-zer)* Device used to deliver a spray or mist of medication into the lungs

KEY TERMS cont'd

Orthotics *(or-THOT-iks)* Art or science of custom designing, fabrication, and fitting of braces

Pharmacology *(farm-uh-KOL-uh-jee)* Study of the actions and uses of drugs

Prosthesis *(pros-THEE-sis)* Artificial device applied to replace a partially or totally missing body part

Prosthetics *(pros-THET-iks)* Art or science of custom design, fabrication, and fitting of artificial limbs

Rehabilitation *(re-huh-bil-i-TAY-shun)* Restoration of normal form and function after injury or illness

Therapy *(THEIR-uh-pee)* Treatment of disease; science and art of healing

Rehabilitative Careers Terminology*

Term	Definition	Prefix	Root	Suffix
Aphasia	Without speaking	a	phas	ia
Audiogram	Record of hearing	audio	gram	
Audiology	Study of hearing		audi	ology
Dysarthria	Difficulty articulating	dys	arthr	ia
Extracorporeal	Pertaining to outside of the body	extra	corpore	al
Hydrotherapy	Water therapy	hydro	therapy	
Myoelectronics	Pertaining to electricity and muscles	myo	electron	ics
Pedorthist	One who corrects child (bones)	ped	orth	ist
Pharmacology	Study of drugs		pharmac	ology
Tracheotomy	Hole in the windpipe		trache	otomy

*A transition syllable or vowel may be added to or deleted from the word parts to make the combining form.

Abbreviations in Rehabilitative Careers

Abbreviation	Meaning
ADL	Activities of daily living
CCC	Certificate of Clinical Competence
COTA	Certification of Occupational Therapy Assistants
CPT	Chest physical therapy
DEA	Drug enforcement agency
DTR	Registered dance therapist
FDA	Food and Drug Administration
OTC	Over the counter
PDR	*Physician's Desk Reference*
Rx	Prescription

Careers

Rehabilitative careers provide a variety of working opportunities (Box 31-1). The **rehabilitation** team includes physicians, surgeons, physical therapists, occupational therapists, social workers, counselors, pharmacists, orthotists, and prosthetists who provide services designed to overcome physical, developmental, behavioral, or emotional disabilities (Table 31-1). The disabilities include impaired muscle strength, physical endurance, sensory or muscle coordination, concentration, and spatial discrimination.

The rehabilitation team works closely with the patient and family members to restore these functions. These occupations require optimism, creativity, persistence, and the ability to work with a variety of people. Additionally, the health care worker in rehabilitation must have strong listening and verbal skills, analytical ability, and patience to meet challenges and solve problems.

BOX 31-1

Rehabilitative Health Careers

- Art therapist
- Audiologist
- Audiometrist
- Corrective therapist
- Dance therapist
- Drug preparation inspector
- Drug preparation utility worker
- Educational therapist
- Horticultural therapist
- Industrial therapist
- Manual arts therapist
- Medication aide
- Music therapist
- Occupational therapist
- Occupational therapy aide
- Occupational therapy assistant
- Orientation therapist for the blind
- Orthoptist
- Orthotic assistant
- Orthotic technician
- Pharmacist
- Pharmacologist
- Pharmacy assistant
- Pharmacy helper
- Physical-integration practitioner
- Physical therapist
- Physical therapy aide
- Physical therapy assistant
- Physiologist
- Prosthetic assistant
- Prosthetic technician
- Recreational therapist
- Speech pathologist
- Teacher of the blind
- Teacher of the deaf
- Teacher of the handicapped
- Teacher of home therapy
- Teacher of vocational training
- Voice pathologist

TABLE 31-1

Rehabilitative Career Educational Cost and Earnings

Career	Educational Cost*	Earnings†
Physical therapist	University of Nevada, doctor of physical therapy degree, 111 graduate credit hours Fees include: Tuition, books, & fees \$30,626 Clinical rotation \$17,726	Median annual salary: Las Vegas, Nev.—\$90,050

*http://pt.unlv.edu/admission.html.
†http://data.bls.gov:8080/oes/datatype.do.

Physical Therapist

Physical therapists (PTs) work to restore function, relieve pain, and prevent **disability** after disease, injury, or loss of a body part. PTs may specialize in many areas of practice, including rehabilitation, community health, sports, industry, research, education, and administration (Fig. 31-1). Additionally, PTs may work for a hospital or other health care facility or practice privately. Admission to the fewer than 30 college programs in physical therapy is competitive. Entry-level practice with a bachelor's degree in physical **therapy** or a related area and completion of certification is being phased out. Master's level preparation is preferred. PTs are licensed by the state.

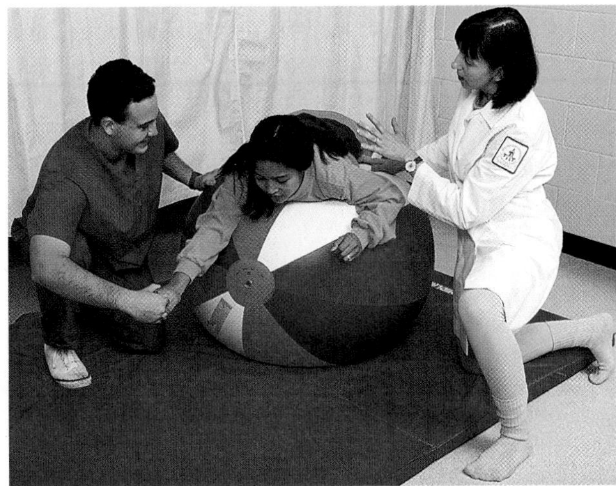

FIGURE 31-1 A physical therapist working with a patient.

Physical therapy assistants provide routine treatments under the supervision of a PT. This work includes application of hot and cold packs, ultraviolet and infrared light treatments, ultrasound and electrical stimulation, and hydrotherapy. Assistants observe patients during treatment and record performance. Accredited programs that prepare physical therapy assistants require 2 years of college-level training and award an associate degree.

BRAIN BYTE

Water's buoyancy makes swimming the ideal exercise for physical therapy and rehabilitation or for anyone seeking a low-impact exercise. An hour of vigorous swimming will burn up to 650 calories. It burns off more calories than walking or biking.

Kinesiotherapists work under the direction of a physician. They help patients strengthen and coordinate body movements with exercise. Kinesiotherapists specialize in maintaining muscle endurance, mobility, strength, and coordination. Their patients include those who are geriatric, have psychiatric needs, have physical or developmental disabilities, are striving for cardiac recovery, have been injured in sports, or have had amputations. Education for the kinesiotherapist includes a bachelor's degree in exercise physiology or physical education that includes an internship of at least 1000 hours of training. Certification is desirable but not required for all employment opportunities. National registration is available through the American Kinesiotherapy Association.

Orientation and mobility instructors or specialists help visually impaired and blind individuals to move about independently. Methods used to improve mobility include use of a cane, sensors, guide dogs, and electronic travel aids to help interpret the environment. A bachelor's degree is minimal for entry-level positions, and a master's degree is preferred. Certification for the orientation and mobility instructor is voluntary. Rehabilitation counseling provides the patient with career guidance and help in locating services that are necessary for successful employment.

Orthotist and Prosthetist

Orthotist and prosthetist practitioner programs usually require a baccalaureate degree. Certification is available through the American Orthotic and Prosthetic Association after successful completion of an approved program, 1 year of experience, and a certification examination. Technicians help to produce the appliances designed by the professional, but they are not responsible for patient assessment. Registration is possible but not required for technicians.

Certified orthotists provide services for patients with disabling conditions of the limbs or spine. They design, fabricate, and fit braces or strengthening apparatus. Additionally, the orthotist supervises support personnel and laboratory activities necessary to develop new devices for straightening a distorted part (orthosis).

Certified prosthetists provide care to patients with partial or total absence of a limb and who use an artificial limb (prosthesis). Responsibilities of the prosthetist include design, material selection, production, instruction on use, and evaluation of the appliance. *Myoelectronics* is the technical term for electromechanical prostheses. Myoelectronic technology amplifies and transfers nerve impulses from the body into electrical current to drive a motor. Parts of the body that have been lost can be replaced with artificial devices. Prostheses can also be specially designed for sports activities, including swimming, skiing, running, and climbing.

Corrective therapists conduct physical exercise programs to prevent muscle deterioration in inactive patients. The corrective therapist teaches the use of braces, crutches, and canes. Elastic stockings may be used for patients with limited mobility to decrease the chance of embolus development (Fig. 31-2). (See Skill List 31-1, Applying Elastic Stockings, p. 501.) Corrective therapists may complete bachelor's or master's degrees.

CASE STUDY 31-1 You notice that you have developed some blue spider veins on your knees. What should you do?

Answers to Case Studies are available on the Evolve website: ***http://evolve.elsevier.com/Gerdin***

Pedorthists modify and provide footwear to patients with imperfectly formed feet. Some conditions that might require specially fitted shoes include arthritis, injury, and congenital defects. Pedorthists follow the prescription of a physician. No education is required for this work, and it can be learned through seminars. Although not required, certification is recommended and based on successful examination by the Board of Certification in Pedorthics.

Health Careers in Practice

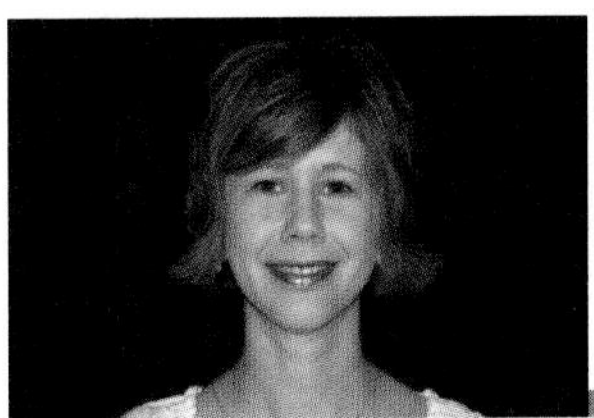

SARAH SPAETHE, OTR/L

REHAB SERVICES MANAGER
THE WESTCHESTER HOUSE

Educational background: Bachelor's degree in occupational therapy from Saint Louis University

A typical day at work and job duties include:

- Arrive at facility around 7:00 AM
- Review each therapist's caseload for the day and make adjustments as needed
- Review the minutes that have been provided to each patient on the previous day, and make adjustments as needed to assure appropriate reimbursement
- Attend patient care meetings to educate families and residents about therapy services
- Attend wound and fall rounds
- Treat patients as needed

The most gratifying part of my job: Spending time with the patients. We treat the geriatric population. I love seeing a patient recover and discharge successfully to home.

The biggest challenge(s) I face in doing my job: The biggest challenge I face is education to families and residents about the restrictions placed upon services by Medicare. Therapists are patient advocates by profession. It is very frustrating to tell people that we cannot provide a piece of equipment or treatment secondary to payment.

What drew me to my career? I volunteered with physically disabled children throughout high school. I thought I would love to work with children as a career. I actually attempted occupational therapy with children. I lasted about 1 year before I knew that my heart was really with the geriatric population, not children.

Something I learned in my early education that I currently use in my career or that caused me to be interested in my career is: I learned about blood pressure and basic exercise in physical education. I need to utilize that information on a daily basis.

Occupational Therapist

Occupational therapy helps patients reach the highest level of independent living by overcoming physical injury, birth defects, aging, or emotional and developmental problems. Occupational therapy uses activities to help a person develop, maintain, or regain skills that enable satisfying and independent living. Specific programs are developed to permit work, leisure, and play activities. Occupational therapists (OTs) use adaptive equipment such as splints, wheelchairs, canes, walkers, and prosthetic devices. They evaluate patients, plan the programs, and supervise or provide treatment. OTs analyze an activity to determine the adaptive skills required for the patient to perform it. OTs may be registered after successful completion of an accredited 4-year baccalaureate program, a minimum of 6 months' clinical training, and a national examination. Master's and doctoral programs are available for specialized practice and top-level employment. Most states require licensure to practice as an occupational therapist.

Occupational therapy assistants may be trained in programs that include a minimum of 2 months of supervised field training. Occupational therapy assistants instruct and assist patients to perform activities of daily living. Assistants help to design and adapt living and working environments to meet the needs of the disabled patient. Certification of occupational therapy assistants is possible after completion of an approved 2-year program. Certification is obtained by passing a national examination. Occupational therapy aides are trained on the job. They assist with transportation, equipment assembly, and maintenance of work areas.

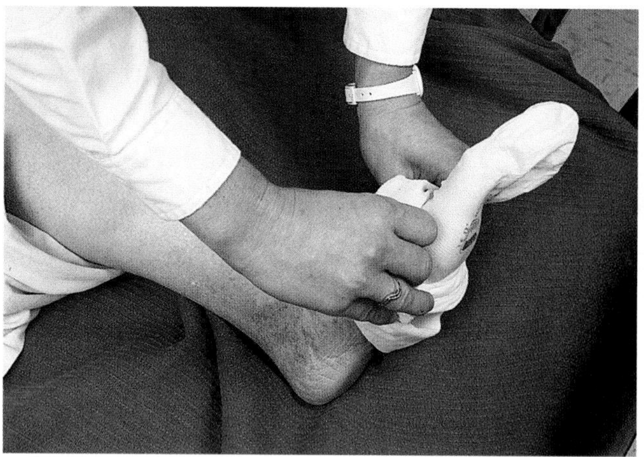
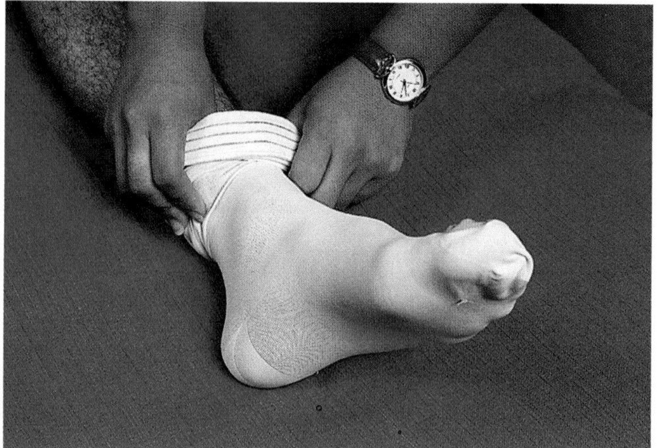

FIGURE 31-2 Elastic stockings help to prevent the development of emboli.

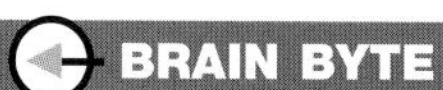

Almost one third of OTs work with children.

Athletic Trainer

Athletic trainers work under the supervision of the team physician in a variety of amateur and professional sports and other settings. High schools, colleges, professional sports teams, and other athletic agencies employ trainers. Many athletic trainers at the high school level also teach classes. The trainer's role includes prevention of injury and emergency treatment. Athletic trainers use methods that include corrective exercise, conditioning, rehabilitation, and nutrition counseling. Often the athletic trainer is also responsible for ordering and maintaining supplies and equipment for the training room.

CASE STUDY 31-2 The patient you have been assigned to help is very overweight. What should you do?

Answers to Case Studies are available on the Evolve website: ***http://evolve.elsevier.com/Gerdin***

The trainer works with the physician, athletes, and coaches and must be able to communicate well. The trainer must also possess manual dexterity and the ability to work in stressful situations. Athletic trainers work long and irregular hours.

Approximately 350 accredited programs for athletic trainers include a minimum of an 1800-hour internship over at least 2 academic years. These programs may also lead to a teaching certification in one of the physical education or related sciences. Most athletic trainers who work for colleges or professional teams have a master's or doctoral degree. Most employers require certification by the National Athletic Trainers' Association Board of Certification.

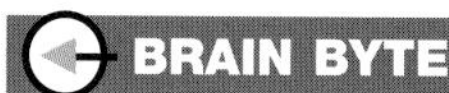

All licensed athletic trainers have a bachelor's degree, and 70% also hold a master's or doctoral degree.

Pharmacist

Pharmacists mix and **dispense** drugs according to prescriptions written by physicians, veterinarians, dentists, and other authorized professionals. They also provide information to the consumer about side effects of medications, food and drug interactions, dosing schedules, and health care supplies. **Pharmacology** prepares the professional as a specialist in the science of drugs. Six of every 10 pharmacists are employed in small community pharmacies. Hospital pharmacists may specialize in the areas of nuclear drugs, poison control, or intravenous therapy. The pharmacist must be good with detail and conscientious about checking and rechecking work. Accuracy, neatness, and cleanliness are important to ensure safe medication. Accredited schooling in pharmacology lasts a minimum of 5 years after a minimum of 1 year of college-level preparation. Two degrees are awarded in pharmacology. The bachelor of science in pharmacology (BS Pharm) or the doctor of pharmacology (PharmD) qualifies an individual to take the licensing examination. Most pharmacy schools offer only the PharmD degree. The doctor of pharmacology degree is the highest level of entry to practice, requiring 6 years of education. About 100 schools of pharmacy exist in the United States. Residency programs are available after graduation in general, clinical, and specialty areas.

Pharmacy technicians assist the pharmacist in processing prescriptions and distribution of medication. Skills of the pharmacy technician include maintaining inventory and packaging, labeling, ordering, and stocking supplies. Pharmacy technicians may attend a 1-year vocational or community college program.

Pharmacy helpers assist the pharmacist by waiting on patients and maintaining the inventory of supplies under the direction of the pharmacist and technician. No standard educational experience is required for a pharmacy helper, and on-the-job training is possible.

The pharmaceutical industry also employs pharmacists for research and product development. These individuals are called pharmacologists or toxicologists. Pharmacologists differ from pharmacists because they work with the clinical science of how the drug works rather than preparing or dispensing medications. Pharmacologists generally earn a pharmacy or medical degree and then specialize in this area.

Another group who works with medications is pharmaceutical industry workers. They produce medicines, remedies, nutritional supplements, and health care products. Some examples of the duties of industry workers are filling and examining vials and ampules and running the machines that fill capsules. Many pharmaceutical companies offer on-the-job training, but employment is competitive. A bachelor's degree in one of the sciences may be required.

Speech and Language Pathologist

Speech and language pathology and audiology provide evaluation, treatment, and research in communication and related disorders. The certificate of clinical competence is the only credential recognized by all states for speech and language pathologists and audiologists. Qualifications for the voluntary certification include successful completion of a master's degree, 9 months of supervised experience, and successful completion of a national examination. More than 47 states require licensure for speech and language pathologists and audiologists. Doctoral preparation is required for research and teaching on the university level.

Researchers in communications disorders have made great advances. These professionals also may be called *speech, language,* or *hearing scientists.* Research has led to the development of better hearing aids, electronic voice boxes, and other technologic devices to assist communication.

Speech pathologists diagnose language problems. They also plan and direct treatment designed to overcome the problems. They treat disorders such as delayed language development, the inability to speak (aphasia), stuttering, and articulation problems. Speech pathologists complete a master's degree and an internship. For employment in a school, speech pathologists must also qualify for a teaching certificate.

CASE STUDY 31-3 You are assigned to care for a patient who cannot speak (mute). What should you do?

Answers to Case Studies are available on the Evolve website: ***http://evolve.elsevier.com/Gerdin***

Audiologists specialize in prevention, identification, assessment, and rehabilitation of hearing disorders. This work includes prescribing and dispensing hearing aids. Audiologists test hearing and determine the level of hearing function. They serve as consultants to the government in areas of noise pollution and environmental influences on hearing.

Audiometrists screen hearing under the supervision of the audiologist. This work includes fitting earphones, providing instruction, and recording the results of testing. Audiometrists may be trained on the job.

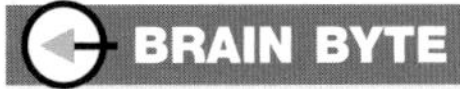

Hearing loss affects 3 of every 1000 children, making it the most common birth defect.

Respiratory Therapist

Respiratory therapists (RTs) evaluate the patient to administer respiratory care and operate life support equipment under the supervision of a physician (Fig. 31-3). The RT monitors the respiratory equipment and observes the patient's response to treatment. Some treatments performed by RTs include oxygen administration, incentive spirometry, tracheotomy care, and mechanical ventilation (Fig. 31-4). (See Skill List 31-2, Assisting with Incentive Spirometry, p. 501.) Respiratory therapists are trained in vocational programs, community colleges, and universities. Certification

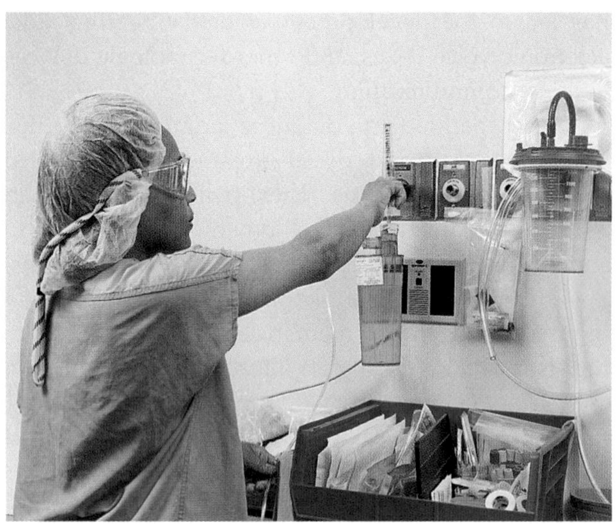

FIGURE 31-3 The rate of oxygen flow is ordered by the physician and is determined by the method of administration.

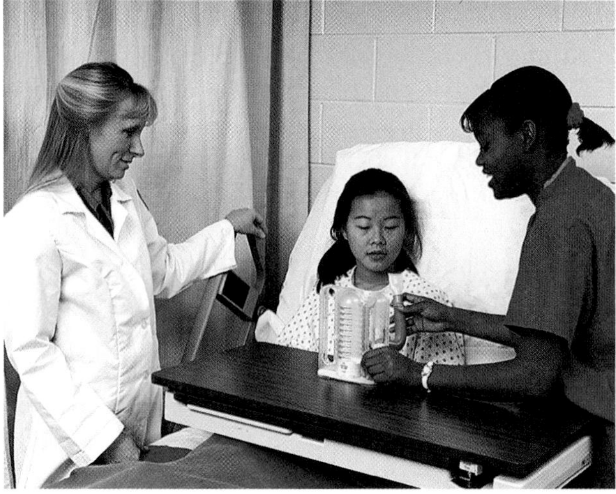

FIGURE 31-4 An incentive spirometer is used to help improve the depth of each inspiration.

and registration are possible after completion of a program approved by the American Medical Association in addition to 1 year of experience. All states except Alaska and Hawaii require licensure.

Respiratory therapy technicians administer routine respiratory care under the supervision of an RT. Technician programs are usually found in community colleges and are 1 year long. Respiratory therapy assistants do not give direct care to patients but help by cleaning and storing equipment.

Other Rehabilitative Personnel

Industrial rehabilitation specialists include vocational rehabilitation, manual arts, and horticultural therapists. Under the supervision of a physician, therapists in manual arts work to prevent physical deterioration of skills. Areas of training include woodworking, photography, metalworking, agriculture, electricity, and graphic arts. Employment as a manual arts therapist requires a bachelor's degree in the area of instruction plus experience.

Rehabilitation teachers work with blind and visually impaired adults. The visually impaired may need to learn Braille and how to organize the home for independent living (Fig. 31-5). Use of community resources and management of activities may be taught by the rehabilitation teacher.

Art therapists use art activities as a method for nonverbal expression and communication to understand emotional conflicts and to promote personal growth. Entry-level education includes master's degree preparation in art and psychology with clinical training. Art therapists plan activities, provide instruction, and observe and record behavior. Most art therapists are employed in psychiatric clinics, but they also may work in extended care facilities or schools. National registration is possible for art therapists.

Dance and movement therapy uses movement to improve the emotional and physical rehabilitation of an individual. Dance therapy is a form of psychotherapy. It differs from educational and recreational dance by the focus on nonverbal behavior and use of movement as a method of intervention. Registered dance therapists must complete graduate-level preparation and examination. Although licensure is not required, most dance therapists are licensed in a related field such as psychology.

Recreational therapists plan, organize, and direct medically approved recreation programs in hospitals and other institutions. The recreational therapist must design programs according to the abilities of the patient and record observations regarding the success of the activities. Educational programs for recreational therapists are available in community colleges and universities. Advanced degree preparation is necessary for top-level positions.

Music therapists plan, organize, and direct music activities and learning experiences for patients. The music therapist analyzes the patient's reaction to activities and records the findings. A bachelor's degree is the minimum for entry-level positions, and a master's degree is preferred for most employment opportunities.

Radiation therapy is the use of radiation to treat or relieve the pain of cancer and other diseases. The radiation technologist helps to plan and administer the treatment in addition to providing support for the patient. Education and training in this area may be

a b c d e f g h i j
1 2 3 4 5 6 7 8 9 0

k l m n o p q r s t

u v w x y z Capital sign Numeral sign

A

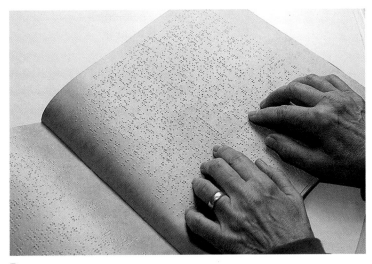

B

FIGURE 31-5 **A & B,** Braille uses the fingertips moving from right to left across a page. (From Sorrentino SA: *Mosby's textbook for nursing assistants*, ed 7, St. Louis, 2008, Mosby.)

completed in a 2-year community college or 4-year university. Some 1-year hospital-based programs are available for graduates of a radiography program. The American Registry of Radiological Technicians certifies radiation therapists.

Dialysis technicians set up and run artificial kidneys for patients requiring assisted filtering of wastes from the blood. The dialysis technician must be familiar with sterile technique and follow instructions for the procedure exactly. Some of the job duties include monitoring vital signs and performing the venipuncture to start the dialysis. Dialysis technicians may be trained on the job.

The perfusionist, or extracorporeal circulation technician, manages the heart-lung machine during surgery and respiratory failure. The perfusionist works under the direction of the surgeon to regulate blood circulation and composition. During the extracorporeal circuit, the perfusionist may administer blood products, anesthetic agents, and drugs under the direction of the surgeon or anesthesiologist. The perfusionist monitors the oxygen and carbon dioxide content of the blood and may induce hypothermia by cooling the blood if so directed. Perfusionists are trained in programs, usually associated with a medical school, after a minimum of 1 year of college work in the basic sciences. Programs last from 1 to 2 years. Most perfusionists have been trained in a related health field such as medical technology, respiratory therapy, or nursing. Several states require licensure for the perfusionist. Certification through the American Board of Cardiovascular Perfusion is possible after completion of acceptable education and training.

Content Instruction

Pharmacology

Pharmacology is the study of drugs, their actions, **dosages**, side effects, indications, and contraindications. Drugs are organic and inorganic materials that may be used for treatment or therapy in illness and injury. Prescription and administration of drugs are under the supervision of the Food and Drug

TABLE 31-2
Common Drug Types and Actions

Drug Type	Action
Analgesic	Relieves pain
Anesthetic	Diminishes sensation
Antacid and acid reducer	Relieves excess stomach acid
Antibiotic	Combats infection
Anticholinergic	Blocks action of acetylcholine
Anticoagulant	Inhibits formation of clots
Anticonvulsive	Controls tremors and seizures
Antidepressant	Relieves mental depression
Antidiarrheal	Reduces diarrhea
Antiemetic	Reduces nausea
Antihistamine	Relieves allergic reactions
Antihypertensive	Reduces blood pressure
Antiinflammatory agent	Reduces inflammation
Antineoplastic agent	Destroys new growth
Antipyretic	Reduces fever
Antitussive	Reduces coughing
Bronchodilator	Opens respiratory tract
Central nervous system depressant	Reduces action of central nervous system
Central nervous system stimulant	Relieves fatigue, elevates mood
Coagulant	Causes blood clotting
Decongestant	Constricts nasal membranes
Desensitization agent	Reduces allergic reactions
Diuretic	Reduces fluid in body
Emetic	Induces vomiting
Hormones and hypoglycemics	Balance hormonal components
Hypnotic	Produces sleep
Laxative	Induces fecal excretion
Sedative	Diminishes responses to stimuli
Sulfonamide	Cures bacterial infections
Vaccines and immunizations	Build immunity to infections
Vasodilator	Dilates blood vessels
Vitamins and minerals	Supplement inadequate diet

Administration of the federal government. Medications may be administered by licensed health care practitioners and by certain assistants under the supervision of a physician. Physicians, veterinarians, dentists, and their authorized agents, such as physician assistants and nurse practitioners, may prescribe medications. Enforcement of the drug laws is the responsibility of the Drug Enforcement Administration. The Controlled Substance Act of 1970 was enacted to regulate drugs capable of causing dependence. Medications that may be sold without a prescription are called *over-the-counter (OTC) drugs*.

Medications have generic, chemical, and trade names. The chemical name is based on the composition of the substance. The generic name is the common name of the drug, as consumers know it. The manufacturer owns the trade name. For example, the chemical name of a common drug that reduces fever (antipyretic) is acetylsalicylic acid. The generic name is aspirin. The drug may be bought over the counter under several brand- or trade-name labels. The trade name is registered and patented with the U.S. government. Drugs are classified according to the primary action that results in the body when used (Table 31-2).

Some common drug references used in pharmacology include the *U.S. Pharmacopoeia-Dispensing Information* (USP-DI) and the *Physician's Desk Reference*

TABLE 31-3
Drug Administration Methods

Route	Description
Buccal	Inside the cheek; rapid administration
Inhalation	Breathed in the lungs; useful in dilating bronchial tubes
Internal	Inserted into a body opening (orifice); rapid absorption
Inunction	Applied topically; used mostly for dermatology conditions
Oral	Given by mouth; easy to administer; slow absorption
Parenteral	Injection; may be given into any layer of tissue—intradermal, intramuscular, intravenous, subcutaneous
Sublingual	Under the tongue; rapid absorption

(PDR). The USP-DI is produced by a private group called the United States Pharmacopeial Convention, whereas the PDR is a collection of inserts from medications produced by pharmaceutical companies. The PDR is cross-referenced in sections that list the drugs by their manufacturer, brand name, generic name, and drug classification.

The dispensing of drugs must be correct to ensure the safety of their use. Prescriptions are valid when written on a printed form containing the name and address of the patient, date of the prescription, the superscription (Rx), list of ingredients (inscription), directions for preparation (subscription), directions for use (sig.), and physician's signature. The medication is labeled with the patient's name, medication name, dosage, method of administration (route), and intervals for administration. Latin abbreviations and terms are used for prescriptions. Drugs may be administered by several routes (Table 31-3). Three systems of measurement are used to calculate dosages (Table 31-4).

Some medications are prepackaged or put into individual doses for convenience and accuracy before distribution. Techniques of medical asepsis are used during prepackaging to prevent contamination of medications. A laminar flow hood, which moves air in a parallel movement, may be used for some preparations to ensure cleanliness. All medications prepared for unit dosage are labeled with the drug name, amount, strength, dosage form, expiration date, and pharmacy control number.

TABLE 31-4
Conversion Units for Medications

Apothecary Units	Metric Units	Household Units
15-16 minims (min)	1 mL (cc)	
1 fluid dram	4 mL (cc)	1 teaspoon or 60 drops (gtt)
	16 mL	1 tablespoon
1 fluid ounce (oz)	30 mL	
1 quart (qt)	1000 mL (1 L)	
1/60 grain (gr)	1 mg	
1 gr	0.065 g	
15 gr	1 g	
2.2 lb	1 kg	
Examples	Because 1 kg = 2.2 lb, change pounds to kilograms by dividing the number of pounds by 2.2.	
	120 lb/2.2 (lb/kg) = 54.05 kg	
	Because 1 oz = 30 mL, change ounces to milliliters by multiplying the number of ounces by 30.	
	8 oz × 30 mL/oz = 240 mL	

Speech Pathology

Nearly 10 million people in the United States have speech and language disorders. Each year 60,000 people in the United States lose the ability to speak (aphasia) because of stroke or head injury. The number of cases of laryngeal cancer increases by 8000 each year.

Speech disorders may result from congenital problems, illness, or injury. Some common speech disorders include difficulty with articulation (dysarthria), delayed speech, aphasia, cleft palate speech, stuttering,

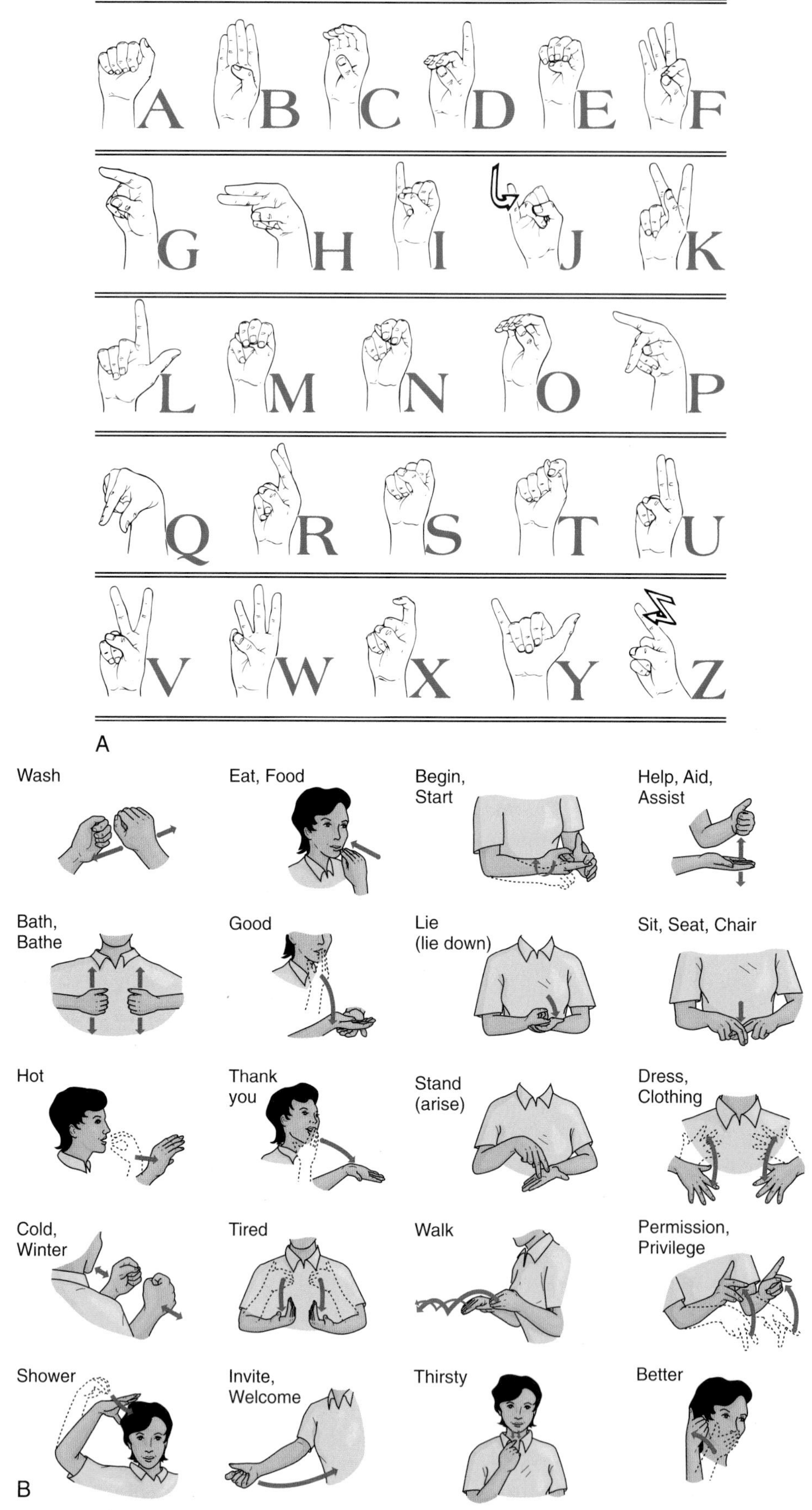

FIGURE 31-6 **A & B,** The manual alphabet is used as a form of communication by most persons who do not hear. (**A,** Courtesy the National Association for the Deaf, Silver Spring, Md.; **B,** From Sorrentino SA: *Mosby's textbook for nursing assistants*, ed 7, St. Louis, 2008, Mosby.)

and voice problems. Speech problems may be detected with tests such as the Wepman Auditory Discrimination Test (ADT), which requires discrimination between similar sounding words. If the speech disorder is severe or permanent, manual or sign language can be learned for communication purposes (Fig. 31-6).

Hearing

More than 17 million people in the United States have hearing loss in one or both ears. Almost half of these people are older than 65 years of age. Hearing may be tested by using an audiometer (Fig. 31-7). Audiograms measure the ability to hear pure tones in each ear. A complete audiogram tests both bone conduction and air conduction. The bone conduction test measures the ability to hear a sound transmitted through bone, whereas the air conduction test determines the ability to hear sounds transmitted through the air. The results of the two tests may help determine whether hearing loss is due to an inability to conduct the sound (conductive hearing loss) or is due to the inner ear or nerve that sends sound signals to the brain (sensorineural hearing loss).

The flexibility of the eardrum may be measured with a tympanogram. This test measures the amount of sound reflected from the tympanic membrane at various levels of air pressure.

CASE STUDY 31-4 Your patient is deaf. What should you do?

Answers to Case Studies are available on the Evolve website: *http://evolve.elsevier.com/Gerdin*

Respiratory Therapies

Breathing treatments include the intermittent positive pressure breathing procedure that increases the concentration of oxygen in the lungs. Pursed-lip breathing is taught to prevent collapse of small air passages in the lungs. The procedure involves exhaling at a slow rate with lips shaped as for whistling to keep the pressure even. Chest physical therapy includes postural drainage and percussion. RTs may use percussion on the chest to loosen secretions or to determine the location of fluid or air in the respiratory system. Using a vibrator or striking the body with the fingers or hands to cause vibrations accomplishes percussion.

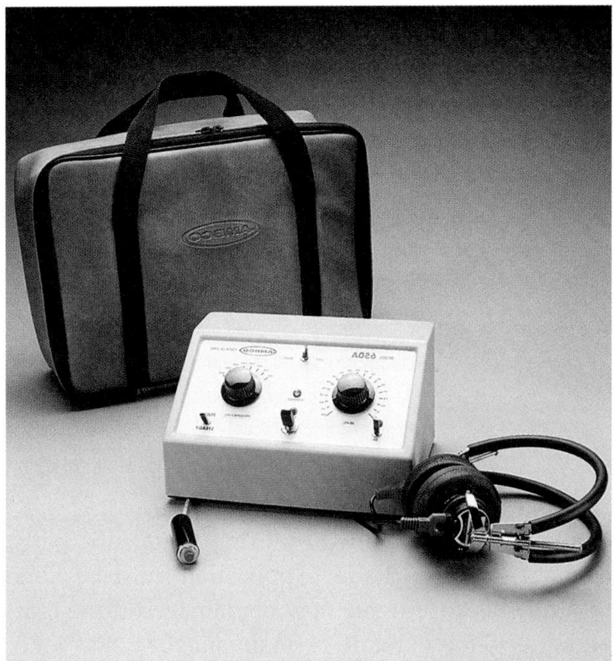

FIGURE 31-7 An audiometer is used to test hearing. (Courtesy AMBCO Electronics, Tustin, Calif.)

The amount of oxygen and carbon dioxide and the pH value of the blood can be measured by using a blood gas analyzer. Respiratory personnel administer gases following the order of a physician. Gases that are used medicinally include oxygen, compressed air, and some air mixtures. The Department of Transportation regulates the manufacture, testing, transportation, and marking of medical gas cylinders. The storage of cylinders is regulated to prevent fire and explosion of the gases. The cylinders containing medical gases are labeled by color to prevent confusion. Flow-regulating devices (flow meters) determine the amount of gas administered from the cylinders.

Oxygen may be delivered by several methods, including nasal cannula or prongs, mask, and tent (Fig. 31-8). Some masks are modified to allow insertion of medication. Humidifiers and nebulizers are used to administer water or medication into the lungs. **Nebulizers** are atomizers or devices that throw a spray of fluid. Humidifiers place moisture into the air that is breathed.

Performance Instruction

Application of Heat and Cold

Heat and cold applications are used in physical therapy to allow increased movement of joints. Heat

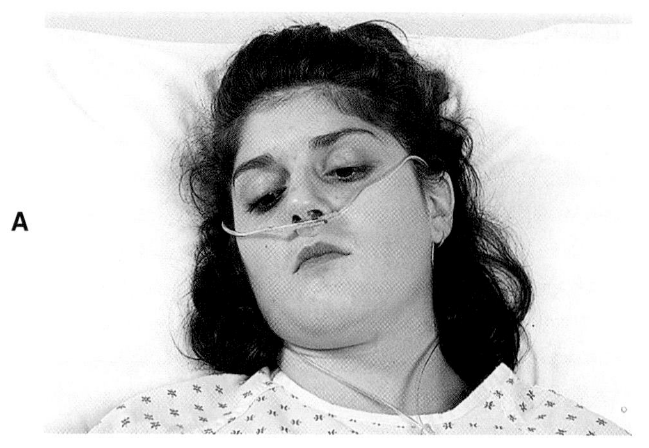

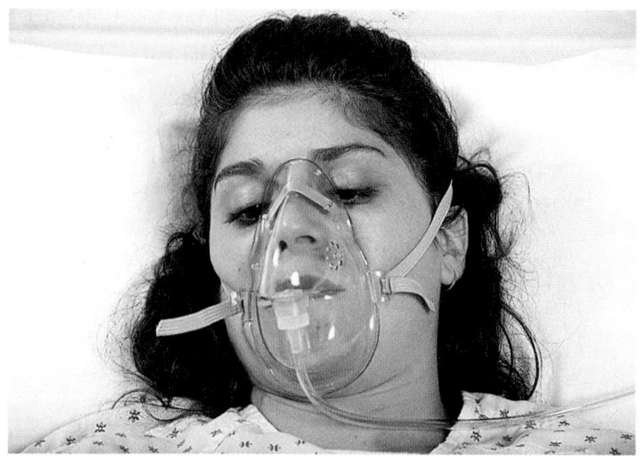

FIGURE 31-8 Methods of administration. **A,** Nasal cannula or nasal prongs. **B,** mask.

and cold may be applied by using Aquamatic pads, ice bags, or water baths. Application must be done carefully because tissue may be damaged if the temperature is too extreme or maintained for too long. The skin on the area of application is checked frequently for redness, paleness, or blistering throughout the treatment (Fig. 31-9).

Crutch Walking

Several gaits or methods of using crutches are possible. The type of injury and area that is not to bear weight during ambulation determine the method used. Crutches must be measured for proper fit while the patient is wearing walking shoes. Some examples of crutch gaits include the four-point, two-point, three-point, and tripod. (See Skill List 31-3, Teaching Crutch Walking, p. 502.)

Medication Calculations

Medications may be given or administered only in a health care facility by licensed personnel. In some cases the medication dosage must be calculated with a conversion formula (see Table 31-4). Accuracy of the conversion should be verified with another worker if possible. Chapter 7 provides more information about math conversions.

Testing Hearing

To test hearing, the patient is seated in a quiet room wearing the earphones of an audiometer. The machine is set to test each ear separately to detect sounds at 20 dB and higher at a frequency of 1000 Hz. The procedure can be repeated at higher and lower frequencies. The patient indicates when the sound has been heard by raising a hand.

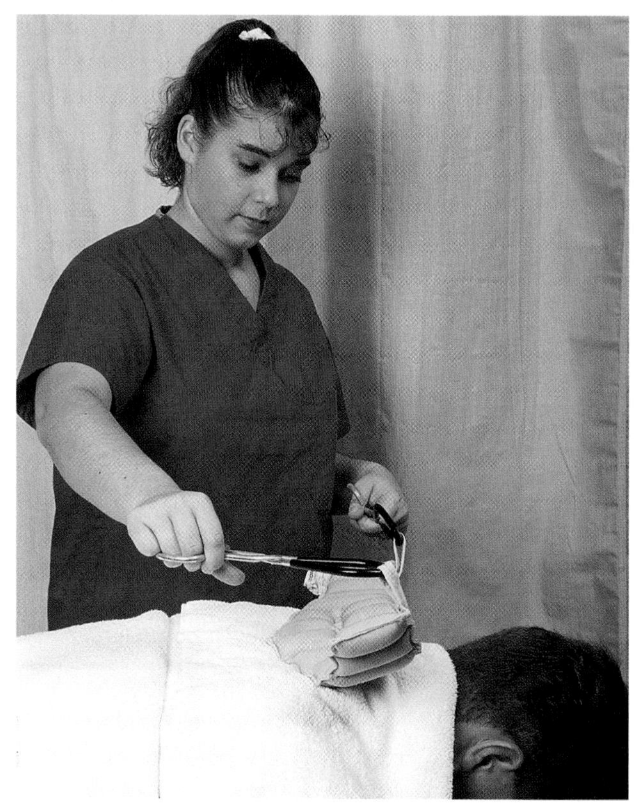

FIGURE 31-9 Applications of heat and cold should never touch the skin directly.

Body Mechanics for Patients with Disabilities

The rehabilitative therapist often works with patients who have disabilities, including disabilities of limited movement, sight, or hearing. Special consideration body mechanics techniques can prevent injury to the worker or patient. Patients and health care workers may also use an assistive device to perform activities of daily living (Fig. 31-10).

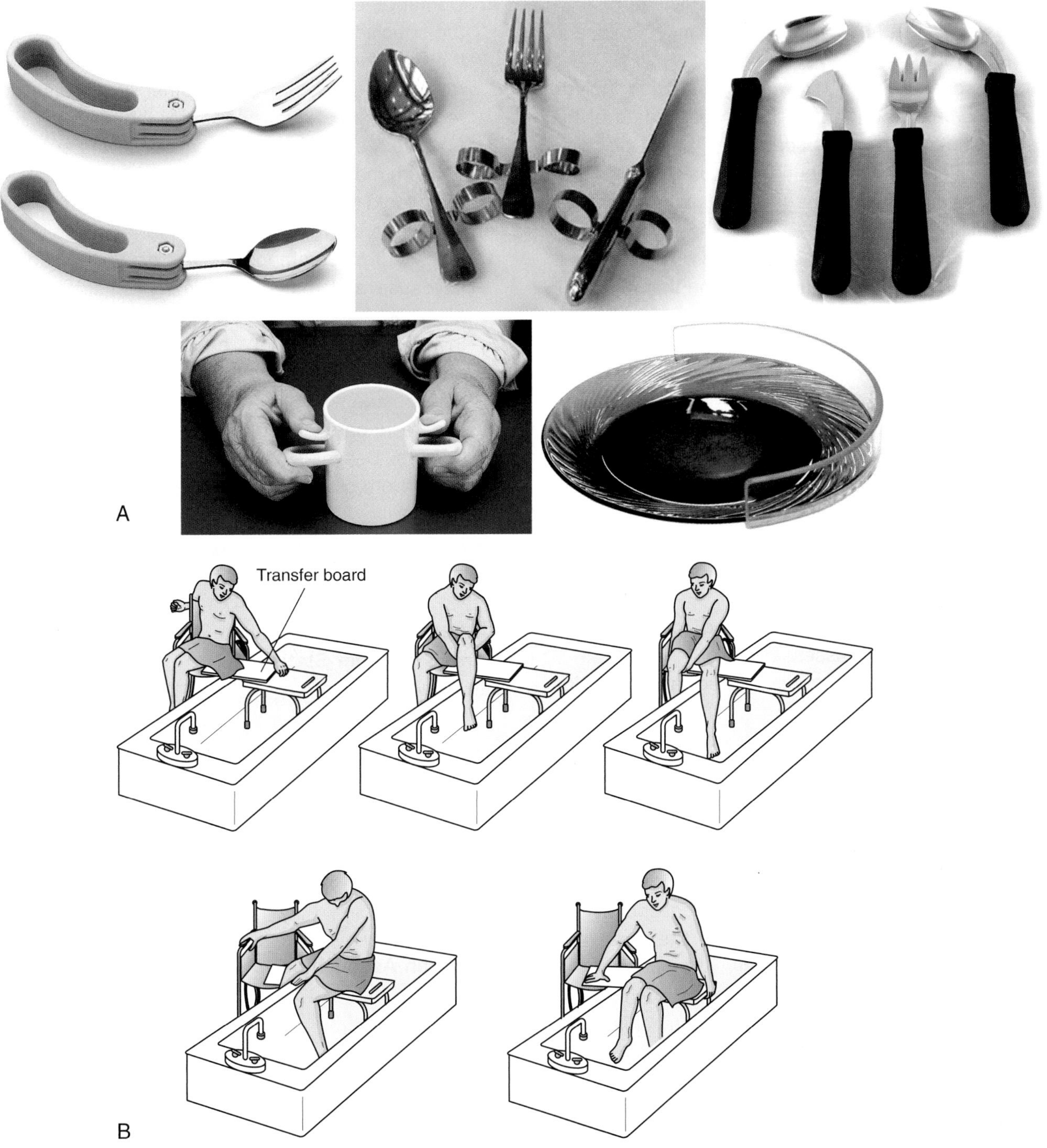

FIGURE 31-10 **A & B,** Patients with disabilities can learn to perform activities of daily living independently by using assistive devices. (From Sorrentino SA: *Mosby's textbook for nursing assistants*, ed 7, St. Louis, 2008, Mosby.)

Summary

- The function of the rehabilitative health care team is to provide services designed to overcome disabilities.
- The role of the PT is to restore function, relieve pain, and prevent disability after illness or injury. The orthotist designs and makes braces. The OT helps patients live independently.
- Five methods or devices used to improve activities of daily living include the use of canes, elastic stockings, guide dogs, braces, and prosthetic limbs.
- Two types of hearing loss are conductive and sensorineural hearing loss.

- Five commonly used drugs types include analgesics, antacids, antihistamines, decongestants, and sedatives.
- Components of a legal drug prescription include the name and address of the patient, date of the prescription, the superscription (Rx), list of ingredients (inscription), directions for preparation (subscription), directions for use (sig.), and physician's signature.
- Three rehabilitative treatments are respiratory therapy, athletic training, and radiation therapy.

Review Questions

1. Describe the function of the rehabilitative health care team.
2. Describe the role of each member of the rehabilitative health care team.
3. Describe the benefits of the wheelchair, crutches, Braille, sign language, and similar devices for the person with disabilities.
4. Describe two types of hearing loss and two methods used to assess hearing.
5. List 10 common categories of drugs and the action of each.
6. List the information needed to write a legal prescription.
7. Describe incentive spirometry, nebulizer, and percussion treatments.
8. Choose one career from Box 31-1. Research the cost of education and annual earnings in local institutions. Write a paragraph describing the factors that might explain why the local and national economic figures vary.
9. Use each of the following terms in one or more sentences that correctly relate their meaning: dispense, dosage, and frequency.

Critical Thinking

1. Investigate and compare the cost of various types of treatments related to rehabilitative health care.
2. Contact the local city building inspector to obtain the specifications for construction of facilities for the disabled. Measure a public facility such as a restroom to determine whether it meets the requirements of accessibility for the disabled.
3. Analyze a common activity of daily living such as eating a meal or changing clothes. Prepare a plan that would allow adaptation of the activity to meet the needs of an individual with varied disabilities.
4. Investigate a common speech disorder, including its cause and methods of improvement for the disorder.
5. Investigate the cost of educational preparation and job outlook for various rehabilitative health care personnel.
6. Create a career ladder for rehabilitative health careers. Describe why it is or is not possible to move from one level to another in the field.

Explore the Web

Career Information

Bureau of Labor Statistics
http://www.bls.gov/

Salary.com
http://salary.com

Professional Associations

American Physical Therapy Association (APTA)
http://apta.org

American Association for Respiratory Care (AARC)
http://www.aarc.org/

National Athletic Trainers' Association (NATA)
http://www.nata.org/

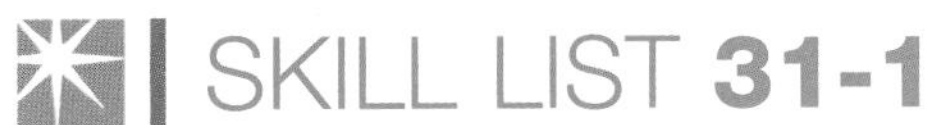

SKILL LIST 31-1 Applying Elastic Stockings

1. Maintain medical asepsis by using the guidelines provided in the Standard and Transmission-Based Precautions, including good handwashing technique and use of gloves as needed.
2. Verify physician's orders for use of antiembolic or elastic stockings, which are used to prevent the development of blood clots in the legs.
3. Identify the patient and explain the procedure.
4. Raise the bed to a comfortable working height.
5. Position the patient supine.
6. Expose the leg to be covered with the stocking while draping other parts of the body with linens.
7. Gather the stocking into one hand so that the toe of the foot can be inserted directly into the toe of the stocking.
8. Slip the stocking over the foot while supporting the foot in one hand and moving the stocking with the other. Adjust the stocking as needed so that the heel of the foot fits into the heel of the stocking.
9. Pull the stocking over the remainder of the leg, making sure it is not twisted or wrinkled. Twisting or wrinkling of the stockings may cause discomfort or cut off circulation to an area of the leg.
10. Repeat the procedure for the other leg.
11. Lower the bed. Position the patient for safety and comfort.
12. Record the time of stocking application. Antiembolic stockings are removed at intervals to allow free circulation of blood to the legs.

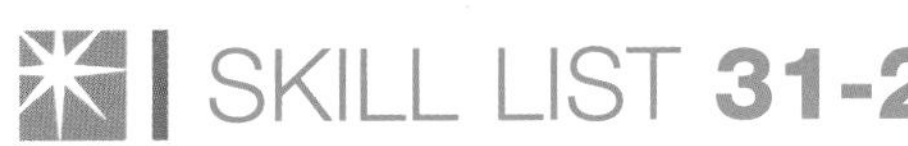

SKILL LIST 31-2 Assisting with Incentive Spirometry

1. Maintain medical asepsis by using the guidelines provided in the Standard and Transmission-Based Precautions, including good handwashing technique and use of gloves as needed.
2. Identify the patient and explain the procedure. Incentive spirometry is used to increase the breathing depth.
3. Instruct the patient to inhale deeply until the ball is raised to the top of the chamber and to hold the ball in that position for 6 seconds.
4. Instruct the patient to repeat this process 10 times.
5. The patient should repeat the procedure several times daily according to the physician's orders.

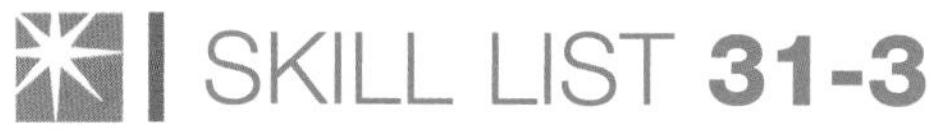

SKILL LIST 31-3 Teaching Crutch Walking

1. Maintain medical asepsis by using the guidelines provided in the Standard and Transmission-Based Precautions, including good handwashing technique and use of gloves as needed.
2. Identify the patient and explain the procedure.
3. Measure the crutches for proper fit. The crutch length should be measured with the patient wearing walking shoes. The height is measured from 2 inches (5 cm) outside the tip of the toe and 6 inches (15 cm) ahead of this mark. The distance from this mark to 2 inches (5 cm) below the axilla is the proper crutch length.
4. Teach the patient the four-point crutch gait sequence of right crutch, left foot, left crutch, right foot. There are several crutch gaits possible. The four-point gait is slow but stable. The patient must be able to move both legs separately and bear weight on each leg.
5. Teach the patient the two-point crutch gait sequence of right crutch and left foot followed by left crutch and right foot simultaneously. This method is faster but requires greater balance.
6. Teach the patient the three-point crutch gait sequence of simultaneously moving both crutches and the weaker extremity, followed by the stronger extremity. This is a rapid gait but requires that the arms be strong enough to support the entire body weight.
7. Teach the patient the tripod crutch gait sequence of both crutches forward followed by both legs swinging forward.
8. Instruct the patient to alternate methods to reduce fatigue and soreness.

CHAPTER 32

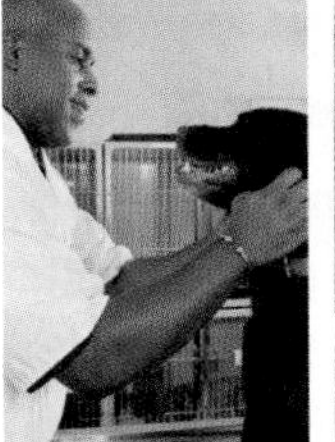
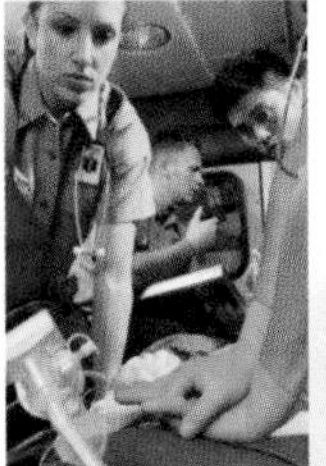
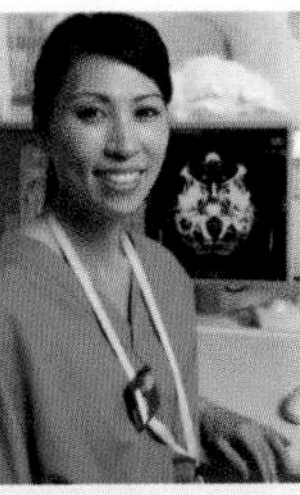

Emergency Health Careers

LEARNING OBJECTIVES

- Define at least 10 terms related to emergency health care.
- Specify the role of the emergency medical technician and emergency department personnel, including personal qualities, levels of education, and credentialing requirements.
- Identify three levels of care that have been developed to provide first aid.
- Identify at least six types of external wounds and first-aid treatment for each.
- Identify at least three types of burns and first-aid treatment for each.
- Describe at least five ways in which poisoning may occur and first-aid treatment for each.
- Describe at least five causes of shock and the physical reaction to and first-aid treatment for each.
- Identify three types of fractures and first-aid treatment for each.
- Describe the effects of extreme cold and heat on the body and first-aid treatment for each.
- Describe the signs, symptoms, and treatment for a stroke and seizure activity.

KEY TERMS

Aspiration *(as-per-AY-shun)* Act of inhaling foreign matter, usually emesis, into the respiratory tract

Aura *(ARE-uh)* Subjective sensation or motor phenomenon that precedes and marks the onset of a seizure

Cardiopulmonary *(kar-dee-o-PUL-mun-ayr-ee)* Pertaining to the heart and lungs

Consciousness *(KON-shus-ness)* Responsiveness of the mind and to the impressions made by the senses

KEY TERMS cont'd

Critical *(KRIT-ih-kul)* Pertaining to a crisis or danger of death

Endotracheal intubation *(end-o-TRAKE-ee-ul in-too-BAY-shun)* Placing a tube within or through the trachea

Hemorrhage *(HEM-uh-ruj)* Abnormal external or internal bleeding

Mottled *(MOT-uld)* Spotted with patches of color

Resuscitation *(ree-sus-ih-TAY-shun)* Restoration of life or consciousness of a person who is apparently dead by using artificial respiration and cardiac massage

Seizure *(SEE-zhur)* Sudden attack of a disease; uncontrolled muscle movements of epilepsy

Shock *(shok)* Condition of acute failure of the peripheral circulation

Tourniquet *(TUR-nik-et)* Instrument used to compress a blood vessel by application around an extremity

Toxin *(TOKS-in)* Poison produced by animals, plants, or bacteria

Emergency Health Careers Terminology*

Term	Definition	Prefix	Root	Suffix
Anaphylactic	Condition of not being protected against disease	an	aphylact	ic
Cardiopulmonary	Referring to the lungs and heart	cardio	pulmon	ary
Cyanoderm	Blue skin	cyan/o	derm	
Hematemesis	Vomiting of blood	hemat	eme	sis
Hemorrhage	Copious loss of blood		hemo	rrhage
Hypothermia	Condition of being below normal temperature	hypo	therm	ia
Midline	Median plane	mid	line	
Pneumothorax	Pertaining to the lungs and chest	pneumo	thorax	
Semiconscious	Partially aware of sensations	semi	consc	ious
Ventral	Abdomen; front side		ventr	al

*A transition syllable or vowel may be added to or deleted from the word parts make the combining form.

Abbreviations for Emergency Health Careers

Abbreviation	Meaning
ACLS	Advanced cardiac life support
AED	Automated external defibrillator
AHA	American Heart Association
AKA	Above knee amputation
ARC	American Red Cross
EMT-Basic	Emergency medical technician-basic
EMT-I	Emergency medical technician-intermediate
EMT-P	Emergency medical technician-paramedic
ER	Emergency room
Fx	Fracture

Careers

Accidents are one of the five leading causes of death in the United States. They account for 50% of the fatalities of those 15 to 24 years of age. Injuries can result from automobile and home accidents, falls, fires, explosions, natural disasters, and industrial mishaps. Snow, water, and other athletic sports also account for injuries that require emergency care. Common injuries caused by accidents include bone fractures, cuts, poisoning, reactions to heat and cold, problems associated with medical conditions, and loss of vital functions.

The goal of modern emergency care is immediate aid, or first aid, at the scene of injury rather than just the transportation of the victim to a medical facility. Levels of care have developed to provide this immediate care (Table 32-1). These include the bystanders or

TABLE 32-1
Emergency Health Career Educational Cost and Earnings

Career	Educational Cost*	Earnings†
Paramedic	Oklahoma City Community College, associate degree, 68 credit hours Fees include: Tuition, books, & fees - $5712	Median annual salary: Oklahoma City, Okla.—$28,490

*http://www.occc.edu/admissions/Tuition-Fees.html#educational.
†http://data.bls.gov:8080/oes/datatype.do.

BOX 32-1

Emergency Health Careers

- Ambulance attendant
- Emergency medical technician
- Emergency medical services coordinator
- First-aid attendant
- Flight nurse
- Flight surgeon
- Hospital entrance attendant
- Paramedic

first responders with knowledge of first aid and cardiopulmonary resuscitation (CPR), emergency medical technicians (EMTs), and advanced emergency personnel (Box 32-1). Emergency medical services (EMS) are present in many communities. The EMS system is a coordinated response by all levels of practitioners to accidents and sudden illness. In most areas of the United States, EMS are initiated by the use of the 9-1-1 telephone call. Personnel answering 9-1-1 calls are trained to determine the type of rescue personnel needed, the location of the emergency, and other pertinent information. In some instances EMS personnel may even be able to direct the caller on methods for giving aid to the victim.

Emergency Medical Technician

EMTs work under the supervision of a physician to provide care to the acutely ill or injured person in the prehospital setting. They respond to medical emergencies, give immediate care, and transport the victim to the hospital. They also maintain the rescue vehicles and equipment. Some EMTs are employed by ambulance companies, emergency centers, and industry. Four classifications of EMTs are recognized by the National Registry of Emergency Medical Technicians: the First Responder, EMT-Basic, EMT-Intermediate, and EMT-Paramedic (EMT-P).

All EMTs must be alert to details and able to manipulate small objects skillfully. The job is physically demanding and requires heavy lifting. The work is usually arranged in shifts and includes irregular hours.

The role of the EMT-First Responder is to provide care in cases of acute illness and injury until more qualified personnel are available. Skills such as CPR, first aid for fractures and bleeding, treatment of shock, and assistance with childbirth are included in the training (Fig. 32-1).

EMT-Basic personnel perform all of the skills of the EMT-First Responder. In addition, the EMT-Basic may care for the person at an accident scene and provide transport in an ambulance.

BRAIN BYTE

About 80% of automobile accidents are linked to distracted driving, such as texting, which increases the risk of crashing by 20-fold.

In addition to the training of the EMT-Basic, the EMT-Intermediate (EMT-I) may establish intravenous lines, assess trauma victims, and apply inflatable antishock garments.

The EMT-P, or paramedic, provides advanced life support. The paramedic must be skilled in all the duties of the other EMT personnel, as well as in monitoring electrocardiograph readings and defibrillation. EMT-Ps may be employed by fire and police departments or act as community volunteers. Paramedics may administer medications and perform endotracheal intubation.

Some states vary in their requirements for emergency medical technician training, which may limit an EMT's opportunities to move to other areas. In some

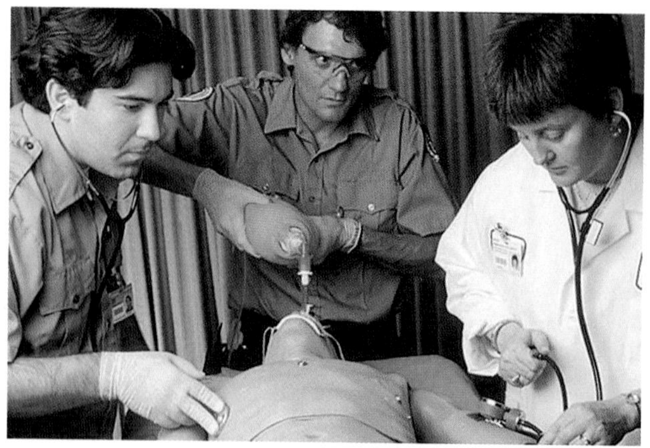

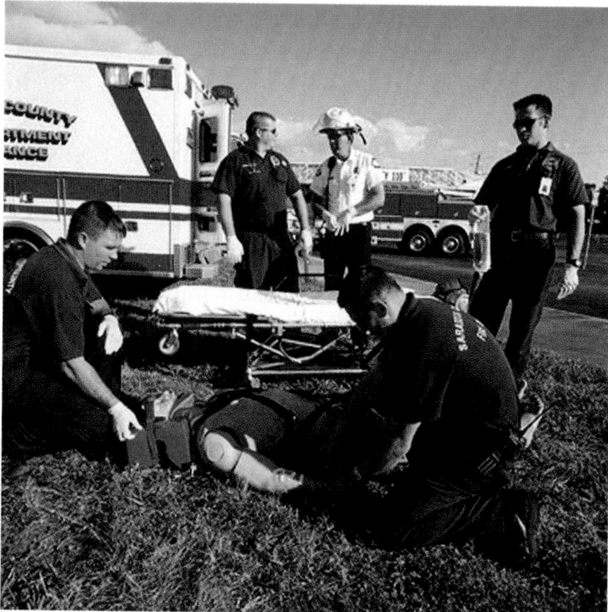

FIGURE 32-1 The Human Patient Simulator is used as a learning tool for emergency medical technicians. The lifelike manikin physically represents the patient. Clinical features such as palpable pulses and heart sounds, monitored parameters, electrocardiogram, and pulmonary artery catheter bring the patient to life. Sophisticated physiologic models of the body systems simulate normal and pathophysiologic responses to drugs, mechanical ventilation, and other therapies. (Courtesy Medical Education Technologies, Sarasota, Fla.)

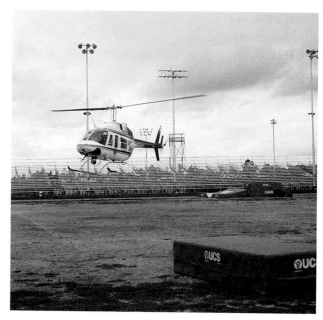

FIGURE 32-2 The helicopter is used in emergencies to transport victims.

EMT personnel may be categorized into four levels. When this type of naming system is used, the lowest level is the EMT-First Responder. These individuals have training in basic first aid and might be firefighters, policemen, or others who are the first to respond to an emergency. The first level of the emergency medical technician training system is the EMT-1, which is the same as the EMT-Basic. The EMT-Intermediate is divided into two levels (EMT-2 and EMT-3), depending on the training received. The EMT-4 level is the EMT-Paramedic.

CASE STUDY 32-1 Your friend says he is taking a basic EMT class so he can be a paramedic. What should you say?

Answers to Case Studies are available on the Evolve website: ***http://evolve.elsevier.com/Gerdin***

states, applicants must be at least 18 years of age and have a high school diploma. Standards for the educational requirements of EMTs are set by the U.S. Department of Transportation. Thirty-eight states require registration with the National Registry of Emergency Medical Technicians for certification. Training also includes a supervised internship. Certification of EMTs is required by all states. Proof of continuing education is required for recertification.

Other Emergency Personnel

Flight rescue professions have evolved as a career opportunity with the use of helicopters to transport victims to emergency facilities (Fig. 32-2). The emergency rescue team usually includes a nurse and a paramedic. It may also include a respiratory therapist.

The minimum requirement for flight nursing includes being a registered nurse with several years

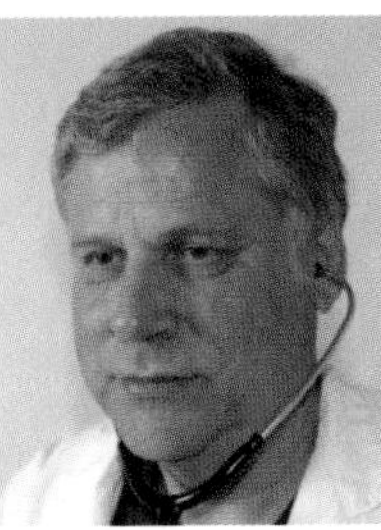

ROBERT T. WEBB, MD

EMERGENCY PHYSICIAN
MEDICAL CENTER HOSPITAL, ODESSA, TEXAS

Educational background: Bachelor of arts, University of Texas (1972); MD, University of Texas Southwestern Medical School (1976); internships in internal medicine and anesthesiology, Emory University, Atlanta, Georgia (1976-1978)

A typical day at work and job duties include: On a typical day, I start seeing emergency patients as soon as I arrive at work and do not stop until 10 or 11 hours later.

The most gratifying part of my job: Being able to change the course of someone's illness for the better.

The biggest challenge(s) I face in doing my job: Keeping up with all the new information and technology of medicine.

What drew me to my career? My mother was a nurse, and I admired her altruistic dedication to her work.

of critical care experience. Advanced certified life support (ACLS) and critical care certification (CCRN) are often required of the registered nurse. Most emergency rescue facilities provide clinical and classroom instruction covering the specific training relating to flight and air rescue. Flight paramedics are also required to hold ACLS certification and have prior field experience. National Registry Paramedic Certification and previous flight experience are preferred in most employment opportunities. Flight respiratory therapists must be certified and have critical care experience. It is preferred that candidates for flight rescue be registered respiratory therapists.

On arrival at the hospital, the victim is admitted by the emergency personnel. Treatment is continued by emergency nurses and physicians who specialize in emergency and trauma care. Emergency medicine was recognized as a board-certified specialty for physicians in 1979.

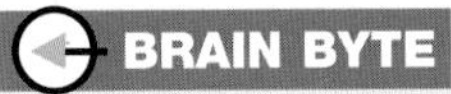

A 2005 patient survey found the average emergency department wait time to be 3.7 hours, with the lowest average in Iowa (2.3 hours) and the highest average in Arizona (5.0 hours).

Content Instruction

Emergency Procedures

First aid is the immediate care given to the victim of injury or sudden illness. The purpose of first aid is to

TABLE 32-2
Emergency Assessment and Treatment

Emergency	What to Do	Why
Triage	Remove victim from immediate danger. Check level of consciousness. Establish an airway if needed. Check pulse and breathing. Treat severe bleeding. Treat poisoning. Treat burns. Treat for the signs and symptoms of shock; apply a blanket and do not give any beverages. Treat fractures. Treat other injuries as needed.	It should be assumed that neck and back injuries have occurred in all accidents; move the victim only if in immediate danger. Severe loss of blood can lead to shock and death within minutes. Alcohol may cause greater injury or prevent medical personnel from providing treatments immediately.

sustain life and prevent death. It includes the prevention of permanent disability and the reduction of time needed for recovery. First aid provides basic life support and maintenance of vital functions.

Certification in first aid is awarded by several accredited agencies, including the American Red Cross and the American Heart Association (AHA). Content of the Red Cross course includes basic first aid for injuries, illness, and CPR procedures.

BRAIN BYTE

In Seattle, where CPR training is common and EMS response is short, the survival rate for witnessed cardiac arrest is about 30%.

Basic first-aid training includes prevention, assessment, and treatment of illness and injury. *Triage* is the term used for setting priorities for care of the victim or victims. First-aid training teaches treatment of wounds, poisoning, burns, shock, fractures, temperature alterations, illness caused by medical conditions, and other injuries.

Emergency Assessment and Treatment

The first-aid rescuer assesses the scene of injury or illness to determine the necessary action (Table 32-2). The first priority of the rescuer is to remove the victim from any immediate danger (Fig. 32-3). The level of consciousness of the victim is the second consideration. The EMS system is activated at the earliest moment, and then hands-on CPR is started. In most areas of the United States, the 9-1-1 emergency number may be used to summon help. When reporting an incident, the rescuer states the location, his or her name, the number of victims involved, and the nature of the incident. The rescuer waits for the EMS to disconnect the phone first. Because the rescuer may be visiting in the victim's home, all homeowners should place their name and address on each phone.

If there is more than one victim, the unconscious victim takes priority over the conscious one. If all victims are breathing and have a pulse, bleeding is the next consideration, then burns and other injuries.

BRAIN BYTE

For sudden collapse in a victim, the health care provider should call 9-1-1 and then use and an automated external defibrillator or begin CPR.

Wounds

Wounds result when tissue is damaged externally or internally (Table 32-3). An example of an internal wound is a contusion, or bruise. Six types of external wounds result in different bleeding situations. These wound classifications are abrasion, incision, laceration, puncture, avulsion, and amputation.

Abrasions result from the scraping of skin or mucous membrane from the surface of the body. Bleeding from an abrasion is minimal, but infection may result. An incision is a cut made with a surgical instrument, knife, or glass. It results in a wound with straight edges. Bleeding is rapid and heavy. Lacerations are irregularly shaped cuts made with a sharp

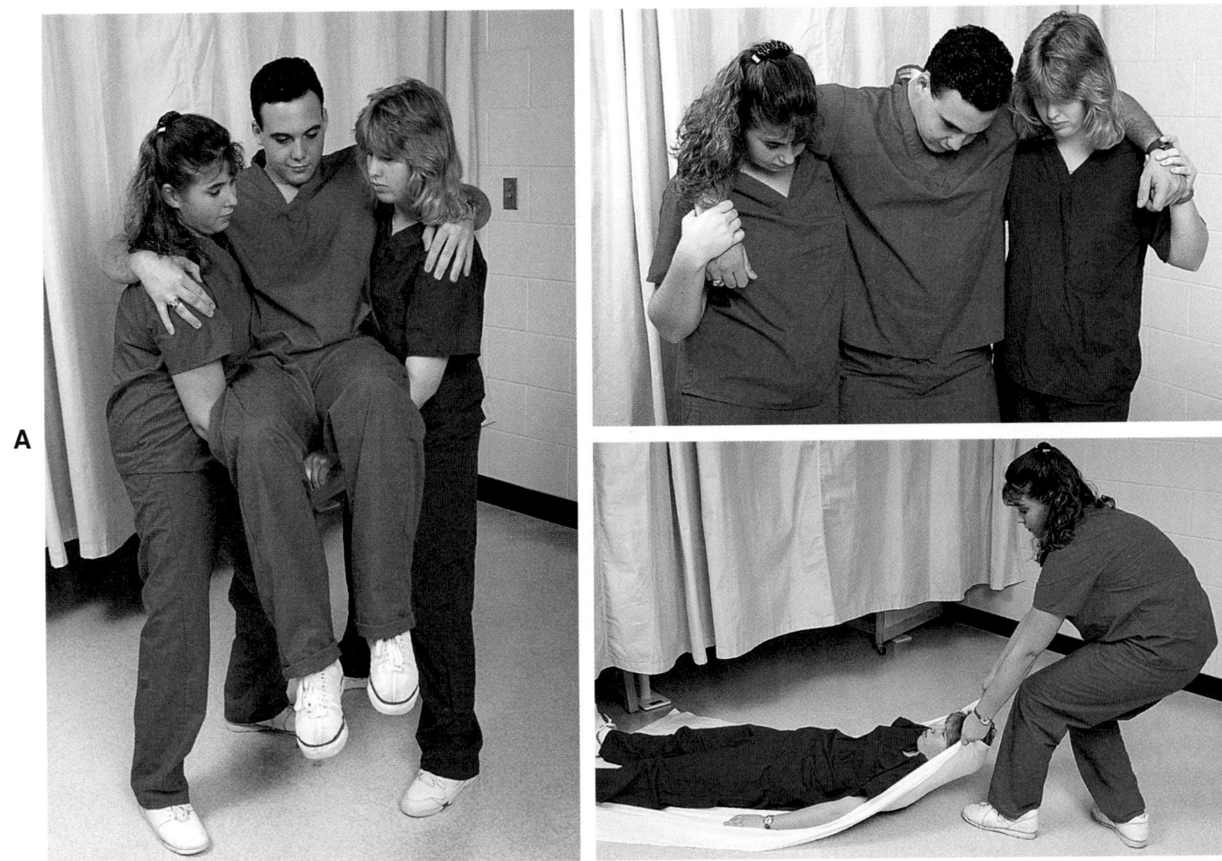

FIGURE 32-3 If the victim of an emergency must be moved, triage determines the correct method. **A,** The two-man carry. **B,** The two-man assistance. **C,** The one-man transfer.

TABLE 32-3
Wounds

Emergency	What to Do	Why
Bleeding wound	Apply direct pressure to the wound using the cleanest dressing or hand available.	Most bleeding can be stopped by direct pressure to the wound.
	Do not remove the dressing.	Dressing removal may interrupt clot formation.
	Elevate the injured area.	Elevation reduces the blood pressure and flow to the area.
	Apply pressure to the pressure point closest to the wound.	Direct pressure, elevation, and pressure on the artery control bleeding in 90% of all cases.
	Apply a tourniquet above the level of the wound only as a last resort; use only if loss of life may occur from further blood loss. **Once applied, a tourniquet must never be removed.**	A tourniquet may damage tissues beyond repair.
	Cool any avulsed tissue or parts and transport them with the victim. **Do not place tissues directly on ice.**	Many parts can be reattached if preserved from further tissue damage.

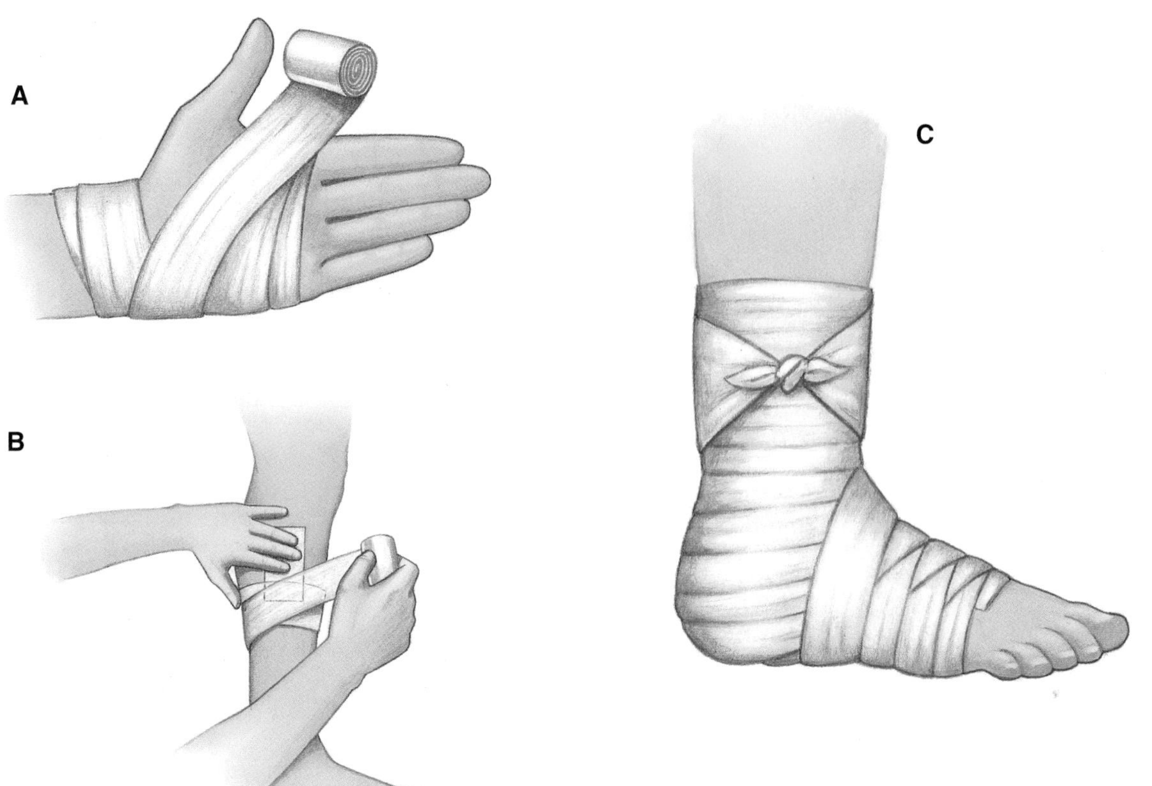

FIGURE 32-4 Methods of bandaging vary with the areas of injury. **A,** A simple figure eight. **B,** A dressing held in place with wrapping toward the heart. **C,** The tie is placed to locate the area of injury.

object and, of the various wounds, lacerations generally bleed the most. When bleeding has been controlled, bandages protect the wound from infection (Fig. 32-4).

Puncture wounds are made when an object pierces the skin. The skin may close around the area and limit the bleeding. Punctures provide a high risk of infection. An avulsion is the traumatic tearing away of part of the body. Bleeding is rapid and heavy. The body part may be reattached or reinserted in some instances. An amputation is the surgical severing or cutting away of part of the body.

Bleeding occurs from all three types of blood vessels. Arterial bleeding is bright red and pulses as the heart beats and is the most serious type. Venous blood is darker in color and does not pulse. Capillary bleeding oozes at the surface of the skin. Shock and loss of consciousness can result from loss of blood in a short amount of time.

Burns

Burns may result from exposure to heat, chemicals, or radiation (Table 32-4). The severity of a burn is determined by the location, depth, and size (Fig. 32-5). Injury to the face, arms, legs, and genitals are the most critical. Burns that cover more than 10% of the body surface generally require hospitalization. Burns are classified into three degrees according to their depth.

First-degree burns affect only the outer layer of skin tissue. The skin becomes red and discolored, and some slight swelling may occur. Healing of first-degree burns is generally rapid. Examples of a first-degree burn are sunburn and a burn caused by immersing part of the body briefly into hot water.

A second-degree burn is one that breaks the surface of the skin and injures the underlying tissue. Second-degree burns may result from a severe sunburn and exposure to hot liquids or heat. The appearance of blisters commonly indicates a second-degree burn. The skin is red or **mottled** in appearance. The skin may become wet when plasma is lost through the damaged skin. This type of burn causes greater pain and swelling.

Third-degree burns are deep enough to damage the nerves and bones. Tissue burned to the third degree is charred and white. A third-degree burn may cause less pain because the nerves are damaged.

TABLE 32-4
Burns

Emergency	What to Do	Why
First-degree burn	Immerse affected area in cool water.	Open wounds or ointments may increase the risk of infection.
	Apply a dressing to the area.	
Second-degree burn	Immerse affected area in cool water.	
	Do not open blisters or apply ointments.	
	Elevate the affected area.	Elevation reduces swelling.
	Seek medical attention if the affected area is large.	
Third-degree burn	Do not remove any clothing adhering to the burn.	Removing clothing can lead to tissue damage and fluid loss.
	Cover the burn with a clean, dry dressing.	Dressing the wound reduces pain and risk of infection.
	Elevate if possible.	
	Do not apply ointments, water, or butter.	This application may increase the risk of infection.
	Seek medical attention as soon as possible.	Third-degree burns must be treated to prevent infection and permanent damage to tissues.

A

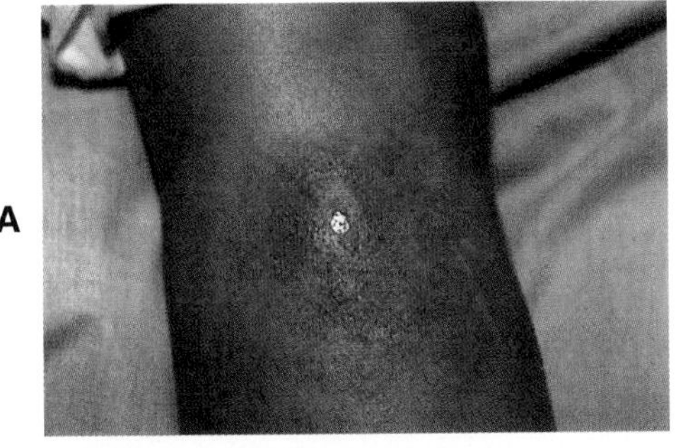

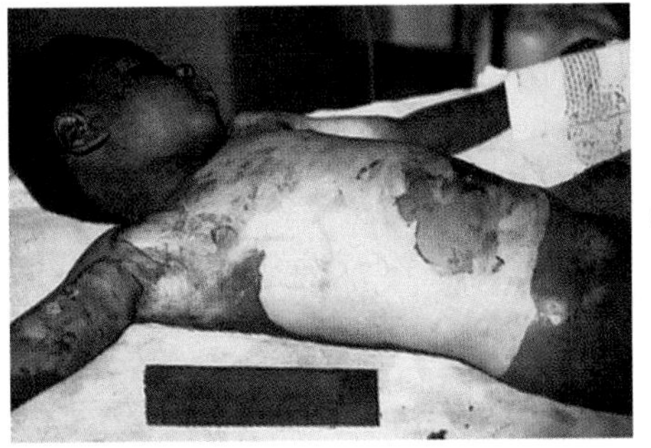

C

B

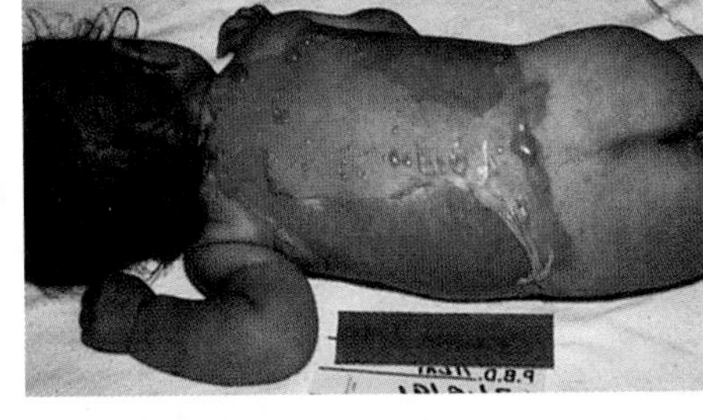

FIGURE 32-5 Thermal burns are those caused by contact with hot liquids, objects, electricity, or fire. They are classified according to the depth of damage to the skin. **A,** First-degree burns are minor, involving only the outer layers of the skin (epidermis). **B,** Second-degree burns affect the deeper layers of the epidermis and dermis and are painful. **C,** Third-degree burns are those that affect not only the skin but also the muscle and bone. (Courtesy St. John's Mercy Medical Center, St. Louis, Mo.)

TABLE 32-5
Poisoning

Emergency	What to Do	Why
Ingestion	Save the suspected source of poison.	Emergency medical services personnel can estimate type and amount of toxin ingested.
	If at home, give the victim water or milk (if the victim is conscious without convulsions).	
	Contact poison control or the emergency department for a suggested treatment; if vomiting is suggested, give syrup of ipecac (vomit inducer) and then water.	If unconscious, the victim may be in danger of aspiration (breathing of vomitus into the lungs).
	Do not induce vomiting if poison is an acid, alkali, or petroleum product.	Tissue damage may occur as the substance passes through the esophagus again. A counteractive treatment may be administered.
	If the poison is a medicine, do not give anything by mouth without professional advice.	
Inhalation	Move the victim to fresh air.	
	Establish an airway; loosen clothing.	Using the head-tilt chin-lift method to open an airway avoids injury to the spinal column.
	Begin mouth-to-mouth artificial respiration if breathing is absent; give one breath every 3 s (about 100/min).	
Contact	Flood affected area with water for at least 10 min; cleanse with soap; do not attempt to neutralize the toxin with acids or alkalis.	
	Remove contaminated clothing and jewelry.	Clothing and jewelry will continue to poison the skin if left in place.
	Flush a contaminated eye from the inner to the outer aspect for at least 20 min; do not force the eye open.	Flushing from the inner to the outer aspect prevents contamination of the other eye.

Third-degree burns may result from exposure to fire, hot water, hot objects, or electricity.

Poisoning

Poisoning may occur in several ways, and most poisoning occurs in the home (Table 32-5). Poison can be ingested, inhaled, absorbed, injected, or obtained by radiation. Ingestion is the taking in of a substance by eating or drinking. Signs and symptoms of poisoning include discoloration or burns on the lips, unusual odor, vomiting (emesis), or presence of a suspicious container.

Shock

Shock is the response of the cardiovascular system to the presence of adrenalin, resulting in capillary constriction (Table 32-6). It may result in inadequate circulation to the body tissues, lowered blood pressure, and decreased kidney function. Shock can result from trauma, electrical injury, insulin shock, **hemorrhage**, or as a reaction to drugs. It may occur in conjunction with other injuries or illness such as respiratory distress, fever, heart attack, and poisoning. Anaphylactic shock is the response of the body to an allergen such as a medication.

TABLE 32-6
Inadequate Circulation Resulting from Shock

Emergency	What to Do	Why
Shock	Eliminate cause if possible.	
	Keep the victim lying down with feet slightly elevated (8 to 12 in).	Elevating the legs allows blood to accumulate around the heart and brain.
	Maintain the airway.	
	Cover the victim with a blanket.	Covering the victim helps maintain body temperature that has been lowered by reduced circulation.
	Do not give any fluids to the victim.	Victims of traumatic injury may require surgery; fluids can be a significant risk in such cases.

TABLE 32-7
Fractures

Emergency	What to Do	Why
Closed fracture	Splint the fracture in the position found.	Immobilization reduces pain and risk of injury.
	Seek medical attention as soon as possible.	Fractures must be set to prevent deformity.
Open fracture	Stop the bleeding if necessary; do not replace a protruding bone in the tissues.	
	Immobilize the fracture to reduce pain and further injury.	Movement may damage tissues.

Early signs and symptoms of shock include pale and clammy skin, weakness, and restlessness. The pulse and respiratory rate are rapid, and vomiting may occur. Late signs of shock include apathy, unresponsiveness, dilated pupils, mottled skin, and loss of consciousness. Shock may result in death if the condition is not reversed.

Fractures

Breakage of a bone is called a *fracture* (Table 32-7). Fractures can be classified as closed or open (Fig. 32-6). Simple, or closed, fractures do not penetrate the skin. In open, or compound, fractures the bone breaks through the skin and is exposed. Open fractures present a greater chance of infection.

Other injuries to the bones and muscle tissue include muscle strains, sprains, and dislocation. Muscle strains result from injury to the muscle tissue, usually from overuse. Muscle strain causes pain and possibly cramping on movement. Sprains result from injury to the ligaments, or the attachments between the muscle and bones. Sprains result in a rapid swelling and pain when the joint is moved. Dislocation occurs when a bone moves out of a joint. Signs and symptoms of dislocation include swelling, pain, and discoloration.

Temperature Alteration

The human body works well at a specified temperature (Table 32-8). If the temperature varies too much, the body cannot function. Exposure to heat can result in muscle cramping, which results from an electrolyte imbalance caused by loss of salt from sweating. It causes pain and inability to use the muscle. Exposure to heat can also cause heat exhaustion or heat stroke.

Signs and symptoms of heat exhaustion include perspiration (diaphoresis) and pale and clammy skin, even though the body temperature is normal. The victim may feel weak and nauseated.

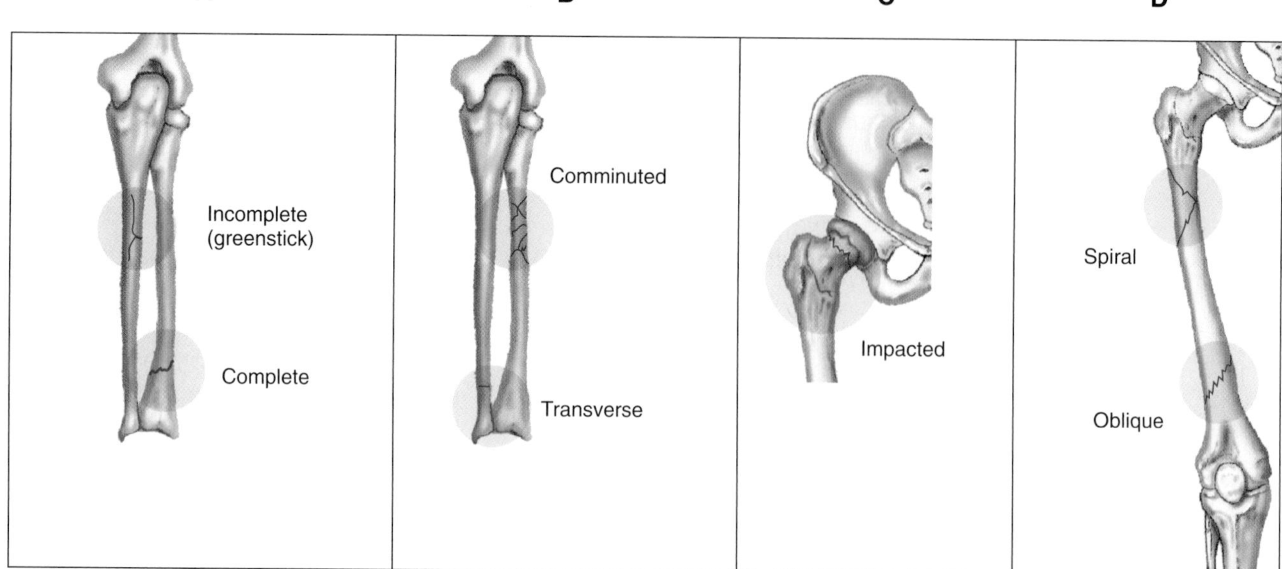

FIGURE 32-6 Types of fractures. **A,** Incomplete and complete (greenstick). **B,** Comminuted and transverse. **C,** Impacted. **D,** Oblique and spiral. (From Sanders MJ: *Mosby's paramedic textbook*, ed 2, St. Louis, 2000, Mosby.)

TABLE 32-8
Temperature Alteration

Emergency	What to Do	Why
Heat cramps	Massage the affected muscle area.	Massage increases circulation and brings oxygen to the tissues.
	Administer small amounts of salty water.	Salt helps retain water; lack of water usually causes heat cramps.
Heat exhaustion	Move victim to a cooler area.	
	Sponge the skin with cool water.	The reduction of temperature is the best treatment.
	Seek medical attention.	
Heat stroke	Move victim to a cooler area.	
	Immerse in cool water or apply ice packs.	
	Monitor vital signs; seek medical attention.	Heat stroke results in life-threatening increase in body temperature and may cause death if not treated immediately.
Hypothermia	If necessary, remove victim from cold water.	
	Remove wet clothing.	Wet clothing retains cold temperatures.
	Cover the victim with a warm blanket or immerse in water.	
	Give warm fluids if the victim is conscious.	
	Monitor vital signs; seek medical attention.	
Frostbite	Bring victim inside.	Continued exposure to cold increases the tissue damage.
	Cover the affected area with a blanket or cloth or immerse in slightly warm water; **do not rub**.	Rubbing may damage the frozen tissue and increase the risk of gangrene infection.
	Give warm fluids if the victim is conscious.	
	Discontinue warming when skin becomes flushed.	
	Elevate and cover the affected area loosely with a dry dressing.	Swelling occurs as the tissues recover.

TABLE 32-9
Miscellaneous Injuries

Emergency	What to Do	Why
Nosebleed	Have victim sit up or lie down with head and shoulders raised.	Raising the head decreases the blood flow to the area.
	Lean the head forward slightly.	
	Apply direct pressure against the bleeding nostril at the midline.	Most bleeding can be stopped with direct pressure.
	Apply a cold compress to the face and nose.	The reduced temperature decreases blood flow to that area.
Near drowning	Remove the victim from the water.	
	Assess respirations; if heartbeat is absent, begin cardiopulmonary resuscitation.	
	Keep the victim as cool as possible. Reduction in body temperature decreases the need for oxygen.	
Penetrating eye injury	Do not rub or rinse the injured eye.	
	Do not remove foreign objects.	
	Keep victim lying flat.	
	Cover both eyes loosely with clean dressing, paper cups, or a similar device that does not place pressure on the eyes.	Movement of the eye may cause further damage; both eyes are covered because the eyes move together when just one is covered.
Insect and snake bites	Keep the victim lying flat with the affected part higher than the level of the heart.	Raising the area of the bite slows circulation to and from that area.
	Apply a band that constricts part of the circulation above the level of the bite.	The constricting should not cut off circulation because tissue damage could occur.
	Apply an ice pack to the area of the bite.	Ice can reduce circulation of blood and toxins through the body.
	Seek medical treatment of bites from poisonous snakes and insects.	Toxin damage may not be evident.

In heat stroke the skin is dry and flushed. The pulse is fast and strong. The internal temperature can rise to 106° F or more, resulting in death of brain tissue. Death may result from heat stroke if it is not treated quickly.

Exposure to cold temperatures can result in frostbite or hypothermia. Frostbite occurs when the water in the body tissues freezes. When the tissue does not get oxygen because of the freezing, the tissue will die. The tissues of the nose, ears, fingers, and toes are the most susceptible. Early signs and symptoms of frostbite include redness and tingling. As damage progresses, the tissue becomes pale and numb.

Hypothermia is an abnormal lowering of body temperature, usually resulting from immersion in cold water or being stranded in subzero weather. Signs and symptoms include shivering, numbness, confusion, paleness, and eventual loss of consciousness.

Miscellaneous Injuries

Other injuries include those to the eyes, nose, jaw, neck, and chest and to those who are drowning (Table 32-9). These injuries may require special treatment techniques. Any object that penetrates the body should not be removed until professional medical help is available.

Bites can occur from animals or insects. Bites caused by animals and humans require medical

TABLE 32-10
Aquatic Injuries

Emergency	What to Do	Why
Marine injuries	Treat all victims of aquatic injury for the signs and symptoms of shock.	
	If possible, remove any materials from puncture and stings from the wound.	Projectiles within toxin continue to poison the wound.
	Soak the wound in warm water for 20 min.	Water will help remove toxins.
	Pain may be relieved with vinegar or diluted ammonia and an application of baking soda paste.	Other home remedies include a paste of meat tenderizer and water.
	Bites are treated to control the bleeding.	
	Seek medical attention if the wound is severe or if there is an allergic reaction.	

attention to ensure prevention of infection. Snake or insect bites require medical attention if the venom is poisonous.

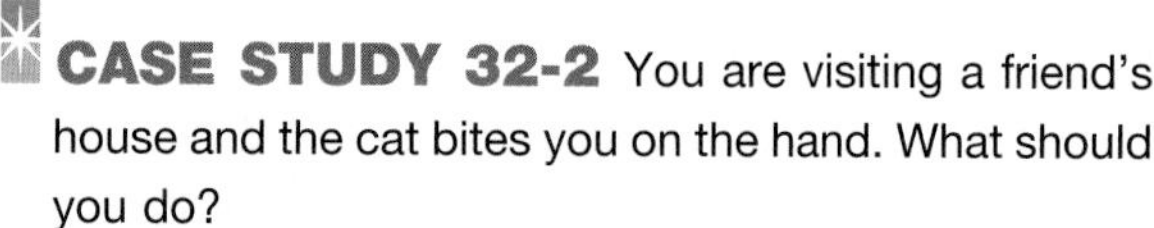

CASE STUDY 32-2 You are visiting a friend's house and the cat bites you on the hand. What should you do?

Answers to Case Studies are available on the Evolve website: ***http://evolve.elsevier.com/Gerdin***

Marine Injuries

With the increase in the numbers of people pursuing marine sports such as skin and scuba diving, safety and first-aid measures for this particular area have become more important (Table 32-10). Most injuries by marine life and during diving are caused by the victim, because aquatic life is rarely aggressive. The Divers Alert Network provides insurance and consultation for members regarding marine injuries throughout the world.

In scuba diving, air embolism and decompression illness resulting from rapid ascent are major concerns. A diver should never rise to the surface faster than the air bubbles and must breathe continuously during descent and ascent and take a precautionary decompression stop at 15 feet for 3 minutes at the end of all dives. In addition, divers should always have a "buddy" who is within sight at all times. Treatment of decompression sickness and air embolism requires immediate, specialized advanced life support techniques of a recompression chamber to restore the normal composition of air in the blood.

Aquatic life differs from one ocean location to another, so consultation with local health care professionals and divers is important in determining treatment (Fig. 32-7). The three main types of marine injuries are stings, punctures, and bites. Sea urchins, stingrays, or spiny fish that are stepped on or touched might cause puncture wounds. Stings from jellyfish or coral may occur when touched. Aquatic life may be venomous (designed to kill prey) or poisonous (causing harm if eaten because of **toxins** in the tissues). Some aquatic animals, including fish, bite when threatened or if food is held in the diver's hand.

Medical Conditions

First aid may be necessary in the case of illness caused by a sudden medical condition such as a stroke or a **seizure** activity (Table 32-11). Strokes, or cerebrovascular accidents, occur from spontaneous rupture of a blood vessel or clot formation in the brain. Signs and symptoms may include loss of consciousness, paralysis, difficulty breathing, slurred speech, loss of bladder control, and unequal pupil size. The condition may threaten the victim's life.

Seizure, or uncontrolled muscle activity, may be preceded by an **aura** and may occur in several patterns. Convulsions are the uncoordinated movement of groups of muscles usually resulting from poisoning (drug overdose) or elevated temperature. Coordinated seizure activity may occur in individuals with epilepsy. The International Classification of Epileptic Seizures divides seizures into two types on the basis of the area of the brain from which they originate. Partial seizures start in a specific area of the brain and

TABLE 32-11
Medical Conditions

Emergency	What to Do	Why
Stroke	Assess and establish vital functions.	Strokes often affect vital functions.
	Activate emergency medical services system.	Medical attention is a priority.
	Treat the victim for the signs and symptoms of shock.	
	Position the victim on the affected side.	Secretions may block the airway.
Seizure	Prevent the victim from self-injury by cushioning the head and arms if possible; do not restrain the victim.	The victim does not recognize the damage done by movement; restraining may lead to injury.
	Observe and monitor vital functions; do not insert anything into the mouth.	Respirations may stop during a grand mal seizure, but they could resume in the clonic phase; items placed in the mouth may cause further injury and obstruction of the airway.
	Assist the victim to lie on the side or abdomen as seizure activity subsides.	

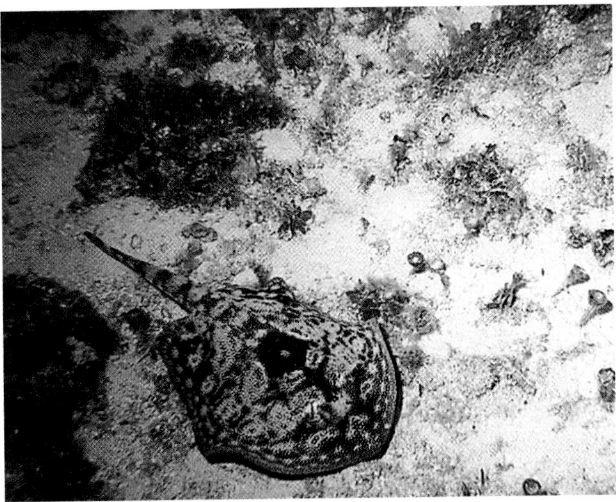

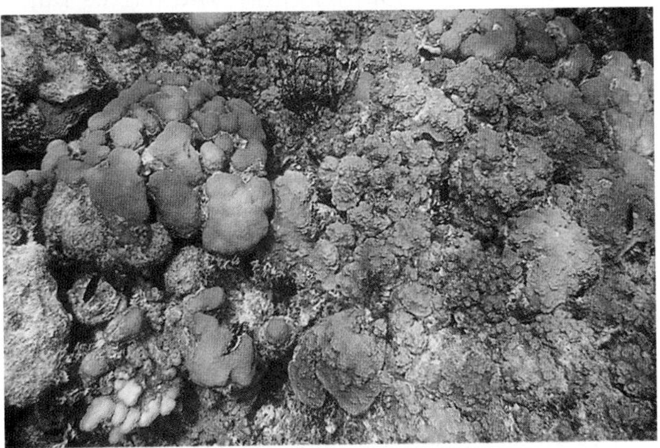

FIGURE 32-7 Aquatic life can contribute to marine injuries.

may cause motor or sensory symptoms such as automatic actions, hallucinations, or twitching of muscle groups. Tonic-clonic (grand mal), absence (petit-mal), and myoclonic seizures involve larger areas of the brain and are categorized as general. Uncontrolled movement of the body and loss of consciousness may occur with generalized seizures.

Performance Instruction

All emergency workers use substance isolation precautions to prevent the spread of microorganisms. This includes the use of gloves when body fluids are touched or breaks are present on the skin. Body fluids include blood, urine, vomitus, feces, and any materials contaminated by these substances. The hands are washed thoroughly after the gloves are removed. Masks, goggles, or face shields may be worn if splattering of body secretions is possible. Barrier devices such as resuscitation masks are used to administer mouth-to-mouth breathing.

Some of the methods of emergency care may be performed by bystanders or first responders trained in first aid. These include the assessment of the type and severity of injuries or triage. If the victim is unresponsive, gasping, or not breathing, CPR or emergency cardiovascular care is initiated (Table 32-12). The American Heart Association (AHA) established

TABLE 32-12
2010 Cardiopulmonary Resuscitation Guidelines Changes

Action	New Guidelines
Recognition	Begin CPR if victim is unresponsive with no breathing or only gasping
Sequence	Perform with compressions before establishing airway and rescue breathing (C-A-B)
Compression rate	At least 100/min (adults, children, and infants)
Compression depth	At least 2 inches, allowing complete recoil between compressions
Untrained bystander	Hands only (compressions only)
Ratio*	30:2 Compression/ventilation
Ventilations*	1 second/breath

*Trained health care provider.

the most common procedure for CPR based on effectiveness research. The 2010 revision places more emphasis on effective chest compressions, changing the sequence to C-A-B for all victims except newborns. Chapter 7 provides more information about the procedure for performing CPR.

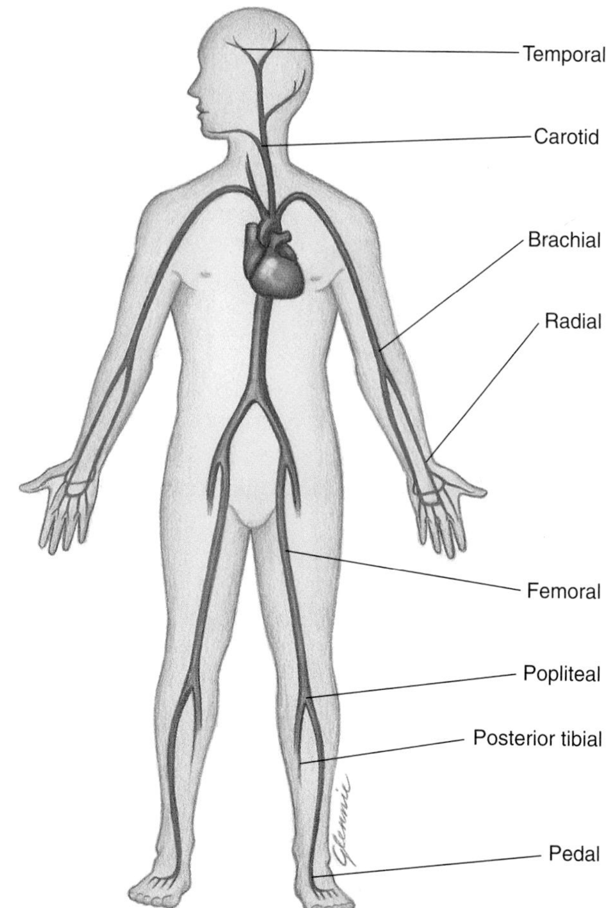

FIGURE 32-8 Pressure on artery points may be used to stop bleeding in 90% of bleeding wounds.

CASE STUDY 32-3 Your friend tells you he does not want to take a CPR class because he does not want to be sued or legally liable if the victim is not revived. What should you say?

Answers to Case Studies are available on the Evolve website: ***http://evolve.elsevier.com/Gerdin***

After establishing the order of treatment of victims involved in the emergency, bleeding is treated first. Most bleeding from wounds can be stopped with a combination of direct pressure and elevation of the wounded area. Pressure may also be placed on the major arteries that supply the affected area (Fig. 32-8). In only the most extreme cases, when death resulting from bleeding is probable, a **tourniquet** may be used. The application of a tourniquet damages the tissues below the area where applied, so it is not recommended unless all other methods have failed to stop bleeding.

Treatment for burns varies with the type and amount of tissue damage. A first-degree burn causes the skin to redden and is treated by applying cool water to the area (Fig. 32-9). Second-degree burns result in blisters and may also be treated with cool water and elevation of the area affected. Third-degree burns cause extensive damage to the skin and tissues beneath it. Clothing and material that adheres to a third-degree burn should not be removed. The burned area may be covered with a clean, dry cloth of dressing and elevated to reduce swelling. Advanced medical treatment is necessary as soon as possible in the case of a third-degree burn. Ointments and other materials are not applied to any burn without medical direction.

Poisoning by ingestion may result from household materials, medications, and other items. The victim of poisoning should be given milk or water if fully

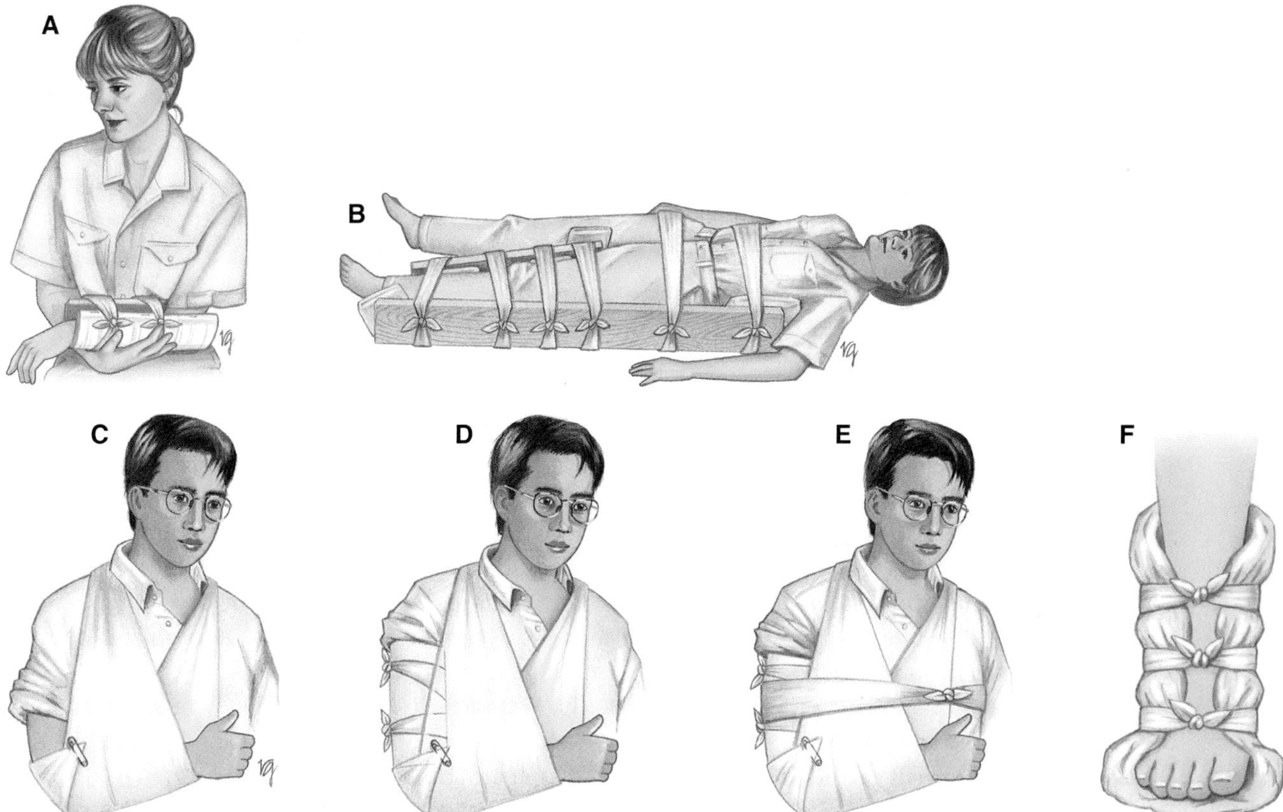

FIGURE 32-9 Fractures may be splinted with materials on hand to immobilize joints. **A,** Rolled newspaper may be used as a splint. **B,** Femoral fractures must be splinted above the hip joint to prevent movement. **C,** Slings may support dislocations, as well as fractures. **D & E**, Fractures of the humerus must be splinted and immobilized. **F,** Household items such as a pillow may be used to immobilize a joint.

conscious and without convulsions. No liquids are given to an unconscious person. Vomiting should not be encouraged unless medically directed to do so because the substance may further damage the body during vomiting if caustic. Because treatment of poisoning depends on the type of poison ingested, advanced medical attention should be sought as soon as possible. Other types of poisoning that may need treatment include inhalation and contact poisoning.

All victims of trauma should be treated for shock. The victim is encouraged to lie down with the feet and legs slightly elevated. The victim may be lightly covered with a blanket. No fluids are given to a victim of trauma unless they are specifically indicated, as in poisoning.

The main focus of the treatment of fractures is immobilization of the injured area (see Fig. 32-9). A closed fracture does not penetrate the skin. An open fracture may require the stopping of bleeding before immobilization. All fractures should be treated with advanced medical support as soon as possible.

Heat cramps may appear in muscles. The affected area may be massaged to bring oxygen to the area, and a small amount of slightly salty water may help to increase the fluid balance in the body. Heat exhaustion and heat stroke are more severe reactions to exposure to heat. The victim should be moved to a cooler area and sponged with cool water. Medical attention for heat exhaustion is necessary as soon as possible. In heat stroke the victim's body temperature should be lowered as soon as possible with cool water or ice packs. Heat stroke is life threatening, and advanced medical attention should be sought as soon as possible.

Hypothermia and frostbite can result with exposure to cold temperatures. The victim of hypothermia should be treated by removal to a warm area if possible. Wet clothing is removed and a warm blanket applied. If the victim is fully conscious, warm fluids may help increase body temperature. Frostbite results in tissue damage because of freezing of body fluids. To prevent further damage, the affected area should not be rubbed. A warm blanket may be applied to the affected area. If the victim is conscious, warm fluids may be given to raise body temperature. Advanced medical attention may be necessary for both hypothermia and frostbite injuries.

Other miscellaneous emergencies that may occur include nosebleeds, drowning, eye injuries, and insect or snake bites. A nosebleed may be treated by having the victim sit or lie down with the head and shoulders raised. With the head slightly forward, the victim may apply direct pressure to the nostrils at the midline. A cold compress on the nose may also help stop bleeding. Victims of drowning are removed from the water as soon as possible and artificial respiration started. First responders should not remove objects that penetrate the eye. Additional damage to the eye may be prevented by loosely covering both eyes to prevent movement of the injured area. Eye injuries require advanced medical treatment as soon as possible. Insect and snake bites may be treated by the application of cold to and elevation of the affected area. A restricting band may be placed between the bite and the heart to slow the poison's spread as long as it does not cut off all circulation to the area. Ice placed on the bite may also reduce the poison's circulation from the area. Advanced medical attention is necessary for many snake and insect bites.

CASE STUDY 32-4 You are taking a walk and you notice another person is walking by a swarm of bees. He has already been stung at least one time and is swatting at the bees. What should you do?

Answers to Case Studies are available on the Evolve website: ***http://evolve.elsevier.com/Gerdin***

Some medical conditions that may require emergency care include stroke and seizures. The stroke victim should be monitored for vital signs while emergency personnel are responding. The person may be placed on the affected side to promote easier breathing and prevent aspiration. Response to seizure activity involves protecting the victim from injury by removing articles that might be in the way of movement or providing a cushioned area when possible. Nothing should be inserted into the victim's mouth, nor should any restraint be applied to stop movement. When the seizure activity has stopped, the person may be turned on one side to promote easier breathing.

Summary

- The role of the emergency personnel is to provide immediate care resulting from illness or injury.
- Three levels of care that have been developed to provide immediate care are the bystander or first responder, EMT, and advanced emergency personnel.
- External wounds include abrasions, punctures, and incisions.
- Burns may be classified as first, second, or third degree.
- Poisoning may occur by ingestion, absorption, injection, inhalation, or radiation.
- Five causes of shock include trauma, electrical injury, insulin shock, hemorrhage, and as a reaction to drugs.
- Three types of fractures are incomplete, comminuted, and impacted.
- The effect of extreme heat is heat exhaustion or heat stroke. Extreme cold may lead to frostbite and hypothermia.
- The signs and symptoms of stroke include loss of consciousness, paralysis, difficulty breathing, slurred speech, and unequal pupil reaction to light. The signs and symptoms of seizure include uncontrolled muscle activity, aura, and loss of consciousness.

Review Questions

1. Describe the members of the emergency health care team, including education, role, and credentialing requirements.
2. Describe the purpose of the emergency health care team.
3. Define first aid and list its three components.
4. Describe six types of external wounds.
5. Describe three ways used to determine the severity of burns and the three degrees of burns.
6. Describe five ways that poisoning may occur.
7. Describe the effect that shock has on the body and list five causes.
8. Describe three types of fractures and treatment for each.
9. Describe the effects of extreme cold and heat on the body.
10. Choose one career from Box 32-1. Research the cost of education and annual earnings in local institutions. Write a paragraph describing the

factors that might explain why the local and national economic figures vary.

11. Use each of the following terms in one or more sentences that correctly relate their meaning: consciousness, critical, hemorrhage, shock, and tourniquet.

Critical Thinking

1. Investigate and compare the cost of various types of emergency care treatments.
2. Research and describe five common medications used in emergency health care.
3. Investigate and compare the cost of education for five emergency health care professionals.
4. Describe the certification requirements for first aid and cardiopulmonary resuscitation.
5. Research and report the poisonous plants, reptiles, and insects local to the area.
6. Use the Internet to research the Good Samaritan law of the state. Describe the criteria that must be met (acting in good faith) for the law to apply.
7. Create a career ladder for emergency health careers. Describe why it is or is not possible to move from one level to another in the field.

Explore the Web

Career Information

Bureau of Labor Statistics
http://www.bls.gov/

Salary.com
http://salary.com

Professional Associations

American Heart Association (AHA)
http://www.americaheart.org

National Association of Emergency Medical Technicians (NAEMT)
http://www.naemt.org/

CHAPTER 33

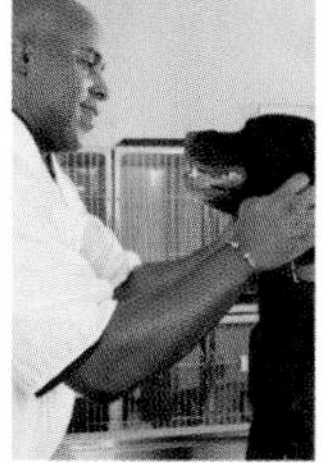
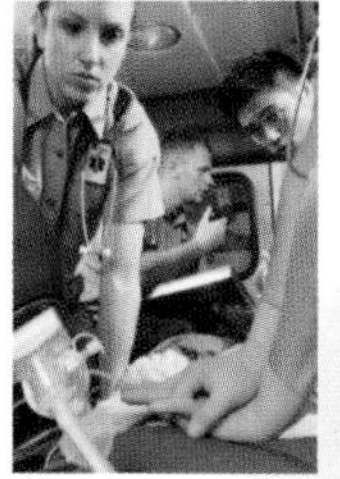
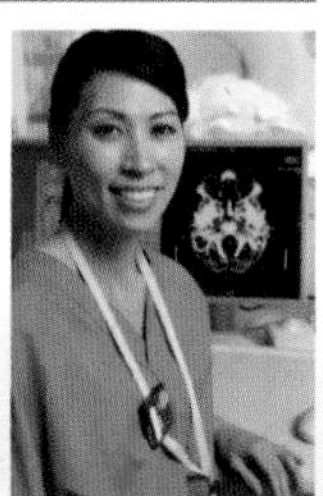

Information and Administration Careers

LEARNING OBJECTIVES

- Identify at least 10 terms related to health care information and administration.
- Specify the role of selected information and administrative health care workers, including personal qualities, levels of education, and credentialing requirements.
- Identify three personal characteristics needed in an efficient health occupations clerk.
- Identify at least five forms used as part of the medical record.
- Describe at least three methods of payment for health care.

KEY TERMS

Administration *(ad-min-ih-STRAY-shun)* Management; performance of executive responsibilities and duties

Benefit *(BEN-uh-fit)* Financial help in time of illness, retirement, or unemployment

Chart Collection of written materials relating to the health care of a patient

Confidential *(kon-fuh-DEN-shul)* Private and secret; may be protected by law

Customary *(KUS-tum-ay-ree)* Fee charged by similar practitioners for a service in the same economic and geographic area

Deficient *(deh-FISH-unt)* Lacking some important part

Dictation *(dik-TAY-shun)* Speaking words to be written by another person; may be recorded

Incident *(IN-si-duhnt)* An individual occurrence or event occurring in connection with something else; a reportable variance

Insurance *(in-SHUR-ins)* Payment by contract by one party to another in which the second party guarantees the first party against financial loss from a specific event

KEY TERMS cont'd

Reasonable *(REE-sun-uh-bul)* Fee that considers both the usual fee charged by a practitioner for a particular service and the fee charged by other practitioners for the same service

Transcribe *(tran-SKRIBE)* To make a written copy of dictated or recorded matter

Health Information and Administration Terminology*

Term	Definition	Prefix	Root	Suffix
Abduction	Move away	ab	duc	tion
Adduction	Move toward	ad	duc	tion
Arthritis	Inflammation of the joint		arthr	itis
Arthrodesis	Fixation of the joint		arthr/o	desis
Cervical	Pertaining to the neck		cervic	al
Hypertrophy	Above normal amount of growth	hyper	troph	y
Myelogram	Picture of the bone marrow		myelo	gram
Neuralgia	Painful nerve		neur	algia
Osteopathy	Disease of the bone	osteo	path	y
Terminology	Study of words		termin	ology

*A transition syllable or vowel may be added to or deleted from the word parts to make the combining form.

Abbreviations for Information and Administration Careers

Abbreviation	Meaning
ART	Accredited records technician
CAAHEP	Commission on Accreditation of Allied Health Education Programs
CEO	Chief executive officer
CPT	Current procedure terminology
CTS	Carpel tunnel syndrome
HUC	Health unit coordinator
RHIT	Registered health information technician
RRA	Registered records administrator
RSI	Repetitive stress injury
URC	Usual, reasonable, customary

Careers

Even though health care administrators and information personnel often do not have direct contact with the patients, they are of critical importance to the quality of care delivered (Table 33-1). Health care managers need to be organized to work quickly and accurately. Good communication skills are necessary to provide information and leadership in the health care setting. Administrators must be able to form and maintain good working relationships with those in subordinate positions. Although administrators and information personnel may not have direct contact with the patient, they are subject to confidentiality and other Health Insurance Portability and Accountability Act (HIPAA) guidelines. More information about these guidelines is found in Chapter 2. With the exception of high-level managers, most health information and administrative service personnel work regular hours. Some examples of careers in **administration** include health care facility managers, supervisors, medical secretaries, unit coordinators, and medical records (health information) personnel (Box 33-1).

Part of the responsibility of the health care administrator is to meet legal regulations. The Joint Commission accredits about 88% of hospitals in the United States. In 1997 they began considering the facility's performance goals data as well as the standards for staff and equipment when granting approval. The new program considers patient outcomes as part of the data. The initiative is called *ORYX*, and it is being expanded into use by other types of agencies accredited by the Joint Commission such as home care, behavioral health, ambulatory and lab facilities.

TABLE 33-1
Information and Administration Career Educational Cost and Earnings

Career	Educational Cost*	Earnings†
Registered health information technician (RHIT)	Bishop State Community College, associate degree, 77 credit hours Fees include: Tuition, books, & fees $8393	Median annual salary: Mobile, Ala.—$28,450

*http://www.bscc.cc.al.us/tuition.html.
†http://data.bls.gov:8080/oes/datatype.do.

BOX 33-1

Information and Administration Careers

Administrator, drug and alcohol facility
Administrator, hospital
Biological photographer
Biophysicist
Chemist, food
Chief of nuclear medicine
Clerk, medical records
Coordinator of rehabilitation services
Coroner
Credentialing specialist
Dietary manager
Dietitian, research
Director, counseling
Director, community health nursing
Director, diagnostics clinics
Director, nursing registry
Director, nursing service
Director, occupational health nursing
Director, outpatient services
Director, pharmacy service
Director, placement
Director, radiology
Director, school of nursing
Director, speech and hearing
Director, volunteer services
District advisor
Executive director, Nurses Association
Food and drug inspector
Health information technician
Health physicist
Health unit coordinator
Hospital registration staff
Information scientist
In-service coordinator, auxiliary personnel
Instructor, psychiatric aides
Laboratory manager
Librarian
Librarian, special
Library technical assistant
Manager, dental laboratory
Medical physicist
Medical records administrator
Medical records technician
Medical staff services technician
Medical staff services coordinator
Medical technologist teaching supervisor
Nurse, consultant
Nurse, evening supervisor
Nurse, head
Nurse, instructor
Nurse, supervisor
Nursing home administrator
Patient resource agent
Photographer, scientific
Public relations representative
Radiology administrator
Rehabilitation center manager
Secretary, medical
Supervisor, artificial breast fabrication
Supervisor, central supply
Supervisor, hearing aid assembly
Supervisor, laundry
Utilization review coordinator
Ward clerk
Ward service supervisor

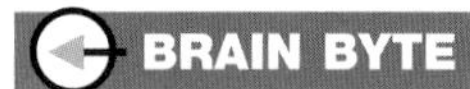

BRAIN BYTE

The Joint Commission was formerly called the Joint Commission on Accreditation of Healthcare Organizations.

Heath Service Managers

Administrators and managers are necessary in all health care facilities, including clinics, health maintenance organizations, hospitals, home care agencies, private practices, rehabilitation agencies, hospice services, long-term medical day care, and ambulatory care settings. The top executive is often referred to as the chief executive officer (CEO). Administrators develop and expand services with authority given to them by the governing board or agency owner. Administrators manage the facility budget, programs, and personnel. They are responsible for relations with other agencies and organizations.

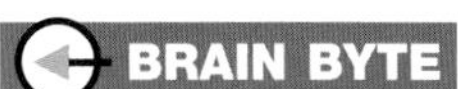

BRAIN BYTE

An Internal Revenue Service report showed that salaries for CEOs of nonprofit hospitals ranged from $490,000 to $16.4 million in 2006.

Administrators coordinate services, hiring, and training of personnel (Fig. 33-1). Administrators may be responsible for establishing the policies and procedures of the facility. The CEO must demonstrate public relations skills as well as leadership ability. Long, irregular hours are often required for public speaking and travel.

Positions for health managers who have obtained 4-year bachelor's degrees are available in small institutions, but master- or doctoral-level preparation is preferred for employment in large facilities. Employment opportunities for managers will grow the fastest in residential care facilities and practitioner's offices and clinics. More than 70 colleges and universities offer accredited master's programs that specialize in health care administration. Master's-level preparation is also available in long-term care administration, public health, public administration, or business administration. Other managers may study business, public administration, or human resources administration before becoming employed in the health care industry. An internship is required by many administrative programs, and postgraduate residents and fellows may occupy middle-management positions as part of the educational program. Although regulations vary from state to state, licensing is usually required for administrators of long-term care facilities. Duties of the health care manager may include hiring and coordination of personnel, budget preparation and implementation, and public relations.

Medical staff services personnel are responsible for maintaining the credentialing of all physicians and

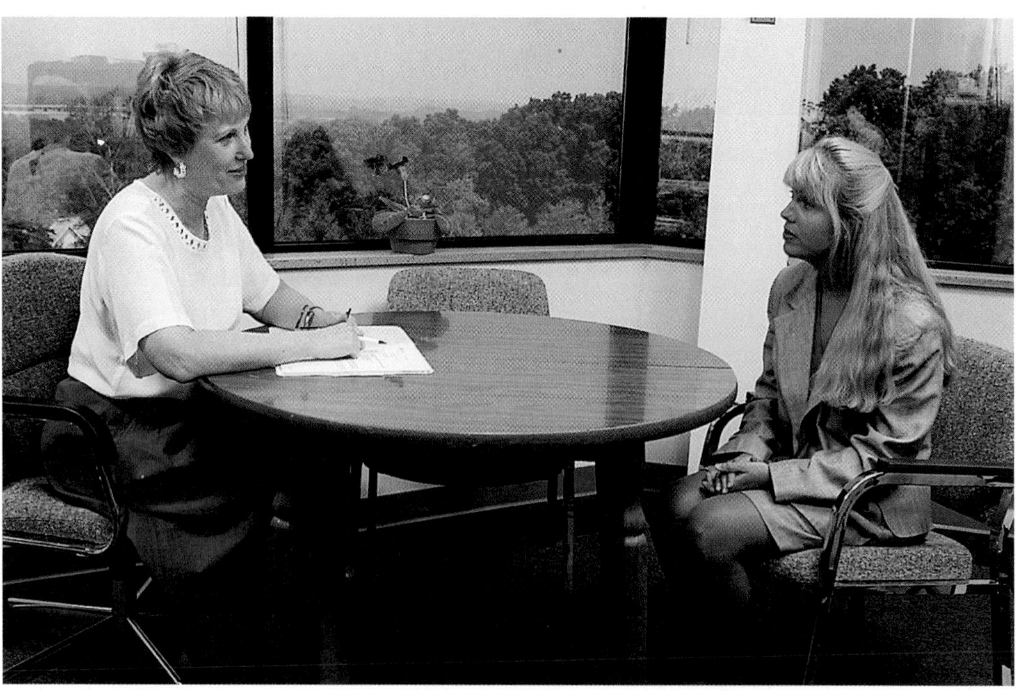

FIGURE 33-1 Administrators often participate in hiring decisions.

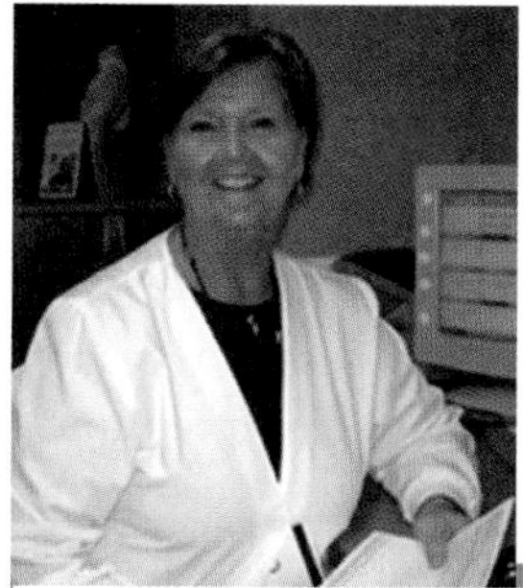

MICHELLE E. GOMBERT RNC, MSN, ARNP

DIRECTOR OF PERINATAL SERVICES (CONSULTANT AND TRANSITIONAL LEADER)
ADVENTIST HEALTHCARE SYSTEM, FLORIDA HOSPITAL ALTAMONTE

Educational background: Nineteen years of education, including college, graduate school, and postgraduate nurse practitioner residency. Professional degrees and certifications include registered nurse certification (RNC), bachelor of science in nursing (BSN), master of science in nursing (MSN), advanced registered nurse practitioner (ARNP), and certified nurse administrator advanced (CNAA).

A typical day at work and job duties include:

- Clinical Nursing Rounds with professional and ancillary nursing staff
- Clinical Patient Care Rounds with care providers
- Unit Manager/Patient Satisfaction Rounds with patients and families
- Facilities/Unit Safety and Compliance Rounds
- Strategic planning meetings
- Staff interviews, evaluation, counseling, and discipline
- Staff meetings, education, and communication

The most gratifying part of my job: Staff and patient and family interactions leading to positive changes in the delivery of quality and satisfying patient care.

The biggest challenge(s) I face in doing my job: As a consultant and transitional leader, I have to "hit the ground running" and experience limitations of time and resources to impact the changes and enhancements I identify as needed in a given work situation.

What drew me to my career? A strong desire to become involved in people's lives and impact the quality of their health and well-being in a positive way, most specifically the well-being of mothers and their newborns.

Something I learned in my early education that I currently use in my career or that caused me to be interested in my career is: I learned early in my life that observing and assessing could teach me much about my fellow human beings and allow me to plan an approach that would maximize the achievement of a positive outcome. This practice continues to serve me well in the work I do and the outcomes I am able to achieve.

Other comments: It is an honor and a privilege to come into a patient's and his or her family's life when they are vulnerable and in need of our care and compassion. It is a sacred duty we take on when we provide care and comfort for our patients, and we must protect their trust and faith in us as we strive to provide the highest quality patient care.

allied health practitioners in a healthcare facility. They maintain the records of licensing, continuing education, and training. They are responsible for reviewing and implementing federal standards. The National Association of Medical Staff Services awards the Certified Provider Credentialing Specialist.

Patient representatives, or advocates, help patients understand the health care policies and procedures of the facility, obtain services, and make informed decisions about their care. The work of the patient representative is varied on the basis of the needs of the current patients. Some duties might include assisting with the drafting of a living will or resolving a conflict between the facility staff and patient. Hospitals and other facilities set their own requirements for the education and experience background of this individual.

BOX 33-2

Health Care Pre-employment or Student Background Check*

- Character and personal references
- Court records
- Credit records
- Criminal records/wants and warrants search
- Driving records and vehicle registration
- Drug test results
- Education and employment verification
- Fingerprint search
- Immunization record
- Incarceration or sex offender records
- Medical records
- Past employer interviews
- Social security number
- State licensing records
- Worker's compensation and bankruptcy records

*Background checks vary greatly. Students in health care programs may be required to pay for background checks.

Many patient representatives have a master's degree in a health-related field.

Human resource and labor relations personnel recruit, screen, and hire qualified employees and match them to appropriate jobs. They may also provide training and development opportunities to increase employee satisfaction and decrease turnover. They may interview prospective employees, explain benefits of employment, and supervise background checks before hiring occurs (Box 33-2). In 2004 the Joint Commission mandated that criminal background checks be performed on any person who interacts with patients. This includes staff, students, and volunteers. The Fair Credit Reporting Act defines the guidelines for requesting or requiring background checks. In some cases human resource personnel may act as mediators or arbitrators to resolve employment disputes. The education required for human resources varies with the duties and level of responsibility required. A bachelor's degree is a typical entry level, but master's degrees in human resources administration are available. Certification is available for the Certified Employee Benefits Specialist, and the Society for Human Resource Management offers two levels of certification for more senior personnel.

Health care risk managers supervise programs to reduce the number of accidents and incidents involving patients and staff members. Risk factors may be environmental or behavioral. Risk management may include establishing policies and procedures as well as reviewing documents such as patient charts and employee incident reports. For example, placement of signs warning that the floor is wet may reduce the risk of falling. Employees complete incident reports when an error or adverse event (reportable variance) occurs. Reportable incidents include any event that is not consistent with the organization's procedures and routine care. Methods recommended by the Joint Commission to reduce the risk of error are the "do not use" list of abbreviations and the annual National Patient Safety Goals (Table 33-2). The National Patient Safety Goals were designed to address specific areas of patient safety such as medication errors. The risk manager may communicate with legal representatives when a complaint about care is made. Certification and licensure are available for the risk manager.

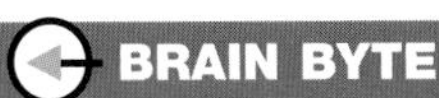

The estimated national cost of preventable medical errors causing injury (lost income, U.S. household production, disability, and health care costs) is $17 billion to $29 billion annually.

Support Personnel

Health services clerks or office managers may have the duties of receptionist, accountant, and assistant. The clerk or manager is responsible for the smooth operation of the services. The clerk must be dependable and take initiative in making sure the office runs well. It is important that the office personnel arrive on time and give the impression of being ready to give eager and efficient care. The clerk working in a private office locates and organizes the charts of patients who are expected to visit that day.

Hospital registration staff record and manage the admission of patients. Admission staffs convey the first impression of the facility. The admitting clerk should be calm, patient, pleasant, and efficient. Duties of the admissions clerk include preregistration interviewing; verifying insurance; arranging transportation; and, in some instances, assigning beds for the hospital stay (see Appendix II, Fig. II-6, Preadmission Form, p. 593). To complete insurance forms, the clerk must first verify the type of insurance and obtain the correct form (see Appendix II, Fig. II-7, p. 594). The clerk may complete some information by using

TABLE 33-2
The Joint Commission's Official "Do Not Use" List[1]

Do Not Use	Potential Problem	Use Instead
U (unit)	Mistaken for "0" (zero), the number "4" (four) or "cc"	Write "unit"
IU (International Unit)	Mistaken for IV (intravenous) or the number 10 (ten)	Write "International Unit"
Q.D., QD, q.d., qd (daily)	Mistaken for each other	Write "daily"
Q.O.D., QOD, q.o.d, qod (every other day)	Period after the Q mistaken for "I" and the "O" mistaken for "I"	Write "every other day"
Trailing zero (X.0 mg)*	Decimal point is missed	Write X mg
Lack of leading zero (.X mg)		Write 0.X mg
MS	Can mean morphine sulfate or magnesium sulfate	Write "morphine sulfate" or "magnesium sulfate"
MSO4 and MgSO4	Confused for one another	

[1]Applies to all orders and all medication-related documentation that is handwritten (including free-text computer entry) or on preprinted forms.
*Exception: A "trailing zero" may be used only where required to demonstrate the level of precision of the value being reported, such as for laboratory results, imaging studies that report size of lesions, or catheter and tube sizes. It may not be used in medication orders or other medication-related documentation.

information contained in the patient's record. Signatures of the patient and spouse, if any, are necessary to authorize release of medical information during care. The forms must be completed accurately because the code used for reimbursement for services is determined in part by use of the insurance forms. (See Skill List 33-1, Assisting the Patient with Insurance Forms, pp. 538–539.) Clerks may also assist with completion of forms for death and birth records. Most clerks learn their responsibilities on the job, but managers usually have a college degree in a health-related field.

CASE STUDY 33-1 You are given a list of patients to call to let them know their lab results are negative. You are told to leave a message if possible. What should you say?

Answers to Case Studies are available on the Evolve website: ***http://evolve.elsevier.com/Gerdin***

The medical secretary is employed by institutions and private facilities, such as a doctor's office, to assist in administration of services. Duties of the medical secretary include taking **dictation**, using transcription skills to compile reports and charts, assisting the physician with medical reports, articles, and conference proceedings, and preparing correspondence (Fig. 33-2). (See Skill List 33-2, Preparing a Business Letter, p. 539.) For this occupation, knowledge of medical terminology supplements the associate degree or vocational training of a general secretary. Secretaries also may file records by using a variety of systems that may be narrative or numerical. The charts may be cross-referenced and marked with a locator card when removed to ensure easy retrieval. If the secretary is also responsible for keeping the budget records, a fee schedule must be established. Although the American Medical Association provides the Current Procedure Terminology code, which gives a schedule for fees for services, the practitioner may have one that differs. The federal government has a system of determining payment for services on the basis of time, skill, expenses of maintaining a practice, and malpractice costs. This system is called the *resource-based relative value scale* and is replacing the usual, **reasonable**, and **customary** practices of the past. All patients are given a receipt for payment if cash or a check is used for payment. Bills are then issued each month for patients with outstanding debt to the practitioner (Fig. 33-3).

The health unit coordinator performs nonclinical activities for the nursing unit. Nonclinical activities are those that do not involve direct contact with the patient. The coordinator's duties include assembling and maintaining patient charts, transcribing physician's orders, and acting as receptionist and secretary on the unit. Part of maintaining the chart includes determining if any part of the chart is missing. The person responsible for that part of the chart is then

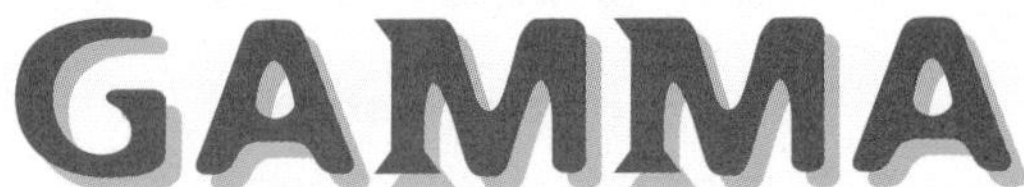

A DIVISION OF THE MERCY HOSPITAL SYSTEM

February 19, 2010

Ms. Miller
Nursing Coordinator
Horizon Medical Center
11204 Sunset Drive
St. Louis, MO 63179

Dear Ms. Miller:
Reference Line (if any)

Body of Letter

Closing,

Susan Williams
Director of Radiology

enclosure

FIGURE 33-2 Business correspondence reflects the relationship of the health care worker with the patient.

notified to correct the **deficiency**. Health unit coordinator and management certification is available on completion of a 2-year college program. The health unit manager coordinates the nonclinical activities for several units. The duties of the manager include establishing policies and procedures for unit coordinators, managing personnel, and preparing the budget.

Medical Records Personnel

Medical records personnel organize, analyze, and generate data relating to patient records. The greatest use of medical records personnel is in hospitals, although other employment opportunities are available in medical offices and health maintenance organizations. Medical records and health information technicians are projected by the U.S. Department of Labor to be one of the fastest growing occupations through 2010.

Registered records administrators (RRAs) or Health Information Managers are responsible for management of the information system. They create policies and procedures to ensure adequate departmental efficiency. Additionally, the RRA may be responsible for employee evaluation and budget preparation. Education for the RRA is a 2-year college certificate or 4-year college or university degree. Supervised clinical experience is required in an accredited program. In 1991 the American Medical Records Association became the American Health Information Management Association.

The Commission on Accreditation of Allied Health Education Programs has accredited 184 programs for

45-613 Eye-Ease®
45-713 20/20 Buff
Made in USA

Daily Record of Charges and receipts
July 18, 2010

Patient	Charges / Adjustments	Receipts: Cash	Receipts: Check	Memo of Charges by type of Service rendered: office visit	Lab	X-ray	Ecg	Medication	Non-Office visit	Receipt. No.
Brown, John	35.00		35.00	35.00						1051
Black, James	122.00		50.00	40.00	42.00	40.00				1052
Doe, Jane.	75.00			35.00			40.00			
Smith, Robert	35.00		35.00		20.00			15.00		1053
Goode, Alice	35.00	35.00		35.00						1054
Jones, Mary	98.00			30.00		50.00		18.00		
Small, Joseph	40.00	20.00					40.00			1055
Biggs, Barney (home)	45.00								45.00	
Mail										
White, Willie			45.00							
Green, Gordon			55.00							
Blue Shield (Check totalling $ 113.38										
Sampson, Sam			43.88							
Vinson, Vera	<10.50>		69.50		<10.50>					
Medicare (Check totalling $ 100.05										
Grey, Gertrude	<12.25>		47.75			<12.25>				
Reddy, Ruth	<17.70>		52.30	<5.50>			<12.20>			
Totals for the day	444.55	55.00	433.43	169.50	51.50	77.75	67.80	33.00	45.00	

FIGURE 33-3 Records for charges and payments are used to provide accurate billing. (From Cooper MG, Cooper DE, Burrows NJ: *The medical assistant*, ed 6, St. Louis, 1993, Mosby.)

CASE STUDY 33-2 Your patient asks to have his medical records because he is unhappy with his treatment. What should you say?

Answers to Case Studies are available on the Evolve website: ***http://evolve.elsevier.com/Gerdin***

health information technicians. The registered health information technician may also specialize in coding by completing a voluntary certification program. The accredited record technician performs the technical functions of medical records maintenance. This includes organizing, analyzing, and evaluating records, using established standards under the direction of an RRA. In a small facility the records technician may have the full responsibility of the medical records department. Health information technicians may be educated in a 2-year program or through an independent study program offered by the American Health Information Management Association. Completed over 3 years, the independent study program must include supervised clinical experience.

The medical transcriptionist, also called *medical stenographer*, listens to and types information to provide a permanent record from a variety of audio equipment. Most health care providers use digital or analog dictating equipment. However, the use of the Internet and speech-recognition software has provided quicker return of documents. Knowledge of medical terminology and computer skills such as keyboarding and word processing are required for accurate transcription of the records. Additionally, the medical records clerk must evaluate the records for completeness and accuracy. Medical records clerks or transcriptionists may sometimes learn on the job because the duties performed are limited in number. Associate degree programs in transcription are offered through some community colleges and vocational programs. Certification is voluntary and provided through the American Association for Medical Transcription. Medical transcription employment opportunities are projected to grow faster than average through 2010. This field may provide flexibility in the hours worked or employment from home.

Health Information and Communication

One of the fastest growing fields in the health care industry is the management of information.

Communication of health-related information is the function of several disciplines, including health science librarians, educators, in-service personnel, public relations personnel, biomedical photographers, illustrators, and writers.

Health science librarians provide access to information by practicing professionals, researchers, and students. The librarian locates information in journals, books, computer resources, and audiovisual media. Librarians may also be responsible for planning, budgeting, and purchasing the resources. Librarians must have good organizational and communication skills to store the information logically and to teach others how to locate desired information. Specialties in health library science include reference, collection development, acquisitions (purchasing), serials (periodicals), and education. Other librarians may function as catalogers, audiovisual technicians, or medical historians. Clinical librarians may accompany the physician on hospital rounds to assess information needs of specific patients. The minimum level of education for health science librarians is a master's degree. Certification is available and must be maintained through a yearly examination.

Educators teach new and experienced health personnel at all employment levels. Health educators may specialize in fields of practice such as personal, community, consumer, environmental, or public health. Most public schools require standard teacher certification, which includes a bachelor's degree in education, for employment as a health educator. A master's degree is required for many positions.

CASE STUDY 33-3 You are asked to pay for a background check before applying for a job. What should you say?

Answers to Case Studies are available on the Evolve website: ***http://evolve.elsevier.com/Gerdin***

Public health educators plan, organize, and direct health education programs for group and community needs. They determine and set goals for the health needs of the community. They prepare and distribute teaching materials in schools, industries, and community agencies. Public health educators may have a bachelor's or master's degree.

Public health educators may work with community health providers to design ways to increase the use of public health resources. The health educator may be responsible for orientation of new employees of the public health department, as well as for educational programs to inform personnel of new developments in the health field. Public health educators may be responsible for development of brochures, pamphlets, and other teaching materials for educating the community.

Public relations representatives plan and conduct programs to create a favorable image of the agency. Public relations includes sending press releases to news media and planning new advertising strategies. Minimal educational requirements include a bachelor's degree in public relations. The education for public relations provides skills in journalism and public speaking. Public relations specialists often work long and irregular hours to be available when special events occur. Media relations and marketing may be part of public relations services.

Biological photographers document life-related health events with a variety of production equipment. This may include producing slides, photographs, prints, transparencies, videotapes, and computer graphics. Photomicrography is taking photographs through a microscope. Electron microscopy can record images without the use of light. Biophotographers often specialize in one area such as animal, plant, or surgical photography. The education is usually 2 to 4 years of college for training in photography and basic sciences, especially biology. Certification and registration are available through the Biological Photographers Association.

Medical illustrators are specialized artists who use a variety of visual materials to communicate vital information regarding the biosciences. Illustrators provide sketches, paintings, drawings, computer images, and three-dimensional models. Advanced functions of medical illustrators include production of instructional models of artificial body parts. Medical illustrators must be talented artists with education in anatomy, art, and general medicine. The five accredited schools available for this area of specialization require applicants to have a bachelor's degree for admission.

Medical writers create and edit technical material for educational and marketing materials. Individuals with a master's degree are preferred for employment as medical writers. Doctoral-level education in health science and related writing areas is available. Many medical writers first enter the health professions as technicians, scientists, or engineers in an area of interest. Job opportunities for the medical writer are available in universities and private industries such as pharmaceutical companies.

Public health statisticians gather, analyze, and present public health data used to uncover trends in health and in the causes of disease. Statisticians may be employed by voluntary organizations, government, or health departments to plan health care services. A doctorate in public health, which includes biostatistics training, is necessary for this profession.

Content Instruction

Office Management

Orderliness of equipment and supplies used in the work area provides a secure environment for maintaining the confidentiality of patient records. Various systems may be used to record appointments and billing information. This information may be kept in written form or stored in computerized systems. Filing may be numeric, alphabetical, or both (Fig. 33-4). Cross-referencing of records in several locations may be necessary for prompt retrieval. Any filing system must be up to date to be useful. (See Skill List 33-3, Filing Forms, p. 539.)

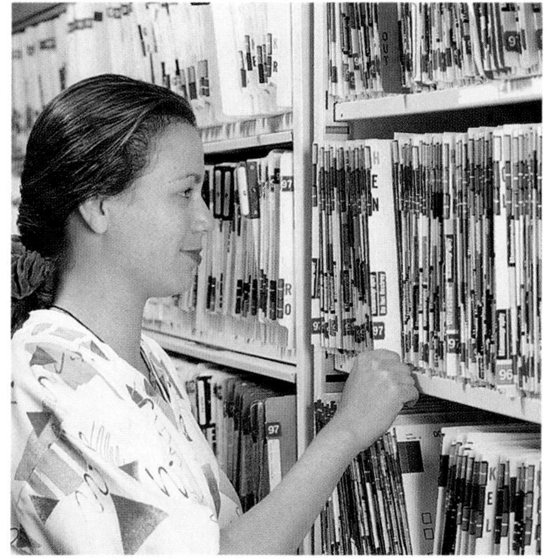

FIGURE 33-4 Many different filing systems work well if items are filed promptly and in the correct location. (From Kinn ME, Woods M: *The medical assistant*, ed 8, Philadelphia, 1999, Saunders.)

CASE STUDY 33-4 Your employer e-mails the surgery schedule that includes the patient names and procedures to everyone on staff. What should you do?

Answers to Case Studies are available on the Evolve website: ***http://evolve.elsevier.com/Gerdin***

Most agencies maintain an appointment procedure that includes a card given to the patient, a confirmation telephone call, and a daily log (Fig. 33-5). Records of daily appointments usually cover at least 1 year to enable planning in advance. Appointment records are often written in pencil so that they can be erased in the case of a cancellation. Patients who are kept waiting because of overbooking or errors in scheduling appointments may become dissatisfied with the service. Some facilities charge patients a percentage of the fee if they miss appointments or fail to provide advance notice (no-show). The patient must be made aware of such a policy before the appointment date. When making an appointment, the clerk records information such as the date, time, and purpose of the visit, as well as the referring individual, if any. Many offices call the individual to confirm the appointment 1 or 2 days before the scheduled date. (See Skill List 33-4, Scheduling an Appointment, p. 540.)

Jonesville Medical Center

John Jones, MD
1000 Center Street
Jonesville, ST 22222

❖ ❖ ❖

Your next appointment is:

________________ at ____________ o'clock

Please notify the office at least 24 hours in advance if you are unable to keep the appointment.

FIGURE 33-5 After the necessary information is gathered, some offices provide the patient with a card as a reminder of the next visit.

In addition to scheduling appointments, the clerk or office manager is responsible for scheduling laboratory tests and other procedures. The patient must be consulted regarding convenient locations and times of additional appointments. The clerk should also inform the patient of the approximate time necessary for the testing and when the results will be available. The clerk can help ensure the best possible care for patients who are sent to other agencies by properly planning the visit and by maintaining a positive relationship with the other agency's personnel.

Records Management

Many forms are used to provide information about the health care patient. When placed in a folder or

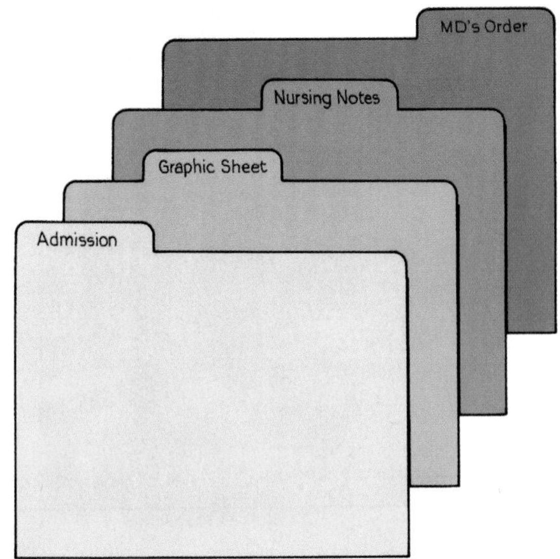

FIGURE 33-6 The medical record may be made up of several different forms, and the types of forms may vary according to the care needed.

notebook, the information is considered to be the chart, or medical record (Fig. 33-6). In many facilities, the chart is kept electronically using computers.

If the patient is able to understand and complete the forms without assistance, he or she may do so. The clerk or health care worker may complete some forms during an interview or when the care is given. Minors may not give legal consent for treatment except in special situations determined by the laws of the state. The clerk must explain all forms regarding payment, release of information, and other nonmedical concerns to the patient in a way that can be easily understood. (See Skill List 33-5, Completion of Forms by the Patient, p. 540.)

Records management is the responsibility of each health care worker. The medical record for a patient is used in all aspects of health care. The chart contains the medical history and physical assessment, test results, surgery reports, and notes about the patient's condition and course of treatment (Box 33-3). Any form that is part of the chart is important because it contains information necessary to provide the best care possible. Not all charts contain all possible forms. Outpatient, obstetric, and other specialized charts may vary. The chart is considered the legal record, and information on the chart is considered confidential. Confidential information may not be given to anyone other than those authorized by the patient and health care practitioner managing the care. With authorization, information from the medical record may be used for billing, education, planning, and research.

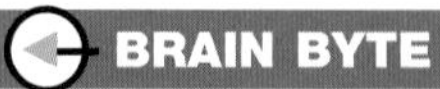

E-mail to or about a patient is a part of the electronic health record.

Records must be accurate, legible, complete, and organized to provide efficient care (Box 33-4). Some medical information may be assembled in verbal form by using medical transcription dictation and speech recognition equipment and software. The oral record must be **transcribed** or written in permanent form to become part of the legal record. The dictating practitioner should ensure accuracy by checking the record that is transcribed from verbal information. Information that a clerk transcribes or copies from one written record to another is checked by authorized personnel.

Methods of Payment

In the United States more than a billion dollars a day is spent on health care. Health care costs account for more than one tenth of the national economy. Methods of payment for health costs have changed with growth of the industry. Payment may be made on a fee-for-service basis or through a prepaid benefit package. Fee-for-service payment requires that money be received at the time of service. A prepaid benefit package may be obtained through insurance or a health maintenance organization. The fee for services in a prepaid system is not based on the type of treatment.

Insurance is payment in advance for services in the event that they are necessary. Insurance may be obtained through groups, privately, or from government benefits (Table 33-3). Group insurance benefits may be obtained through benefit programs arranged by the employing agency. Private insurance packages are obtained from the insurance company directly. In the United States the federal Medicare and Medicaid programs provide health insurance for many individuals. State laws vary, but all provide worker's compensation and disability programs.

An insurance company may not pay a certain part of the cost of treatment as a condition of its terms. The amount that must be paid by the patient before the insurance company begins to pay is called the

BOX 33-3

Inpatient Chart Order

1. Fact sheet (information sheet)
2. Diagnosis-related group (DRG) worksheet
3. Emergency room record
   a. Paramedic transport record
   b. Nursing notes
4. Death
   a. Autopsy report
   b. Autopsy release
   c. Release of body
5. Discharge summary (typed)
6. History and physical (typed)
7. Consultation(s) (typed)
8. Physician orders
9. Progress notes
10. Dialysis progress notes
11. Operative procedures
    a. Consent for procedure
    b. Consent for transfusion
    c. Preoperative checklist
    d. Operative record
    e. Anesthesia record
    f. Operative report (typed)
    g. Postanesthesia record
    h. Pathology report(s)
12. Outside laboratory report(s)
13. Laboratory reports (computerized)
14. Radiograph
15. Electrocardiogram
16. Holter monitor echo report
17. Nutritional progress notes
18. Social service notes
19. Respiratory therapy
    a. Progress notes
    b. Continuous therapy notes
    c. Arterial blood gases
    d. Pulmonary function report
    e. Ventilator flow sheet
20. Physical therapy
    a. Continuous therapy notes
21. Speech therapy
22. Graphic record
23. Medication sheets
24. Intravenous flow
25. Intake and output sheet
26. Cardiac arrest sheet
27. Nursing Kardex care plan
28. Nursing Kardex treatments
29. Nursing assessment sheet
30. Nursing flow sheet
31. Diabetic flow sheet
32. Nurses notes
33. Miscellaneous
    a. Consents
    b. Releases
    c. Transfers
    d. Records from other facilities
34. Discharge instruction sheet

deductible. Some insurance packages require that a percentage of each transaction be paid by the insured (copayment). Individuals may have coverage from more than one insurance program. Without insurance, the patient is responsible for full payment of the cost of care. Inability to pay may lead health care workers to refuse uninsured, nonemergency treatment and to offer less than optimal health care.

Not all procedures and treatments are covered by insurance companies. Billing codes are used to designate the type of treatment and to determine whether coverage is allowed. Diagnostic-related groupings have been established by the federal government to determine a usual, reasonable, and customary fee for services for Medicare recipients. Many insurance companies use this fee structure to determine the allowable payment. Health care providers in private practice and other agencies may establish a different fee schedule for services.

Performance Instruction

All patients who visit the health care facility are greeted by name and asked to log in their time of arrival (Fig. 33-7). Some patients may need help with completion of the forms necessary for care. If it is the first visit, the clerk or receptionist may make the patient feel more comfortable by introducing the practitioner.

The clerk or receptionist uses the telephone to obtain and give information to patients and other

BOX 33-4

Guidelines for Charting*

1. Print in black ink.
2. All entries must be timed, dated, and signed.
3. Charts should be done in sequential, consecutive order.
4. Leave no blanks between notes or at the end of a line.
   Correct: 9:30 AM c/o pain rt hand, rt leg. Able to sit up in bed unassisted. J. Smith, SNA
5. Chart in accurate, clear, and brief manner. Avoid unnecessary words such as *and*, *the*, and *a*.
6. Use only standard abbreviations. Refer to The Joint Commission's Official "Do Not Use" List (see Table 34-2) for abbreviations to avoid.
7. Use the patient as the subject of each statement. The word *patient* is assumed, not written.
8. Be objective, not subjective. Record information and treatments that can be seen, heard, felt, smelled, or measured.
9. Avoid words that interpret or make judgments, such as *seems*, *appears*, and *normal*.
   Incorrect: 9:50 AM Appears to be in pain when moving.
   Correct: 9:50 AM Facial grimace and wincing noted on movement.
10. Document each treatment and activity, even if it is part of routine care.
   Correct: 9:55 AM Side rails up.
11. Use a direct quote to express the patient's reaction to care.
12. Sign each note at the time it is written, using first initial, last name, and professional designation.
   Correct: J. Smith, SNA
13. Correct errors by making one line through the mistake, writing "ERROR" above it. Initial the change.
   ERROR *JS*
   Correct: 10:00 AM c/o pain rt ~~forearm~~ wrist.
14. Do not write above or below the line to insert a forgotten word.
   Incorrect: 10:10 AM Urine clear, ^small amount. Stool ... *yellow*
15. Record that unusual treatments or activities were reported to supervising personnel.
   Correct: 10:15 AM c/o severe pain rt elbow. Team leader notified.
16. Do not chart activities and treatments performed by other health personnel.

*The chart is the medical and legal record of health care. Legally, services not charted were not performed.

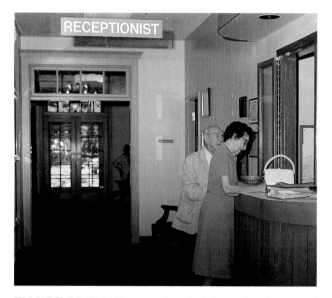

FIGURE 33-7 At the reception desk the patient is greeted and asked to sign the log.

health care professionals. Good communication skills are necessary to perform these duties well (Fig. 33-8). Some people may not welcome information regarding billing, records, and scheduling, so the health services clerk must be able to work well with various and sometimes difficult personalities. Courtesy and efficiency are necessary at all times regardless of the responses of others. The importance of the call must be determined by the clerk to decide whether it is an emergency or routine call. Good communication skills include stating the name of the facility and personal title when answering the call, as well as speaking slowly and clearly. All information gathered should be repeated to ensure accuracy. Information received and given during telephone calls is always confidential. A well-timed and caring sense of humor may be helpful in dealing with difficult telephone conversations.

TABLE 33-3
Types of Health Insurance

Type	Description
Group or private	Open to company employees and their dependents; coverage usually includes medical and hospital care; may require deductible or copayment
Blue Cross and Blue Shield	Open to employees of prepaid companies or to individuals at higher rate; may require deductible or copayment; in some states, Blue Cross and Blue Shield are separate agencies
Medicare	Federal program through Social Security Act to provide health care to those older than 65 years of age; provides specified fee for services; may require deductible
Medicaid	State program to supplement Social Security Act to provide health care to those who cannot afford it; eligibility varies state to state; usually no deductible but varies with coverage
Worker's compensation	Required in all states to provide insurance for employees injured on the job; not all doctors accept worker's compensation, but those who do must register each year; coverage includes all services necessary to treat industrial injury; no deductible or copayment
CHAMPUS*	A cost-sharing program in which federal government pays part of charges; remainder paid by recipient of the care; provides benefits for those in the uniformed services and their dependents

*Civilian Health and Medical Program of the Uniformed Services.

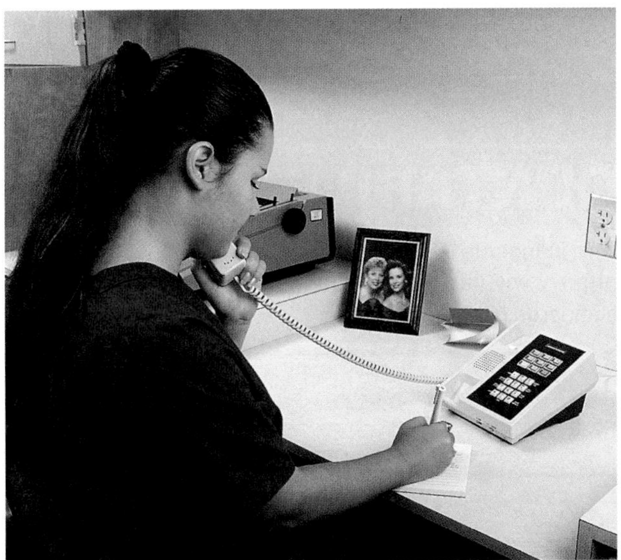

FIGURE 33-8 The foundation of good telephone etiquette is built on courtesy, accuracy, and thoroughness.

Summary

- The role of the health information and administration health care team is to manage the budget and maintain patient records. Health information administrators manage personnel by hiring and training workers.
- Three personal characteristics of an efficient clerk are the ability to work with varied personalities, courtesy, and efficiency.
- Five forms used on the medical record include the admission report, graphic sheet, nursing record, laboratory report, and physician orders.
- Three methods of payment for health care include fee-for-service, individual, and group insurance.

Review Questions

1. Describe the role of health information and administrative health care workers.
2. List at least five occupations in health information and administrative health care and include the personal qualities, levels of education, and credentialing requirements for these workers.
3. List five forms that make up part of the medical record.
4. Describe three methods used to pay for health care services.
5. Define insurance and the possible consequences of lacking adequate insurance and the inability to pay for health care services.
6. Describe the funding structure relating to diagnostic-related groupings.

7. List five rules for maintaining an accurate medical record.
8. Choose one career from Box 33-1. Research the cost of education and annual earnings in local institutions. Write a paragraph describing the factors that might explain why the local and national economic figures vary.
9. Use each of the following terms in one or more sentences that correctly relate their meaning: benefit, customary, insurance, and reasonable fee.

Critical Thinking

1. Investigate and compare the cost of education for at least three of the health care information and administrative health care workers.
2. Establish and maintain a filing system for classroom notes or club activities.
3. Use the Internet to research the ORYX rating of a local hospital or health care facility. Describe the quality of care provided by the information.
4. Investigate the requirement of preemployment background checks by a local health care facility.
5. Create a career ladder for health information and administration careers. Describe why it is or is not possible to move from one level to another in the field.

Explore the Web

Career Information

Bureau of Labor Statistics
http://www.bls.gov/

Salary.com
http://salary.com

Professional Associations

Joint Commission Quality Check
http://www.qualitycheck.org/consumer/searchQCR.aspx

National Association Medical Staff Services (NAMSS)
http://www.namss.org/

American Health Information Management Association (AHIMA)
http://www.ahima.org

STANDARDS AND ACCOUNTABILITY

See Evolve website: National Consortium on Health Science and Technology Education, National Health Science Career Cluster Models, Health Informatics Pathway Standards & Accountability Criteria; also available at http://www.healthscienceconsortium.org/healthcare_standards.php.

SKILL LIST 33-1 Assisting the Patient with Insurance Forms

1. Gather all equipment and supplies, including the correct form and a pen. A clipboard may be used to provide a writing surface if desired.
2. Obtain the correct form for the patient's insurance coverage. The format of forms may differ, although the information required is fairly consistent.
3. Copy available information from the patient's registration slip and insurance identification card neatly and accurately. Follow the order described on the form. The patient who is not required to complete the same information more than once will be impressed by your competence and courtesy.

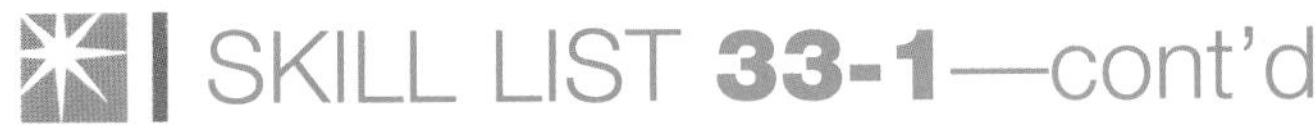

SKILL LIST 33-1—cont'd
Assisting the Patient with Insurance Forms

4. Interview the patient for any corrections and missing information in the following categories:
   Insured: The patient's policy information or relationship to the insured is required.
   Other insurance: Some coverage may be excluded or added if the patient or patient's spouse has an additional policy.
   Signatures: The patient's (and spouse's) signature is required to authorize the release of medical information as needed during care.
   Medical information: The nature of the complaint (signs and symptoms), length of duration, first time of treatment, history of prior illnesses and injuries, and care provider identification number are noted.
   Coding of treatment: Correct codes for the diagnosis and treatment determine the billing and must be completed carefully.
   Financial agreement: The method of payment for services excluded in the insurance coverage must be designated in the record of patient care.
5. Verify all information before completing the interview.
6. The care provider's identification information may be completed by the assistant but requires the signature of the professional.

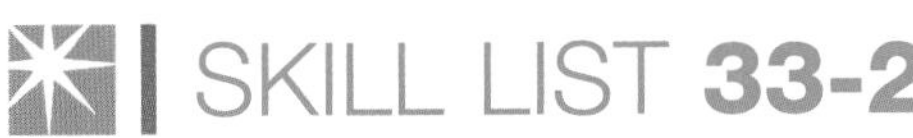

SKILL LIST 33-2
Preparing a Business Letter

1. Select the appropriate stationery for the letter required. The letter must be correct in content and uniformly displayed to look professional. Paper that is 8½ × 11 inches is standard for business letters.
2. Type the letter following the format preferred by the health care professional. Although there may be more than one acceptable letter format, a professional appearance includes the addressee information, date, salutation, body, closing, signature, and enclosures when needed.
3. Proofread the letter for accuracy and format.
4. Address an envelope to accompany the letter.

SKILL LIST 33-3
Filing Forms

1. Establish a filing system by alphabetic or numeric order. Files should be maintained so that an item can be found immediately.
2. File items immediately after use. Filing trays may be necessary if time does not permit immediate placement in files, but they should be emptied daily.
3. Place an "out" card (or placeholder) in the location of a file that is removed from the system. Another employee may seek the chart and waste time looking if it has been removed.
4. Establish rules for filing and cross-referencing files. All employees should use the same rules and system for locating and placing files.

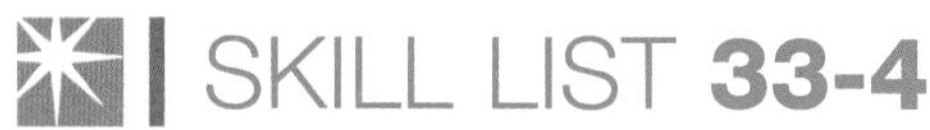

SKILL LIST 33-4 Scheduling an Appointment

1. Obtain and write down all pertinent information when the appointment is made, including the full name; address; telephone number; purpose of the visit; and referring person, if any.
2. Assign the earliest time available that meets the patient's needs. Schedules should be realistic for needed services and should allow for emergency treatment.
3. Enter the required information, including the time and the patient's full name, telephone number, and reason for visit in the appointment book in pencil. Using pencil permits appointments to be changed neatly if conflicts occur.
4. Prepare an appointment card to be given or sent to the patient. A visual reminder may ensure that the patient does not make a conflicting appointment.
5. Call the patient to confirm the appointment 1 or 2 days before it is scheduled. Confirming appointments helps ensure that both the patient and health care practitioner keep to the schedule.

SKILL LIST 33-5 Completion of Forms by the Patient

1. Seat the patient in a comfortable chair away from distractions. Patient records should be kept confidential.
2. Ask the patient about each item on the form. Explain any items that are unclear. Terminology that is common to health care personnel may not be understood by the patient.
3. Allow the patient to answer completely. Information that is not immediately familiar may require time for recall.
4. Verify insurance coverage and expiration date by checking the insurer's card.
5. Obtain the patient's signature to guarantee payment by an insurance program or by the patient. Insurance providers will not supply information or payment without a release signature from the patient.
6. Code forms with the appropriate payment number for billing. The coding may determine the amount, promptness, and acceptability of the coverage.
7. Terminate the interview by informing the patient how, when, and by whom the service will be rendered.

CHAPTER 34

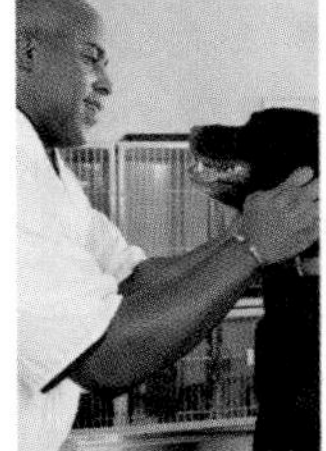

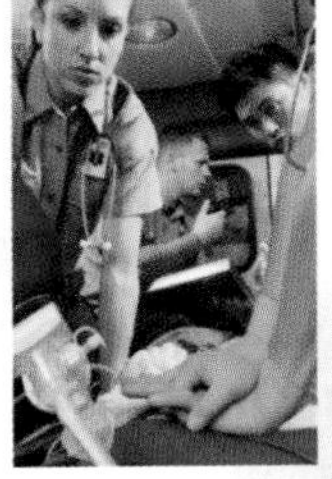

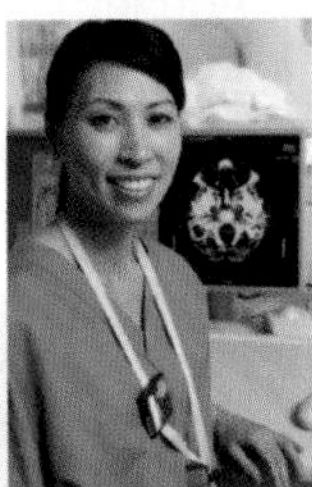

Environmental Careers

LEARNING OBJECTIVES

- Define at least eight terms relating to environmental health care.
- Describe the function of the environmental health care team.
- Specify the role of the environmental health care team members, including personal qualities, educational requirements, responsibilities, and credentialing requirements.
- Identify at least five areas of pollution control that are monitored and regulated by environmental health services.
- List at least five health conditions that are affected by environmental pollution.
- Describe the natural recycling process or chain of life in an ecosystem.

KEY TERMS

Biosphere *(BIE-us-fere)* Part of the universe, including the air (atmosphere), earth (lithosphere), and water (hydrosphere), in which living organisms exist

Decibel *(DES-ih-bul)* Unit used to express ratio of power between two sounds

Ecosystem *(EE-ko-sis-tum)* Living organisms and nonliving elements interacting in a specific area

Hydrocarbon *(HIE-dro-kar-bun)* Organic compound made of hydrogen and carbon only

Mutagen *(MYOO-tuh-jen)* Physical or chemical agent that induces genetic mutation or change

Particulate *(par-TIK-yoo-lut)* Composed of separate particles or pieces

Pesticide *(PES-tih-side)* Poison used to destroy pests of any kind

Pollution *(puh-LOO-shun)* Condition of being defiled or impure

Environmental Terminology*

Term	Definition	Prefix	Root	Suffix
Aquatic	Pertaining to the ocean		aquat	ic
Asepsis	Pertaining to absence of pathogens	a	sep/s	is
Biomedical	Pertaining to medicine and life	bio	medic	al
Biosphere	Pertaining to the earth and air	bio	sphere	
Ecology	Study of environment		ec	ology
Hydrocarbon	Pertaining to hydrogen and carbon	hydro	carbon	
Hydrosphere	Pertaining to water	hydro	sphere	
Lithosphere	Pertaining to the earth and rock	lith/o	sphere	
Mutagen	Originating mutation	muta	gen	
Ultrasonic	Pertaining to sound beyond the range (of human hearing)	ultra	son	ic

*A transition syllable or vowel may be added to or deleted from the word parts to make the combining form.

Abbreviations for Environmental Careers

Abbreviation	Meaning
CBET	Certified biomedical equipment technician
CLES	Clinical laboratory equipment specialist
CRES	Certified radiological equipment specialist
CO	Carbon monoxide
CST	Certified surgical technologist
dB	Decibel
EMF	Electromagnetic field
EPA	Environmental Protection Agency
ORT	Operating room technologist
pH	Potential or partial concentration of hydrogen ions

Careers

Environmental careers create a supportive environment for the patient. Support services or ancillary health workers are necessary in all aspects of health care (Table 34-1). Most ancillary workers are not seen by the person receiving the service (Box 34-1). Many of the assistant-level environmental workers provide care in other career areas by maintaining the equipment and supplies necessary for optimal care. In addition to the specific skills and knowledge necessary in each specialty area, ancillary workers must know basic medical terminology and principles of asepsis.

Nutrition Services

Dietitians provide nutritional counseling and services in a variety of settings. They supervise food operations to meet the patients' needs and provide counseling on nutrition. Dietitians manage the nutritional services of the health care system. The goals of the dietitian include promotion and maintenance of health, prevention and treatment of illness, and assistance in rehabilitation through nutritional education and diet. Dietitians may specialize in clinical, community, management, business, education, or consulting services. Dietitians must successfully complete a minimum of 4 years in a bachelor's degree program in dietetics, nutrition, or food systems management. Part of the dietitian program includes an internship in the health care industry. A master's or doctoral degree is preferred in many employment opportunities. Registration is available after successful completion of an accredited program and examination.

Dietary technicians complete a 2-year associate degree program. They plan menus and supervise the production of food. Food service workers or dietary assistants prepare and deliver the meal trays to patients or prepare the dining area (Fig. 34-1). They may also help the patient select a menu and process the order. Food service workers may prepare food and beverages. Collecting the empty meal trays and washing the dishes are also duties of the food service worker. On-the-job training is available for some of the entry-level dietary positions.

Dietitians are assisted by others in the facility to distribute meal requisitions to patients early in the day (Fig. 34-2). The type of meal plan is determined by the physician's order, preferences, and special

TABLE 34-1
Environmental Career Educational Cost and Earnings

Career	Educational Cost*	Earnings†
Dietitian	University of Kentucky, bachelor's degree, 128 credit hours Fees include: Tuition $4305/semester Fees $477/semester	Median annual salary: Lexington, Ky.—$51,110

*http://www.uky.edu/Registrar/feesgen.htm.
†http://data.bls.gov:8080/oes/datatype.do.

BOX 34-1

Environmental Health Careers

Dietetic consultant
Dietetic intern
Dietetic technician
Dietitian, chief
Dietitian, clinical
Dietitian, teaching
Ecologist
Food service worker
Food management aide
Health equipment servicer
Industrial hygienist
Industrial safety health teacher
Medical coordinator, pesticides
Microbiologist, public health
Pollution control engineer
Public health dentist
Public health educator
Public health service officer
Safety manager
Sanitarian
Sheltered works director

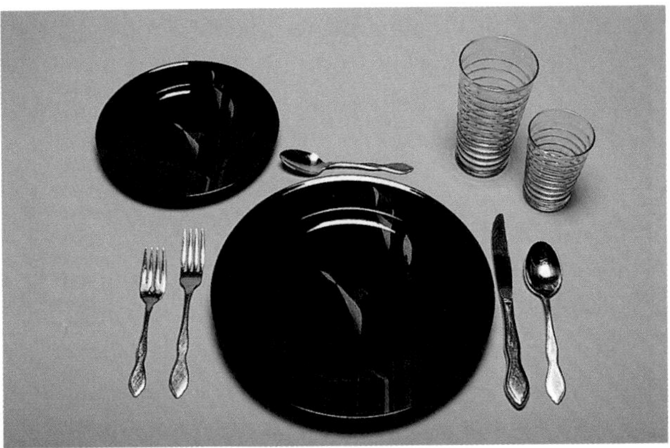

FIGURE 34-1 Using the proper place setting can make food more appealing to patients.

needs of the patient. When the diet menus are completed, they are collected, and the amount of food portions necessary to complete the meals may be determined and prepared. In some cases, the meals may be served using "a la carte" room service. Patients are allowed to request their meals and snacks from a personal diet menu at any time. (See Skill List 34-1, Planning Menus, and Skill List 34-2, Preparing the Dining Area, p. 555.)

Weight-reduction specialists counsel patients to lose weight using dietary and activity guidelines. These individuals may be called *nutritionists, dietary*

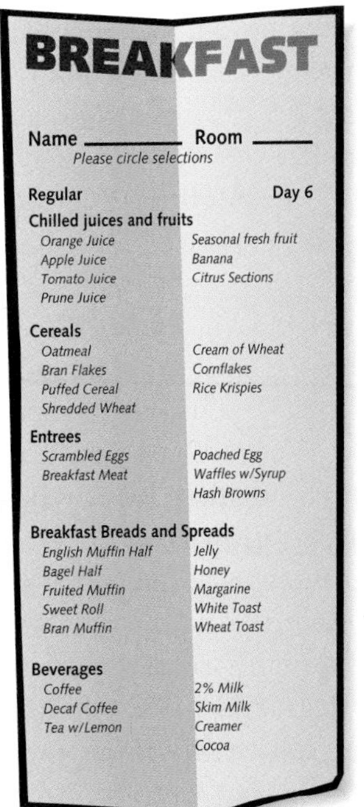

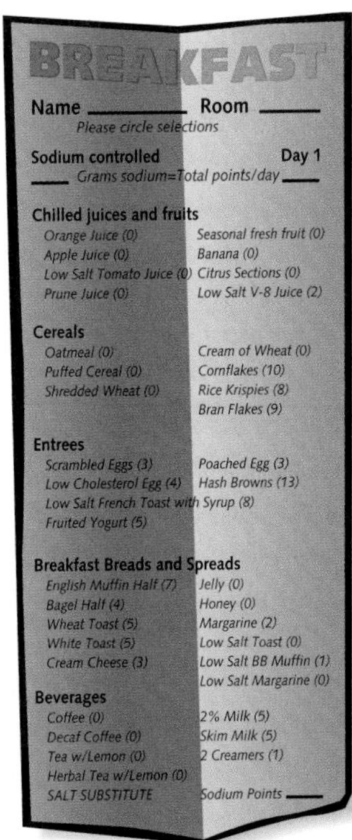

FIGURE 34-2 Planned meal requisitions allow a variety of food choices within the limits of the individual diet.

consultants, or *weight counselors*. The person giving weight-loss counseling must be outgoing, sincere, and patient. Weight-loss programs vary greatly, as do the qualifications of these specialists. Some weight-loss centers hire individuals who have gone through a weight-loss program and have had some training sponsored by the organization. Weight-loss specialists in private practice may be registered dietitians. Licensing for diet counselors is either in place or under consideration in 31 states.

The food scientist-technologist evaluates the safety of food processing and ingredients in the industry setting. This worker also develops new foods and new methods for producing known foods. Food scientist-technologists complete a minimum of 2 years of college. Bachelor's degrees are available in the area of food technology.

CASE STUDY 34-1 You are caring for a patient on a restricted diet for diabetes. You notice there is an empty candy wrapper in the trashcan after the family visits. What should you do?

Answers to Case Studies are available on the Evolve website: ***http://evolve.elsevier.com/Gerdin***

Environmental Control

The pollution control engineer analyzes contamination problems to establish methods and equipment to prevent pollution. Engineers review data from potential sources of contamination such as industrial plants. They calculate the pollutants being produced and may recommend denial of operating permits in plants that cause excessive amounts of pollution. A bachelor's degree is minimal for entry-level employment as a pollution control engineer.

The environmental engineer modifies facilities for environmental protection. The responsibilities include recommending methods for insect and rodent control and providing for safe disposal of radioactive waste materials. The environmental engineer researches factors concerning population growth, industrial planning, and natural environments. The duties of an environmental engineer include recommendation of equipment to meet the standards set by government agencies. A master's degree is recommended for entry-level employment as an environmental engineer.

Industrial hygienists conduct health programs in manufacturing plants and government agencies. Hygienists identify, control, and eliminate health hazards and diseases in the workplace. Responsibilities of an industrial hygienist include collection and analysis of dust, gases, and other possibly harmful substances. Consideration is given to ventilation, radiation, noise, exhaust, lighting, and other items that may affect the workers' health. Industrial hygienists prepare reports and recommend actions to eliminate potential hazards. Employment may be possible with a bachelor's degree, but master's-level preparation is preferred.

Safety engineers are employed in all work environments. They identify existing and potential hazards in conditions and practices. Additionally, safety engineers develop, implement, and evaluate methods to control hazards. Most safety engineers are employed by manufacturing, insurance, construction, or government agencies.

Health and regulatory inspectors enforce laws and regulations concerning employment hazards. Inspectors work for the local, state, or federal government. Health inspectors regulate consumer products such as food, drugs, and cosmetics. They also regulate quarantine for imported products and for people from other countries. Environmental health inspectors ensure that food, water, and air meet government standards. Health inspectors may specialize in such areas as dairy, food, waste, and air or in institutional or occupational health.

Radiation monitors, also called *health physics technicians*, test air, soil, water, floors, walls, and other areas of human contact for radiation. Most radiation monitors have at least 2 years of college education with a degree in nuclear technology. Most employers train radiation monitors on the job in the specific procedures used to detect radiation. Certification is available through the National Registry of Radiation Protection Technologists.

Ecologists analyze and regulate the quality of the environment as it is affected by living organisms. Some areas of specialization include air pollution analysis, water quality analysis, soil analysis, forest ecology, aquatic ecology, plant ecology, and animal ecology. Most ecologists work in the habitat to be studied, such as the forest, large city, ocean, and so forth. Ecologists earn a baccalaureate degree in one of the major sciences with emphasis on courses in the area of specialization. Most ecologists are employed by the government or private industry such as petrochemical companies.

Sanitarians plan, develop, and execute environmental health programs. Their work includes organizing waste disposal procedures for schools and

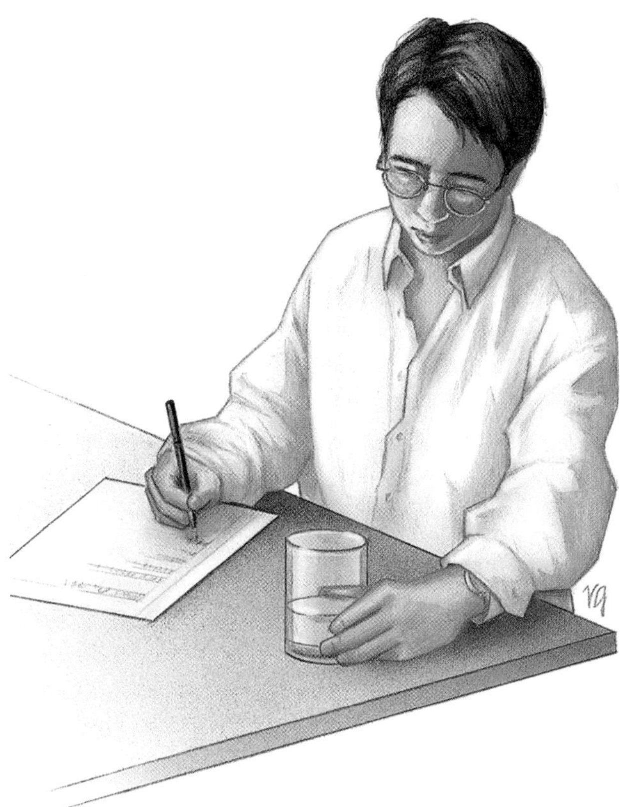

FIGURE 34-3 Water may be analyzed for its quality, bacterial content, or other pollutant content.

governments and for community, industrial, and private organizations. Sanitarians set and enforce standards concerning food, sewage, and waste disposal. Bachelor's preparation in environmental science is minimal for entry-level appointments. Advancement requires a master's degree in public health. Sanitation engineers may be educated in civil engineering.

Environmental health technicians collect and analyze air and water samples under the supervision of the sanitarian (Fig. 34-3). Training for the environmental health care technician is available in postsecondary vocational programs. Training may also be offered in the community college and result in an associate degree. Certification is available for the environmental health technician through the National Environmental Health Association. Environmental health assistants perform routine tasks under the supervision of the sanitarian. Environmental health assistants learn on the job.

Public health microbiologists conduct tests and study the relationship of people to organisms that cause pollution, disease, or epidemics to prevent the same problems in the future. Microbiologists in public health usually work for some level of government. Some examples of the work done by microbiologists include testing foods, monitoring the sludge from sewage treatment, and identifying organisms that cause widespread disease. Microbiologists must have at least a bachelor's degree in biological or life science. However, most microbiology study is completed on the graduate level. Some states require public health microbiologists to be licensed. Certification as a Specialist in Public Health may be granted by the Academy of Microbiology. (See Skill List 34-3, Using the Epidemiological Approach, p. 556.)

Other Support Service Personnel

Other support service personnel are found in all areas of the health care facility. Departments of support personnel include sterile supply, central service, biomedical engineering, laundry, security, and maintenance operations. Ancillary services also include grounds keeping, housekeeping, and other personnel necessary to run a large institution. Under the supervision of the infection-control nurse, housekeeping staff may be responsible for cleaning hospital units on a daily basis (concurrent) and terminal cleaning of all parts of the health care environment. Concurrent cleaning includes disinfecting contaminated objects and disposing of soiled articles used by an infected patient using a method that prevents the spread of the pathogen. On-the-job training is available for many entry-level support services positions.

Some 2-year colleges work in cooperation with local hospitals to offer a degree in biomedical equipment technology. On-the-job training may be possible in some areas. These biomedical equipment technicians work with the biomedical engineering staff to service and maintain equipment in the facility. Duties of the equipment technician include installing, calibrating, and inspecting and maintaining electrical, mechanical, hydraulic, and pneumatic equipment. The equipment includes electrocardiogram, blood gas analysis, radiologic, anesthetic, and other apparatus. Voluntary certification of technicians by the Society of Biomedical Equipment Technicians is available in three areas of specialization. Areas of certification are certified biomedical equipment technician, clinical laboratory equipment specialist, and certified radiologic equipment specialist.

The surgical technician, or operating room technologist (ORT), works under the direction of the surgeon. The duties of the ORT include maintaining

Health Careers in Practice

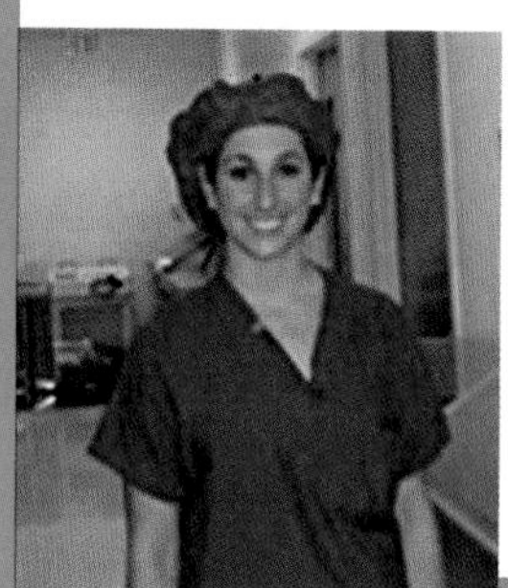

MELISSA SUBIC

CERTIFIED SURGICAL TECHNOLOGIST (CST)
BEAUMONT HOSPITAL

Educational background: Associate degree of applied science from Macomb Community College

A typical day at work and job duties include:

- When I arrive at work, I am assigned to an operating room. I then find out what surgeries are assigned to that room for the day.
- I then gather all the supplies and equipment needed in preparation for the surgery.
- I open the supplies in the operating room using aseptic technique.
- After the supplies are opened, I perform the surgical hand scrub and put on the sterile gown and gloves.
- I begin the set up of the sterile field and the back table, which consists of all surgical drapes, supplies, and instruments needed for the surgery.
- I count all items used in the surgery—such as sponges, needles, and instruments—with the circulator to ensure nothing will be left in the patient at the end of the case.
- When the patient comes into the operating room, I assist the surgeon with the application of the sterile drapes after the patient is put to sleep.
- During the surgery, I pass surgical instruments to the surgeon, monitor the sterile field, assist the surgeon with suctioning of blood and retracting of tissue, anticipate and obtain anything the surgeon may need during the surgery.

The most gratifying part of my job: My job is very exciting, never boring, and I know I potentially can help save a person's life. Also, it feels good to have the knowledge to do any surgical case that comes in and know I can help ensure that the surgeon has everything he or she needs to do the best possible job and to ensure a good patient outcome.

Continued

BRAIN BYTE

According to the Centers for Disease Control and Prevention (CDC), 46 million inpatient surgeries were performed in the United States in 2006.

the sterile field and passing instruments to the surgeon during an operation. The role may include cleaning and restocking the operating rooms. Knowledge of surgical procedures is necessary to anticipate the needs of the surgeon. Most ORTs complete a vocational or hospital-based training program lasting 9 to 12 months. In some states the ORT may serve as the circulator or primary nonsterile member of the surgical team. Certification is available through the Association of Surgical Technologists and may result in a higher salary for the certified surgical technologist.

CASE STUDY 34-2 You are caring for a patient who is scheduled for knee surgery. He points to his right knee when talking about it, but the chart refers to the left knee. What should you do?

Answers to Case Studies are available on the Evolve website: ***http://evolve.elsevier.com/Gerdin***

Central service or sterile supply technicians sterilize, assemble, clean, and store diagnostic and surgical equipment (Fig. 34-4). Training of central service technicians includes isolation, aseptic, and decontamination techniques. Training is available through vocational and 2-year college programs or on the job. (See Skill List 34-4, Housekeeping: General Rules, p. 556.)

The biggest challenge(s) I face in doing my job: Being able to use critical thinking skills in an emergency trauma or in stressful situations.

What drew me to my career? This career is very interesting and never boring because I am rarely doing the same thing. Also, I am always learning new things, and it is a very hands-on job.

Something I learned in my early education that I currently use in my career or that caused me to be interested in my career is: All the things I learned early in school are now applied to my job in different ways. Anatomy and physiology are extremely important. When you get into college, you are building on the things you learned in high school, and you always use anatomy and physiology in your job. Also, medical terminology and microbiology are important classes to know and understand. A class in health occupations in high school helps provide a basic understanding of certain things, such as sterile technique, from which to build skills.

Other comments: Becoming a surgical technologist has been convenient for me in terms of the way my program at Macomb Community College is set up in a clinical career ladder. In the first portion of the clinical ladder you are learning all the surgical instruments and how to reprocess them and also doing clinicals in a sterile processing department at a hospital. This semester really gives you the backbone of knowledge of instrument identification you need to work in the operating room. On completion of the first semester, I received a certificate as a central processing distribution technician. I was then able to get a job at a hospital in the sterile processing department. The next two semesters are surgical technology classes and clinicals where you are scrubbed into real surgeries, working side by side with a real surgical technologist working as a member of the surgical team. Also, during this time there is a classroom portion for learning textbook information. After you have 3 years experience working as a surgical technologist, you can do the third piece of the clinical career ladder and obtain a certificate or a bachelor degree in applied science specializing in the role of first assist. This is what I am currently pursuing. First assist helps the surgeon perform the actual surgery and also learns to close the wound or suture the patient and works under the surgeon's supervision.

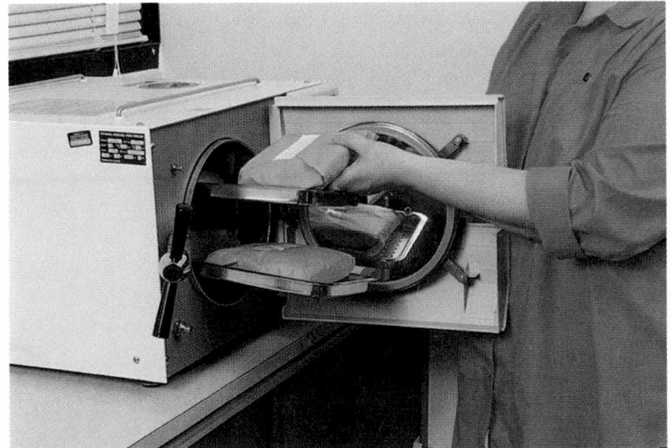

FIGURE 34-4 The autoclave sterilizes instruments by using steam under pressure to kill all microorganisms, including viruses and spores. (From Bonewit-West K: *Clinical procedures for medical assistants*, ed 7, St. Louis, 2008, Saunders.)

Central supply assistants inventory, receive, store, and distribute the equipment and products necessary in large health care institutions (Fig. 34-5). The educational requirement for the central supply clerk is minimal, because the work is repetitive. On-the-job training is possible for central supply assistants.

Content Instruction

Environmental Resources and Hazards

The earth has a limited supply of air, water, and land. These resources are constantly being used and reused (recycled). The **biosphere** is the air, crust of the earth,

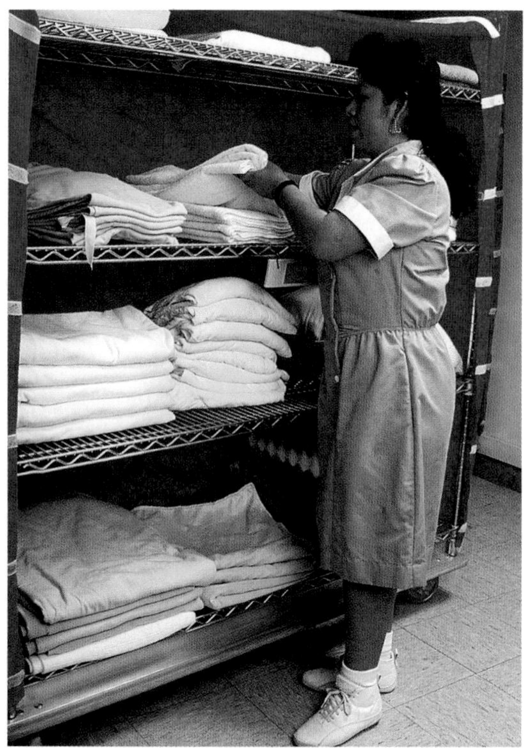

FIGURE 34-5 Central supply assistants help with the distribution of linens for the health care facility.

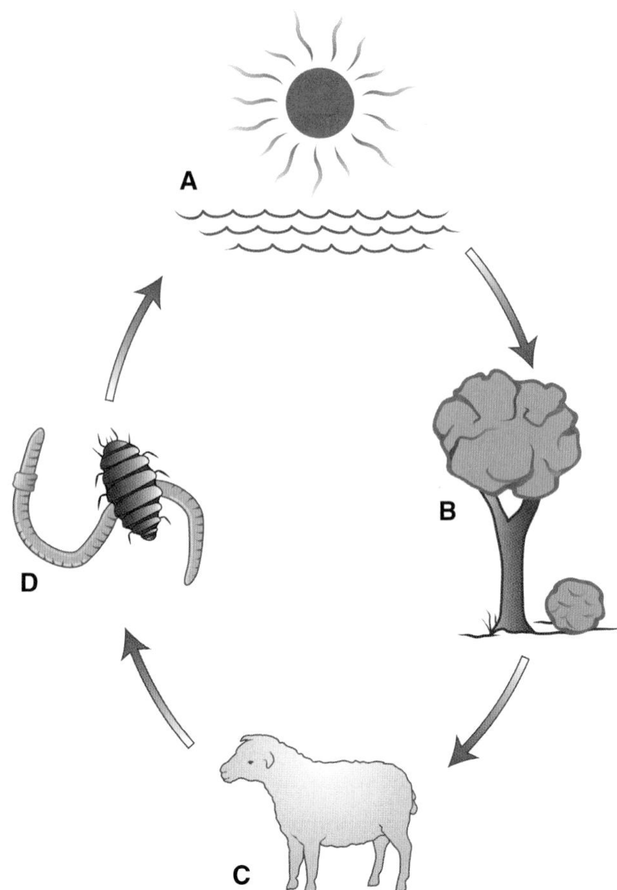

FIGURE 34-6 The chain of life ecosystem. The chain of life is composed of the following elements. **A,** Sunlight, water, oxygen, carbon dioxide, organic compounds, and nutrients found in the ecosystem. **B,** Plants or "producers" on land and in water convert carbon dioxide and other nutrients from the ecosystem in carbohydrates through photosynthesis, releasing oxygen. **C,** Herbivores (cows, sheep), carnivores, and other "consumers" feed on the producers and on each other. **D,** "Decomposers" such as bacteria, fungi, and insects break down dead producers and consumers, thereby returning their compounds into the ecosystem for reuse.

and water. It is made up of **ecosystems**, or the living and nonliving parts of the environment that support a chain of life in a selected area (Fig. 34-6). Ecology is the study of living organisms and how they relate to their environment. Humans produce more waste than can be recycled through natural processes. Pollution of the water, air, and land now endangers life as it is known. The goal of the public health programs that control the environment is to protect life and preserve the resources necessary for it. The Environmental Protection Agency is the federal agency that sets and regulates the standards for environmental factors.

Many diseases and health conditions are linked to environmental conditions. Emphysema and other lung disorders may be caused or worsened by air pollution. Lead poisoning has resulted from paint and gasoline additives. Because of government programs to reduce the blood level of lead in the population, it has decreased in adults since 1970. The CDC reports that 250,000 U.S. children between the ages of 1 and 5 have elevated lead levels in their blood. Carbon monoxide from car exhaust is linked to heart disease. As a waste product of manufacturing, mercury has been linked to nerve disorders. Lung cancer has been known to result from exposure to asbestos fibers, which, in the past, were used for insulation. Chemicals found in the environment act as **mutagens** and cause many cancers.

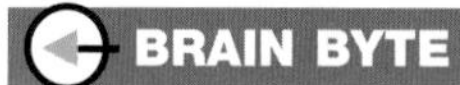

BRAIN BYTE

Elevated blood lead levels in children are due mostly to ingestion of contaminated dust, paint, and soil.

Air pollution is composed of dust and soot (**particulates**), carbon monoxide, **hydrocarbons**, and nitrogen oxides. The American Lung Association reported in 2010 that more than 175 million Americans live in counties with unhealthy levels of air pollution. Thinning of the protective ozone layer of the

TABLE 34-2
Air Pollution Facts

Body System	Effect of Air Pollution
Respiratory	Ozone reduces the body's ability to remove toxins and infectious agents
Sensory	Chemicals in air pollution irritate the eyes
Nervous	Carbon monoxide in air pollution disturbs coordination and concentration
Cardiovascular	Carbon monoxide in air pollution takes the place of red blood cells on the hemoglobin molecule, reducing the blood level of oxygen
Smog Index Rating	**Smog Index Meaning**
0-50	Good
51-100	Moderate
101-199	Unhealthy—people with heart or respiratory problems are encouraged to limit activity
200-299	Very unhealthy—older people and those with heart or respiratory problems are encouraged to stay inside
300+	Hazardous—everyone should avoid outdoor activities

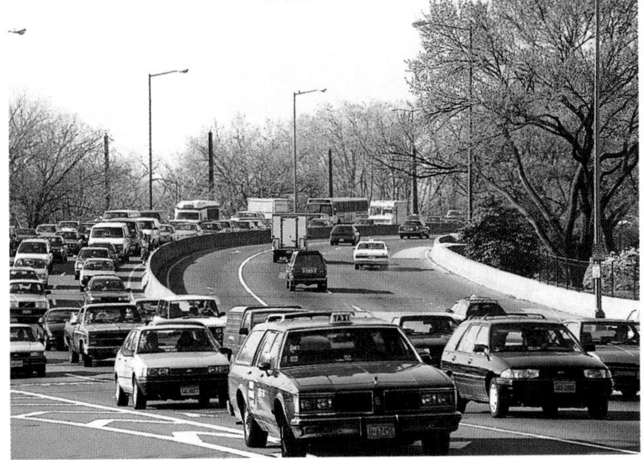

FIGURE 34-7 Pollution of the air, caused partly by automobile exhaust, has become a significant health factor.

atmosphere has resulted from the contaminants released from automobile exhaust, aerosol propellants, and painting materials (Fig. 34-7). The decrease in the ozone layer has increased the intensity of ultraviolet rays reaching the surface of the earth, leading to a higher incidence of skin cancer. Much of the air pollution in cities results from the burning of fuels such as oil. Air pollution in rural areas is caused by agricultural, mining, and lumbering activities. The physical effects of air pollution have been documented (Table 34-2).

Sound is a form of energy measured by pitch and loudness. Pitch, or the quality of the sound that is heard, is determined by the speed of the vibrations against the eardrum. Loudness is the intensity of the sound waves or how hard the sound waves strike the eardrum. Loudness of sounds is measured in **decibels** (dB) (Table 34-3). The lowest sound level that can be heard by the healthy human ear under quiet conditions is 1 dB. According to the American Speech-Language Hearing Association, the number of Americans with hearing loss has doubled in the past 30 years. One third of these hearing losses are noise-induced hearing losses or are linked to environmental causes and could be prevented.

Inside the cochlea of the ear, microscopic hairs move back and forth, stimulating nerve fibers that transmit sound to the brain. The hairs can be damaged when too great a force is created by loud sounds. The ear protects itself by changing the loudness of the sound with the ossicles, or small bones of the ear. If the sound is too loud, this cannot be done. Hearing loss caused by exposure to noise in cities has been reported. Excessive noise exists in homes and offices, as well as in traffic and outdoor environments. Environmental noise in homes results from appliances, tools, and music equipment.

At sound levels of about 40 dB, noise disturbs a sleeping person, and above 50 dB it disturbs conversation. At levels above 85 dB, stress reactions caused by noise may be expected. Damage to the ear that results in hearing loss occurs at 80 dB. At about 120 dB, the ear feels pain, and small animals die when exposed to 165 dB. Other adverse effects of excessive noise include cardiovascular, endocrine, and neurologic reactions that are similar to exposure to continuous stress. When a "temporary threshold shift" or muffling, bussing, or fullness is felt after exposure to noise, damage to the ear has been done.

TABLE 34-3
Sources and Effects of Noise

Sound	Noise Level (dB)	Effect
Firecracker, balloon pop, shotgun blast	150	Pain, hearing loss from unprotected exposure
Jet engine (near)	140	Pain, hearing loss from unprotected exposure
Jet takeoff (100-200 ft), stockcar races	130	Pain, hearing loss from unprotected exposure
Thunderclap (near), nightclub	120	Sensation felt
Power saw, rock music band, snowmobile, leaf blower, car horn, video arcade	110	More than 1 min unprotected exposure risks permanent hearing loss
Garbage truck	100	More than 15 min unprotected exposure risks hearing loss
Motorcycle, shop tools, lawnmower, subway	90	Very annoying
Electric razor	85	Hearing damage occurs
Traffic noise, garbage disposal, telephone ring	80	Annoying, interferes with conversation
Vacuum cleaner, hair dryer	70	Interferes with telephone conversation
Normal conversation, typewriter, sewing machine	60	Comfortable
Office, air conditioner, rainfall, refrigerator, air conditioner	50	Comfortable
Whisper, quiet library	30	Very quiet
Normal breathing	10	Just audible
	0	Threshold of normal hearing

Water is tested for its quality, bacteria, and pollutants. The quality is determined by the water temperature, turbidity, odor, animal and plant life, pH, and presence of debris. Water can be contaminated directly by industrial plants, oil discharges, **pesticides**, fertilizers, and heat from plants producing electricity. Water can also be polluted when chemicals and waste seep into the ground water, which supplies wells and springs. Standards for acceptable drinking water are set by the federal government.

In 2008 Americans produced 250 million tons of solid waste. That represents 4.5 lb of trash for each person daily. Eighty-three million tons of this was recycled or composted. Waste may be incinerated or stored in landfills. Although the number of landfills is declining, the average size is increasing (Fig. 34-8). This waste includes materials such as plastic containers, cans, and paper products that do not break down easily into recyclable compounds. When stored, the waste produces a reservoir for disease-causing organisms. Disposal of radioactive and other hazardous waste materials has become a concern of the environmental health services (Fig. 34-9).

Controversy still exists regarding the possible harmful effect of electromagnetic fields generated by power lines, computers, hair dryers, and other electrical devices. Electromagnetic fields are low-frequency energy emissions. Some research has associated exposure to electromagnetic fields to cancers such as leukemia, miscarriages, and birth defects.

BRAIN BYTE

According to the World Health Organization (WHO), 13 million deaths could be prevented every year by making our environments healthier worldwide.

Work-related injuries and illnesses are the concern of public health personnel. The National Institute for Occupational Safety and Health has identified 10 leading causes of work-related disorders and injuries (Box 34-2). Some agents that lead to lung damage include silica dust and asbestos. Cancers induced by work-related exposure to agents include liver, larynx, blood, and bone. Cardiovascular disease is aggravated in the workplace by exposure to solvents, carbon monoxide, noise, and psychosocial stress.

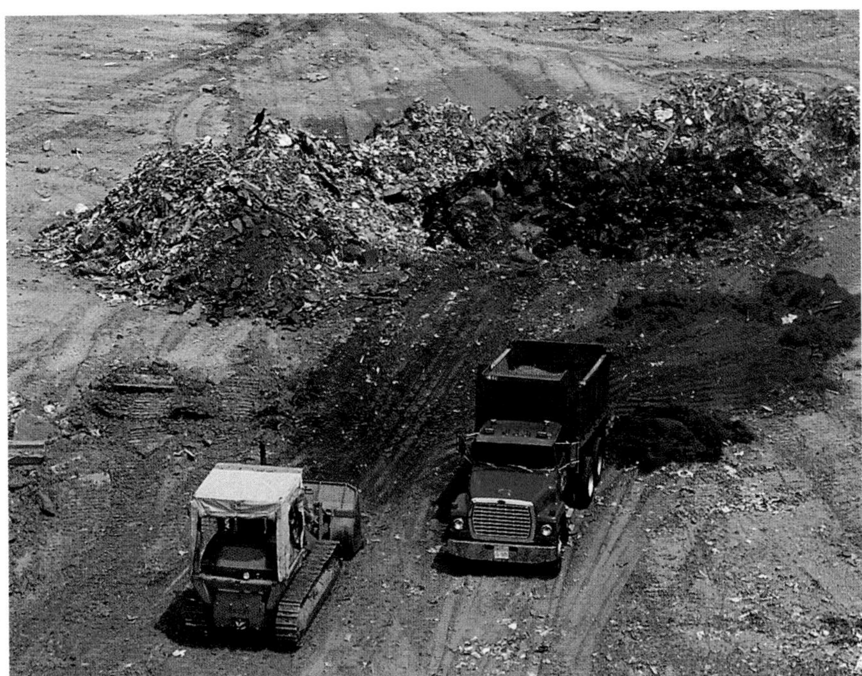

FIGURE 34-8 Disposal of waste in public landfills provides a reservoir for disease-causing organisms.

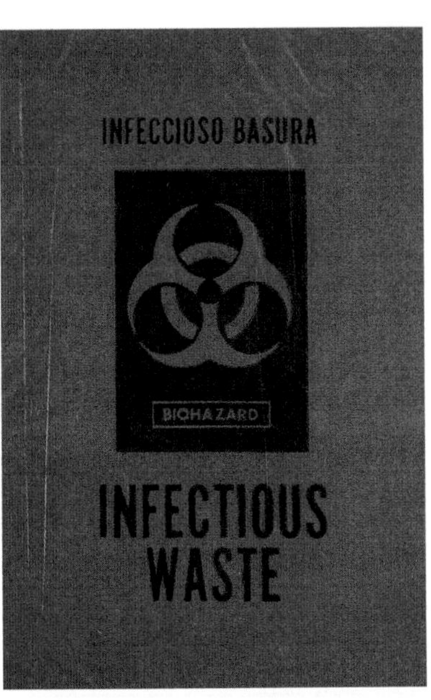

FIGURE 34-9 A biohazard symbol.

BOX 34-2

Ten Leading Work-Related Diseases and Injuries

1. Occupational lung diseases
2. Musculoskeletal injuries
3. Occupational cancers other than lung cancer
4. Severe traumatic injury
5. Cardiovascular disease
6. Disorders of reproduction
7. Neurotoxic disorders
8. Noise-induced hearing loss
9. Dermatology conditions
10. Psychological disorders

From the National Institute for Occupational Safety and Health.

Performance Instruction

Food Preparation

Food may be prepared by a food service worker under the supervision of the dietary department. Medical asepsis may be maintained by using good handwashing technique, as well as wearing nets to contain the hair and gloves to protect the food. Recipes may be used to measure the ingredients to make food items. All prepared food is stored appropriately to prevent contamination until it is used. The menus must meet individual patient medical needs as well as provide a balanced 24-hour diet. The counters and equipment in the kitchen area are cleaned and disinfected to prevent contamination of food items. (See Skill List 34-5, Preparing Meals, p. 556.)

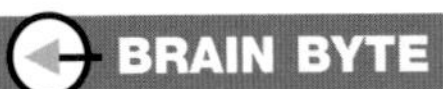

BRAIN BYTE

The CDC used data from frequent-shopper cards to identify the source of a salmonella outbreak in 2010.

Water Analysis

Water analysis involves the collection of a water specimen to determine the presence of pollution in the form of animal or plant waste. Some of the tests performed in water analysis include determination of the turbidity, odor, presence of microorganisms, and pH. Water that is suitable for one purpose, such as swimming, might not be acceptable for another, such as drinking. (See Skill List 34-6, Analyzing Water, p. 557.)

Instrument Maintenance

When the operative or medical procedure is completed, it is the task of the surgical technician, central supply worker, or other designated personnel to clean and prepare the instruments or equipment for further use. Medical asepsis is maintained throughout the cleaning procedure by using good handwashing techniques and wearing disposable gloves. Contaminated materials are removed from the instruments by rinsing them in cold water first because warm water may cause some materials to harden. Rinsing the instruments is followed by scrubbing them with a brush in warm, soapy water. Small instruments may be cleaned in an ultrasonic cleaner that uses vibration at high frequency to remove debris (Fig. 34-10). Instruments are dried well with a clean cloth or in a hot-air oven. Some instruments may require oiling according to the manufacturer's instructions. Surgical instruments are arranged in trays to make a set needed for a specific operation, such as an eye, abdominal, or dental procedure. Other instruments may be wrapped and then sterilized by using steam or chemicals (Fig. 34-11). Soiled water and materials used in cleaning are disposed of in an appropriate manner to avoid contamination of the cleaning area. Chemicals that sterilize may be used to decontaminate some instruments and the cleaning area. (See Skill List 34-7, Cleaning Instruments; and Skill List 34-8, Wrapping Packages for Sterilization, pp. 557–558.)

Terminal Cleaning

Terminal cleaning or environmental infection control includes the methods used to prevent the spread of infections in a health care facility. Infections in a patient that start in the hospital are called *nosocomial infections* and kill about 90,000 patients in the United States each year. Patients with infections may be isolated and their rooms terminally cleaned when they are discharged to protect another patient or health care worker. Terminal cleaning generally includes removing everything that is detachable. The remaining surfaces including the lighting, air ducts, walls, and all surfaces are cleaned with disinfectant. The removable objects are sanitized or disinfected before they are returned to the room after it has been cleaned. Personal protective clothing is worn during terminal cleaning of isolation rooms.

CASE STUDY 34-3 You notice some used tissues, a razor, and wet linens on the bathroom floor after a patient has been shaved for surgery. What should you do?

Answers to Case Studies are available on the Evolve website: ***http://evolve.elsevier.com/Gerdin***

CASE STUDY 34-4 You are the nursing assistant for a patient that has been discharged. You are asked to prepare the room for terminal cleaning. What should you do?

Answers to Case Studies are available on the Evolve website: ***http://evolve.elsevier.com/Gerdin***

Summary

- The function of the environmental health care team is to create a supportive environment for the patient.
- The role of members of the environmental health care team includes providing nutrition and a clean environment.
- Five areas of pollution control that are monitored by the environmental health care team are air quality, water quality, sound, food, and waste management.
- Five health conditions that are affected by environmental pollution include emphysema, heart disease, lung cancer, lead poisoning, and nervous system disorders.
- The chain of life in an ecosystem starts with the sun. A producer makes food for a consumer. When it dies, the compounds that make the consumer are returned to the soil by a decomposer.

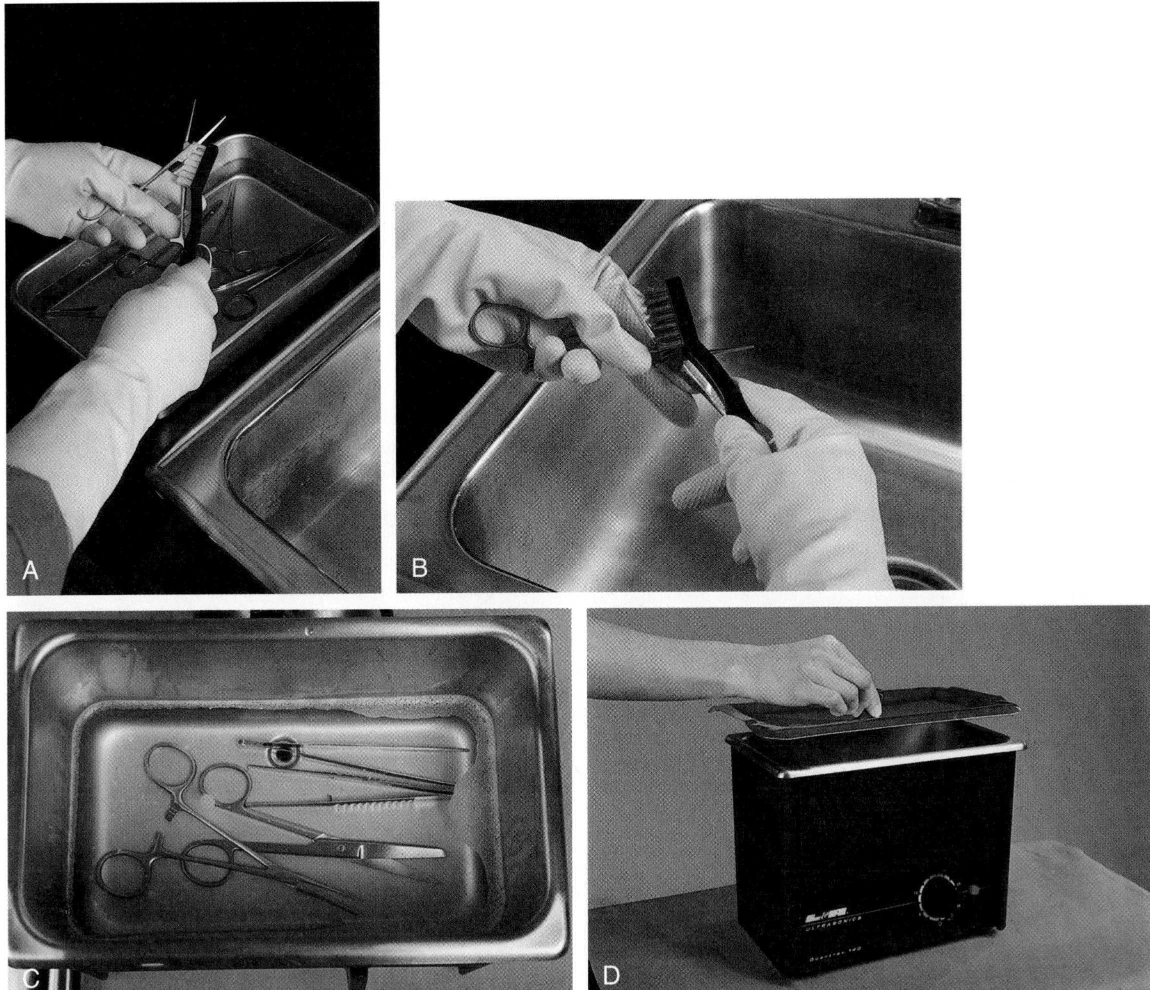

FIGURE 34-10 **A-D,** Instruments are washed thoroughly before being placed in the ultrasound. (From Bonewit-West K: *Clinical procedures for medical assistants*, ed 7, St. Louis, 2008, Saunders.)

Review Questions

1. Describe the role of at least three members of the environmental health care team.
2. Describe the function of the environmental health care team.
3. Describe the role of agencies that control the quality of the air, water, noise, food, and soil.
4. Describe the effects of atmospheric, water, noise, food, and soil pollution on the health of the community.
5. Identify the chain of life of an ecosystem in the local community.
6. List the departments and functions of the federal government's environmental health services.
7. Choose one career from Box 34-1. Research the cost of education and annual earnings in local institutions. Write a paragraph describing the factors that might explain why the local and national economic figures vary.
8. Compare and contrast concurrent and terminal cleaning.
9. Use each of the following terms in one or more sentences that correctly relate their meaning: decibel, ecosystem, hydrocarbon, particulate, pesticide, and pollution.

Critical Thinking

1. Investigate and compare the cost of various types of environmental health care services.
2. Keep a log of particulate values from local weather reports for 1 week. Investigate the cause of the most prevalent types of particulates in the area.
3. Test the noise level production of various sites in the environment. Record observations about the feeling various noises produce.

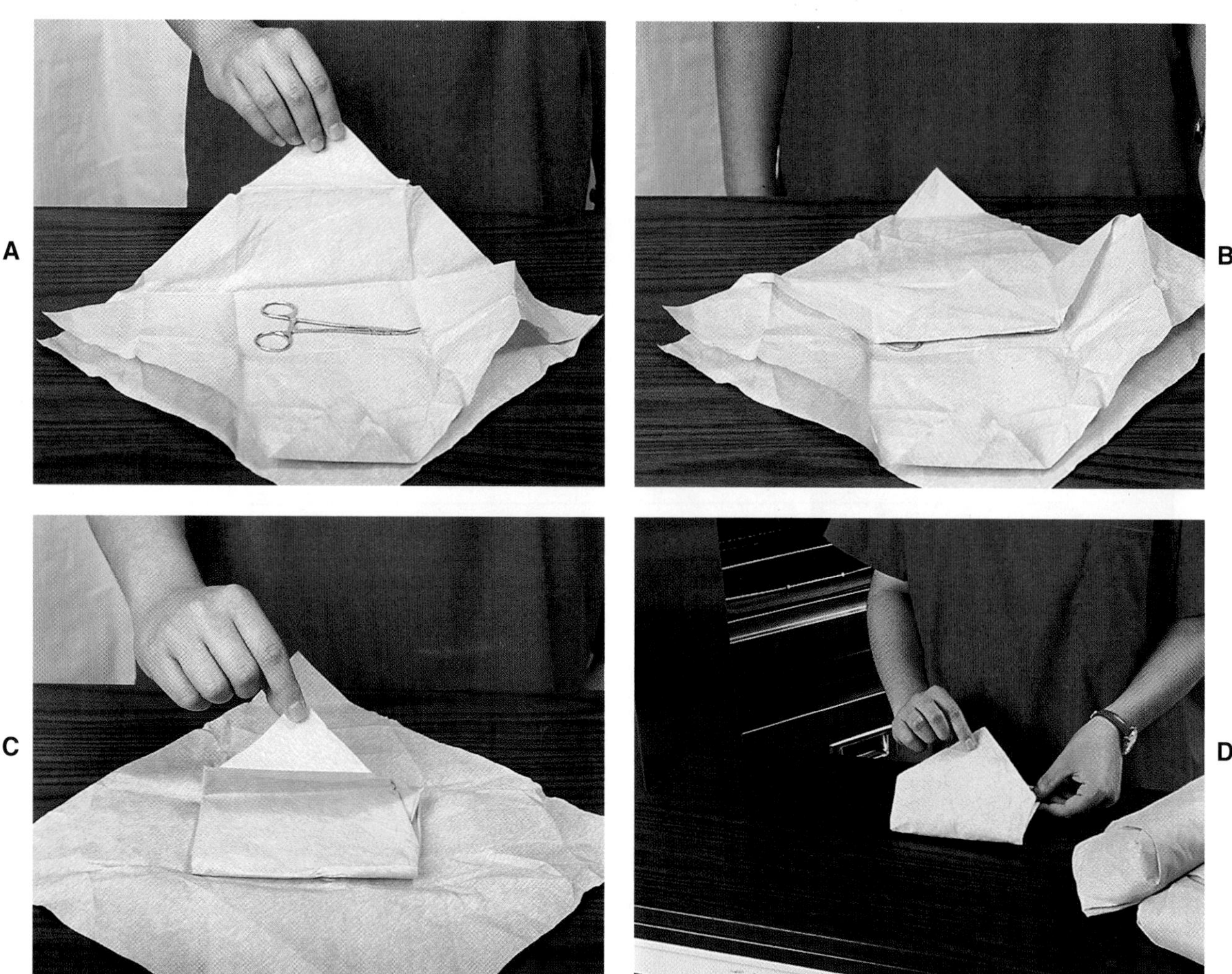

FIGURE 34-11 **A-D,** A wrapper must be selected so that no area of the items to be sterilized remains uncovered. Many items are wrapped twice to provide easier use after sterilization.

4. Investigate the services provided by environmental health care agencies in the community.
5. Create a pamphlet that includes selections for a 24-hour normal and a 24-hour therapeutic diet.
6. In 2010 the CDC traced frequent-shopper cards used to buy groceries to locate the origin of a salmonella outbreak. Investigate and write a paragraph describing how the source was found and the role the shopping cards played.
7. Create a career ladder for environmental careers. Describe why it is or is not possible to move from one level to another in the field.
8. Investigate and describe a health care facility program of recycling and waste management for cost containment and environmental protection.

Explore the Web

Career Information

Bureau of Labor Statistics
http://www.bls.gov/

Salary.com
http://salary.com

Professional Associations

American Dietetic Association
http://www.eatright.org/

Association of Surgical Technologists
http://www.ast.org/

STANDARDS AND ACCOUNTABILITY

See Evolve website: National Consortium on Health Science and Technology Education, National Health Science Career Cluster Models, Support Services Pathway Standards & Accountability Criteria; also available at http://www.healthscienceconsortium.org/healthcare_standards.php.

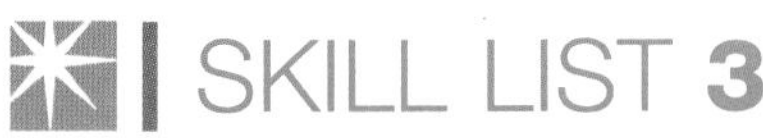

SKILL LIST 34-1 Planning Menus

1. Maintain medical asepsis by using the guidelines provided in the Standard and Transmission-Based Precautions, including good handwashing technique and use of gloves as needed.
2. Distribute meal requisitions (menus) early in the day. The type of meal requisition is determined by the physician's diet order and special needs of the patient.
3. Collect meal requisitions when completed. Patients may need assistance with completion of meal forms.
4. Determine the number of meals needed according to the number of patients (census). Tally the number of food portions required for each of them. Establish a schedule for the food preparation. Salads and fresh fruits should be prepared as late as possible to ensure freshness.

SKILL LIST 34-2 Preparing the Dining Area

1. Maintain medical asepsis by using the guidelines provided in the Standard and Transmission-Based Precautions, including good handwashing technique and use of gloves as needed. The hands should be washed after cleaning the surfaces of the table and chairs because the utensils for setting the table are cleaner than the furniture.
2. Arrange the chairs for easy access. Patients may require enough space for access by a wheelchair. Use separate cloths to clean the top of the table and chairs. Separate cleaning cloths are used for the table and chair seats because the tabletop is generally cleaner than the chairs.
3. If desired, spread a tablecloth.
4. Select the correct flatware, dinnerware, and glassware. Handle utensils by the stem. Utensils should be handled so that the area that touches the mouth is not touched by the hands.
5. Set the places correctly. A proper place setting provides all materials necessary for the patient to eat the meal and helps to create a pleasant environment to encourage eating.
6. If necessary, assist the patient with opening containers, cutting food, placing a napkin, and eating.
7. When the meal is finished, thoroughly clean the area and return used items to the designated location.

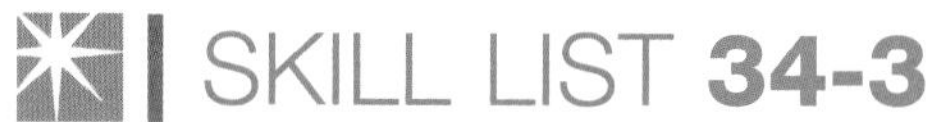

SKILL LIST **34-3**
Using the Epidemiologic Approach

1. Identify the health problem, disease, or illness. The person, place, and time are necessary to identify and solve the problem, just as the signs and symptoms of disease are necessary to determine the condition.
2. Identify the source of the problem by interviewing the affected individuals, checking public records, and making observations.
3. Plan a method to prevent the problem from recurring. Methods of prevention may include changing the environment to eliminate the causative agent or educating the affected population about methods of prevention.

SKILL LIST **34-4**
Housekeeping: General Rules

1. Maintain medical asepsis by using the guidelines provided in the Standard and Transmission-Based Precautions, including good handwashing technique and use of gloves as needed.
2. Establish and maintain a cleaning schedule. A clean and sanitary facility provides a safe and comfortable environment for the patient.
3. Place contaminated waste in the designated container immediately. Clean all contaminated equipment and supplies and return them to the designated location. Use the appropriate container for disposal of biohazardous waste.
4. Disinfect all work surfaces.
5. Handle contaminated linens as little as possible.
6. Report any exposure to contaminated materials to the supervisor immediately.
7. Maintain the patient's privacy and confidentiality while providing care at all times.

SKILL LIST **34-5**
Preparing Meals

1. Maintain medical asepsis by using the guidelines provided in the Standard and Transmission-Based Precautions, including good handwashing technique and use of gloves as needed.
2. Assemble equipment and supplies necessary for the recipe.
3. Measure the ingredients as required for the number of portions necessary.
4. Prepare the food according to the recipe.
5. Store the food appropriately until the time of use.
6. Clean the countertops and equipment with disinfectant.
7. Return the equipment and supplies to the designated storage area.

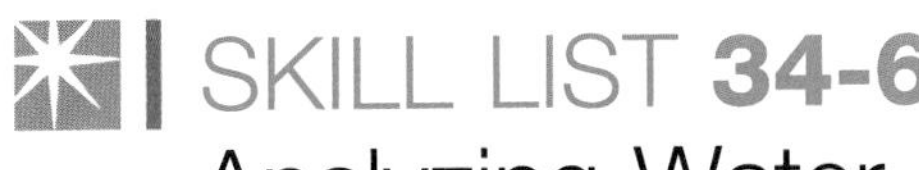

SKILL LIST 34-6 Analyzing Water

1. Maintain medical asepsis by using the guidelines provided in the Standard and Transmission-Based Precautions, including good handwashing technique and use of gloves as needed.
2. Collect a water sample in a sterile container to prevent contamination from other sources. Elements of the water that may indicate pollution include the presence of animal and plant life.
3. Observe and record the temperature of the water. Water temperature varies with the climate, oxygen content, and depth of the water sample.
4. Observe and record the turbidity of the water. The turbidity or clarity of the water can be determined by the amount of light that passes through it or by use of a Secchi disk. Water with high turbidity may be unacceptable for use by humans.
5. Observe and record the odor of the water. Odor may result from chemicals, organisms, or organic materials in the water. Odor does not necessarily indicate pollution of the water, but it is undesirable.
6. Using a microscope, observe the water and record the presence of life forms in the sample. The animals and plants that live in a body of water are indicators of its oxygen and other contents.
7. Observe and record the uses of the water sample area. Water may be used for recreational or industrial purposes. Litter in the water may indicate pollution from inappropriate use.
8. Measure and record the pH of the water sample. Litmus paper can be used to indicate the concentration of acid or alkaline materials in the water sample. The acidity of the water determines whether algae will grow and relative quantity of minerals or hardness of the water.
9. Prepare and incubate a streak culture plate to determine the presence of microscopic bacteria in the sample. Record the results.
10. Determine the acceptability of the water sample for its intended use. Drinking water should have a neutral pH, be free of microorganisms, have no odor, and be at an appropriate temperature.

SKILL LIST 34-7 Cleaning Instruments

1. Maintain medical asepsis by using the guidelines provided in the Standard and Transmission-Based Precautions, including good handwashing technique and use of gloves as needed. If the instruments are contaminated with body secretions, wear gloves to prevent the spread of microorganisms.
2. Remove all contaminating materials from the instruments by rinsing them in cold water. Contaminating materials may be more difficult to remove if warmed beforehand.
3. Scrub instruments with a brush in warm, soapy water. If necessary, place small instruments in a sonic cleaner for cleaning by vibration. Dry instruments thoroughly by using a towel or hot-air oven. Oil instruments according to the manufacturer's instructions. Arrange instruments on trays, or return them to the designated area. Instruments may be stored on trays for convenient use, for example, in abdominal, eye, or dental procedures.
4. Dispose of soiled water and linens appropriately, because pathogens can be carried on moist surfaces.

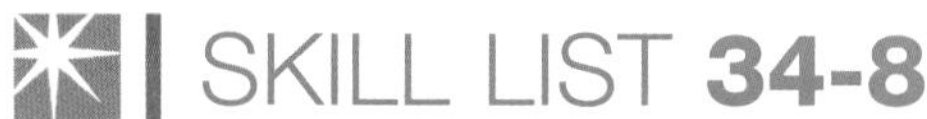

SKILL LIST 34-8 Wrapping Packages for Sterilization

1. Maintain medical asepsis by using the guidelines provided in the Standard and Transmission-Based Precautions, including good handwashing technique and use of gloves as needed. Wrapping packages for sterilization is a clean procedure requiring that the hands and instruments be as free from microorganisms as possible.
2. Select clean instruments for sterilization. Instruments may be arranged into sets for convenient use in particular procedures.
3. Select a wrapping towel or drape that is large enough to cover all contents completely. Drapes for autoclave sterilization may be made of cotton or specialized disposable material. Draping materials must allow penetration by the pressurized steam or gas.
4. Place instrumentation and sterilizing indicator diagonally in the center of the wrapping materials. The outside indicating tape does not ensure that the inner contents have been sterilized.
5. Fold the corners of the draping material into the center of the tray. The near edge is folded first, sides next, and the far edge last. The package should be neat and tight, with no exposed edges of the wrapping materials. Tuck the last edge into the pocket formed by the first three sides.
6. Seal the package with indicator tape. Secure tape so that the package will not be pulled open when the tape is removed.
7. Label the tape with the date and time of sterilization, contents, and the initials of the preparer. Items are not considered sterile indefinitely.
8. Place the package in the appropriate location for articles requiring sterilization.

CHAPTER 35

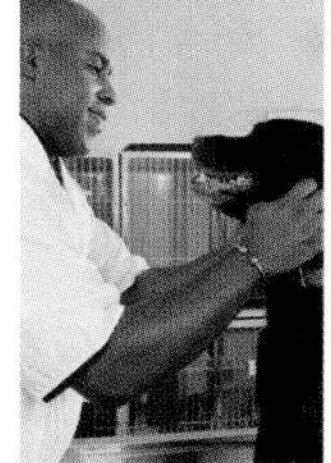
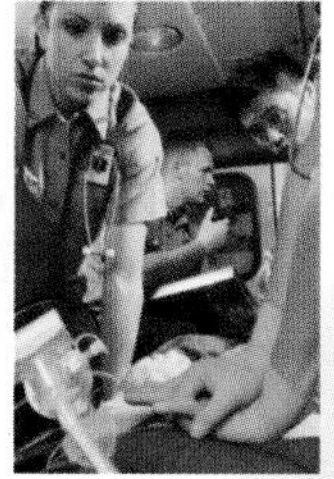
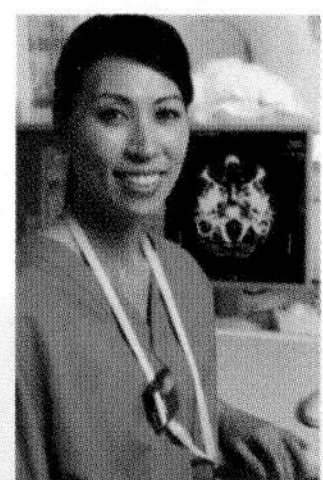

Biotechnology Research and Development Careers

LEARNING OBJECTIVES

- Define at least 10 terms relating to biotechnology.
- Identify the function of the biotechnological health care team.
- Describe the role of at least five of the biotechnological health care team members, including personal qualities, levels of education, and credentialing requirements.
- Describe the structure, function, and method of replication of DNA.
- Describe three research techniques used by biotechnologists.
- Describe at least three ethical concerns that have been raised since the beginning of DNA research.

KEY TERMS

Agarose *(ah-ga-ROZ)* A type of media made of sugar molecules taken from seaweed and used for electrophoresis

Artificial insemination *(art-uh-FISH-ul in-sem-ih-NAY-shun)* Injection of semen into the uterine canal, unrelated to sexual intercourse

Bioinformatics *(bi-o-in-for-mat-iks)* Collection, classification, and analysis of biological information such as molecular and genetic data

Biologic *(BI-oh-la-gik)* A drug, vaccine, or antitoxin that is made from living organisms

Deoxyribonucleic acid (DNA) *(dee-ok-see-rie-bo-noo-KLAY-ik AS-id)* Large nucleic acid molecule that makes up chromosomes

Electrophoresis *(ee-lek-tro-fore-EE-sis)* Movement of charged suspended particles through a medium in response to an electric field

Enzyme *(en-ZIME)* Protein that acts as a catalyst in the cell

Eugenics *(yoo-JEN-iks)* Study of the methods for controlling the characteristics of humans

KEY TERMS cont'd

Fermentation *(fer-men-TAY-shun)* Chemical change that is brought about by the action of an enzyme or microorganism

Forensics *(fore-EN-ziks)* Pertaining to the courts of law

Monoclonal antibody *(mon-o-KLO-nal AN-tee-bod-ee)* Identical cells or cells originating from the same cell

Selective breeding *(seh-LEK-tiv bree-ding)* Choosing the parents of offspring to enhance development of desired traits

Biotechnology Terminology*

Term	Definition	Prefix	Root	Suffix
Antibody	Against substances	anti	body	
Biodiversity	Variety of life	bio	divers/it	y
Biotechnology	Study of technology and life	bio	tech/n	ology
Congenital	Born with	con	gen/it	al
Dystrophy	Painful or difficult growth or nutrition	dys	troph	y
Endocrine	To secrete inside	endo	crine	
Eugenics	Pertaining to new origins	eu	gen	ics
Genetic	Pertaining to the origin		gen/et	ic
Neoplasm	New growth	neo	plasm	
Transgenic	Pertaining to cross origins	trans	gen	ic

*A transition syllable or vowel may be added to or deleted from the word parts to make the combining form.

Abbreviations for Biotechnology Careers

Abbreviation	Meaning
AIDS	Acquired immune deficiency syndrome
CBER	Center for Biologics Evaluation and Research
CF	Cystic fibrosis
DNA	Deoxyribonucleic acid
ELISA	Enzyme-linked immunosorbent assay
FDA	Food and Drug Administration
GM	Genetically modified
HIV	Human immunodeficiency virus
MD	Muscular dystrophy
NIH	National Institutes of Health

Careers

Biotechnology applies scientific and engineering techniques to the manipulation of the genes of living organisms. Biotechnology includes a broad range of improvements that may be applied to plants or animals and their products (Box 35-1). More than 111 vaccines and **biologics** have been approved by the U.S. Department of Agriculture (USDA) for improving the health of livestock, poultry, and companion pets. In 2009, 80% to 90% of all soybean, corn, and cotton crops in the United States were bioengineered. Most of the genetic engineering was to allow the plant to produce its own insecticide or resist herbicides used to kill weeds.

Biotechnologists research medical disorders and create drugs and proteins that can affect the cell. According to the March of Dimes organization, 1 in 150 live births have a chromosomal abnormality. Biotechnologists also directly alter or change the cells of living things to discover and improve genetic traits (Box 35-2). More than 200 therapies and vaccines have been created to treat cancer, diabetes, HIV/AIDS, and autoimmune disorders.

BRAIN BYTE

Biotechnology is a $38 billion a year industry and has produced more than 160 drugs and vaccines.

BOX 35-1

Biotechnology Timeline Highlights*

1870-1890	Plant breeders crossbreed cotton, developing hundreds of varieties with superior qualities. Farmers first inoculate fields with nitrogen-fixing bacteria to improve yields. William James Beal produces first experimental corn hybrid in the laboratory.
1919	First use of the word *biotechnology* in print.
1930	U.S. Congress passes the Plant Patent Act, enabling the products of plant breeding to be patented.
1941	*Genetic engineering* term used by microbiologist A. Jost.
1942	Microorganisms used to produce penicillin.
1946	U.S. Congress provides funds for plant collection and preservation.
1961	Registration of the first biopesticide: *Bacillus thuringiensis*.
1974	Recombinant DNA Advisory Committee of the National Institutes of Health (NIH) started to oversee genetic research.
1976	DNA base pairs sequence for a specific gene is defined.
1977	First human gene placed in bacteria.
1978	Human insulin produced in bacteria.
1979	Human growth hormone made.
1981	Transgenic animals made using mice. Fish cloned.
1982	Biotech human insulin produced in modified bacteria approved by Food and Drug Administration (FDA).
1983	The polymerase chain reaction technique is conceived. First whole plant grown from biotechnology: petunia.
1985	Genetic fingerprinting used in a courtroom as evidence. Gene-therapy experiments in humans approved by NIH.
1986	Hepatitis B vaccine produced. Interferon produced. Transgenic tobacco plant approved by Environmental Protection Agency.
1988	Transgenic mouse patented.
1990	The Human Genome Project started. Successful gene therapy treatment performed. Transgenic dairy cow used to produce human milk proteins for infant formula.
1992	Technique developed for testing embryos in vitro for genetic abnormalities.
1993	Bovine somatotropin approved by FDA to increase dairy-cow milk production.
1994	FLAVR SAVR tomato approved by FDA. Gene for breast cancer is discovered.
1995	Baboon-to-human bone marrow transplant is performed.
1997	Dolly the sheep cloned from adult cell.
2003	GloFish become available as pets.
2004	Pet kitten cloned.
2006	Vaccine to prevent cervical cancer and genital warts approved by FDA.
2008	Genetic Information Nondiscrimination Act becomes law.

*Modified from the Biotechnology Industry Organization, http://www.bio.org/speeches/pubs/er/timeline.asp.

Biotechnologist

Scientists have been using natural techniques of biotechnology such as **fermentation**, **selective breeding**, and **artificial insemination** for many years. This emerging field began to take form as a separate discipline in the early 1980s with the development of cloning and recombinant **deoxyribonucleic acid** (DNA) techniques of gene manipulation (Box 35-3). Other personnel are filling positions to design, manufacture, and operate the equipment necessary to make these techniques possible (Table 35-1). Personnel in biotechnology must show great creativity and logical thought and must be able to work independently and as part of a team. The work takes great concentration

TABLE 35-1
Biotechnology Career Educational Cost and Earnings

Career	Educational Cost*	Earnings†
Forensic science technician	Southern Wesleyan University, bachelor's degree, 82 credit hours Fees include: Tuition $9100/block of 12-18 hours Fees $315/block Books $300-$700/semester	Median annual salary: Concord, S.C.—$48,520

*http://www.swu.edu/financial_aid/tuition_fees.htm.
†http://data.bls.gov:8080/oes/datatype.do..

BOX 35-2

Biotechnology Careers

Biochemist
Biochemistry technologist
Biomedical engineer
Biomedical equipment technician
Biophysicist
Biotechnologist
Cytologist
Dairy technologist
Dental equipment installer and servicer
Electromedical equipment repairer
Food technologist
Forensic science technician
Genetic counselor
Geneticist
Medicolegal investigator
Microbiologist
Physiologist
Poultry scientist
Radiologic equipment specialist
Radiologic equipment tester
Staff toxicologist
Veterinary bacteriologist

BOX 35-3

Genetics Pioneer Profile

Barbara McClintock was often considered an eccentric and a maverick during her career in the field of genetics. She entered Cornell University in 1919 and had her work in the field ignored and discarded for the following 30 years. She overcame many obstacles of birth; women were not considered to be credible scientists. In fact, she was not allowed to join the research department of her choice at Cornell because women were excluded from it.

In 1931 McClintock published research that proved chromosomes formed the basis of inheritance in corn (maize). In 1944 DNA was discovered, providing a broader basis for research in heredity. The structure of DNA as a double helix was not discovered by Crick and Watson until 1953.

McClintock formed experiments that led to her concept of "jumping genes," or the movement of genes on chromosomes (recombination). Her theory went against the accepted "Central Dogma of Crick," which stated that DNA is transcribed to RNA to translate to protein. Her work was ignored, and the concept was later claimed by two other scientists. Barbara McClintock was recognized for her work as a pioneer cytogeneticist in 1983 with the awarding of the Nobel Prize in Medicine.

and perseverance because the results might not be available immediately.

Because of the competitive nature of the field, most biotechnology laboratories use elaborate safety and security systems. Safety guidelines for the transfer and manipulation of DNA have been established by the National Institutes of Health (NIH). Some of these precautions include the use of laminar flow hoods to vent and filter air, strict sterilization, and careful planning to ensure all microorganisms are harmless. To date no incident of a safety problem has been documented.

Biotechnologists also face criticism within their own profession. Many researchers believe that too much money is being spent duplicating work. For example, more than a dozen laboratories worked in competition rather than in cooperation to identify a gene that causes breast cancer.

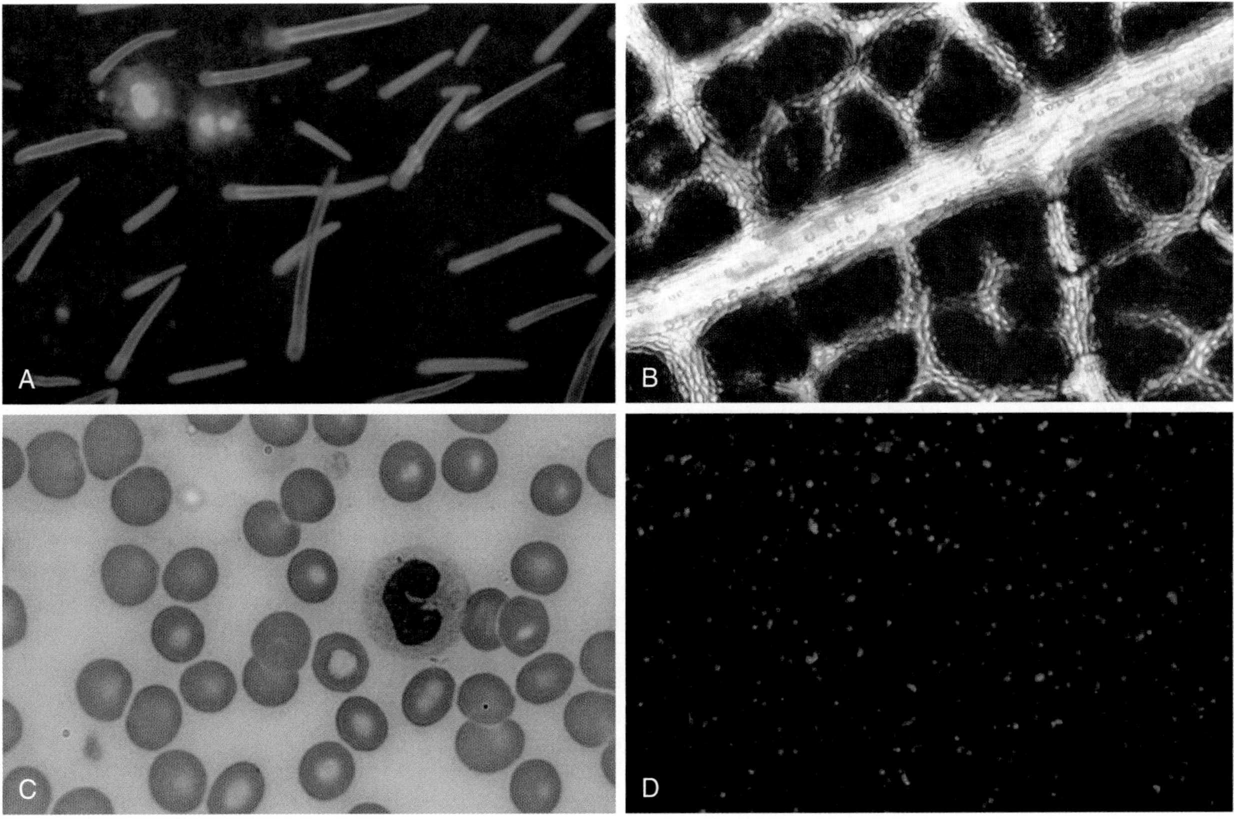

FIGURE 35-1 Microscopic Cells. **A,** Plant hairs. **B,** Plant. **C,** Blood. **D,** Yeast.

Biotechnologists face a unique challenge as professionals in the health care field. Unlike any other area of health care practice throughout history, biotechnology has made many complex advances faster than they can be communicated to the public. More than 1400 biotechnology companies exist in the United States, most working in therapeutic and diagnostic areas of the field. Biotechnologists also face ethical concerns about the control of human characteristics (**eugenics**) and the safety of organisms produced by gene manipulation. Some concerns include the counseling of couples to not have children if a faulty gene is present, insurance carriers refusing to cover offspring born after detection of a known genetic defect, and selection of offspring before implantation based on favorable traits such as gender. Some controversial genes are being researched, such as those that may influence characteristics such as obesity, violence, and hyperactivity.

Biotechnologists may work in many fields of practice including research, **forensics**, immunology, and teaching. Health professionals from other disciplines may specialize in the field of biotechnology. Biotechnologists may also work for regulating agencies such as the Food and Drug Administration (FDA) and NIH.

CASE STUDY 35-1 Your friend tells you he believes that genetically modifying food is wrong and he does not eat any of it. What should you say?

Answers to Case Studies are available on the Evolve website: ***http://evolve.elsevier.com/Gerdin***

Medical biotechnologists work with the production of antibodies for diagnosis or treatment of disease. Immunologists have used the skills of biotechnology to produce **monoclonal antibodies** for the treatment of many disorders, such as cancer and AIDS. Other medical biotechnologists work to produce methods and products to treat diabetes, blood diseases, and heart disease (Fig. 35-1).

Research biotechnologists supervise the work of associates and assistants in industry and health care to find better products and solutions to disorders. One product of genetic research is the development of transgenic animals. Through the process of genetic

Health Careers in Practice

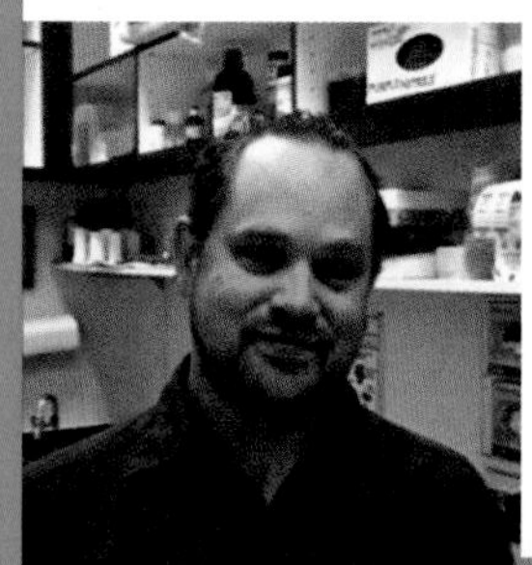

JEREMY E. ELLIS, PhD

LABORATORY MANAGER AND RESEARCH ASSOCIATE
AN INDEPENDENT CLINICAL, DIAGNOSTIC, AND RESEARCH LABORATORY

Educational background: Bachelor of science in microbiology, Arizona State University (4 years); PhD in developmental and cellular biology, University of California, Irvine (8 years)

A typical day at work and job duties include: My time at work is split nearly evenly between managing the clinical diagnostics laboratory and medical research. I am responsible for ensuring that the laboratory:

- is functioning properly
- is dealing with problems
- is stocked with reagents
- is complying with all of the state and federal regulations that govern our business

In addition to these managerial tasks, I am responsible for:

- developing new diagnostic tests
- developing the new diagnostic tests into production tests
- identifying new areas of research
- writing scientific publication material
- performing basic science studying new and emerging infectious diseases

The most gratifying part of my job: Bringing cutting edge genetic and molecular biology based technologies to the public is challenging and rewarding.

The biggest challenge(s) I face in doing my job: The state and federal regulations are by far the largest challenge. Before any project can be started, all of the scientists are required to come together and discuss what regulations we must comply with and proceed from there.

What drew me to my career? I have always been interested in biology and the underlying mechanisms that govern life. I also have felt that as technology moves forward there is an ever-increasing gap between what is accessible by the common individual and what is technically feasible. I feel that I am uniquely suited to bridge that gap and create cutting edge technologies that are accessible for the common person.

Something I learned in my early education that I currently use in my career or that caused me to be interested in my career is: In high school I learned about how everything is interrelated and there are common themes throughout biology and physics. This concept helps me perform tasks from simple chemistry to the creation of transgenic animals.

transfer, animals that contain new genetic information can be bred. One example is the manipulation of the Shiverer mouse. These mice are naturally born with a condition that prevents production of myelin sheath on nerves and is soon fatal. The species has been genetically altered to produce the myelin. Other mice have been genetically engineered to produce monoclonal antibodies and yet others to carry the gene for muscular dystrophy to allow research in that area.

CASE STUDY 35-2 Your friend tells you that moving genes from one species to another is morally wrong. What should you say?

Answers to Case Studies are available on the Evolve website: ***http://evolve.elsevier.com/Gerdin***

Biotechnologists in medicolegal forensics use biological samples from a crime scene such as hair, skin,

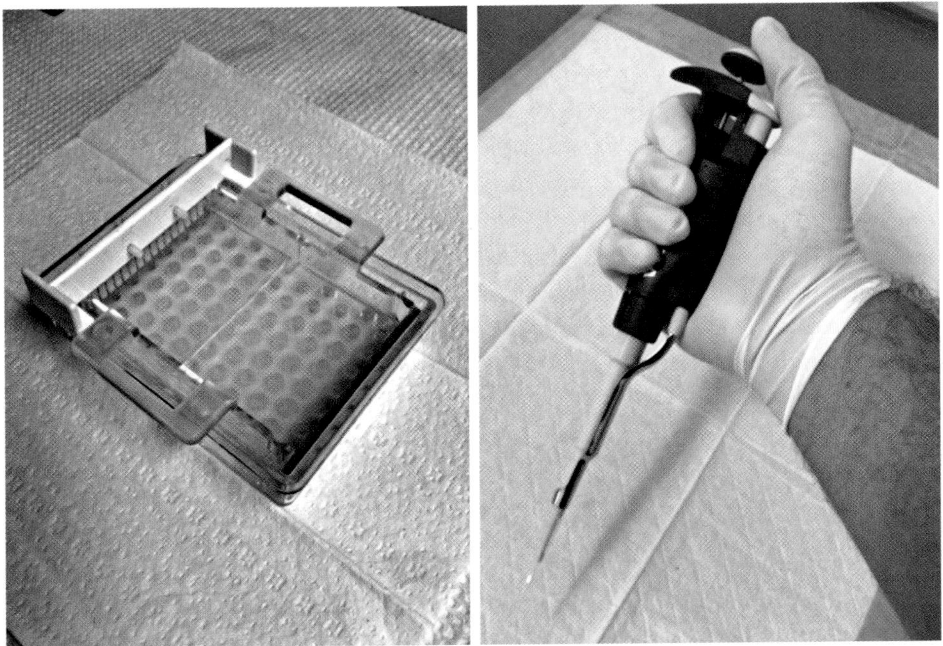

FIGURE 35-2 Electrophoresis is used to separate DNA fragments.

and blood to identify suspects. Because each person has unique DNA segments, DNA fingerprinting makes this possible. These segments can be separated in a process called **electrophoresis**, which uses the natural electrical charge of molecules to separate them (Fig. 35-2). The biotechnologist can then take photographic images of DNA fragments that are unique to each person. Forensic science technicians may hold an associate or bachelor's degree.

Most biotechnologists complete a minimum of a master's degree but usually hold a doctoral degree in biotechnology or a related field such as biochemistry or genetics. Biotechnologists are not currently licensed.

Associates in biotechnology (biotechnicians) perform complex procedures of DNA extraction and cloning. They may be responsible for using computer technology to analyze the data gathered. Research associates usually hold a master's degree in biotechnology or a related field.

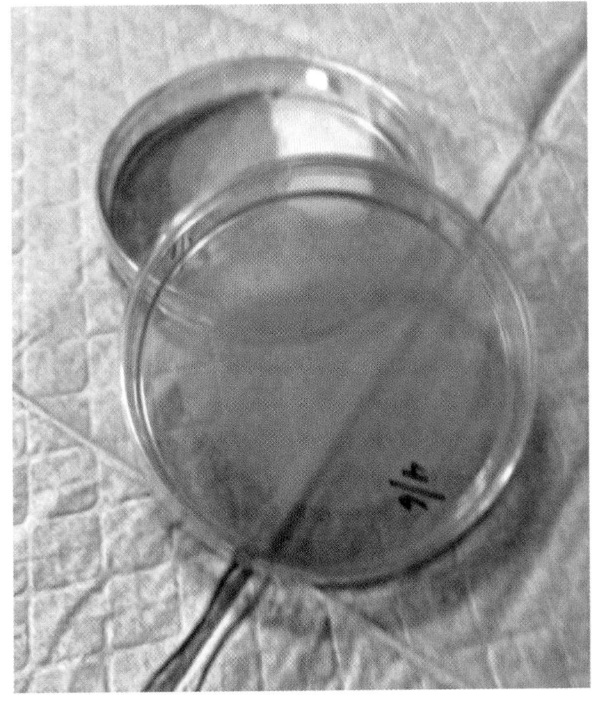

FIGURE 35-3 Genes can be combined in Petri dishes using bacteria or enzymes.

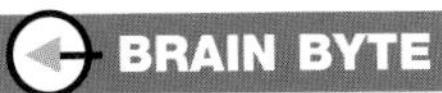

BRAIN BYTE

The FDA, Environmental Protection Agency (EPA), and USDA regulate the biotechnology industry.

Assistants in biotechnology perform the routine work of gene manipulation, including combining bacteria with nutrients or **enzymes** in Petri dishes, photographing projects, and performing simple tests (Fig. 35-3). They also perform laboratory duties such as cleaning and sterilizing glasswork. Assistants in biotechnology usually hold a bachelor's degree in biotechnology or a related field such as biochemistry or molecular biology.

Geneticists study patterns of inheritance and develop methods to influence genetic information.

Geneticists may work as counselors for individuals with a family history of genetic abnormalities. Some of the techniques used by geneticists include isolation of genes and genetic manipulation. They may also use computers to create models of proteins, drugs, and genes to design drugs or therapies. Some areas of specialization for geneticists include human, medical, molecular, cell, or population genetics. Geneticists may also specialize in genetic engineering. Geneticists are usually required to hold a doctoral degree for employment in research, teaching, or administration. Licensure and certification are not required for geneticists.

Support Personnel

Biomedical engineers, or bioengineers, design, develop, and help maintain instruments and machines that are used to monitor and treat disease in health care. Some examples of technological devices include lasers, pacemakers, and artificial hearts and kidneys.

Another development is the use of biosensors, or biological structures that recognize other structures such as enzymes, antibodies, and receptors. The biosensor converts the information to a voltage charge, sound, or light emission. The glucose meter that patients with diabetes use to check their blood for sugar is a type of biosensor. The enzyme glucose oxidase binds with the blood that produces an electrochemical reaction in the meter to indicate the sugar level.

Technology has led to the development of robotic surgical instrumentation that can be used to visualize the surgery site from a distance. This type of surgery may possibly allow telecommunication of surgical skills in the future. Specialties for biomedical engineers include medical, clinical, and rehabilitation practice. They may also work in research to design new devices.

Most biomedical engineers work for hospitals. Education and training for this emerging field vary greatly. Most biomedical engineers hold at least a 4-year university degree. Some areas of study are engineering biophysics, bioinstrumentation, biothermodynamics, biotransport, biomechanics, and biomedical computers. Biomedical engineers working in health care must be registered. Licensing as a professional engineer is preferred. Voluntary certification is available.

Biomedical equipment technicians and repairers inspect and adjust the equipment used in health care. The equipment includes such items as heart monitors and radiologic equipment. The education for biomedical equipment repairers is usually an associate degree in that area. An apprenticeship may be required. Voluntary certification is available on passing an examination and documentation of experience.

Bioprocess engineers design and operate the equipment used to ferment organisms used in biotechnology. They may also collect and purify the products for use. Some examples of products produced by fermentation include insulin and human growth hormone.

Content Instruction

Cell Genetics

The genetic information of humans is found in the nucleus of each cell in 23 pairs of chromosomes (Fig. 35-4). DNA is a molecule that, by the sequencing

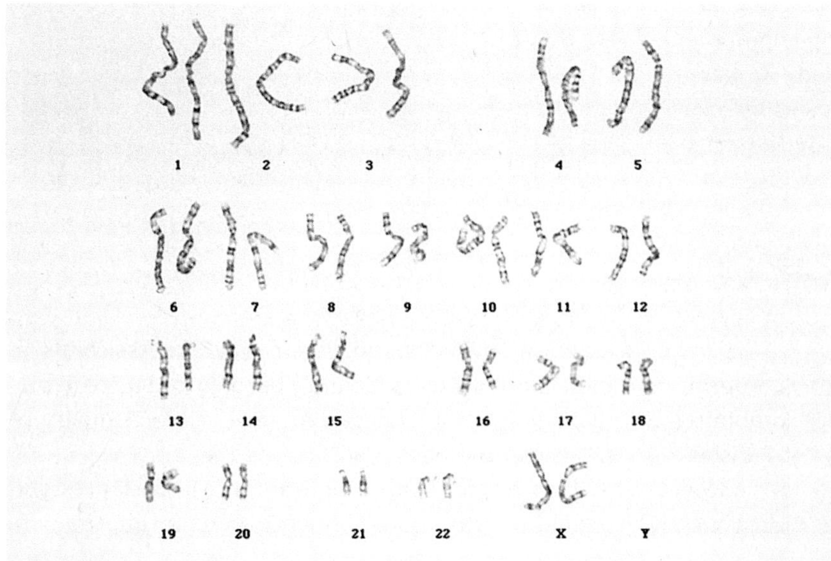

FIGURE 35-4 The karyotype may be used to show genetic abnormalities. (Courtesy Ward's Natural Science Establishment, Rochester, N.Y.)

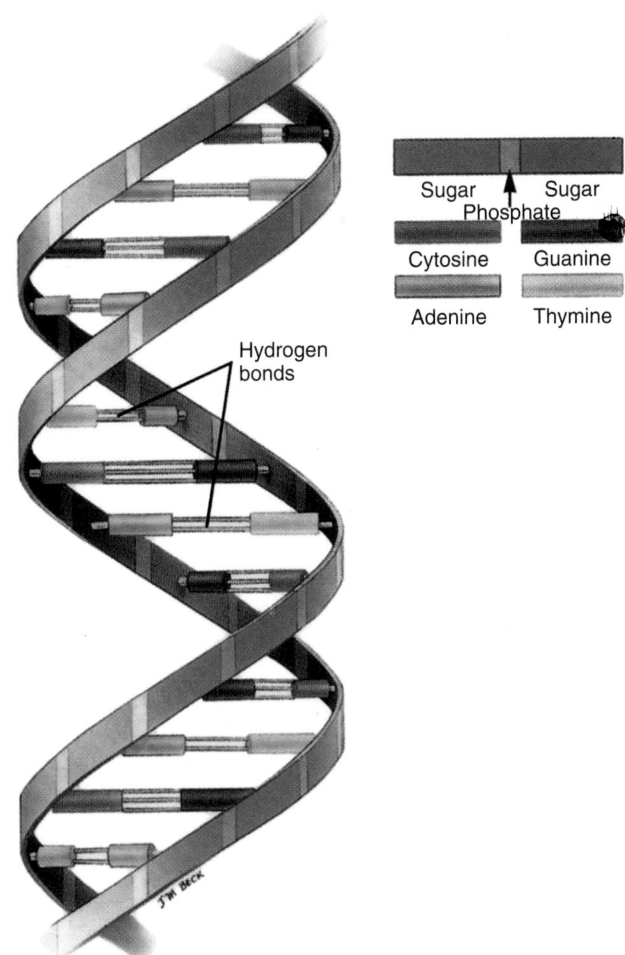

FIGURE 35-5 DNA holds the individual genetic code for each person. Each strand of DNA is made up of a series of nucleotides. The sequence of nucleotides determines which protein is synthesized. (Courtesy Joan M. Beck.)

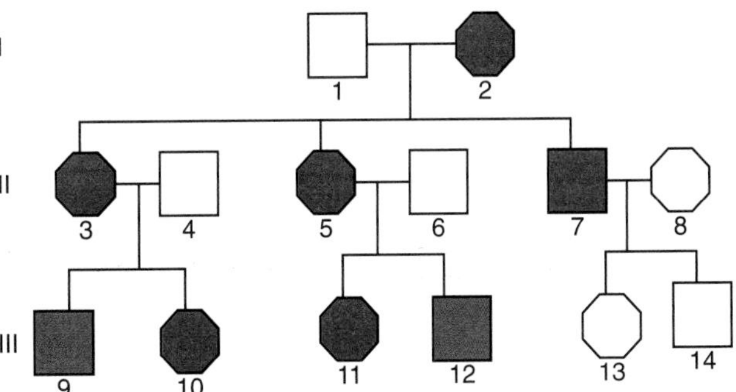

FIGURE 35-6 In a pedigree diagram, the females are shown as circles and the males as squares. The individuals who are shaded have the same mitochondrial DNA.

of its components, determines of the characteristics of living things. Nucleic acid is made of a nitrogenous base that is attached to a sugar and phosphate. Each strand of DNA is formed in a double helix of chains of these nucleotides. Each human chromosome is made up of 50 to 250 million base pairs (Fig. 35-5). Replication is the process by which DNA makes copies of itself. During replication, the double helix of DNA uncoils and opens. Nucleotides join each side of the DNA strand to make new copies.

A chromosome is a long chain of DNA. On the chromosome, sections of DNA carry messages called *genes*. The gene found on the DNA chain conveys its message by making proteins. DNA unfolds and breaks into two strands. Special units of three nucleotides, called *messenger ribonucleic acid (RNA)*, translate the DNA to form a message. The new messenger (mRNA) strand leaves the nucleus and joins with more nucleotide segments called *transfer RNA (tRNA)*. The tRNA carries amino acids that combine to form a protein. The protein then directs a body function or makes up a structural characteristic.

BRAIN BYTE

RNA transcripts or messages have been discovered in what was previously considered to be "junk DNA" or non-functioning "dark matter."

A single gene, such as that for cystic fibrosis, is made up of 6100 base pairs. Some genes are expressed at one stage of development and no other. The human genome contains an estimated 30,000 genes. Most genes are around 3000 bases in length but vary in size. Ninety percent of the DNA sequence or genome does not contain a code for proteins.

Mitochondrial DNA (mtDNA) is DNA that is found in the mitochondria of the cell. The mother of the organism contributes most or all of the mtDNA. Mitochondrial DNA contains 37 genes that affect the proteins involved in cellular respiration or the use of energy in the cell. The mtDNA of an organism is the same as its mother because there is no connection with the father's mtDNA. Mutations of mtDNA can cause several disorders, including Kearns-Sayre syndrome and exercise intolerance. Kearns-Sayre syndrome may cause the loss of function of the heart, eye, and muscle movement. Mitochondrial DNA has become an important tool in forensics and determining lineage or ancestry because there is more of it in the cell than nuclear DNA (Fig. 35-6).

The Human Genome Project (HGP), formally begun in 1990, was established with goals including the identification and sequencing of all the human chromosomes. This process is called *gene mapping* (Table 35-2). Computerization of the sequencing techniques allowed biotechnologists to identify gene

TABLE 35-2
Mapped Genes

Chromosome Number	Genetic Information Influenced
1	Rh blood type—blood protein
	Thyroid-stimulating hormone—metabolism
	Amylase—starch digestion
2	Myosin—coats neurons
	Antibodies—fight infection
	Glucagon—sugar storage
3	Rhodopsin—light-sensitive pigment
4	Huntington disease—neurotransmission defects
	Alcohol dehydrogenase—breaks down alcohol in body
	Red hair color
6	Major histocompatibility complex—antibodies
	Several reproductive hormones
7	Collagen production
	Trypsin—digestive enzyme
	Cystic fibrosis
9	ABO blood grouping
10	Hexokinase enzyme—hemolytic anemia
11	Hemoglobin—sickle-cell anemia or thalassemia
	Insulin
	Parathyroid hormone
	Albinism
12	Phenylketonuria
14	Antibody production
15	Tay-Sachs disease—neurologic disorder
16	Chymotrypsinogen—protein digestion
17	Neurofibromatosis—nerve tissue tumors
	Growth hormone
18	Tourette syndrome—neurologic disorder
19	Familial hypercholesterolemia
	Brown hair color
	Green-blue eye color
20	Adenosine deaminase—immunodeficiency disease
X	Duchenne muscular dystrophy
	Red-green color blindness
	Hemophilia

sequences at a much faster rate than in the past. Researchers involved in this project have identified at least 18 genes involved in insulin-dependent diabetes. This HGP was completed in 13 years with the identification of approximately three billion chemical base pairs that make up human DNA. Scientists also identified the location of a gene called *BRCA1*, which causes 5% of all breast cancers. At least one gene that makes people susceptible to allergies and asthma also has been identified. In all, more than 80 genetic diseases can now be identified with genetic testing (Table 35-3). In addition to diagnostic testing, the information from DNA can be used for newborn screening, prenatal screening, carrier identification, and forensic identification. The function of about 50% of the genes discovered by the project is not known. Some scientists involved in the project have now begun the study of human proteins (proteomics).

Products that may serve as pharmaceuticals are being developed with biotechnology techniques in the emerging discipline called *pharmacogenomics*. Some genetically modified foods in development include

TABLE 35-3
Types of DNA Tests*

Disease	Description
Adult polycystic disease	Multiple kidney growths
Alpha-1-antitrypsin deficiency	Can cause hepatitis, cirrhosis of the liver, emphysema
Amyotropic lateral sclerosis (ALS, also called "Lou Gehrig" disease)	Fatal degeneration of the nervous system
Charcot-Marie-Tooth disease	Progressive degeneration of muscles
Cystic fibrosis	Lungs clog with mucus; usually fatal by 40 years of age
Duchenne/Becker muscular dystrophy	Progressive degeneration of muscles
Familial adenomatous polyposis	Colon polyp by age 35 years, often leading to cancer
Fragile X syndrome	Most common cause of inherited mental retardation
Gaucher disease	Mild to deadly enzyme deficiency
Hemophilia	Blood fails to clot properly
Huntington disease	Lethal neurological deterioration
Multiple endocrine neoplasia	Endocrine gland tumors
Myotonic dystrophy	Progressive degeneration of muscles
Neurofibromatosis	Café au-lait spots to large tumors
Retinoblastoma	Blindness; potentially fatal eye tumors
Sickle cell disease	Sickle cell anemia
Spinal muscular atrophy	Progressive degeneration of muscles
Tay-Sachs disease	Lethal childhood neurological disorder
Thalassemia	Mild to fatal anemia

*More than 900 genetic tests are available.

edible vaccines, therapeutic proteins, and antibodies produced by plants. For example, the ProdiGene company (College Station, Texas) is developing vaccines and insulin to be produced by corn plants. CropTech is trying to grow plants that produce enzymes and anticancer proteins. Other researchers are developing bananas grown to contain the hepatitis B vaccine.

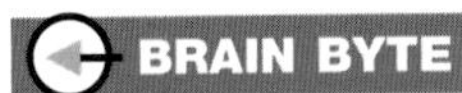
BRAIN BYTE

About 70% of processed foods contain genetically modified plants.

Research advances in molecular biology and genomic technologies have resulted in a large database of biological information. **Bioinformatics** combines the disciplines of biology, computer science, and information technology to study this information. Examples of bioinformatic activities include gene mapping, DNA analysis, and protein analysis.

Techniques of Biotechnology

Some of the techniques of biotechnology include gene cloning and gene splicing or recombinant DNA. Biotechnologists have been cloning plants for many years. This process involves removing a small number of meristem or growing plant cells and, by manipulation with hormones, creating a complete new plant. A similar process has been used to produce cattle by separating the cells of an in vitro embryo to create several embryos with exactly the same genetic information. Genetically identical tadpoles have also been cloned from the stomach lining cells of a single donor. Sea urchins have been reproduced by chemical manipulation of cells from one individual. In 1993 scientists split an early stage human embryo that was defective into single cells. Each was then coated in an artificial gel and continued to develop for several days before being discarded.

CASE STUDY 35-3 Your friend tells you that she is going to get her dog cloned so she will never lose him. What should you say?

Answers to Case Studies are available on the Evolve website: ***http://evolve.elsevier.com/Gerdin***

Gene splicing, also called transgenics, involves moving genes from one location to another in the same or a different organism. An enzyme is used to "cut" a section of DNA open, allowing another to take its place. Free-floating rings of DNA called *plasmids* from an organism such as *Escherichia coli (E. coli)* can be used to introduce new genetic information. This process is called *transformation*, or *recombinant DNA*, as the genetic message in the organism is changed in the process. More than 80 specific enzymes, called *restriction enzymes*, have been identified to cut DNA at specific locations.

One example of the application of gene manipulation is the production of human growth hormone by *E. coli*. In the past, human growth hormone was harvested from pituitary glands donated at the time of death. It takes 80 to 100 pituitary glands to treat one child for 1 year. Most treatment plans last 8 to 10 years. The shortage of donated pituitaries and cost of the process have made the treatment difficult. Through the process of recombinant DNA, the common bacteria *E. coli* has been given the genetic direction to make the human growth hormone. Fermentation processes allow large quantities to be produced. The quality of the hormone produced is consistent and economical.

Some other applications of biotechnology research include the use of early detection pregnancy tests and the enzyme-linked immunosorbent assay technique, which can be used to detect the presence of HIV and other viruses.

BOX 35-4

Categories of Gene Therapy Studies*

- Bacterial and fungal diseases
- Behaviors and mental disorders
- Blood and lymph conditions
- Cancers and other neoplasms
- Digestive system diseases
- Diseases and abnormalities at or before birth
- Ear, nose, and throat diseases
- Eye diseases
- Gland and hormone related diseases
- Heart and blood diseases
- Immune system diseases
- Injuries, poisonings, and occupational conditions
- Mouth and tooth diseases
- Muscle, bone, and cartilage diseases
- Nervous system diseases
- Nutritional and metabolic diseases
- Respiratory tract (lung and bronchial) diseases
- Skin and connective tissue diseases
- Symptoms and general pathology
- Urinary tract, sexual organs, and pregnancy conditions
- Viral diseases

*More than 236 gene therapy studies have been approved by the National Institutes of Health.

CASE STUDY 35-4 Your friend tells you that she heard there is a cloned human infant living in Florida. What should you say?

Answers to Case Studies are available on the Evolve website: ***http://evolve.elsevier.com/Gerdin***

More than 3000 people have been treated with one of several techniques called gene therapy (Box 35-4). Gene therapy is used to treat diseases such as heart disease, cystic fibrosis, infectious disease, and cancer. In cancer therapy, genes may be inserted into a tumor by using a virus to "infect" the cell with new information. Treatment with gene therapy is expensive. The cost of one treatment may range from $150,000 to $300,000. The Center for Biologics Evaluation and Research regulates human gene therapy products. Gene therapy is available only in a research setting.

Performance Instruction

Electrophoresis

To determine a genetic "fingerprint," the DNA must first be removed from the nucleus of the cell. This is accomplished by using a detergent to break the cell membranes open. An enzyme is then used to separate the DNA strands into segments. The DNA is then removed by using a centrifuge to separate the heavier cell part away from it. Once removed, the DNA may be placed in a solution for electrophoresis (Fig. 35-7). An agarose gel bed is prepared, through which the DNA will move. Templates are used during the preparation to make "wells," or spaces in which the DNA samples are placed. The electrical current of the electrophoresis technique draws the DNA through the gel. Once completed, the gel bed may be dyed to compare the bands from each DNA sample.

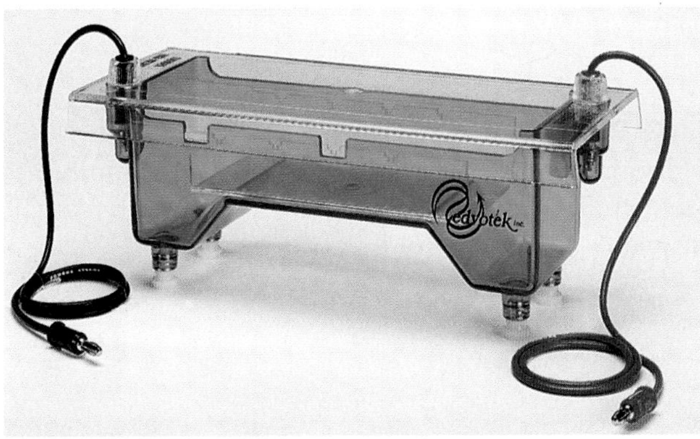

FIGURE 35-7 Electrophoresis uses a slight charge to separate DNA into a pattern that is unique to each individual. (Courtesy of Edvotek, Bethesda, Md.)

Electrophoresis may also be used to separate proteins on the basis of their size. (See Skill List 35-1, Extracting DNA; Skill List 35-2, Preparing Agarose Gel for Electrophoresis; and Skill List 35-3, Using a Micropipette, pp. 572–573).

Summary

- The function of the biotechnology team is to apply scientific and engineering techniques to the manipulation of genes.
- The role of the biotechnologist is to use gene manipulation to improve animal and plant products.
- The structure of DNA is a double-helix. It provides the genetic code for making proteins. It replicates by splitting in half and duplicating each side.
- Three research techniques used by biotechnologists are gene cloning, gene splicing, and gene therapy.
- Three ethical concerns that have been raised regarding DNA research include possible control of human characteristics, safety of the created organisms, and discrimination based on the genetic makeup of individuals.

Review Questions

1. Describe the duties, educational preparation, lines of authority, and credentialing of five biotechnology health care personnel.
2. Describe the method and use of the techniques of cloning, genetic engineering, and gene therapy.
3. Describe three ethical concerns regarding DNA research.
4. Choose one career from Box 35-2. Research the cost of education and annual earnings in local institutions. Write a paragraph describing the factors that might explain why the local and national economic figures vary.
5. Use each of the following terms in one or more sentences that correctly relate their meaning: electrophoresis, eugenics, forensics, and selective breeding.
6. Write a paragraph that describes the relationship of the following terms: chromosome, deoxyribose, DNA, gene, helix, nucleic acid, and phosphate.

Critical Thinking

1. Investigate and compare the cost of various types of biotechnology tests and procedures.
2. Research and report the cost of education for two biotechnology professionals.
3. Identify a "scare story" from the media regarding biotechnology. For example, the media reported the impending extinction of monarch butterflies because of pollen of genetically engineered corn. It was also reported that genetically engineered corn that was accidentally introduced into grain used in tacos caused allergic reactions. Investigate and report the facts of the story chosen.
4. Investigate and report the incidence of researchers failing to report "adverse events" involving gene therapy trials to the NIH. For example, the FDA stopped research by scientists at Tufts University in 2000 because it was believed they did not report the deaths of two volunteers being treated with gene therapy to grow new blood vessels.
5. Investigate and describe the uses of bioinformatics, including evolutionary studies and gene relationships to disease.
6. Use the Internet to investigate and describe the categories of genetic testing.
7. Create a career ladder for biotechnology careers. Describe why it is or is not possible to move from one level to another in the field.
8. Write a paragraph and prepare an effective oral presentation describing the origin of one eponym from Table 35-3.

Explore the Web

Career Information

Bureau of Labor Statistics
http://www.bls.gov/

Salary.com
http://salary.com

Professional Association

National Center for Biotechnology Information (NCBI)
http://www.ncbi.nlm.nih.gov/

STANDARDS AND ACCOUNTABILITY

See Evolve website: National Consortium on Health Science and Technology Education, National Health Science Career Cluster Models, Biotechnology Research and Development (R & D) Pathway Standards & Accountability; also available at: http://www.healthscienceconsortium.org/healthcare_standards.php.

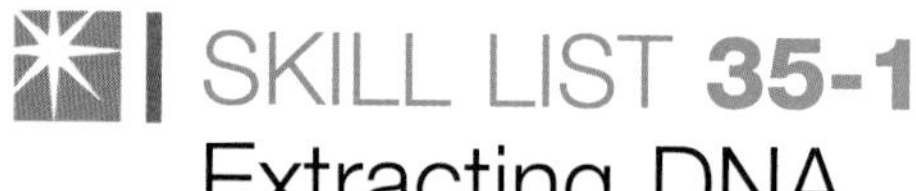

SKILL LIST 35-1 Extracting DNA

1. Maintain medical asepsis by using the guidelines provided in the Standard and Transmission-Based Precautions, including good handwashing technique and use of gloves as needed. The NIH has established safety guidelines for the handling and transfer of DNA.
2. Prepare a culture of nonpathogenic bacterial broth. Acceptable nonpathogenic bacteria, solution qualities, and percentages should be obtained by a qualified instructor or laboratory personnel.
3. Place a small amount of bacterial broth into a test tube and add a small amount of dishwashing solution to it. The dishwashing solution disrupts the cell membrane, opening the cells.
4. Place the test tube in a hot water bath for 15 minutes.
5. Use an eye dropper to pour a small amount of alcohol on top of the solution.
6. Carefully move a glass rod through the alcohol into the bacteria solution and turn it gently.
7. Continue to move the rod gently through the alcohol into the solution. The fiberlike DNA strands will "spool" around the glass rod for collection.
8. This DNA may be treated and stained to verify components of deoxyribose or phosphates.
9. Clean all materials and return them to the designated location for storage.

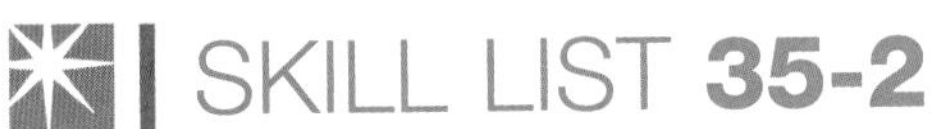

SKILL LIST 35-2
Preparing Agarose Gel for Electrophoresis

1. Maintain medical asepsis by using the guidelines provided in the Standard and Transmission-Based Precautions, including good handwashing technique and use of gloves as needed.
2. Prepare an electrophoresis gel bed for use by taping the ends of the box to form a square.
3. Dilute the concentrated buffer with distilled or deionized water according to the manufacturer's instructions.
4. Weigh the agarose powder to obtain the concentration required by the experiment being performed.
5. Add the weighed powder to the diluted buffer solution.
6. Heat the mixture, swirling gently, to dissolve the agarose completely.
7. Cool the hot agarose to 50° C.
8. Pour the cooled agarose into the gel bed. Use a pipette to line the edges of the gel bed. Allow 2 to 3 minutes for the gel to solidify.
9. Place templates (combs) into the designated location in the electrophoresis gel bed to form wells.
10. Allow the gel to set or harden before use.

SKILL LIST 35-3
Using a Micropipette

1. Maintain medical asepsis by using the guidelines provided in the Standard and Transmission-Based Precautions, including good handwashing technique and use of gloves as needed.
2. Unlock the pipette by pulling the control button out and turning it to adjust the volume setting. Micropipettes may range from small volumes such as 0.5 to 2500 µL.
3. Lock the volume setting in place by pushing the control button down.
4. If dispensing a liquid against the inside dry surface of a vessel, prerinse the pipette tip with water before using it. Do not prerinse the tip if a liquid is already present in the vessel.
5. Press the control button down to the first stop.
6. Hold the pipette in a vertical position and immerse the pipette 2 to 3 mm into the liquid to be dispensed.
7. Allow the control button to glide back slowly, pulling the liquid into the pipette.
8. Touch the tip of the pipette to the side of the vessel while pulling it out.
9. Wipe off any external droplets of fluid from the tip with a lint-free tissue.
10. Hold the tip of the pipette against the wall of the vessel or on the surface of the liquid in the vessel where it is to be dispensed.
11. Slowly press the control button to the first stop, releasing the fluid. Wait 1 to 3 seconds.
12. Continue to press the control button down to the second stop to remove any remaining fluid.
13. While continuing to hold the control button down, remove the pipette by sliding the tip along the side of the vessel.
14. Remove the pipette by pressing the control button down to the final stop.
15. Clean the pipette by wiping it with a soap solution or isopropanol.
16. Rinse the pipette with distilled water and lubricate the piston slightly with silicone grease.
17. Return the pipette to the designated storage area.

APPENDIX I

Common Prefixes, Word Roots, and Suffixes

Word Root Examples

Root	Meaning	Example	Meaning
A			
aden	gland	adenoma	tumor of the gland
adren	adrenal gland	adrenalectomy	removal of the adrenal gland
angi	vessel	angiogram	picture (radiograph) of a vessel
appendic	appendix	appendectomy	removal of the appendix
arter	artery	arteriosclerosis	hardening of the artery
arthro	joint	arthritis	inflammation of the joint
aur	ear	auricle	pertaining to the ear
B			
bio	life	biology	study of life
blephar	eyelid	blepharospasm	uncontrolled muscle contraction of the eyelid
bronch	bronchus	bronchitis	inflammation of the bronchus
bucc	cheek	buccal	pertaining to the cheek
C			
calc	stone	renal calculus	kidney stone
carcin	cancer	carcinoma	tumor that is cancerous
cardio	heart	cardiology	study of the heart
cephal	head	encephalitis	inflammation on the inside of the brain
cerebr	brain	cerebrospinal	pertaining to the spine and brain
cervix	neck	cervical	pertaining to the neck
cheil	lip	cheilorrhaphy	suture of the lip
chole	bile	cholecystectomy	removal of the bile sac (gallbladder)
chondr	cartilage	chondrectomy	removal of cartilage
col	colon	colocentesis	surgical puncture of the colon
colpo	vagina	colporrhaphy	repair of the vagina
cost	rib	intercostal space	space between the ribs
cranio	skull	craniotomy	incision into the skull
cut	skin	cutaneous	pertaining to the skin
cysto	bladder	cystoscopy	examination of the bladder
cyt	cell	cytology	study of the cell

Word Root Examples—cont'd

Root	Meaning	Example	Meaning
D			
dactyl	finger	dactyledema	swelling of the finger
dent	tooth	dentiform	shape of a tooth
derm	skin	dermatitis	inflammation of the skin
dors	back	dorsolateral	pertaining to the side and back
dyn	pain	acrodynia	pain in the extremities
E			
emesis	vomiting	hematemesis	vomiting of blood
endarter	inside lining	endarterectomy	removal of the inside lining
enter	intestine	enteritis	inflammation of the intestines
erythro	red	erythrocyte	red blood cell
G			
gastr	stomach	gastritis	inflammation of the stomach
gen	originate, born	congenital	born with
gingiv	gums	gingivitis	inflammation of the gums
gloss	tongue	subglossal	below the tongue
glyc	sweet, sugar	glycogen	formed of sweet, sugar
gyne	woman	gynecology	study of woman
H			
helio	sun	heliotherapy	sun treatment
hemo	blood	hemogram	picture (radiograph) of the blood
hepato	liver	hepatomegaly	enlargement of the liver
histo	tissue	histoma	tumor of the tissue
hydro	water	hydrotherapy	water treatment
hypno	sleep	hypnotic	pertaining to sleep
hyster	uterus, womb	hysterectomy	removal of the uterus, womb
L			
laparo	abdomen	laparotomy	incision into the abdomen
later	side	lateral	pertaining to the side
lingua	tongue	sublingual	below the tongue
lip	fat	lipoid	resembling fat
lith	stone	lithotomy	incision into a stone
M			
mamm	breast	mammography	picture (radiograph) of the breast
manus	hand	manipulation	move about with the hands
mast	breast	mastitis	inflammation of the breast
meningo	membrane	meningitis	inflammation of the meninges
metra	uterus	myometrium	muscle of the uterus
myco	fungus	mycology	study of fungus
myelo	marrow	myelogram	picture of the bone marrow
myo	muscle	myoma	tumor of the muscle
myring	eardrum	myringotomy	incision into the eardrum

Continued

Word Root Examples—cont'd

Root	Meaning	Example	Meaning
N			
naso	nose	nasal	pertaining to the nose
nephr	kidney	nephrology	study of the kidney
neuro	nerve	neuralgia	painful nerves
noct	night	nocturia	urination at night
O			
ocul	eye	ocular	pertaining to the eye
odont	tooth	odontology	study of teeth
onco	mass, tumor	oncology	study of mass, tumor
oophor	ovary	oophorectomy	removal of the ovary
ophthalm	eye	ophthalmologist	one who studies the eye
orch	testicle	orchitis	inflammation of the testicle
orchido	testicle	orchidectomy	removal of a testicle
orth	straight, correct	orthopedics	dealing with straightening of bones
oss	bone	ossicle	small bone
osteo	bone	osteoarthritis	inflammation of the bone and joints
oto	ear	otoscope	instrument to view the ear
P			
pan	complete, all	panhysterectomy	complete removal of the uterus
path	disease	pathologist	one who studies disease
pedes	foot	pedicure	foot grooming
pepsi, pept	digest	peptic	pertaining to digestion
pharynx	throat	pharyngitis	inflammation of the throat
phlebo	vein	phlebitis	inflammation of the vein
phob	fear	phobia	fear of
phren	diaphragm, mind	phrenic	pertaining to the diaphragm
pleura	rib, side	pleuritis	inflammation of the rib, side
pnea	breathing	bradypnea	slow breathing
pneumo	air, lung	pneumonectomy	removal of the lung
pod	foot	podiatry	diagnosis and treatment of the foot
procto	rectum	proctoscopy	examination of the rectum
pseud	false	pseudocirrhosis	false condition of the liver
psora	itch	psoriasis	skin condition characterized by itching
psych	mind	psychology	study of the mind
pulmon	lung	pulmonary	pertaining to the lung
pyelo	kidney, pelvis	pyelonephrectomy	removal of the kidney
pyo	pus	pyuria	pus in the urine
Q			
quadr	four	quadriceps	four heads (muscle)
R			
ren	kidney	renal	pertaining to the kidney
retr	back, behind	retrograde	situated behind
rhin	nose	rhinoplasty	plastic repair of the nose

Continued

Word Root Examples—cont'd

Root	Meaning	Example	Meaning
S			
salping	fallopian tube	salpingectomy	removal of the fallopian tube
sarc	flesh	sarcoma	tumor of the flesh
sebum	oil	sebaceous	pertaining to oil
sedat	quiet, calm	sedation	calmed with medication
somni	sleep	insomnia	lack of sleep
splen	spleen	splenectomy	removal of the spleen
spondyl	vertebrae	spondylitis	inflammation of the vertebrae
stoma	mouth	stomatitis	inflammation of the mouth
T			
thorac	chest	thoracentesis	surgical puncture into the chest
thorax	chest	thoracotomy	incision into the chest
thromb	clot	thrombitis	inflammation of a clot
tox	poison	toxin	poisonous
trachea	windpipe	tracheotomy	incision into the windpipe
trophy	growth, nutrition	hypertrophy	greater than normal amount of growth
tympano	eardrum	tympanitis	inflammation of the eardrum
U			
utero	uterus	uteropexy	fixation of the uterus
V			
valv	valve	valvotomy	incision into a valve
vaso	vessel	vasectomy	removal of a vessel
vena	vein	venipuncture	puncture into a vein
ventr	front, abdomen	ventral	pertaining to the abdomen
vesic	bladder	vesicotomy	incision into the bladder
viscera	organ	visceral	pertaining to organs
vit	life	vital	pertaining to life

Prefix Examples

Prefix	Meaning	Example	Meaning
A			
a-	without	atrophy	without growth
ab-	away from	abduction	move away from
acro-	extremities	acromegaly	enlargement of the extremities
ad-	toward	adduction	move toward
ambi-	both	ambidextrous	able to use both hands
an-	without	anorexia	without appetite
ante-	before	antenatal	before birth
anti-	against, opposing	antiemetic	against emesis (vomiting)
astr-	star	astrocyte	star-shaped cell
auto-	self	autohemotherapy	transfusion using blood from self

Continued

Prefix Examples—cont'd

Prefix	Meaning	Example	Meaning
B			
bi-	two, both	bilateral	both sides
brachy-	short	brachymorphic	pertaining to a short form
brady-	slow	bradycardia	slow heart rate
C			
capit-	head	biceps	two head (muscle)
con-	with	congenital	born with
contra-	against	contraception	against conception
cryo-	cold	cryotherapy	treatment with cold
cyan-	blue	cyanoderm	blue skin
D			
dys-	bad, out of order	dyspepsia	digestion that is bad (indigestion)
dys-	painful	dyspnea	painful respiration
E			
ecto-	on the outside	ectopic	on the outside of the normal location
en-	inside	encephalotomy	incision into the inside of the head (brain)
end-	inside	endocardium	inside of the heart
epi-	upon, in addition to	epigastric	upon the stomach
erthro-	red	erythrocyte	red cell
eu-	normal	eupnea	normal breathing
ex-	out, away from	exogenic	produced away from
H			
hemi-	half	hemiplegia	paralysis of half of the body
hyper-	above, more than	hyperglycemia	above the normal amount of sugar in the blood
hypo-	under, beneath	hypoglycemia	under the normal amount of sugar in the blood
I			
inter-	between	intercostal	between the ribs
intra-	within	intravenous	within the vein
L			
leuk-	white	leukopenia	decrease in number of white blood cells
M			
melan-	black	melanoma	black tumor
micro-	small	microencephaly	small brain
N			
neo-	new	neoplasm	new tissue
P			
para-	beside, by the side	paraplegia	paralysis beside
peri-	around, about	periodontal	around a tooth
poly-	many, much	polydactyl	many fingers

Continued

Prefix Examples—cont'd

Prefix	Meaning	Example	Meaning
post-	after, behind	postnatal	after birth
pre-	before, in front of	prenatal	before birth
pro-	in front of	prolapse	an organ's slipping in front of its usual position
S			
semi-	half	semicomatose	half conscious
sub-	under	subglossal	under the tongue
supra-	above, over	supracostal	above the ribs
T			
tachy-	fast	tachycardia	fast heart rate

Suffix Examples

Suffix	Meaning	Example	Meaning
A			
-ac	pertaining to	cardiac	pertaining to the heart
-al	pertaining to	cervical	pertaining to the neck
-algia	pain	neuralgia	pain of the nerve
-ar	pertaining to	muscular	pertaining to the muscles
-asthenia	weakness, lack of	myasthenia	muscle weakness
C			
-cele	tumor or swelling	cystocele	tumor of swelling of the bladder
-centesis	surgical puncture	arthrocentesis	surgical puncture into a joint
-cle	small, little	ossicle	small bone
-crine	to secrete	endocrine	to secrete inside
D			
-desis	surgical union or fixation	arthrodesis	fixation of a joint
E			
-eal	pertaining to	esophageal	pertaining to the esophagus
-ectasis	expansion	nephrectasis	enlargement of the kidney
-ectomy	removal of	chondrectomy	removal of a rib
-emia	blood condition	anemia	blood condition of too few cells
-esthesia	sensation	anesthesia	lack of sensation
G			
-genic	originating from	carcinogenic	originating from cancer
-gram	record	angiogram	record of a vessel
-graphy	recording	mammography	recording of a breast
I			
-iasis	condition resulting	lithiasis	condition resulting in a stone
-ic	pertaining to	enteric	pertaining to the intestines

Continued

Suffix Examples—cont'd

Suffix	Meaning	Example	Meaning
-ist	one who practices	neurologist	one who practices study of nerves
-itis	inflammation of	myositis	inflammation of the muscle
L			
-lysis	loosening, destruction of	hemolysis	destruction of red blood cells
M			
-malacia	softening	adenomalacia	softening of the gland
-megaly	enlargement	cardiomegaly	enlargement of the heart
O			
-oid	like, resembling	lipoid	resembling fat
-ologist	specialist in the study of	radiologist	specialist in the study of radiographs
-ology	study of	pathology	study of disease
-oma	tumor	adenoma	glandular tumor
-orrhea	discharge	rhinorrhea	discharge from the nose
-osis	condition of	nephrosis	condition of the kidney
-ostomy	opening into	colostomy	opening into the colon
-otomy	incision into	arthrotomy	incision into a joint
-ous	pertaining to, containing	sebaceous	pertaining to oil
P			
-pathy	disease of	osteopathy	disease of the bone
-penia	decrease, deficiency	leukopenia	deficiency of white blood cells
-pexy	surgical fixation	nephropexy	surgical fixation of the kidney
-phobia	fear	photophobia	fear of light
-plasty	surgical repair	rhinoplasty	surgical repair of the nose
-plegia	paralysis	hemiplegia	paralysis of half of the body
-ptosis	drooping	blepharoptosis	drooping eyelid
R			
-rrhexis	breaking, bursting	cardiorrhexis	breaking of heart
-rrhaphy	suture	herniorrhaphy	suture of a swelling
S			
-sclerosis	hardening	atherosclerosis	hardening of the vessels
-scopy	look, observe	cystoscopy	look into the bladder
-spasm	involuntary contraction	cardiospasm	involuntary contraction of the heart
-stasis	halting	hemostasis	halting the flow of blood
-stenosis	narrowing	arteriostenosis	narrowing of the artery
U			
-ular	pertaining to	valvular	pertaining to a valve
-uria	presence of (a substance) in urine	hematuria	blood in the urine

APPENDIX II

Medical Charts, Graphs, and Forms

Working Copy

BARNES-JEWISH HOSPITAL

Nursing Shift Assessment C-6

Requested by: CAROL

789651458 X
Collins, Phil

S.S.
Dr.
Unit: Bed:

Search Interval From: 05-Dec-2010 at 07:00
To: 06-Dec-2010 at 14:51

Patient Assessment

		Monday 12/06 07:00
N/S	**NEUROSENSORY STANDARD** Alert and awake. If asleep awakens to name. Verbal appropriate, clear, and understandable. Swallows without coughing. Oriented to time, place, person and situation. Behavior is appropriate to situation. Moves all extremities well, ambulates with steady gait.	Within Normal Limits
RESP	**RESPIRATORY STANDARD** Respirations are even and unlabored. Nailbeds and mucous membranes are pink. Patent airway. Lung sounds clear to auscultation. No cough noted	Within Normal Limits
CARD	**CARDIOVASCULAR STANDARD** Regular palpable pulses. Skin pallor within patient's norm. Skin warm and dry. No edema.	Within Normal Limits
SKIN	**SKIN INTEGRITY STANDARD** Skin and mucous membranes intact without notable lesions or impaired integrity. Mucous membranes moist and pink. Braden Score greater than 17.	* Exception as noted below
	Braden Risk Assessment	Mobility: Slightly Limited (3) Sensory: Slightly Limited (3) Moisture: Occasionally Moist (3) Activity: Walks Occasionally (3) Nutrition: Adequate (3) Friction/Shear: Potential Problem (2) Total Score 17
	Casts, Splints, Braces Type: Fiberglass Cast Site: Right Lower Leg	Maintains correct anatomical position No pressure areas noted Distal extremity pink warm to touch Palpable distal pulse Capillary Refill <3 seconds Sensation normal Able to move distal phalanges.
	VASCULAR ACCESS STANDARD IV SITE: Site free of redness, swelling, pain, bleeding, drainage, IV patent, dressing occlusive and intact.	
NUTR	**NUTRITION STANDARD** Tolerating prescribed diet without nausea and vomiting. Eating at least 75% of each meal without difficulty. Feeds self.	Within normal limits
	Diet Type	Regular
GI	**GASTROINTESTINAL STANDARD** Abdomen soft. Bowel sounds active all 4 quadrants. No pain with palpation. Having bowel movements within patient's normal pattern, consistency, and color.	Within Normal Limits
GU	**GENITOURINARY STANDARD** Continent of urine. Urine clear and yellow to amber color.	Within Normal Limits
PSYCH	**PSYCHOSOCIAL STANDARD** Accepts situation and facial expressions are appropriate. family support available and patient receives visitors. Able to communicate without assistance.	Within Normal Limits
EDU	Health Status Teaching	
	Tests/Procedures/Therapies	
	Medication Teaching	
	Nutrition Teaching	
	Medical Equipment Teaching	
HMGT	Equipment	
Charted By		cl

Signatures:
cl C. Logan, RN

Printed: 06-Dec-2010 at 14:51

A

FIGURE II-1 **A**, Charting by exception. (Courtesy Barnes-Jewish Hospital, BJC Health System, St. Louis, Mo.)

VITAL SIGN / I & O / PAIN RECORD

Date ______________ **INTAKE** *KEY:* **C**ontinent / **I**ncontinent **OUTPUT**

	Parenteral				Oral / Tube Feedings			Urine		Other				
To Count:					Amt	Amt	Amt	Amt	Amt	Amt	Amt	Amt	Amt	Amt/Freq
2300					120									
2400								325		Chest Tube 75				
0100		50												
0200														
0300														
0400														
0500														
0600														
8 hr Sub Totals	50				120			8 hr Sub Totals 325		75				
8 hr Total Parenteral					8 hr total Oral/tube									
					8 hr Shift Intake			8 hr Shift's Output						
To Count:														
0700					650									
0800								500						
0900														
1000		50								75				
1100														
1200														
1300														
1400														
8 hr Sub Totals	50				650			8 hr Sub Totals 500		75				
8 hr Total Parenteral					8 hr total Oral/tube									
					8 hr Shift Intake			8 hr Shift's Output						
To Count:														
1500					650			600						
1600														
1700										75				
1800														
1900		50												
2000														
2100														
2200														
8 hr Sub Totals	50				650			8 hr Sub Totals 600		75				
8 hr Total Parenteral					8 hr total Oral/tube									
					8 hr Shift Intake			8 hr Shift's Output						
Twenty-four hour Total								Twenty-four hour Total						

FLUID EQUIVALENTS			
1 oz	30cc	8 oz (1 cup)	240cc
4 oz (1/2 cup)	120cc	12 oz (soda-1 can)	360cc
6 oz (3/4 cup)	180cc		

ADDRESSOGRAPH / LABEL

VITAL SIGN / I & O / PAIN RECORD

SLM-1000-035 (6/2000) 10 BACK

B

FIGURE II-1, cont'd B, Intake and output summary. (Courtesy Barnes-Jewish Hospital, BJC Health System, St. Louis, Mo.)

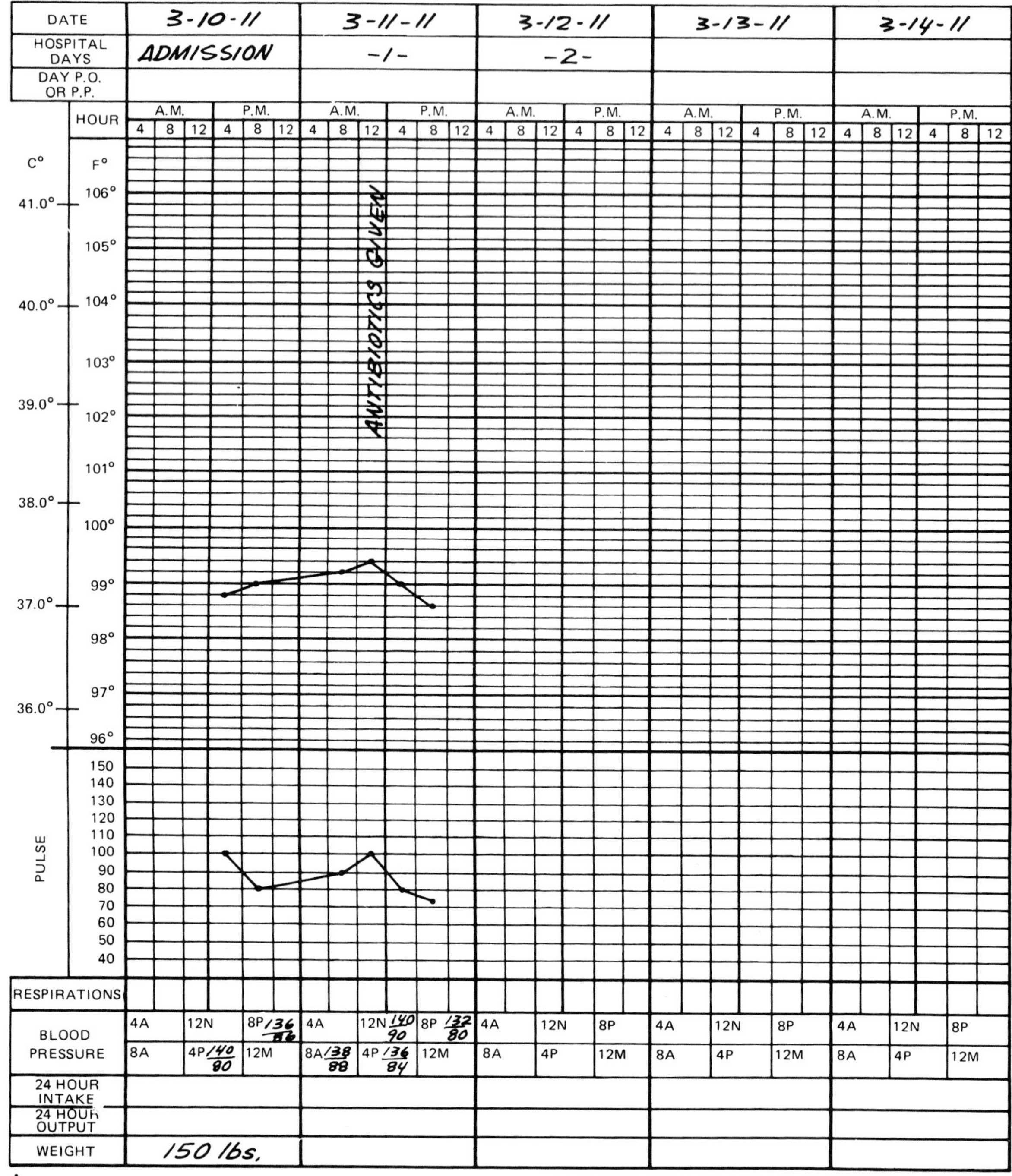

FIGURE II-2 **A**, The graphic sheet is used to record vital signs during a patient's hospital stay.

DATE: 3-11-11

		7-3	3-11	11-7	
SKIN	COLOR: PINK	—	—		
	PALE	B SMITH, RN	R DAVIS - RN		
	JAUNDICE	—	—		
	CYANOTIC	—	—		
	MOISTURE: WARM	—	R. DAVIS - RN		
	DRY	—	—		
	COOL	—	—		
	DIAPHORETIC	SLIGHT - B SMITH	R. DAVIS - RN		
LEVEL OF CONSCIOUSNESS	ALERT & COOPERATIVE	B. SMITH	R. DAVIS - RN		C/O HEADACHE, MD NOTIFIED 13:00 - R. DAVIS - RN
	RESPOND TO PAINFUL STIMULI	—	—		
	RESPOND TO VERBAL STIMULI	—	—		
	ALERT & UNCOOPERATIVE	—	—		
	COMATOSE	—	—		
	INCOHERENT	—	—		
	SLURRED SPEECH	—	—		
ABDOMEN	BS – PRESENT	B. SMITH	—		
	BS – ABSENT	—	—		
	FLAT – SOFT	B. SMITH	—		
	DISTENDED	—	—		
	NG TUBE	—	—		
	COLORS	—	—		
RESPIRATORY	O_2 – VIA/RATE	—	—		
	TRACH CARE	—	—		
	IPPB/UPDRAFT	—	—		
	TRI FLOW	—	—		
	COUGH & DEEP BREATHE	—	—		
		—	—		
IV'S	IV TYPE & FLOW RATE	—	B. SMITH		IV INSERTED PER MD ORDER BS, RN
	SITE/CONDITION	—	B. SMITH		IV INSERTED 14:30 - B. SMITH, RN
	IMED	—	—		
	HEP LOCK	—	—		
	IV DSG	—	—		
	IV TUBING	—	—		
ELIMINATION	VOIDING QS	B. SMITH	R. DAVIS - RN		
	FOLEY PATENT	—	—		
	COLOR	—	—		
	CATH CARE/TAPED	—	—		
	FOLEY DC	—	—		
	STOOL	$\bar{c}$ FORMED	—		
		BRN			
SAFETY PRECAUTIONS	SEIZURE PRECAUTIONS				
	SIDE RAIL UP				
	RESTRAINTS CHECKED				

B

FIGURE II-2, cont'd **B**, Nurse's notes provide a quick and effective way to document the care provided (front).

Continued

Section	Item	7-3	3-11	11-7	NURSE'S NOTES
HYGIENE	BATH	B.SMITH, RN	—		
	MOUTHCARE	B.SMITH	—		
	PERICARE	—	—		
	HS CARE	—	—		
DIETARY	DIET/TYPE	GOOD/REG	POOR/REG		17:30 c/o STOMACH ACHE - R. DAVIS - RN
	TUBE FEEDING	—	—		
	HS SNACK	—	—		
ACTIVITIES	BED REST	—	—		
	BRP	—	—		
	TURNING	—	—		
	CHAIR	—	—		
	AMBULATION	B.SMITH	R.DAVIS		
TREATMENTS	ENEMA'S – TYPE/NO.	—	—		
	DOUCHE – TYPE/NO.	—	—		
	SCRUBS/PREPS	—	—		
	K-PADS	—	—		
	SITZ BATH	—	—		
	TRACTION: TYPE	—	—		
	OTHER:	—	—		
SPECIMENS	URINE	—	—		
	STOOL	—	—		
	SPUTUM	—	—		
	OTHER: SPECIFY	—	—		
		—	—		
DRESSINGS	SUTURE LINE	—	—		
	DRAINS/DRAINAGE	—	—		
	DRESSING CHANGED	—	—		
TED'S	PRESENT	—	—		
	OFF X 30 MIN. AM PM	—	—		
VISITS	PHYSICIAN VISIT AM PM	10:00 B.S.			
	ORDERS NOTED	10:15 B.S.			
	INITIALS RN/LPN	B.SMITH, RN	R.DAVIS-RN		
ADDITIONAL NOTES					

C

FIGURE II-2, cont'd **C**, Nurse's notes provide a quick and effective way to document the care provided (back).

ADMISSION NURSING ASSESSMENT

STATUS UPON ADMISSION

Admission Notes

Date of admission ____/____/____ Time ________ a.m. p.m.

Transported by ____________________

Accompanied by ____________________

Age ______ Sex ________ Weight ________ Height: ______ Ft. ______ In.

Vitals: T ________ P ________ (❑ Reg ❑ Irreg) R ________ B/P ____/____

Attending physician notified? ❑ No ❑ Yes, date/time ____/____/____ ________ a.m. p.m.

Diagnosis: ____________________ Date last chest x-ray or PPD ____/____/____

Allergies

Meds ____________________

Food ____________________

Other ____________________

Skin Condition

Using the diagrams provided, indicate all body marks such as old/recent scars (surgical and other), bruises, discolorations, abrasions, pressure ulcers, or questionable markings. Indicate size, depth (in cms), color and drainage.

RIGHT LEFT

COMMENTS: ____________________

SPECIAL TREATMENTS & PROCEDURES: ____________________

PAIN

(As described by resident/representative)

Frequency:
- ❑ No pain
- ❑ Less than daily
- ❑ Daily, but not constant
- ❑ Constant

Location: ____________________

Intensity:
- ❑ No pain
- ❑ Mild pain
- ❑ Distressing pain
- ❑ Severe pain
- ❑ Horrible pain
- ❑ Excruciating pain

Pain on admission:
❑ No ❑ Yes, describe ____________________

CURRENT STATUS

General Skin Condition

Check all that apply.
❑ Reddened ❑ Pale ❑ Jaundiced
❑ Cyanotic ❑ Ashen
❑ Dry ❑ Moist ❑ Oily ❑ Warm ❑ Cold
❑ Edema, site ____________________

Physical Status (describe if applicable otherwise indicate NA)

Paralysis/paresis-site, degree ____________________

Contracture(s)-site, degree ____________________

Congenital anomalies ____________________

Prosthesis: ____________________

Other ____________________

Functional Status

TRANSFERS-ABLE TO TRANSFER
- ❑ Independently
- ❑ 1 person assist
- ❑ 2 person assist
- ❑ Total assist

WEIGHT BEARING-ABLE TO BEAR
- ❑ Full weight
- ❑ Partial weight
- ❑ Non-weight bearing

AMBULATION-ABLE TO AMBULATE
- ❑ Independently
- ❑ 1 person assist
- ❑ 2 person assist
- ❑ With device
  Type ____________________
- ❑ Wheelchair only
- ❑ Wheelchair/propels self
- ❑ Bedrest

SUPPORTIVE DEVICES USED:
- ❑ Elastic hose
- ❑ Footboard
- ❑ Bed cradle
- ❑ Air mattress
- ❑ Sheepskin
- ❑ Eggcrate
- ❑ Hand rolls ❑ Sling ❑ Trapeze
- ❑ Other ____________________
- ❑ Other ____________________

Drug Therapy

	DRUG	DOSE/FREQUENCY		DRUG	DOSE/FREQUENCY
1			6		
2			7		
3			8		
4			9		
5			10		

NAME-Last	First	Middle	Attending Physician	Record No.	Room/Bed

CFS 5-3HH R1001

ADMISSION NURSING ASSESSMENT
❑ Continued on Reverse

FIGURE II-3 Admission form. (Courtesy Briggs Corp., Des Moines, Iowa. In Sorrentino SA: *Mosby's textbook for nursing assistants*, ed 7, St. Louis, 2008, Mosby.)

Continued

CURRENT STATUS - CONTINUED

Hearing	Right	Left	R & L	Vision	Right	Left	R & L	Communication
Adequate				Adequate				❑ Clear
Adequate w/aid				Adequate w/glasses				❑ Aphasic ❑ Dysphasic
Poor				Poor				Language(s) Spoken:
Deaf				Blind				________

Oral Assessment

Complete oral cavity exam: ❑ Yes ❑ No
If yes, condition ________

Own teeth: ❑ Yes ❑ No
If yes, condition ________

Dentures: Upper ❑ Comp ❑ Part
Lower ❑ Comp ❑ Part
Do dentures fit? ❑ Yes ❑ No

Eating/Nutrition

❑ Dependent ❑ Independent ❑ Needs assist
❑ Dysphagic; reason ________
❑ Adaptive equipment (specify) ________

Type/consistency of diet ________

Food likes ________
Food dislikes ________
Bev. preference ________
HS snack preferred: ❑ Yes ❑ No

Sleep Patterns

Usual bed time ________ a.m./p.m.
Usual arising time ________ a.m./p.m.
Usual nap time ________ a.m./p.m.
Other ________

Bathing/Oral Hyg.	Indep.	Assist	Dep.	General Grooming	Indep.	Assist	Dep.
Tub				Shave			
Shower				Grooming			
Bed bath				Dressing			
Oral hygiene				Shampoo			

Psychosocial Functioning

FAMILY RELATIONSHIPS:
Members visit (frequency) ________

Closest relationship with ________

WHICH WORDS BEST DESCRIBE RESIDENT? ❑ Alert ❑ Angry ❑ Fearful ❑ Noisy ❑ Friendly ❑ Cooperative ❑ Lethargic ❑ ________ ❑ Non-questioning ❑ Combative
ANSWERS QUESTIONS: ❑ Readily ❑ Reluctantly ❑ Inappropriately
MOOD: ❑ Passive ❑ Depressed ❑ Elated ❑ Quiet ❑ Secure ❑ Questioning ❑ Talkative ❑ Homesick ❑ Wanders mentally ❑ Hyperactive ❑ ________

ORIENTED: ❑ Yes ❑ No, if No,
DISORIENTED TO: ❑ Time ❑ Place ❑ Person

COMPREHENSION: ❑ Slow ❑ Quick ❑ Unable to understand
MOTIVATION: ❑ Good ❑ Fair ❑ Poor
PERSONAL HABITS: Smokes? ❑ Yes ❑ No Uses alcohol? ❑ Yes ❑ No

RESIDENT GIVEN EXPLANATION OF/OR INVOLVED IN PLAN OF CARE? ❑ Yes ❑ No
RESIDENT ORIENTED TO FACILITY? ❑ Call light ❑ Bathroom ❑ Mealtime ❑ Activities

Bowel and Bladder Evaluation

Uses: ❑ Toilet ❑ Urinal ❑ Bedpan ❑ Bedside commode
BOWEL HABITS: Continent? ❑ Yes ❑ No Constipated? ❑ Yes ❑ No Laxative used? ❑ Yes ❑ No
Enemas used? ❑ Yes ❑ No Last bowel movement ________ a.m./p.m.
BLADDER HABITS: Continent? ❑ Yes ❑ No Dribbles? ❑ Yes ❑ No Catheter? ❑ Yes, type ________ ❑ No
Urine color ________ Consistency ________ Time last voiding ________ a.m./p.m.

Restorative Programs Indicated

Based on the foregoing assessment, check all that apply.

❑ ROM
❑ Splint or brace assistance
❑ Bed mobility training & skill practice
❑ Transfer training & skill practice
❑ Walking training & skill practice
❑ Dressing/grooming training & skill practice
❑ Eating/swallowing training & skill practice
❑ Appliance/prosthesis training & skill practice
❑ Communication training & skill practice
❑ Scheduled tolieting
❑ Bladder retraining

Comments: ________

Therapy Indicated

❑ Physical
❑ Occupational
❑ Speech
Comments: ________

Completed by:
Signature/Title ________ Date ________

NAME-Last	First	Middle	Attending Physician	Record No.	Room/Bed

ADMISSION NURSING ASSESSMENT

FIGURE II-3, cont'd

2 to 20 years: Boys
Body mass index-for-age percentiles

NAME ______________________

RECORD # ____________

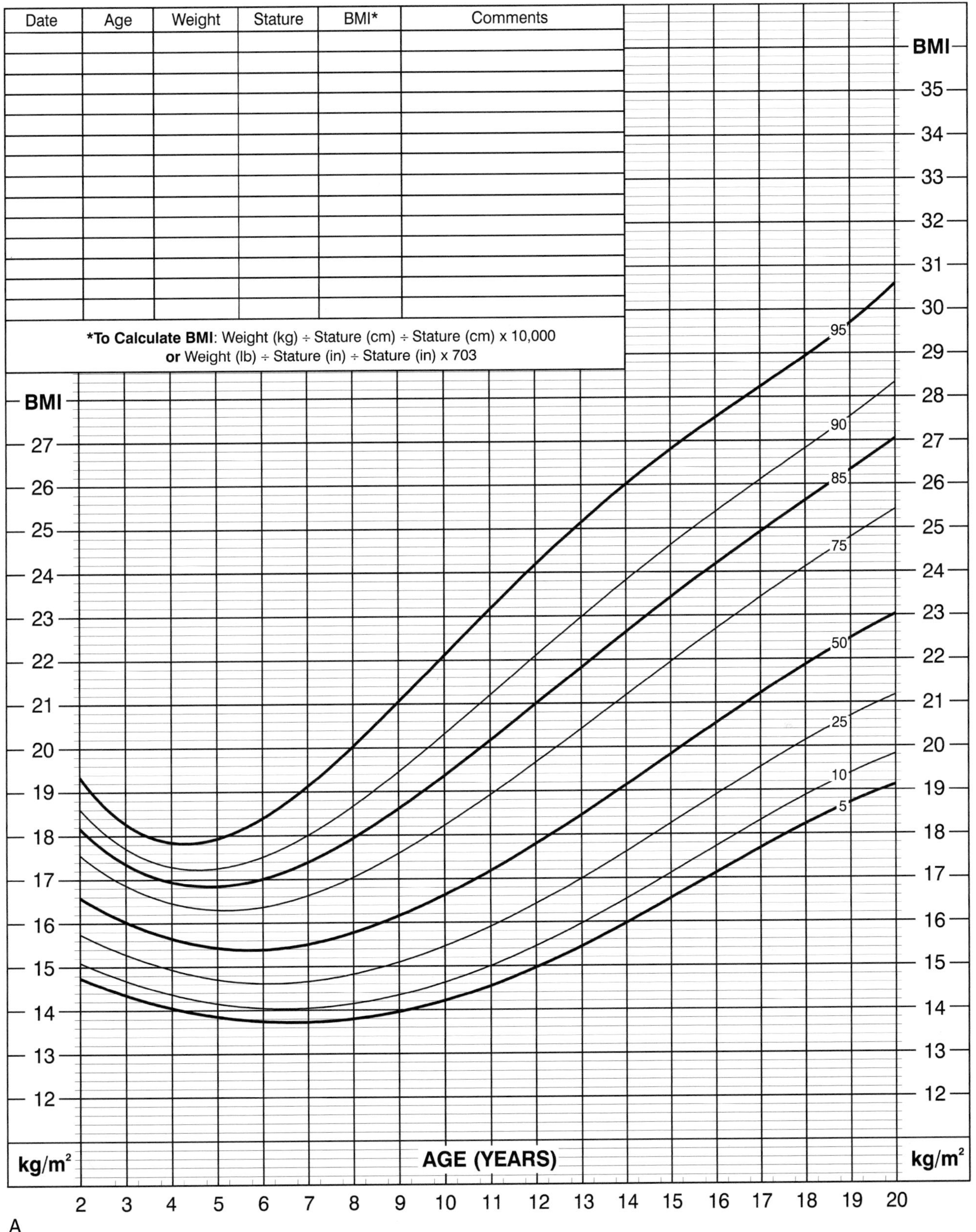

A

FIGURE II-4 Body mass index-for-age percentiles **A**, Boys. (From Centers for Disease Control and Prevention: http://www.cdc.gov/growthcharts/.)

Continued

2 to 20 years: Girls
Body mass index-for-age percentiles

NAME ____________________

RECORD # ____________

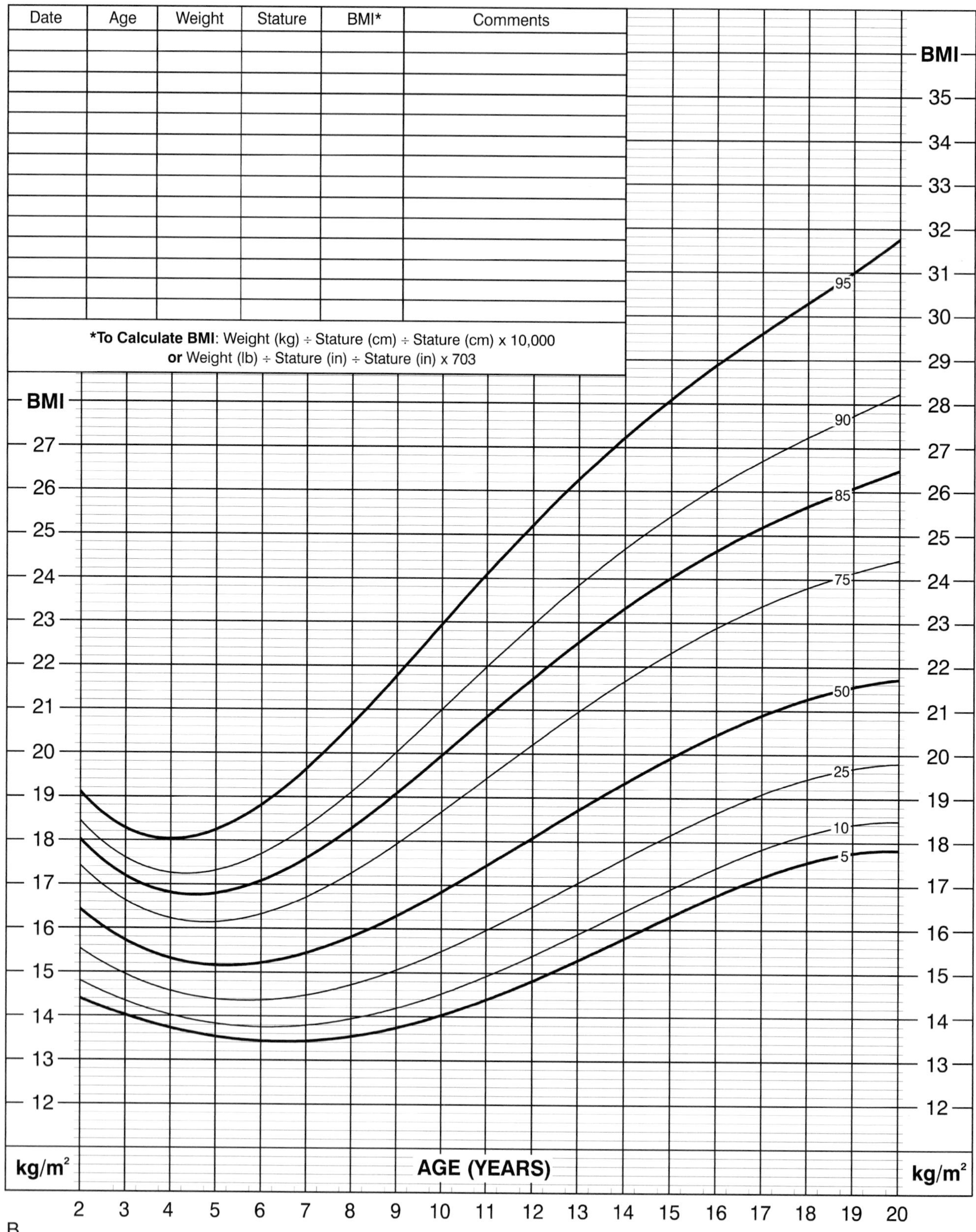

FIGURE II-4, cont'd **B**, Girls. (From Centers for Disease Control and Prevention: http://www.cdc.gov/growthcharts/.)

MEDICAL ALERT

Initial Clinical Examination
(Use this form on initial visit only)

Date ______________________

Patient Name ______________________ Patient # ______________________

Chief Dental Complaint
Oral Habits
Existing Illnesses/Current Drugs Used
Allergies

History Verification - A health (medical and dental) history has been completed and reviewed by:

Dr. ______________________

Initials ______________ Date ______________

Blood Pressure		Pulse
Date Last Dental Exam		
General Physical Condition		
Under Physician's Care Now?		
History of Bleeding?		
Reaction to Anesthetic?		
Existing Xrays	Date	Xrays Required
Existing Prosthesis		
Max.	Date Placed:	Condition:
Min.	Date Placed:	Condition:

Oral, Soft Tissue Examination and TMJ Evaluation	
Area	Description of Any Problem
Pharynx	
Tonsils	
Soft Palate	
Hard Palate	
Tongue	
Floor of Mouth	
Buccal Mucosa	
Lips	
Skin	
Lymph Nodes	
Occlusion	

R. L.

R. L.

TMJ Evaluation

Right ☐ Crepitus ☐ Snapping/Popping

Left ☐ Crepitus ☐ Snapping/Popping

Tenderness to Palpation:

TMJ ☐ Right ☐ Left

Muscles ______________________

Deviation on Closing ____________ Rmm ____________ Lmm

Needs further TMJ evaluation ☐ Yes ☐ No

If Yes, use TMJ evaluation form

Oral Hygiene	☐ Excellent	☐ Good	☐ Fair	☐ Poor
Calculus	☐ None	☐ Little	☐ Moderate	☐ Heavy
Plaque	☐ None	☐ Little	☐ Moderate	☐ Heavy
Gingival Bleeding		☐ Localized	☐ General	☐ None
Perio Exam	☐ Yes	☐ No		

Additional Comments: ______________________

A

FIGURE II-5 Clinical examination form. **A**, Front. (Courtesy Colwell, a Division of Patterson Dental Supply Inc., St. Paul, Minn.)

Continued

Missing Teeth and Restorations

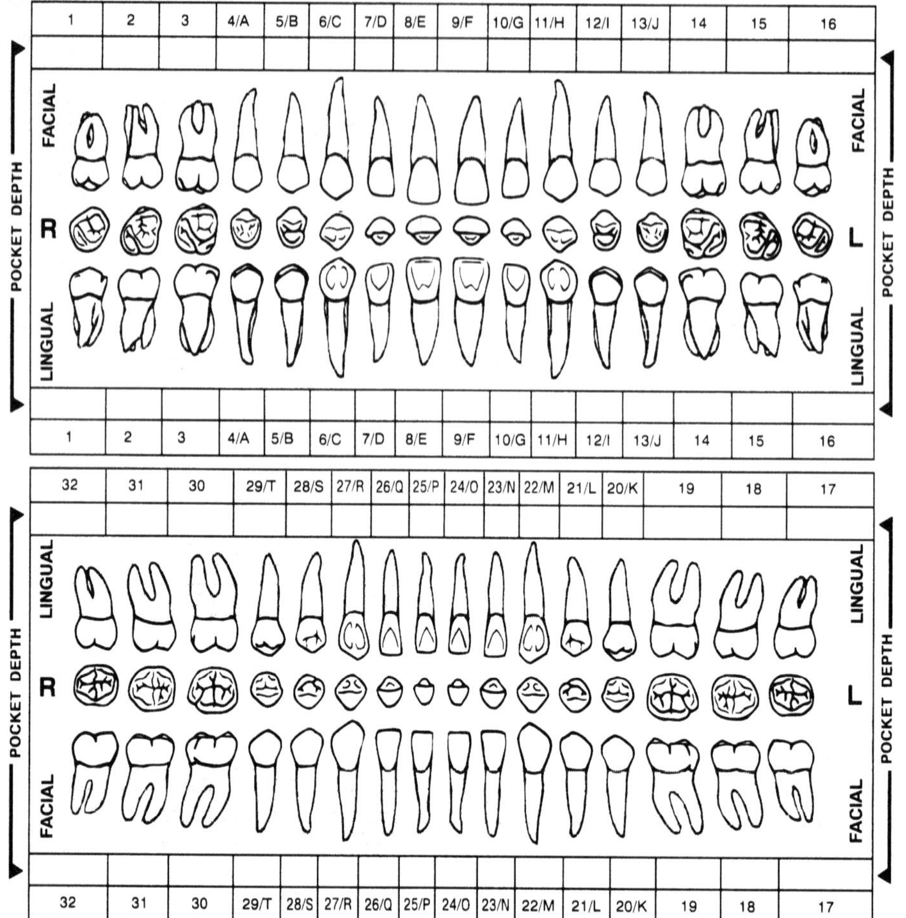

Diagnosis and Treatment Plan

Date	Tooth	Surface	Service Planned

Consent to treatment plan obtained: Date________________ **Dr.**______________________________________

B

FIGURE II-5, cont'd **B**, Back. (Courtesy Colwell, a Division of Patterson Dental Supply Inc., St. Paul, Minn.)

Preadmission Form

Patient Information	Last Name First Middle Address City State Zip County Telephone Social Security # Date of Birth Maiden Name Reason for Admission OB/GYN Patients: Date of last menstrual cycle OB/GYN's name OB Due Date Religion (optional) Notify clergy ____ yes ____ no Telephone Spouse's Name Social Security #
Employment Information	Occupation Employer Address City State Zip Telephone Spouse's Occupation Spouse's Employer Telephone Address City State Zip
Person Responsible for Payment	Name (if other than yourself) Address City State Zip County Telephone Relationship to Patient Occupation Employer Employer's Address City State Zip Telephone How long employed?
Emergency Contact	Name (relative or friend) Address City State Zip Telephone
Insurance Information	Subscriber's name Relationship to Policy Holder Subscriber's Identification/Member Number Effective Date Type of Policy ____ individual ____ group Group Number Employer (if group policy)
Other Insurance	Insurance company Policy Holder's Name Relationship to Policy Holder Policy Number Effective Date Type of Policy ____ individual _____ group Group Number Employer (if group policy)
Medicare	Name (exactly as shown on card) Claim Number Effective Date
Previous Admissions	Have you ever been admitted to this hospital before? _____ yes _____ no
Accident Information	Date of accident Time of accident Is accident job related? _____ yes _____ no How did accident happen?
Signature	______________________________ Date ________________

FIGURE II-6 The patient may complete the admission form alone or with help from a health care worker.

Medical Benefits Request

Return To: Any Insurance Co.
Any Road
Any Town, USA 12345

Complete section 1-6.

Sign section 7 to have benefits paid to your doctor.

Complete Employee Information on reverse side.

If you have submitted a request for benefits to another plan, including Medicare, attach a copy of the bills you submitted to the other plan and the explanation of benefits you received from the other plan.

Attach itemized bills or ask your health care provider to complete the applicable section on the reverse side. The bills must include:

-patient's name -relationship to employee
-date of service -type of service rendered
-condition being treated

If this information is missing, write it on the bill and sign your name.

If prescription drugs are covered under your plan, submit receipts or a Prescription Drug Record form. Receipts must contain:

-drug name -purchase date -quantity
-dose per/day -strength -physician name
-charge -prescription number -pharmacy name/address
-nature of illness or injury

This information can be copied from the prescription bottle or box.

Incomplete forms will delay payment.

1. Employer Information
Name (as shown on ID card) | Policy/Group Number

2. Employee Information
Social Security Number - - | Name | Birth Date
___Active ___Retired | Address (include zip code) ___Address is new | Daytime Phone ( )
Date if retirement:

3. Patient Information
Social Security Number - - | Name | Birth Date
Relationship to Employee (circle) Self Spouse Child Other | Address (if different from employee)
Sex (circle) Male Female | Full Time Student (circle) Yes No | Expected Graduation Date | School Name | Marital Status
Is patient employed? (Circle) No Yes | Name/Address of Employer
Date of Retirement:

4. Other Coverage Information
Are any family members expenses covered by another group health plan, group pre-payment plan (Blue Cross-Blue Shield, etc.), no fault auto insurance, Medicare or any federal, state or local government plan? (circle)
No Yes
If yes, list policy or contract holder, policy or contract number(s) and name/address of insurance company or administrator:
Insured's Social Security Number | Insured's Name | Insured's Birth Date

5. Claim Information
If claim for a laboratory test or doctor's office visit, state diagnosis or nature of illness: | Is claim related to employment? (circle) No Yes
Is claim related to an accident? (circle) No Yes | If yes, date | Time | am pm
Description of Accident:

6. Release
To all providers of health care:
You are authorized to provide Any Insurance Company, and any independent claim administrators and consulting health professionals and utilization review organizations with whom Any Insurance Company has contracted information concerning health care advice, treatment or supplies provided the patient (including that relating to mental illness and/or AIDS/ARC/HIV). This information will be used to evaluate claims for benefits. Any Insurance Company may provide the employer named above with any benefit calculation used in payment of this claim for the purpose of reviewing the experience and operation of the policy or contract. This Authorization is valid for the term of the policy or contract under which a claim has been submitted. I know that I have a right to receive a copy of this authorization upon request and agree that a photographic copy of this authorization is as valid as the original.
Patient's or Authorized Person's Signature____________________ Date ____________

7. Assignment
I authorize payment of medical benefits to the physician or supplier of service.
Patient's or Authorized Person's Signature____________________ Date ____________
Any person who knowingly and with intent to defraud or deceive any insurance company files a statement of claim containing any materially false, incomplete or misleading information is guilty of a crime.

FIGURE II-7 Accurate completion of insurance forms determines whether claims will be paid promptly.

GLOSSARY

A

abduct to draw away from median plane
abrasion wound characterized by the scraping of skin or mucous membrane from the surface of the body
abscess localized collection of pus in a cavity, formed by destruction of tissue
absorption uptake of substances into or across tissues
academic associated with a school of higher learning such as a university
accessory supplementary, complementary
accommodation focusing of the eye for varied distances
accreditation official authorization or approval
acculturation the process of learning cultural behaviors from one group or person
acetylcholine neurotransmitter between muscles and nerves
acquired not innate; not born with but received from an outside source
active transport movement of materials across cell membrane and epithelial layers requiring energy
acuity sharpness or clearness
acute having a short and relatively severe course
addiction dependency on some habit; may be physical, psychological, or both
adduct draw toward the middle, or median plane
adenohypophysis anterior pituitary
adhere to stick to something
adipose of a fatty nature; fat
adjourn to suspend a session to another time or permanently
administration management performance of executive responsibilities and duties
adolescence period of growth from appearance of secondary gender characteristics to cessation of body (somatic) growth; roughly 12 to 18 years of age
adrenalin epinephrine; hormone that relaxes airways and constricts blood vessels
advocacy pleading the case of another; support
aerobic presence of oxygen
aerosol continuous dispersion of gas; atomization
afferent moving toward a center
agar dried product of algae capable of supporting bacterial growth
agenda list of things to be done or considered, program of work
agoraphobia fear of being in crowded places
agarose type of media made of sugar molecules taken from seaweed
airborne present in the air, may be carried in respiratory droplets
alactasia malabsorption of lactose caused by a deficiency of the enzyme lactase
albuminuria excess protein in the urine
alignment arrangement of a group of points or objects along a line
allergen substance capable of inducing hypersensitive or allergic reaction
allopathic system of medical practice that uses remedies designed to produce effects that differ from those caused by the disease being treated
alloy solid mixture of two or more metals
alternative something different, a substitute for something else
alveoli bony cavities in maxilla and mandible in which the roots of the teeth are attached; site of gas exchange in lungs
ambulatory walking or able to walk
amenorrhea complete loss of menstrual cycle
amino acids chemical compounds needed to build muscle, bone, blood, and antibodies
amputation the severing or cutting away of part of the body
amylase enzyme that is secreted by the salivary glands to begin the chemical portion of the digestive process
anabolism any constructive process by which simple substances are converted by living cells into more complex compounds
anaerobic absence of oxygen
analgesic pain reliever
analytical able or inclined to separate things into parts to study or examine them
analyze to examine a complex whole and compare the components
anaphylactic shock the response of the body to an allergen such as a medication
anatomical position person standing with feet and face forward and hands to the side, used to describe the relationship or location of the parts of the body
ancillary providing support for something
androgen any substance that possesses masculinizing activities
anemia below normal number of red blood cells
anesthesia loss of feeling or sensation
anesthesiology study of medicine to relieve pain during surgery
angina chest pain characterized by the feeling of choking and suffocation
anorexia eating disorder characterized by loss of appetite
antagonist muscle that acts in opposition to the action of another muscle, its agonist
antecubital area in front of the elbow
anterior in front or in the forward part of an organ; toward the head of the body
anthrax an infectious disease of warm-blooded animals (such as cattle and sheep) caused by a spore-forming bacterium (*Bacillus anthracis*), characterized by external ulcerating nodules or by lesions in the lungs
antibody substance produced in the body as a reaction to a specific antigen
anticoagulant substance preventing the coagulation or clotting of blood
antidiuretic substance suppressing the rate of urine formation

antigen substance that causes the formation of antibodies
anti-inflammatory counteracting or suppressing inflammation
antiseptic substance that deters the growth of microorganisms
anuria complete suppression of excretion by kidneys; absence of urine
anus opening to the rectum between the buttocks
anxiety a feeling of fear or apprehension
apathy lack of feeling or emotion; indifference
apex narrowed and pointed end; tip
aphasia inability to speak
apical pertaining to, or located at, the apex of the heart
apiculture study of bees
apnea cessation of breathing
apocrine sweat gland that is attached to hair follicles
apparatus set of materials or instrument for a specific operation
apprehensive anxious or fearful about the future; uneasy
aptitude general suitability; ability to learn
arrhythmia variation in the normal pattern of the heartbeat
arteries blood vessels that carry blood away from the heart
articulation place of junction between two bones, joint; enunciation of words and syllables, how sounds are spoken
artificial insemination injection of semen into the uterine canal, unrelated to sexual intercourse
asbestos a chemical-resistant mineral form made of magnesium silicate that separates into long flexible fibers
asepsis freedom from infection; the methods used by health care workers to prevent the spread of microorganisms
aspirate remove by suction
aspiration act of inhaling foreign matter, usually emesis, into the respiratory tract
assertiveness technique to reduce the inner stress caused by inaccurate communication or lack of communication
assimilation the merging of cultural traits from different cultural groups
assisted reproductive technology treatment of sperm and eggs to increase the chance of reproduction
astringent causing contraction, usually locally after topical application
asymmetry lack of sameness on both sides of the body in size, shape, and relative position
asymptomatic showing or causing no subjective evidence (symptom) of a condition or disease
atrophy wasting away; decrease in size
atrium chamber of the heart
attitude mental position or feeling with regard to a fact or situation
audiology science of hearing
auditory pertaining to the sense of hearing
aura subjective sensation or motor phenomenon that precedes and marks the onset of a seizure
auscultation listening to sounds produced in the body cavities using a stethoscope
autoclave machine that uses steam under pressure to sterilize materials
autoimmune directed against the body's own tissue
autonomic involuntary
autonomic nervous system portion of the nervous system that regulates the activity of the cardiac muscle, smooth muscle, and glands
autopsy examination of parts of dead body to determine cause of death and pathological conditions
autosome any one of 22 paired chromosomes that are not sexual
autotransfusion the collection and transfusion of a person's own blood
aversion desire to avoid something that is disliked
avulsion the traumatic tearing away of part of the body
axilla the space under the arms; armpit

B

baccalaureate a bachelor's degree
bacteria single-celled organism that is neither plant nor animal; the most common cause of human disease and infection; classified by shape (bacilli, cocci, spirilla)
balance ability to maintain a steady position that does not tip
basal metabolic rate minimal energy expended for respiration, circulation, peristalsis, muscle tone, body temperature, and glandular activity of the body at rest
behavior conduct, actions that can be observed
benefit financial help in time of illness, retirement, or unemployment
benign not malignant or cancerous, not recurring
bevel slant or incline
bile fluid that helps digest fat in the small intestine; produced in the liver and stored in the gallbladder
binocular using both eyes
biochemical relating to the chemical substances present in living organisms
biofeedback conscious control of biological functions normally controlled involuntarily
bioinformatics collection, classification, and analysis of biological information such as molecular and genetic data
biologic drug, vaccine, or antitoxin made from living organisms
biological death a death caused by the absence of breathing and heartbeat caused by the loss of cell function
biomechanics study of the mechanical laws and their application to living organisms, especially locomotion
biopsy removal and examination of living tissue
biosphere part of the universe, including the air (atmosphere), earth (lithosphere), and water (hydrosphere), in which living organisms exist
birth canal the passageway for delivery of the fetus
blood pressure pressure of the blood on the walls of the artery, depending on energy of the heart action, elasticity of the walls of the arteries, and volume and viscosity of the blood
bolus the portion of food mixed with saliva that is swallowed
botany study of plant life
bovine pertaining to cattle
bradypnea abnormally slow rate of breathing
braille system of writing that uses raised characters as letters
bronchodilator medication to dilate the bronchi and bronchioles for easier breathing
budget summary of projected income and expenses
bulimia excessive, binge eating that may be followed by self-induced vomiting or purging
bursa saclike cavity filled with fluid to prevent friction

bylaws rules adopted by an organization to regulate its business

C

calculus calcium phosphate and carbonate with organic matter, deposited on the surfaces of teeth; tartar
calibrate to mark or determine gradations or units of measurement
calorie unit of heat
cancellous having a spongy or lattice-like structure
canine pertaining to dogs
capacity holding power
capillaries blood vessels that receive blood from the arteries and carry it to the veins
carbohydrates starches, sugars, cellulose, and gums
carcass dead body of an animal, other than human
cardiac arrest period when the heart has stopped functioning entirely
cardiopulmonary pertaining to the heart and lungs
cardiopulmonary resuscitation (CPR) a combination of mouth-to-mouth breathing and chest compressions that supplies oxygenated blood to the brain
cardioversion restoration of normal rhythm of the heart by electrical shock
career an occupation or profession
caries decalcification of the surface of the tooth followed by disintegration of the inner part of the tooth
carnivore animal that eats animals
carrier an animal that harbors or hosts a microorganism or gene without self-injury
cartilage specialized fibrous connective tissue
catabolism a breaking-down process by which complex substances are converted by living cells into more simple compounds
catalyst substance, usually used in small amounts relative to the reactants, that modifies and increases the rate of a reaction without being consumed in the process
catheter tube for injecting a fluid into or removing a fluid from a cavity such as the bladder or heart
caustic capable of destroying or burning
cautery the application of heat that burns tissue
cavity hollow space
cellulose complex carbohydrate derived from plant walls
Celsius one measurement for temperature; 0 degrees is the freezing point of water, and 100 degrees is the boiling point of water
centrifuge machine that separates lighter portions of a solution, mixture, or suspension by centrifugal force
cerebrospinal fluid fluid contained in the brain's ventricles, intracranial spaces, and central canal of the spinal cord
certification documentation of having met certain standards
ceruminous pertaining to earwax
character distinctive qualities that make up an individual
chart collection of written materials relating to the health care of a patient
chemotherapy treatment of disease by a chemical agent
chiropractic system of therapy based on the theory that health is determined by the condition of the nervous system
cholecystectomy surgical removal of the gallbladder
cholesterol pearly, fatlike steroid alcohol found in animal fats and oils; precursor of bile acids and hormones
chronic persisting over a long period
chyme thick, semiliquid contents of stomach during digestion
cilia (cilium) hairlike projections from the surface of a cell
circumcision the removal of the prepuce of the penis
clarity quality of being clear; lucid
client person who engages the professional services of another
climacteric menopause
clinical death death from the loss of brain activity (for a specified amount of time)
clone genetically identical cells descended from a single cell
clonic pertaining to alternate muscular contraction and relaxation in rapid succession
coagulation process of clot formation
coarctation narrowing of a vessel
coccygeal pertaining to the tail bone
cognitive relating to the process of acquiring knowledge by reasoning
collagen white protein fibers of the skin, tendons, bone, and cartilage (connective tissue)
combustion burning
communicable capable of being transmitted from one person or animal to another
communication exchange of information
compact having a dense structure
compassion sympathy with another's distress and a desire to remove it
compensate to make satisfactory payment or reparation to; recompense or reimburse
complementary making a pair or whole
composition arrangement into proper proportion or relation; qualitative and quantitative makeup of a chemical compound
compound (open) fracture fracture in which the bone breaks through the skin and is exposed
comprehensive covering all areas; inclusive
conception onset of pregnancy; union of sperm and egg (ovum)
condition change from normal function that cannot be cured
confidential private and secret; may be protected by law
confinement restriction or limitation within the boundaries or scope of something
conformation particular shape
confusion loss of orientation
congenital referring to conditions that exist at birth regardless of cause
conscientious meticulous or careful; guided by conscience
consciousness responsiveness of the mind to the impressions made by the senses
consistency constitution or character; description of something's composition
constipation difficult or inadequate passage of fecal material
consumer one who uses goods or services produced by another
contagious capable of being transmitted from one person to another
contaminate to soil, make unclean, or infect with pathogens
continuum uninterrupted ordered sequence
contraceptive agent that prevents conception or pregnancy
contract shorten; reduce in size
contraction shortening or development of tension in muscle tissue
contracture permanent shortening of tendons and ligaments of a joint resulting from atrophy of muscle

contusion an internal wound; a bruise

converge when two eyes move in a coordinated fashion toward fixation on the same near point

convergence coordinated movement of two eyes toward fixation on the same near point

convex evenly curved, resembling part of a sphere

convulsion the uncoordinated movement of groups of muscles usually resulting from poisoning or elevated temperature

coordinate put into order or rank to provide for smooth operation

coronary pertaining to the heart

coroner public officer whose primary function is to inquire about any death that may have occurred from unnatural cause

corpuscle any small mass or body

corrosive able to cause burning damage

creatinine end product of metabolism, found in muscle and blood and excreted in urine

credential document showing that a person is entitled to credit or to exercise official power

criterion an accepted standard used in making decisions or judgments about something

critical pertaining to a crisis or to danger of death

cryotherapy therapeutic use of cold

cultural competence the ability to meet the health care needs of patients while meeting and adhering to their cultural values, beliefs and practices.

culture sum of the social patterns that guide a person's life; the act of belonging to a designated group

customary fee charged by similar practitioners for a service in the same economic and geographic area

cutaneous pertaining to the skin

cystocentesis process in which urine is obtained by a surgical puncture of the urinary bladder with a sterile needle

D

debate discuss a question

debris the scattered remains of something broken or destroyed; rubble or wreckage

decibel unit used to express relative power intensity of sounds

defecation evacuation of waste or fecal material from rectum

defibrillation termination of atrial or ventricular fibrillation usually by electroshock; cardioversion

deficient lacking some important part

deficit difference in amount

deformity distortion of any part or disfigurement of the body

degeneration deterioration; change from higher to lower (less functional) form

degenerative having progressively less function

deglutition act of swallowing

delinquency antisocial or illegal behavior or acts

dementia organic loss of intellectual function

demographic pertaining to the study of people as a group, especially of statistical groupings according to age, gender, and environmental factors

dentition used to designate natural teeth in the mouth

deoxygenate act of depriving of oxygen

deoxyribonucleic acid (DNA) large nucleic acid molecule that makes up chromosomes

dependence addiction to drugs or alcohol

depilatory substance with the ability to remove hair

dermabrasion treatment of severe acne by removing the top layers of scarred skin

dermatitis inflammation of the skin

dermis corium, layer of skin beneath the epidermis

dexterity skill and ease in using body parts; mental skill or quickness

detoxify to treat (an individual) for alcohol or drug dependence, usually in a medically supervised program designed to rid the body of intoxicating or addictive substances

diagnosis methods used to discover cause and nature of an illness

diagnosis-related grouping predetermined payment structure for health care services established by the federal government

dialysis separating particles from a fluid by filtration through a semipermeable membrane

diaphoresis perspiration

diastole dilatation of the heart; resting phase of the ventricles; alternates with systole

diastolic blood pressure during ventricular relaxation

dictation words spoken or recorded to be written by another person

differentiate see or show the differences between two or more things

diffusion process of being widely spread; spontaneous movement of molecules or other particles in solution to reach uniform concentration

dilate stretch beyond normal dimension

dipping act of placing chewing tobacco or smokeless tobacco between the lower lip and teeth

disability lack of ability to function in the manner that most people function physically or mentally

discretionary offering the freedom to make a decision according to individual circumstances

discriminate to make distinctions on the basis of differences

discrimination unfair treatment of one person or group, usually because of prejudice

disease interruption of normal function of the body, usually caused by a factor that can be treated, such as microorganisms

disinfectant substance that kills microorganisms except viruses and spores

dislocation injury in which a bone moves out of a joint

dispense prepare, package, compound, or label for delivery according to a lawful order of a qualified practitioner

distend stretch out; inflate

diuresis increased excretion of urine

divergence simultaneous abduction of both eyes

diversity quality of being different

diverticulum pouch that results from the weakening of the colon wall

dogmatism unwarranted or arrogant positiveness of opinion

domestic relating to the household or the family

domesticated animal that has been trained to live with people

dominant gene trait that appears when carried by only one in the pair of chromosomes

donor a person who supplies living tissue or who furnishes blood for transfusion to another person

dopamine neurotransmitter in the central nervous system

dosage regulation of size, frequency, and amount of medication
duct tube for passage of excretions or secretions
dysarthria difficulty with articulation
dysfunction disturbance, impairment, or abnormality in functioning of an organ
dysphagia difficulty swallowing
dyspnea difficult or labored breathing
dystrophy disorder resulting from defective or faulty nutrition
dystocia abnormal labor
dysuria painful or difficult urination

E

eccrine sweat gland that secretes onto the skin
echocardiography recording the position and motion of the heart walls or its internal structure using ultrasonic waves
ecosystem living organisms and non-living elements interacting in a certain specific area
ectoparasite parasite that lives on the outside of the body, such as a tick
ectopic located away from normal position
edema swelling
efferent moving away from the center
effusion oozing fluids from blood or lymph vessels into body cavities
elasticity quality or condition of being able to stretch and resume original shape
electrocardiogram graphic tracing of the electrical activity of the heart
electrocardiography field of diagnostic health care in which the heart is monitored
electroencephalography field of diagnostic health care in which the brain is monitored
electrolysis destruction of hair by passage of an electrical current through the follicle
electrolyte substance that separates into ions in solution and is capable of conducting electricity
electrophoresis movement of charged suspended particles through a medium in response to an electric field
elongate to become or be made longer
embolism blockage of an artery, usually by a blood clot
embryo the young of any organism at an early stage of development
emesis act of vomiting; vomit
emmetropia normal vision; 20/20 vision
emotive expressing or exciting emotion
empathy ability to understand another person's feelings
endocrine secreting internally into blood or lymph
endometrium the lining of the uterus
endorphin one of the neuropeptides released by the brain that reduces pain
endoscopy visual inspection of a body cavity
endospore form assumed by some bacteria that is resistant to heat, drying, and chemicals; spore
endosseus referring to the inside of the bone
endotracheal intubation placing a tube within or through the trachea
enema liquid instilled into the rectum
engorge fill to capacity
enkephalin pain-relieving pentapeptide released by the brain
entomology study of insects
entry inhibitor molecule that attaches to the surface of a cell such as the human immunodeficiency virus (HIV); prevents HIV from entering the body's T-cell
enzyme protein that accelerates specific chemical reaction
epidemic an outbreak of disease that affects a large number of people in one area
epidemiology the study of relationships of factors that determine the frequency and distribution of disease in a human community
epidermis outermost and nonvascular layer of skin
epilepsy transient disturbances of brain function
eponym name of a person after which a particular place, item, or discovery is named
equilibrium state of balance
equine pertaining to horses
equivalent equal in value
erectile capable of becoming rigid and elevated when filled with blood
equivalent equal in value
ergonomics design of workplace equipment that minimizes fatigue and maximizes productivity
erythrocyte red blood cell or corpuscle
Escherichia coli a microorganism that is nonpathogenic if found in the intestines but pathogenic if found in the urinary tract
essential basic and necessary
esthetic pertaining to sensation, beauty, or improvement of appearance
ethics dealing with what is good or bad; determining moral duty and obligation
ethnocentrism the belief that ones own culture is superior to another
ethnography a branch of anthropology that studies and records various human culture
eugenics study of the methods for controlling the characteristics of humans
eupnea easy or normal breathing
euthanasia the induction of death in a sick, severely injured, or unwanted animal
excretion discharge of waste matter such as urine, feces, or sweat
exocrine secrete outwardly via a duct
exophthalmos abnormal protrusion of the eyeball
expenditure amount of money spent, as a whole or on a particular thing
expiration act of breathing out; exhalation
extract to obtain from a substance by chemical or mechanical action
extremity distal or terminal portion; arm or leg
extrinsic coming from or originating outside

F

fabrication created, invented, made from parts
fat adipose tissue; reserve supply of energy
farrier one who shoes horses
fatigue increased discomfort and decreased efficiency caused by prolonged or excessive exertion; exhaustion
feces excrement discharged from intestines
federal referring to the central unit of government of the United States
feedback a method to determine whether a message was received accurately; a response by the receiver to indicate how the information was understood
feline pertaining to cats
fermentation chemical change that is brought about by the action of an enzyme or microorganism
fertile capacity to conceive or induce conception

fetal pertaining to an unborn baby from 2 months of gestation to birth
fever an elevation of body temperature
fibrillation quivering or spontaneous contraction of individual muscle fibers
fibroid tissue composed of threadlike, fibrous structure
filtration passage of liquid through a filter by gravity, pressure, or suction
fissure cleft or groove; linear ulcer
first aid the immediate care given to the victim of injury or sudden illness
first-degree burn a burn that affects only the outer layer of skin tissue
flaccid weak; soft
flatulence excessive air or gas in stomach or intestines leading to distention of organs
fluoride chemical compound consisting of fluorine and another element
fluoroscope device used to examine deep structures by means of radioactive waves
fluoroscopy immediate visualization of part of the body on a screen using radiography
follicle sac or pouchlike depression or cavity
fomite inanimate or nonliving object that transfers infectious microorganisms
forensic relating to, used in, or appropriate for courts of law or for public discussion or argumentation
formed element solid part of blood; red and white blood cells and platelets
fracture breakage of bone
fray to wear away the edge or surface of cloth or rope by friction
frequency the number of times an event occurs in a given period; in hearing, measure of one cycle per second (hertz)
friction act of rubbing
frostbite exposure to cold that causes the water in the body tissues to freeze
functional having practical application or serving a useful purpose
fungus microorganism that grows in groups or colonies on other organisms; includes yeasts and molds
fusion merging of different elements into a union

G

gastric pertaining to the stomach
gender sex of an individual; male or female
genital reproductive organ
genome complete set of chromosomes with the associated genes
genotype genetic pattern of an individual
geriatric referring to all aspects of aging
gestation development of young from conception to birth, pregnancy
gingiva gum of the mouth; mucous membrane with supporting fibrous tissue
glucose simple sugar
glycosuria presence of sugar in urine
gonad sex glands that produces gametes
gonadotropin any hormone that stimulates the reproductive organs
gout swelling of the joints resulting from a buildup of uric acid caused by some metabolic disorder
grand mal seizure seizure that is preceded by an aura and results in semiconsciousness
grief the process that gradually resolves a sense of loss
grievance complaint; injustice
groin depression between thigh and trunk, inguinal region
growth hormone somatotropic hormone; secreted by the anterior pituitary gland
gustatory pertaining to the sense of taste

H

habit act performed voluntarily without conscious thought
halitosis offensive or bad breath
hallucination imaginary visions
harassment to disturb persistently, torment, bother, or persecute
hay fever seasonal rhinitis, usually caused by pollen in the air
health state of optimal well-being, achieved through prevention of illness and injury
hearing the auditory sense; the primary function of the ear
heat exhaustion condition characterized by perspiration, pale and clammy skin, and weakness
heat stroke condition characterized by dry skin, strong pulse, and a high internal temperature
hematology the study of the components of solid, or formed, elements of blood and blood-forming tissues
hematuria presence of blood in urine
hemodialysis filtration of the blood using an artificial membrane
hemolysis rupture of red blood cells
hemopoiesis process in which blood forms and develops
hemorrhage abnormal external or internal bleeding
herbal consisting of or made with aromatic plants
herbivore animal that eats plants
hereditary passed genetically, from one generation to another
heredity genetic transmission of trait or particular quality from parent to offspring
herniation abnormal protrusion of an organ or other body structure through a defect or natural opening in a covering membrane, muscle, or bone
heterosexual person who is attracted to the opposite sex
hierarchy arrangement into a graded series or levels of differing worth
hirsutism abnormal or excessive hair placement or growth
holistic practice of medicine that considers the person as a whole unit, not as individual parts
homeopathic system of medical practice that uses remedies designed to produce similar effects to those caused by the disease being treated
homeostasis tendency of an organism to maintain the "status quo" or the same internal environment
homosexual person who is attracted to the same sex
hormone chemical substance produced in the body that has specific regulatory effect on the activity of a certain organ
horticultural pertaining to the growing of plants
hospice long-term care facility providing care for the terminally ill
hyperactivity behavior characterized by constant overactivity
hydrate to supply water to in order to restore or maintain fluid balance
hydraulic operated or moved using liquid as the source of power
hydrocarbon organic compound made of hydrogen and carbon only
hydrotherapy application of water for therapeutic purposes
hygiene proper care of the mouth, teeth, and other parts of the body for maintenance of health and the prevention of disease
hyperglycemia abnormally high sugar content in the blood
hyperplasia tissue overgrowth

hypertrophy enlargement or overgrowth of an organ or part caused by an increase in its cells
hypochondria the belief in imaginary illness
hypoglycemia abnormally low sugar content in the blood
hypophysis pituitary gland
hypothermia an abnormal lowering of body temperature

I

imaging storing of an image or visual representation of someone or something
immerse to place or plunge something into a liquid
immunity high level of resistance to certain microorganisms or diseases; security against a particular disease
immunization process of becoming secure against a particular disease or pathogen
immunize secure against a particular disease
immunoassay quantitative determination of antigenic substance by examination of blood
immunohematology specialized branch of immunology that studies and identifies blood groups
immunology the study of how the blood cells prevent disease caused by microorganisms
immunosuppression prevention or diminution of immune response
impair damage
impulse sudden pushing force; activity along nerve fibers
inanimate pertaining to a nonliving article
incentive something that stimulates an action
incident an individual occurrence or event occurring in connection with something else; a reportable variance
incinerate act of burning, cremation
incision wound characterized by a cut made with a surgical instrument, knife, or glass
incubation period of time when an infection shows its effects
incus one of the three auditory bones of the inner ear; called the "anvil"
industry employment or business involving a skill
infarction an area of tissue death (necrosis) caused by loss of oxygen (ischemia) as a result of obstruction of circulation to the area
infection invasion and multiplication of microorganisms in the body tissues
inferior lower than another; bottom part
inflammation localized protective response to injury or destruction of tissue resulting in pain, heat, redness, swelling, and loss of function
informatics study of information processing, computer science
informed consent agreement to surgical or medical treatment with knowledge of facts and risks involved
ingest to take food or medicine into the body by mouth; eat or drink
inhale take into lungs by breathing
initiate cause something, especially an event or process, to begin
initiative enterprise; displaying energy or aptitude
inlay solid filling of gold or porcelain, used in dentistry to fill a defective area
innate (inborn) born with; not acquired; having from birth
inorganic having no organs; not derived from hydrocarbons
inscription the list of ingredients
insemination deposit of seminal fluid within the vagina or cervix
inspire to stimulate to action; motivate
inspiration act of drawing air into the lung; inhalation
insurance payment for health care expenses, which may or may not occur, in return for a specified payment in advance
integer whole number that is positive or negative or zero
integrative combing parts or objects that work together
intercourse sexual union
internship period of initial training under the supervision of a qualified practitioner
interpret to explain the meaning of
interstitial placed between, usually referring to between tissues
intervention any act performed to prevent harm or to improve the mental, emotional, or physical function of a patient
intracranial situated within the cranium
intraocular within the eye
intravenous within a vein or veins
intrinsic situated entirely within or pertaining exclusively to a part
inventory to make a list or catalog of contents
ischemia insufficient blood to a body part caused by functional constriction or actual obstruction of a blood vessel
isolation separation from others of someone with an infection to prevent the spread of microorganisms
isotope one or more forms of an atom with a difference in the number of neutrons

J

Jacksonian seizure a seizure that causes muscle movements on one side of the body
jaundice yellow appearance resulting from bile pigment stored in the skin and sclera of the eyes
jurisprudence science or philosophy of law
jurisprudent understanding the science or philosophy of law

K

keloid sharply elevated, irregularly shaped scar that progressively enlarges
keratinize to make into insoluble protein that composes hair, nails, epidermis, and enamel of the teeth
ketones the presence of sugar and waste products of fat metabolism in urine; may indicate uncontrolled diabetes mellitus
keyboarding skills needed to enter and retrieve data from a computer
kidneys urinary organs that form and eliminate urine
kinesthetic pertaining to muscular sense of balance or movement

L

labyrinth system of communicating canals in the inner ear
laceration type of wound characterized by irregularly shaped cut made with a sharp object
lactation production and secretion of milk by the mammary glands (breasts)
laminar air flow filtered air moving in parallel flow to prevent bacterial contamination and collection of harmful fumes
laparoscopy examination of the internal organs of the abdomen using a scope
laser device that converts electromagnetic radiation of highly amplified

ultraviolet, visible, or infrared radiation frequencies

laxative agent that acts to promote evacuation of the bowel; cathartic

legal deriving authority from or founded on law

legume fruit or seed from a leguminous plant (e.g., beans or peas)

lethargy condition of drowsiness or indifference

leukocyte white blood cell or corpuscle

liable legally responsible

libel communicating something untruthful and harmful about another person in writing

license legal authority to perform a function, usually based on experience and education and an examination

licensure legal authority to perform an activity

ligament band of fibrous tissue that connects bones and supports joints

lingua the tongue

lipoprotein protein that contains lipids

lithotripsy crushing of a stone in, for example, the kidney, followed by washing out of fragments

litigation legal dispute; lawsuit

local infection an infection limited to a small area of the body

logical based on otherwise known statements, events, or conditions

lunula general term for a small crescent or moon-shaped area of fingernail

M

malignant tending to become progressively worse and result in death; characterized by uncontrolled growth; invasive; tending to produce death

malleus one of the three auditory bones of the ear; like a hammer

malpractice failure of professional skill or learning that results in injury, loss, or damage

mammography radiologic view of breasts

mandible bone of the lower jaw

manipulative characterized by controlling or handling

marine pertaining to the sea

marrow soft organic material that fills the cavities of bones

mastication the process of chewing food

matriarchal a society or group with a female as head of the family or tribal line

maxilla irregularly shaped bone that forms the upper jaw

mediastinum mass of tissues and organs separating the two lungs

Medicaid joint federal and state program that provides health care for individuals with low income and limited resources

Medicare federal program that provides financial assistance to those 65 years of age and older and certain specified others as part of the benefits of the Social Security Act

medium substance that transmits impulses or that serves as growth location for microorganisms

megadose overdose; 10 times the recommended dose

megavitamin dose of a vitamin much greater than the required amount to maintain health

melanin dark, shapeless pigment of the skin

melatonin hormone derived from serotonin and secreted by the pineal gland

meninges three membranes that surround and protect the brain and spinal cord

menopause time of life during which menstruation stops permanently

menses normal flow of blood and uterine lining that occurs in cycles in women

menstrual cycle the recurring cycle of change of the reproductive organs induced by hormones in women

menstruation cyclic, physiologic discharge through the vagina of blood and mucosal tissues from the nonpregnant uterus

mental health a state of mind in which a person can cope with problems and maintain emotional balance and satisfaction in living

mental hygiene methods used to preserve and promote mental health

metabolism sum of all the physical and chemical processes by which living organized substance is produced and maintained (anabolism) and the transformation by which energy is made available for the uses of the organism (catabolism)

metastasis transfer of disease from one organ or part to another not directly connected with it

metazoan multicellular worm that causes disease

microbes microorganisms

microorganism microscopic living organism; microbe

micturition passage of urine; urination

milestone a significant point in development

mineral nonorganic solid substance

mobility the ability to move

monoclonal antibody identical cells or cells originating from the same cell

moral relating to principles of right and wrong; standard based on the experience, religion, and philosophy of the individual and the society

morbidity the rate of a sickness in relation to the rest of the population

mortality number of deaths in a given time or place

mortuary funeral home, place where bodies are stored until burial

motion proposal for action

mottling spotting, with patches of color

muscle cramping pain and inability to use the muscle when loss of salt from sweating causes an electrolyte imbalance

mutagen physical or chemical agent that induces genetic mutation or change

mutation permanent change in a gene or chromosome

myalgia muscle pain

mycostatic agent that inhibits the growth of fungus

myelography radiographs of the spinal cord after injection of a contrast medium

myoelectronics electromechanical prostheses

N

nebulizer device used to deliver a spray or mist of medication into the lungs

necrosis an area of tissue death

negligence failure to execute the care that a reasonable (prudent) person exercises

neonate newborn; neonatal period is the first 28 days after birth

neurobiology the study of the brain's relationship to psychosocial behavior

neurohormone hormone that stimulates a neural reaction or mechanism

neurohypophysis the posterior pituitary
neurotransmitter chemical messages, released from the axon of one neuron, that travel to another nearby neuron
neutering surgical sterilization of male animals to prevent unwanted births
nonpathogen microorganism that does not produce disease
nonverbal not involving language to communicate
nucleic acid group of complex compounds found in all living cells and viruses, composed of purines, pyrimidines, carbohydrates, and phosphoric acid
nutrients proteins, carbohydrates, fats, vitamins, and minerals necessary for growth, normal functioning, and maintaining life
nutrition process of taking in nutrients and using them for body function

O

oath solemn pledge
OBRA Omnibus Budget Reconciliation Act; law that requires training for nursing assistants, including competency testing of skill performance
obstetrician medical doctor specializing in delivery of infants
occupation vocation; activity in which one participates
ocular referring to the eyes
olfactory pertaining to the sense of smell
oliguria excretion of diminished amount of urine in relation to fluid intake
opaque substance that cannot be penetrated by visible light
optimal best possible
oral pertaining to the mouth
orchiectomy the removal of the testes
organic pertaining to an organ; having an organized structure; chemical substances containing carbon
organism an individual living thing, plant, or animal
organization a structure through which individuals cooperate systematically to conduct business
organizational development framework of management practice and theory
oropharynx section of the pharynx that contains the palatine tonsils and the lingual tonsils
orthopedic pertaining to the correction or prevention of deformities
orthotics art or science of custom designing, fabrication, and fitting of braces
orthosis device designed for straightening a distorted part
OSHA Occupation Safety and Health Administration; federal agency that establishes and enforces standards of safety for the workplace
ossicle auditory bone of the ear
osteopathic treatment of disease and injury with an emphasis on the relationship between the body organs and musculoskeletal system
osteopetrosis autosomal genetic bone disorder characterized by bones that are too dense
ova eggs
oviducts the fallopian tubes
ovulation release of the egg (ovum) from the ovary
oxidase enzyme that acts as a catalyst
oxygenate to add oxygen to

P

pallor lack of color; paleness
palpation act of feeling with the hand
pandemic epidemic that spreads over a wide geographic area affecting a large part of the population
panic disorder a condition of feeling an unreasonable fear with no known cause
papilla small, nipple-shaped projection or elevation
paralysis loss or impairment of motor function
paranoia the feeling of being persecuted or plotted against by others
paraprofessional worker who assists a professional in the performance of duties
parasite plant or animal that lives on or within another living organism at the expense of the host organism
particulate composed of separate particles or pieces
pasteurized process of heating milk or other liquids to a moderate temperature for a definite time to kill pathogenic bacteria
patent unobstructed opening such as a patent ductus arteriosus in the heart
pathogen microorganism that produces disease
patient person under medical care and treatment
pegboard paper forms, backed with carbon, that are aligned on a set of pegs to allow written information to appear on all sheets
perception process of using the senses to acquire information about the environment
percussion tapping or striking a body part to learn the condition of inner parts by analyzing the sound or to loosen secretions
perfusion the flow of blood through a specific area of the body
perinatal pertaining to the period shortly before and after birth
periodic occurring at regular intervals
periodontal situated or occurring around a tooth
periosteum specialized connective tissue covering all the bones of the body
peripheral pertaining to the extremities or edges; away from the center
peristalsis wave of contraction or wormlike movement of digestive system that propels the contents
peritoneal pertaining to the layer of membrane lining the abdominopelvic walls
peritoneum a flat serous membrane that surrounds the abdominal cavity
permanent dentition the teeth that erupt and take the place of primary dentition; secondary teeth
perseverance steady persistence in adhering to a course of action, a belief, or a purpose; steadfastness
personality set of traits, characteristics, and behaviors that make one person an individual
personnel people working in a unit or in a facility
pesticide poison used to destroy pests of any kind
petit mal seizure a seizure that results in the momentary loss of consciousness marked by staring with rapid blinking
petroleum oily liquid similar to gasoline
pH symbol relating to the concentration of hydrogen ions or acidity of a solution
phagocyte cell that surrounds and destroys microorganisms and foreign particles
pharmacology the study of the actions and uses of drugs
phenotype an individual's physical, biochemical, and physiological configuration; determined by genes

phlebotomy incision into a vein to withdraw blood
phlegm thick mucus secreted by the tissues in the respiratory passages and usually discharged through the mouth
phobia persistent, abnormal dread or fear
photosynthesis process by which plants turn energy from the sun and elements from the soil into food
pigment organic material that gives color in the body
pilus hair
pipette narrow, usually calibrated glass tube into which small amounts of liquid are suctioned for transfer or measurement
placenta an organ, characteristic of mammals during pregnancy, joining mother and offspring
plague disease causing a high rate of death, or mortality
plaque mass adhering to surface of tooth, composed of bacteria, saliva, and organic waste
plasma fluid portion of blood
pneumatic operated or moved using air as the source of power
podiatry branch of medicine concerned with care and treatment of the feet
poison substance that impairs health or destroys life when ingested
polarity specialization of a nerve cell determining the flow of impulses; having opposite effects at two ends such as a magnet
pollution condition of being defiled or impure
polydipsia excessive thirst persisting for long periods
polyneuritis inflammation of many nerves at once
polyphagia excessive eating
polyuria passage of large amount of urine in a given time
population all the inhabitants of a certain region or country
porcine pertaining to pigs, swine
portfolio collection of materials that represent a person's work
postmortem after death
post-secondary pertaining to after high school; college or vocational training
posture position or arrangement of the body parts
poultry domesticated birds kept for eggs or meat sources
practitioner one who has met educational and training requirements to practice health care
precursor one that comes before; substance used to make another structure
prejudice preconceived judgment or opinion
prepuce foreskin that forms a retractable casing
prerequisite something that must be accomplished before attempting another task or course of study
prescription written order for dispensing drugs
primary dentition the teeth that erupt first and are replaced by permanent dentition; deciduous teeth
prime mover muscle that acts directly to bring about a desired movement
prion microscopic protein molecule that may cause disease
profession occupation that requires specialized knowledge and often long and intensive academic training
projectile an item that is hurled or impelled forward
prolactin lactogenic hormone; produced and secreted by the anterior pituitary
prominence protrusion, bump
proprioceptor receptor that responds to stimulus originating in the body itself, especially to pressure, position, and stretching
prospective expected in the future
prostaglandin lipid molecule that has hormone-like effect; tissue hormone
prosthesis an artificial device applied to replace a partially or totally missing body part for functional or cosmetic purposes
prosthetics art or science of custom design, fabrication, and fitting of artificial limbs
protein a group of complex organic compounds that are the main part of cell protoplasm
proteomics study of human proteins
protoplasm cytoplasm; protein and other materials contained in cells
protozoan animal-like, unicellular organism
protrusion something that sticks out from its surroundings
prudent reasonable; wise
psyche the mind
psychic pertaining to the mind; mental
psychology the study of human and animal behavior, both normal and abnormal
psychoneurosis functional disturbance of the mind in which the individual is aware that reactions are not normal
psychosis major mental disorder in which the individual loses contact with reality
psychosocial related to factors of both psychological and social nature
psychosomatic physical symptoms caused by the mind
psychotherapy treatment of discomfort, dysfunction, or diseases by methods designed to understand and cope with one's problems
puberty the period during which the secondary sexual characteristics begin to develop and the capacity of sexual reproduction is attained
pulmonary pertaining to the lungs
pulmonary circulation carrying venous blood from the right ventricle to the lungs and returning oxygenated blood to the left atrium of the heart
pulse heartbeat that can be felt, or palpated, on surface arteries as the artery walls expand with blood
punctuality arriving or completing tasks at the appointed time
puncture wound made when an object pierces the skin
purine colorless crystalline solid made from uric acid
putrid foul, unpleasant
pyloric pertaining to the distal opening of the stomach through which stomach contents are emptied into the intestine
pyramid a structure built on a broad supporting base and narrowing gradually to a point
pyuria pus in the urine

Q

quackery treatment that pretends to cure disease
quadrant one of four regions used to describe location in the abdomen
quarantine period of detention or isolation as a result of disease suspected to be communicable
quantitative expressible by a measurement

R

radiation emission of energy, rays, or waves

radiographic contrast media a chemical that does not permit passage of x-rays
radiography making film records of internal structures by passing x-rays or gamma rays through the body to make images on specially sensitized film; roentgenography
radioisotope a type of chemical element that is radioactive
radiopharmaceutical chemical agent used for treatment or diagnosis
range of motion active or passive movement of muscle groups to the fullest extent possible; used to prevent contracture
rate expression of speed or frequency of an event in relation to a specified amount of time
rational number that can be shown as an integer or fraction
reagent substance used in a chemical reaction to detect, measure, examine, or produce other substances
reality orientation awareness of position in relation to time, space, and person
reasonable fee a fee that considers both the usual fee charged by a practitioner for a particular service and the fee charged by other practitioners for the same service
receptacle container for disposal of used materials
receptor a specific type of cell that responds to a specific stimulus
recessive gene trait that does not appear unless carried by both members of a pair of chromosomes
recipient one who receives from another, such as in a blood transfusion
recombinant genetically engineered DNA prepared by transplanting or splicing genes from one species into the cells of a host organism of a different species, becoming part of the host organism
reflex an involuntary action in response to a stimulus
refraction deviation of light when passing through a medium to another medium of a different density
regenerate to renew or reproduce, such as a lost tissue or part
regeneration natural renewal of a structure, as of lost tissue or part
registration official record of individuals qualified to perform certain services
rehabilitation restoration of normal form and function after injury or illness
remedy medication or treatment that cures disease or relieves pain
remission decrease in symptoms of a disease
renal pertaining to the kidney
repetitive done over and over again
replication making a copy
reservoir place or cavity for storage; alternative host or passive carrier of pathogenic organism
residency period of training in a specific area under the supervision of a qualified health care practitioner
resident microorganism that is always present
resonance an echo or other sound produced by percussion of an organ or cavity of the body; process of energy absorption by an object
resorption loss of bone tissue caused by the action of specialized cells
respiration exchange of oxygen and carbon dioxide between the atmosphere and the cells of the body; ventilation
restoration replacement of part of a tooth, usually with silver alloy, gold, or aesthetic composite material
restrain to limit, restrict, or keep under control
resume brief summary of professional and work experience
resuscitation restoration to life or consciousness of one apparently dead by using artificial respiration and cardiac massage
retardation intellectual slowing
retrieve to bring back or recover
retrovirus large group of viruses containing RNA
rhythm measured movement; recurrence of an action or function at regular intervals
rickettsiae tiny bacteria-like organisms that cannot live outside living tissue
rigor mortis temporary stiffness or rigidity of skeletal muscles occurring after death
ritual established ceremony
roughage indigestible material such as fiber in diet
rural relating to the country life or agriculture

S

salinity relative content of salt
sanitation promotion of hygiene and maintaining cleanliness
sarcoma cancer arising from connective tissues such as bone and muscle
sarcomere repeating units of muscle fibers with the ability to contract
schizophrenia psychotic disorder characterized by withdrawal from reality
sclerosis the hardening of tissue
scope of practice legal limitations of activities or practice of a health career worker
sebaceous pertaining to sebum or a greasy lubricating substance
sebum oil secreted by the sebaceous glands
second-degree burn a burn that breaks the surface of the skin and injures the underlying tissue
secretion process by which glands produce and add chemical substances into the blood
sedentary sitting habitually; inactive habits
sediment substance that settles at the bottom of a fluid
seizure sudden attack of a disease; uncontrolled muscle movements of epilepsy
selective breeding choosing the parents of offspring to enhance development of desired traits
self-actualization becoming the best possible person
semipermeable permitting the passage of certain molecules and not others
senile pertaining to or characteristic of old age
sensation the ability to feel
sensitize to make film react to light by coating it with an emulsion
septal pertaining to a wall separating two cavities such as in the nose or in the heart
sequence order of succession or arrangement
serology the study of antibody reactions in serum, whole blood, or urine
serum fluid portion of blood with clotting proteins removed
shock condition of acute failure of the peripheral circulation
shroud burial garment or dress
simple (closed) fracture fracture that does not penetrate the skin
simultaneous occurring at the same time

sitz bath apparatus to bathe the perineal area with continuous flow of fluid

skeletal pertaining to the framework of the body

slander verbally communicate something untruthful and harmful about another person

sociobiology the study of the relationship of genes to psychosocial behavior

socioeconomic pertaining to the society and the effects on it of production, distribution, consumption of goods, and services

somatic voluntary; pertaining to the body

spasm sudden involuntary contraction of a muscle or group of muscles

spaying the process of surgical sterilization in females to prevent unwanted births

specific gravity weight of a substance compared with an equal volume of another substance (usually water) used as a standard

spectrophotometry measurement of quantity of matter in solution by passing light through a spectrum

sperm the male gamete produced by the testes

sphincter ringlike band of muscle that closes a passage or opening

spinal pertaining to the spine

spirochete spiral bacterium; microorganism

sprain injury to the ligaments or the attachments between the muscle and bones

sputum matter ejected from the respiratory tract through the mouth

Standard Precautions Centers for Disease Control and Prevention guidelines for infection control that are applied to all body fluids of all patients all the time

stapes one of the three auditory bones in the inner ear; called the "stirrup"

statistics numeric data

stenosis narrowing or stricture of a duct or canal

stereotype simplified image used to characterize or describe a group

sterile unable to produce offspring; free from living microorganisms

steroid group name for lipids that contain a specific compound

stethoscope an instrument of various forms and materials used to listen to body sounds (auscultation)

stillborn born dead

stimulus any agent, act, or influence that produces a change in the development or function of tissues; any agent that produces a reaction in a receptor

strain injury to the muscle tissue usually resulting from overuse

strenuous energetic, very active

stoic free from passion, without complaint

subcutaneous beneath the skin

subluxations incomplete or partial dislocations of the spine

subordinate of a lower rank, under the authority of another

subscription directions for preparation

sudoriferous conveying sweat

superior higher than another; above

susceptible likely to be affected with; especially sensitive

swine hogs

synchronous occurring at the same time

syndrome group of signs and symptoms that characterize a condition or disease

synovial pertaining to transparent alkaline fluid contained in joints

systemic pertaining to a group of interdependent parts or organs

systemic circulation general circulation, carrying oxygenated blood from the left ventricle to tissues of the body and returning the venous blood to the right atrium of the heart

systemic infection an infection located throughout the body

systole period of contraction of the ventricles of the heart; alternates with diastole

systolic blood pressure during ventricular contraction

T

tachypnea excessively fast respiration

tactile pertaining to the touch

tax contribution to the support of government, fee, or dues of an organization to pay its expenses

technological resulting from improvements in productivity of machines

telehealth use of technology to provide health care over a distance

telemedicine use of telecommunications technology to provide, improve, or make health care services faster

temperature measurement of the heat production and loss in the body

tendon fibrous cord by which a muscle is attached to a bone

terminal illness or injury for which there is no reasonable expectation of recovery

testosterone an androgenic hormone that causes the appearance of secondary sexual characteristics

tetany prolonged muscle spasm or contraction

thanatology the study of death

therapeutic relating to treatment of disease or disorder by remedial methods

therapy treatment of disease; science and art of healing

theriogenology branch of veterinary medicine dealing with reproduction

thermal pertaining to or characterized by heat

third-degree burn a burn that is deep enough to damage the nerves and bones

thoracic pertaining to the chest

thrill a vibration caused by an abnormal flow of blood; felt over an artery

thrombocyte blood platelet

tolerance the decreasing effect of a drug owing to constant use

tomography specialized use of radiographs to show structures in one plane of the body by blurring the image of other planes

tonic having muscle tone

tonometer instrument that measures tension or pressure

tonus slight, continuous contraction of muscle

tourniquet instrument used to compress a blood vessel by application around an extremity

toxicology study of poisons

toxin poison produced by animals, plants, or bacteria

tracheotomy an alternative opening made into the trachea for the exchange of gases

transaction business deal; communication or activity between two or more people

transcendence being above the limits of material limits and experience

transcribe to make a written copy of dictated or recorded matter

trans fat fatty acid made from vegetable oil that has been treated to increase shelf life; does not occur in nature

transfusion introduction of whole blood or blood component into bloodstream

transgenic animal or plant that contains genes from different species
transient a microorganism that is found temporarily
translucent permitting passage of light but not transparent
Transmission-Based Precautions Centers for Disease Control and Prevention (CDC) guidelines for infection control applied to patients with known or suspected infections
transsexual person who changed his or her biologic sex
transverse situated at right angles, placed crosswise
trauma wound or injury, physical or psychic
triage the term used for setting priorities for care of the victim or victims

U

ulcer open sore or lesion
ultrasonography visualization of deep structures of the body by recording reflections of sound waves directed into the tissues
ultrasound mechanical radiant energy, sound waves beyond the range of the human ear
ultraviolet wavelengths from 5 to about 400 nanometers of the visible light spectrum
umami meaty or savory taste
unit part of a facility, including equipment and supplies, organized to provide specific care
universal occurring everywhere and in all things
universe all matter and energy that exists in the vastness of space
urea white substance found in urine, blood, and lymph; end product of protein digestion
urinal container into which a person may urinate or void urine
urinalysis physical, chemical, or microscopic examination of urine
urination discharge or passage of urine
urologist a physician that specializes in urinary conditions
urticaria vascular reaction of the skin marked by smooth elevated patches that are redder or paler than surrounding skin and itching
utility usefulness, effectiveness; a service provided by a public company, such as supplying gas, electricity, or water

V

vaccination introduction of a microorganism that has been made harmless in order to cause immunity to develop
value rate of usefulness, importance, or general worth
vapor solid or liquid in gaseous state such as steam
vascularity containing blood vessels or indicative of a large blood supply
vector carrier that transfers an infective agent from one host to another; organism that carries or transports a pathogen
veins blood vessels that carry blood back to the heart
venereal pertaining to or resulting from sexual intercourse
venomous toxic fluid secreted by animal life
ventilator machine that produces or assists with breathing
ventral front side, anterior
ventricle small cavity of the brain, lower chamber of the heart
verbal relating to or consisting of words or sounds
vesicle small bladder-like cell or cavity
vessel any one of many tubules in the body that carry fluid
veterinary pertaining to animals and their diseases
vicious mean or uncontrolled
villus one of many tiny vascular projections on the surface of small intestine
virus microorganism that is not really a cell but contains genetic information that can reproduce and cause illness inside a cell of the body
visceral pertaining to any large interior organ in any one of the cavities of the body
viscosity property of a fluid showing density or thickness
vision act or faculty of seeing, sight
vital necessary to life
vitamins organic compounds needed by the body for metabolism, growth, and development
vocational education designed to provide the skills for a particular job or career
void to empty; urinate or defecate
volume the amplitude of sound waves
voluntary under control of the conscious will

W

wheeze whistling sound made during respiration
whelping delivery of puppies by a female dog
withdrawal extreme nervousness, uncontrollable trembling, excessive sweating, and painful cramps that result when a drug (substance) is not taken anymore

X

xiphoid bone at the end of the sternum; shaped like a sword

Z

zoology study of animal life
zoonosis disease carried by animals to humans

INDEX

Page numbers followed by *f* indicate figures; *t*, tables; *b*, boxes.